STUDENT COMPANION

to accompany
Biochemistry: A Short Course
2nd Edition

Frank H. Deis

Nancy Counts Gerber

Richard I. Gumport

Roger E. Koeppe II

W. H. Freeman and Company
New York

ISBN-10: 1-4641-0934-6
ISBN-13: 978-1-4641-0934-8

Printed in the United States of America

Second Printing

W. H. Freeman and Company
41 Madison Avenue
New York, NY 10010
Houndmills, Basingstoke RG21 6XS, England
www.whfreeman.com

Preface,   v

Acknowledgments,   vii

Chapter 1   Biochemistry and the Unity of Life, 1
Chapter 2   Water, Weak Bonds, and the Generation of Order Out of Chaos, 7
Chapter 3   Amino Acids, 15
Chapter 4   Protein Three-Dimensional Structure, 21
Chapter 5   Techniques in Protein Biochemistry, 31
Chapter 6   Basic Concepts of Enzyme Action, 39
Chapter 7   Kinetics and Regulation, 49
Chapter 8   Mechanisms and Inhibitors, 61
Chapter 9   Hemoglobin: An Allosteric Protein, 71
Chapter 10   Carbohydrates, 81
Chapter 11   Lipids, 95
Chapter 12   Membrane Structure and Function, 101
Chapter 13   Signal-Transduction Pathways, 113
Chapter 14   Digestion: Turning a Meal into Cellular Biochemicals, 129
Chapter 15   Metabolism: Basic Concepts and Design, 135
Chapter 16   Glycolysis, 151
Chapter 17   Gluconeogenesis, 165
Chapter 18   Preparation for the Cycle, 171
Chapter 19   Harvesting Electrons from the Cycle, 177
Chapter 20   The Electron-Transport Chain, 189
Chapter 21   The Proton-Motive Force, 201
Chapter 22   The Light Reactions, 211
Chapter 23   The Calvin Cycle, 221
Chapter 24   Glycogen Degradation, 227
Chapter 25   Glycogen Synthesis, 239
Chapter 26   The Pentose Phosphate Pathway
Chapter 27   Fatty Acid Degradation, 257
Chapter 28   Fatty Acid Synthesis, 271
Chapter 29   Lipid Synthesis, 281
Chapter 30   Amino Acid Degradation and the Urea Cycle, 299
Chapter 31   Amino Acid Synthesis, 373
Chapter 32   Nucleotide Metabolism, 323

Chapter 33 The Structure of Informational Macromolecules, 337

Chapter 34 DNA Replication, 353

Chapter 35 DNA Repair and Recombination, 365

Chapter 36 RNA Synthesis and Regulation in Bacteria, 373

Chapter 37 Gene Expression in Eukaryotes, 385

Chapter 38 RNA Processing in Eukaryotes, 393

Chapter 39 The Genetic Code, 401

Chapter 40 The Mechanism of Protein Synthesis, 411

Chapter 41 Recombinant DNA Techniques, 421

Expanded Solutions To Text Problems **439**

Biochemistry has a reputation for being a difficult subject. If you talk to physicians, nutritionists, or health professionals of all sorts, you will often hear that they remember biochemistry as one of their hardest courses. But there are different ways for a subject to be difficult. Some subjects are difficult because the ideas are difficult. Quantum chemistry and differential equations may be difficult in that way. In contrast, the ideas in biochemistry are mostly easy to comprehend. If you compare biochemistry with organic chemistry—biochemistry is made up of a very small subset of reactions, most of which occur in aqueous solution at neutral pH. This eliminates easily 90% of the reactions of organic chemistry. Furthermore most of biochemistry deals with reactions of a small number of building blocks. There are only a few amino acids, nucleotides, and sugars that are used over and over again. The difficulty of biochemistry has more to do with the volume of material, the amount of detail that a student has to learn. In a sense it is similar to the difficulty of learning a foreign language, with vocabulary lists to memorize for each lesson.

Thus it should be obvious that an important part of studying biochemistry is the time spent thinking about the subject. Biochemistry is very time-consuming, and spending only one or two nights studying for an exam is a recipe for disaster. This book is designed to help you cope with the volume of detail in a biochemistry course. It is carefully arranged so that the material matches the content of *Biochemistry: A Short Course,* Second Edition. Each chapter in this Companion consists of an Introduction, Learning Objectives, a Self-Test, Answers to Self-Test, Problems, and Answers to Problems. The Introduction defines the scope of the chapter, setting the stage. The Learning Objectives are presented in the order that the concepts appear in *Biochemistry: A Short Course,* Second Edition. Key words are shown in italics—if you are unfamiliar with any of these words you should look them up and understand what they mean. Self-Test questions are useful for checking how much of the chapter material you have retained after reading and studying, and the Answers are provided in the next section. The Problems often expand on the chapter material and offer an opportunity to think about the wider consequences of the material in the textbook. Answers are also provided for the Problems. Finally, Expanded Solutions to end-of-chapter problems in the text are presented in a separate section of the Companion.

One possible way to study effectively would be: First, attend lectures and take good notes, perhaps record lectures if your professor allows that. It is not unusual for a professor to omit significant amounts of material from the textbook, so it can be a bad idea to start by reading the textbook without knowing which parts you are responsible for. Once that has been ascertained, you might start by reading the Introduction in this Companion and perhaps skimming the Self-Test to get an idea of the scope of the material. Then read the text-book chapter, and return to the Companion for a more serious use of the Self-Test and Problems. Part of what you need to be trying to do is to spend time with the material and get to know it inside out. If you really understand biochemistry you start to see that there is a reason for everything, that there is an internal logic for each metabolic pathway. And if you can see it that way, the material becomes much easier to remember, and in fact it becomes hard to forget. If this Companion helps you to reach that level of understanding, the authors will have accomplished their goal. We welcome readers' comments, especially those drawing our attention to errors in the text. Comments should be sent to:

Dr. Frank H. Deis
Department of Molecular Biology and Biochemistry
Rutgers University
Nelson Laboratories
604 Allison Road
Piscataway, NJ 08854-8082
deis@rci.rutgers.edu

ACKNOWLEDGMENTS

Just as *Biochemistry: A Short Course,* Second Edition is an edited and re-focused version of *Biochemistry* by Jeremy Berg et al., this Student Companion is an edited and re-focused version of the Companion to the Berg textbook. None of the Companion volumes would exist in their present form without the insights and inspiration of the late Dr. Richard I. Gumport. His decades teaching first year medical students in the College of Medicine at the University of Illinois at Urbana-Champaign led him to analyze how students learn a complex subject, and then to create the Companion as a tool for learning. A good deal of the writing in this book is his.

FHD would like to thank the students in his biochemistry courses at Rutgers University; his wife, Louise; and his kind and hard-working editor Amanda Dunning. NCG thanks her colleagues in the Department of Chemistry and Biochemistry at San Francisco State University for their support and feedback and her family for their patience during long hours of writing. REK, II thanks Denise Greathouse, Olaf Andersen, Frank Millett, and his students at the University of Arkansas in Fayetteville.

Frank H. Deis
Nancy Counts Gerber
Richard I. Gumport
Roger E. Koeppe II

December 2011

Chapter 1

Biochemistry and the Unity of Life

This chapter briefly surveys the major constituents of living cells. The word "bio-chemistry" is a combination of biology (living cells) and chemistry, and thus focuses on the chemicals and chemistry present in living cells. No other way of looking at life makes it so clear that all living organisms on Earth are related, and all are descended from a common ancestor. "What is true of *E. coli* must also be true of elephants." All organisms, whether plant or animal, fungus or bacterium, share a rather short list of common building blocks, and very similar ways of metabolizing food and getting things done. This overview will serve as a good introduction to the specifics in coming chapters.

LEARNING OBJECTIVES

When you have mastered this chapter, you should be able to accomplish the following objectives.

Living Systems Require a Limited Number of Atoms and Molecules
(Text Section 1.1)

1. Know that 98% of the atoms in a living organism are carbon, oxygen, and hydrogen.
2. Understand that all known forms of life require water.
3. Describe the composition of fuel molecules and their products after oxidation.
4. Explain the advantage of carbon over silicon as a major constituent of living cells.
5. Know that nitrogen, phosphorus, and sulfur also play important roles in organisms.

There Are Four Major Classes of Biomolecules (Text Section 1.2)

6. Describe and differentiate between the key classes of biomolecules.
7. Explain the various uses of proteins in the cell.
8. Describe the building blocks and structure of proteins.
9. Know the two main kinds of nucleic acids in the cell, and that their main use is in storing information.
10. Describe the building blocks and structure of nucleic acids.
11. Know the names and structures of the four "bases" used in DNA.
12. Understand the uses of lipids in the cell.
13. Explain which classes of biomolecules are used as fuel.
14. Define what carbohydrates are and what the building blocks are for macromolecules such as starch and glycogen.

The Central Dogma Describes the Basic Principles of Biological Information
(Text Section 1.3)

15. Write out Crick's original diagram for the "Central Dogma."
16. Define *replication*, *transcription*, and *translation*.
17. Name the enzymes responsible for replication and transcription.
18. Explain how selective expression of genes is necessary to differentiate one body tissue from another.

Membranes Define the Cell and Carry Out Cellular Functions (Text Section 1.4)

19. Identify the key features that differentiate eukaryotic cells from prokaryotic cells.
20. Describe the basic structure of a biological membrane.
21. Explain where the membranes are in bacterial (or "prokaryotic") cells.
22. Define *plasma membrane, cytoplasm, cytoskeleton, organelle, mitochondrion,* and *endoplasmic reticulum.*
23. Describe the process of endocytosis in eukaryotes.

SELF-TEST

Living Systems Require a Limited Number of Atoms and Molecules

1. True or False: the percentages of elements in living cells match the abundance of elements in the earth's crust.

2. Which element was mentioned as having an essential role for life?
   (a) boron
   (b) aluminum
   (c) sulfur
   (d) helium
   (e) silicon

3. What happens to carbon when it is oxidized (combusted)? What happens to silicon when it is oxidized?

There Are Four Major Classes of Biomolecules

4. Most large biomolecules are generally linear and unbranched. Which large biomolecules are likely to be branched?

5. Which two biomolecule types are mainly used as fuel? Which two are mentioned as informational?

6. Which biomolecules form the membranes that surround the cell?

The Central Dogma Describes the Basic Principles of Biological Information

7. Every cell in an organism contains the same complete set of genes in the DNA. How is it then that some cells turn into skin, others into taste-buds or retina, and others into nerves?

8. DNA polymerase is responsible for the process called _____.

Membranes Define the Cell and Carry Out Cellular Functions

9. Prokaryotes basically have one interior compartment. Eukaryotes, on the other hand, are like a house with many rooms. Name five interior compartments found in eukaryotic cells.

ANSWERS TO SELF-TEST

1. False. Silicon is much more abundant in the Earth's crust than in living cells, and there are many other differences as well.

2. (c) Sulfur.

3. When carbon-carbon bonds are oxidized, much energy is released and a gas is formed, carbon dioxide. When silicon is oxidized, far less energy is released and the silicates formed become stone.

4. Glycogen and certain other carbohydrates are branched. Most other biomolecules are linear. While it is beyond the scope of this chapter, RNA can occasionally be branched and can form a "lasso" shape. And while proteins are strictly linear they can be co-valently cross-linked, so two chains can become attached.

5. The fuel molecules would be lipids and carbohydrates. Nucleic acids are informational, and in some cases carbohydrates can also carry information, serving as recognition sites on the outside of cells.

6. Lipids are the main constituents of cell membranes.

7. As the chapter explains, even though every cell in your body contains the same DNA, and the same set of genes, transcribing those genes into RNA and expressing the information is optional. So different cells choose to express different genes, allowing some to be nerves and some to be muscles, etc. In the processes of development from egg to organism, a given cell may have varying patterns of gene expression through time as well.

8. replication

9. Nucleus, vacuole, mitochondrion, golgi, lysosome, endoplasmic reticulum, chloroplast—see illustrations in chapter.

PROBLEMS

1. Imagine the cell as a house. Which kind of biomolecule would be the encyclopedia on the bookshelf? Which would be the walls and roof of the house? What would be the furniture? What would be the wood pile next to the fireplace? What would be the windows? And what biomolecule would correspond to the people living in the house?

2. Imagine that you are writing a paper—writing with a pen on paper—and you are giving the paper to a secretary to type up. But before you do that you want to photocopy what you have written so you have a copy you can keep. And before you photocopy, you proofread the paper and indicate some deletions and moves. How will the handwritten paper correspond to what gets typed up; will it match exactly? How does this relate to the Central Dogma? What next step would you have to add to make it exactly like the Central Dogma?

3. According to the Central Dogma, can information travel from RNA to DNA? Why do the authors say "the scheme is not as simple as depicted"?

ANSWERS TO PROBLEMS

1. The encyclopedia is DNA—it contains all of the information on how to make the "house" and everything in it, but it cannot read itself. The walls and roof—the best answer would be lipids, since lipids make up the cell membrane. The furniture—probably carbohydrates, since there are carbohydrates (like glycogen) sitting around the cell, and in a pinch they can be "burned" in the "fireplace." The wood pile, carbohydrates or lipids; the "fuel," molecules. The windows would be made of protein, like receptor molecules that allow contact with the outside of the cell. The people are definitely proteins. We need people to read the encyclopedia just as we need proteins (enzymes) to express the genes. Any actions within the cell are probably going to be made by proteins, just as actions within a house are going to be carried out by people.

2. What this story is getting at is that the terms "replication" and "transcription" originated with written information. When you photocopy a manuscript ("replication") you make a perfect copy along with any proofreading instructions ("leave this out" or "move paragraph to end"). A good secretary will not reproduce these instructions

but obey them. So the transcript (the typed version of the manuscript) will be both shorter and "cleaner" than the original; it will be pure message with no proofreading marks. To match the model of the Central Dogma, we have to imagine that the paper must be translated into a foreign language. The message is the same, the words have the same meaning, but everything is different. This is just like when an RNA message is "translated" into amino acids; you have to know the code to see the correspondence.

3. The original form of the Central Dogma did not allow for information to travel from RNA to DNA. Years afterward it was realized that RNA viruses did exactly that, and the RNA message was made into DNA using "reverse transcriptase." Several retro-viruses are known today with RNA genomes including HIV and Rous sarcoma virus.

Chapter 2

Water, Weak Bonds, and the Generation of Order out of Chaos

This chapter covers a variety of extremely important fundamental concepts of biochemistry. Students should take care to be sure that they understand these ideas because they form a foundation for everything that is to come in the rest of the book. The authors begin with a discussion of heat-driven motion in solution. Next they discuss the properties of water, and then they move on to weak interactions. These include ionic forces (unlike charges attract), hydrogen bonds, van der Waals forces, and in water, the hydrophobic effect. These forces underlie all of biochemistry and explain why a given protein will have a characteristic folded shape, why DNA forms a double helix, and why enzymes can attract specific substrates. The chapter ends with a discussion of another important subject, pH and buffers.

LEARNING OBJECTIVES

When you have mastered this chapter, you should be able to accomplish the following objectives:

Thermal Motions Power Biological Interactions (Text Section 2.1)

1. Define what is meant by *Brownian motion*.
2. Relate the *angstrom* to other measures of length such as the meter.
3. Explain what is meant by transient *chemical interactions*.
4. Know the length of a typical noncovalent bond.

Biochemical Interactions Take Place in an Aqueous Solution (Text Section 2.2)

5. Discuss how a water molecule can be considered a dipole, or *polar*.
6. Define the term *hydrogen bond*.
7. Describe the *hydrophobic effect*.

Weak Interactions Are Important Biochemical Properties (Text Section 2.3)

8. List the three kinds of *noncovalent bonds* that mediate interactions of biomolecules and describe their characteristics.
9. Describe how the properties of water affect the interactions between molecules.
10. State the equation for *Coulomb's law* and understand what it means.

Hydrophobic Molecules Cluster Together (Text Section 2.4)

11. Explain the origin of the *hydrophobic effect* between *nonpolar molecules* and give examples of their importance in biochemical interactions.
12. State the *Second Law of Thermodynamics*. Explain what is meant by entropy.

pH is an Important Parameter of Biochemical Systems (Text Section 2.5)

13. Define pH and pK_a.
14. Know and use the *Henderson-Hasselbalch Equation*.
15. Understand how buffers respond to changes in [H^+] or [OH^-] concentration.

SELF-TEST

Thermal Motions Power Biological Interactions

1. The authors state that "transient chemical interactions form the basis for biochemistry and life itself." What are some examples where transient interactions are better than "strong covalent bonds"?
2. Is water the only substance mentioned in the text as exhibiting Brownian motion?

Biochemical Interactions Take Place in an Aqueous Solution

3. What would be the maximum number of hydrogen bonds a water molecule could have? What is the average number of hydrogen bonds per molecule of water? *3*

4. How does the cohesiveness of water relate to the height of a redwood tree?
   H₂O travels upward through tension & cohesion

Weak Interactions Are Important Biochemical Properties

5. How much weaker are the strongest hydrogen bonds than covalent bonds?
   a. half as strong
   b. one-tenth as strong
   c. 1/20 as strong
   d. 1/100 as strong

6. A keto group (C=O) could NOT form a hydrogen bond with:
   a. C-H
   b. N-H
   c. O-H

7. Could two methyl groups exhibit van der Waals forces and attract each other at close range?

8. How can weak bonds cause strong attachments, such as the bonding between the two strands of DNA, or a Gecko walking on the ceiling?

Hydrophobic Molecules Cluster Together

9. For the bonds or interactions in the left column, indicate all the characteristics in the right column that are appropriate.

   (a) electrostatic interaction
   (b) hydrogen bond
   (c) van der Waals bond
   (d) hydrophobic interaction

   (1) requires nonpolar species
   (2) involves charged species only
   (3) requires polar or charged species
   (4) involves either O and H or N and H atoms
   (5) involves polarizable atoms
   (6) exists only in water
   (7) optimal at the van der Waals contact distance
   (8) has an energy between 4 and 20 kJ/mol in H_2O
   (9) has an energy between 2 and 4 kJ/mol
   (10) is weakened in water

10. Biological membranes are made up of phospholipids, detergent-like molecules with long nonpolar chains attached to a polar head group. When isolated phospholipids are placed in water, they associate spontaneously to form membrane-like structures. Explain this phenomenon.

11. If two molecules had a tendency to associate with each other because groups on their surfaces could form hydrogen bonds, what would be the effect of putting these molecules in water? Explain.

12. Which of the following statements is correct? The entropy of a reaction refers to
    (a) the heat given off by the reaction.
    (b) the tendency of the system to move toward maximal randomness.
    (c) the energy of the transition state.
    (d) the effect of temperature on the rate of the reaction.

pH Is an Important Parameter of Biochemical Systems

13. The concentration of water is given in the chapter as 55 moles/liter. How would you calculate the concentration of water?

14. If the pH of 10^{-2} M HCl is 2, and the pH of 10^{-7} M HCl is 7, what is the pH of 10^{-9} M HCl? Remember that adding acid to water lowers its pH.

ANSWERS TO SELF-TEST

1. Biochemistry involves a lot of macromolecules like proteins, DNA, and RNA. The folding of these large molecules is driven by "weak bonds," so we get the DNA double helix and proteins folded up in a way that makes them powerful catalysts. Enzyme substrate reactions are another example, and the formation of lipid bilayer membranes as well. As you learn about biochemistry you will constantly see the importance of these transient interactions.

2. No. Dust particles can be seen "dancing" in air.

3. The oxygen in water has the "sp^3" structure, in other words a tetrahedral arrangement of four electron orbitals. Two of the orbitals are O-H bonds, and two are unshared electron pairs. So H_2O can form four hydrogen bonds with other molecules. The text states that the average number actually seen is 3.4 bonds to neighbors. This is high, and that is why water is cohesive with a high boiling point. Water has a molecular weight of 18, which is close to the molecular weight of methane (16), and yet methane is a gas at room temperature and 1 atmosphere. That is because methane (CH_4) cannot make any hydrogen bonds with itself.

4. The text points out that the process of "transpiration" in plants allows water to be pulled up from the roots to the leaves. Redwood trees can grow to a height of more than 300 feet, which puts a lot of stress on the hydrogen-bonded water column. It is possible that no plant could be 400 or 500 feet tall because transpiration would be impossible and the leaves would dry out and die.

5. c. 1/20. The text says that a covalent C-H bond has an energy of 418 kJ/mol, or 100 kcal/mol. A hydrogen bond will have 8–20 kJ/mol (2–5 kcal/mol) so the ratio of 5/100 is 1/20 for the strongest hydrogen bonds.

6. a. C-H bonds cannot participate in hydrogen bonding.

7. Yes. Any two organic compounds can become induced dipoles and exhibit van der Waals attractions at the appropriate distance.

8. The answer is "strength in numbers." If you have ever looked closely at a zipper, you can see a very tiny bump which fits into a very tiny hole. How can such a thing hold your clothing shut? There are **many** bumps and **many** holes, so the large numbers give a zipper strength.

9. (a) 2, 8 (b) 3, 4, 8, 10 (c) 5, 7, 9 (d) 1, 6

10. When the nonpolar chains of the individual phospholipid molecules are exposed to water, they form a cavity in the water network and order the water molecules around themselves. The ordering of the water molecules requires energy. By associating with one another through hydrophobic interactions, the nonpolar chains of phospholipids release the ordered water by decreasing the total surface area and hence reduce the energy required to order the water. Such coalescence stabilizes the entire system, and membrane-like structures form.

11. Because of the high dielectric constant of water and its ability to form competing hydrogen bonds, the interaction between the molecules would be weakened.

12. b

13. The molecular weight of water is 18, 16 for oxygen and 2×1 for the hydrogens. Thus a mole of water weighs 18 grams. A liter of water weighs 1000 grams, so $1000 \div 18 = 55$ M.

14. The pH of pure water is 7, meaning the H^+ concentration is 10^{-7} or 0.0000001 M. If we add 10^{-9} M HCl to pure water, we are increasing the proton concentration by 0.000000001 M. The sum of the two is 0.000000101 and the pH is now 6.996 instead of 7.0. Students often get pH = 9 for this problem but they have to be ignoring the pre-existing $[H^+]$ concentration.

PROBLEMS

1. Imagine a cell with some other solvent than water which somehow did not allow for Brownian motion. What effect would this have on normal cellular processes?

2. As will be seen in succeeding chapters, enzymes provide a specific binding site for substrates where one or more chemical steps can be carried out. Often these sites are designed to exclude water. Suppose that at a binding site, a negatively charged substrate interacts with a positively charged atom of an enzyme.

    (a) Using Coulomb's equation, show how the presence of water might affect the interaction. What sort of environment might be preferable for an ionic interaction? Note that a numerical answer is not required here.

    (b) How would an ionic interaction be affected by the distance between the oppositely charged atoms?

3. Water molecules have an unparalleled ability to form hydrogen bonds with one another. Water also has an unusually high heat capacity, as measured by the amount of energy required to increase the temperature of a gram of water by 1°C. How does hydrogen bonding contribute to water's high heat capacity?

4. The Second Law of Thermodynamics states that the entropy (disorder) of a system and its surroundings always increases for a spontaneous process. So why does DNA fold up spontaneously? It is evident that DNA folding moves from a disorderly state (randomly unfolded) to an orderly state (double helix). Explain.

5. What is the molarity of pure water? Show that a change in the concentration of water by ionization does not appreciably affect the molarity of the solution.

6. When sufficient H^+ is added to lower the pH by one unit, what is the corresponding increase in hydrogen ion concentration?

7. You have a solution of HCl that has a pH of 2.1. What is the concentration of HCl needed to make this solution?

8. Human blood maintains a very tight pH range (about 7.35–7.45). It accomplishes this homeostasis partly through what is known as the bicarbonate buffering system. Blood has large amounts of bicarbonate, HCO_3^-, a weak acid with a pK_a near physiological pH. As the equilibrium below shows, bicarbonate can pick up H^+ and form carbonic acid. Carbonic acid is degraded by enzymes to form CO_2, which can exit via the lungs.

$$CO_2 + H_2O \longleftrightarrow H_2CO_2 \longleftrightarrow H^+ + HCO_3^-$$

Uncontrolled diabetes can result in ketoacidosis, a condition in which metabolic acids such as β-hydroxybutyric acid (a substance known as a ketone body) build up. β-hydroxybutyric acid has a pK_a below that of physiological pH. A characteristic of ketoacidosis is deep and rapid breathing. Why would ketoacidosis lead to this symptom? Explain.

9. A woman is brought into the emergency room experiencing nausea and vomiting. She is also hyperventilating. She says that she ingested a bottle of aspirin about two hours earlier. Aspirin (acetylsalicylic acid) is converted to salicylic acid in the stomach. Assuming 100% conversion to salicylic acid, calculate the percentage of protonated and unprotonated forms of salicylic acid in her stomach, given a pH of 2.0 for the stomach.

10. Spontaneous processes are those that increase in entropy. Explain how a freezer then can make ice, a process that reduces entropy in the system.

11. It is surprising for some people to think that "clean things" like soaps and detergents can be made from components such as beef fat and ashes. Beef fat contains stearic acid, an 18-carbon carboxylic acid, whereas wood ashes contain potassium hydroxide. When these two substances are mixed and heated, sodium stearate is produced. Sodium stearate is a major component of soap. Explain why soap works. Why is it able to disperse greasy substances in water?

ANSWERS TO PROBLEMS

1. Chemical reactions all occur when molecules collide with each other. Enzymes must collide with substrates in order to find the active site. Without Brownian motion there would be nothing to propel the molecules around, everything would sit still and nothing would ever collide with anything. Such a cell would not be able to live.

2. (a) The magnitude of the electrostatic attraction would be diminished by the presence of water because D, the dielectric constant, is relatively high for water. Inspection of Coulomb's equation shows that higher values of D will reduce the force of the attraction. Lower values, such as those for hydrophobic molecules like hexane, allow a higher value for F. We shall see that many enzyme active sites are lined with hydrophobic residues, creating an environment that enhances ionic interaction.

(b)   Inspection of Coulomb's equation also reveals that the force between two oppositely charged atoms will vary inversely with the square of the distance between them.

3.   When water is heated, considerable energy is required to break the hydrogen bonds. Only after a large percentage of bonds are broken are the molecules more mobile and the temperature raised. This buffering capacity of water is very important to cells, which can resist changes caused by increases in temperature because of water's high heat capacity.

4.   As described in the chapter, all of the "weak forces" commonly involved in biochemistry help in formation of the double helix. Hydrogen bonds allow formation of Watson-Crick base pairs. Van der Waals forces allow "pancake" stacking of base pairs. Ionic forces keep the phosphates distant from each other, and the hydrophobic effect favors putting the flat hydrophobic surfaces of base pairs inside where they don't interact with the surrounding water. But this question is phrased in terms of thermodynamics so we have to remember the equation $\Delta G = \Delta H - T\Delta S$. The entropy term (S) must be unfavorable because obviously the change from two chains with randomly coiled conformation to one precisely formed double helix is a loss of disorder, a gain in orderliness. Thus, because we know that the double helix forms spontaneously in water, there must be a compensating change in heat or enthalpy (H). And indeed a substantial amount of heat is released when the double helix forms. This could be broken down into components, one of which would be the formation of hydrogen bonds mentioned above. The "weak forces" allow bonding which leads to favorable loss of heat energy.

5.   The molarity of water equals the number of moles of water per liter. A liter of water weighs 1000 grams, and its molecular weight is 18, so the molarity of water is

$$M = \frac{1000}{18} = 55.6$$

At 25°C, K_w is 1.0×10^{-14}; at neutrality, the concentration of both hydrogen and hydroxyl ions is each equal to 10^{-7} M. Thus, the actual concentration of H_2O is $(55.6 - 0.0000001)$ M; the difference is so small that it can be disregarded.

6.   Because pH values are based on a logarithmic scale, every unit change in pH means a tenfold change in hydrogen ion concentration. When pH = 2.0, $[H^+] = 10^{-2}$ M; when pH = 3.0, $[H^+] = 10^{-3}$ M.

7.   Assume that HCl in solution is completely ionized to H^+ and Cl^-. Then find the concentration of H^+, which equals the concentration of Cl^-.

$$pH = -\log\left[H^+\right] = 2.1$$

$$\left[H^+\right] = 10^{-2.1}$$

$$= 10^{0.9} \times 10^{-3}$$

$$= 7.94 \times 10^{-3}\,M$$

$$\text{Thus, } \left[H^+\right] = \left[Cl^-\right] = \left[HCl\right] = 7.94 \times 10^{-3}\,M$$

8. The breathing is the body's attempt to return to normal pH. If β-hydroxybutyric acid builds up, it loses its H⁺ and increases the concentration of H⁺ in the blood. This drives the equilibrium to the left, as the H⁺ combines with bicarbonate, generating carbonic acid, which degrades to CO_2 and H_2O. The CO_2 is expelled via the lungs.

9.

$$pH = pK_a + \log \frac{[A-]}{[HA]}$$

$$2 = 3 + \log \frac{[A-]}{[HA]}$$

$$-1 = \log \frac{[A-]}{[HA]}$$

$$\frac{[A-]}{[HA]} = 0.1 \qquad 10^{-1} = 0.1$$

Let x = % A^-

$1 - x$ = % HA

$$\frac{x}{1-x} = 0.1$$

$$x = 0.09$$

$$\%A^- = 9\%$$

% HA (protonated) = 91%

10. A freezer increases the entropy around it. Work is required to lower the entropy of the water in making ice, and this process occurs at the expense of a freezer moving electricity around and generating heat. Entropy can be made to decrease locally, but only at the expense of useful work. The work causes the entropy of the universe to increase.

11. Soap contains an ionic end that interacts with water and a long nonpolar chain that interacts with nonpolar items such as grease. The soap surrounds the grease particle, creating a micelle. The charged portions interact with the solvent, enabling the micelle to disperse in the solvent and be washed away.

Amino Acids

Chapter 3

Amino acids are the building blocks of proteins. A true understanding of biochemistry starts with a thorough knowledge of the 20 common amino acids. It is essential that you learn the names, symbols, and properties of these amino acids at this point, as they will recur throughout the text in connection with protein structures, enzymatic mechanisms, metabolism, protein synthesis, and the regulation of gene expression. Amino acids are ionizable, and it is important to understand the pK_a values provided. One argument for the importance of amino acids is the fact that if certain amino acids are lacking in the diet, severe nutritional diseases can result. Humans can synthesize only 11 of the 20 required amino acids. The remaining nine amino acids are called "essential" amino acids. These must be included in the diet just like vitamins.

LEARNING OBJECTIVES

When you have mastered this chapter, you should be able to accomplish the following objectives.

Proteins Are Built from a Repertoire of 20 Amino Acids (Text Section 3.1)

1. Distinguish between the *Fischer projection* and *stereochemical* rendering of molecules.
2. Know that proteins only contain L *amino acids.*
3. Draw the structure of an amino acid and indicate the following features, which are common to all *amino acids: functional groups, side chains,* and *ionic forms.*

Amino Acids Contain a Wide Array of Functional Groups (Text Section 3.2)

4. Classify each of the 20 amino acids according to the side chain on the α *carbon* as *aliphatic, aromatic, sulfur-containing, aliphatic hydroxyl, basic, acidic,* or *amide* derivative.
5. Give the name and one-letter and three-letter symbol of each amino acid. Describe each amino acid in terms of *size, charge, hydrogen-bonding capacity, chemical reactivity,* and *hydrophilic* or *hydrophobic* nature.
6. Describe the way that interactions between *pH* and *pKa* affect the *ionization state* of any given amino acid or its side chain in a protein.

Essential Amino Acids Must be Obtained from the Diet (Text Section 3.3)

7. List the nine essential amino acids for adult humans.
8. Describe the cause and symptoms of *kwashiorkor.*

SELF-TEST

Proteins Are Built from a Repertoire of 20 Amino Acids

1. Is the amino acid shown below D or L? Is naturally occurring Glycine D or L?

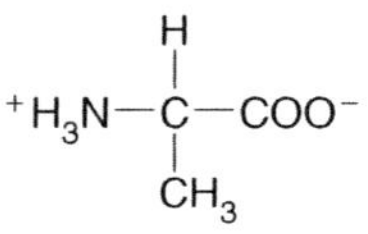

$$^+H_3N-\overset{\overset{\displaystyle H}{|}}{\underset{\underset{\displaystyle CH_3}{|}}{C}}-COO^-$$

Amino Acids Contain a Wide Array of Functional Groups

2. (a) Examine the four amino acids given below:

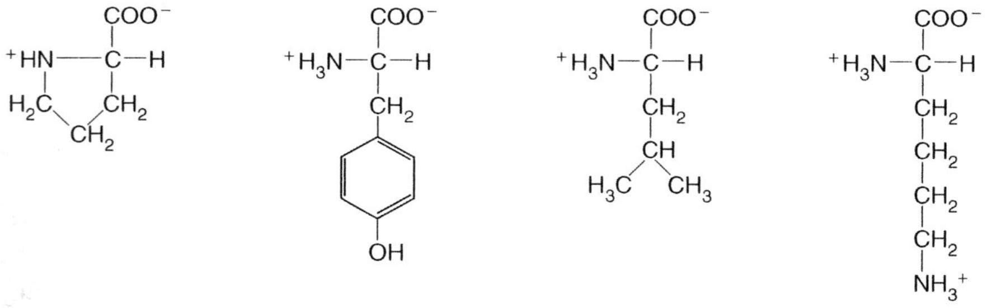

A   B   C   D

Indicate which of these amino acids are associated with the following properties:
- (a) aliphatic side chain
- (b) basic side chain
- (c) three ionizable groups
- (d) charge of +1 at pH 7.0
- (e) pK ~10 in proteins
- (f) secondary amino group
- (g) designated by the symbol K
- (h) in the same class as phenylalanine
- (i) most hydrophobic of the four
- (j) side chain capable of forming hydrogen bonds

(b) Name the four amino acids.

(c) Name the other amino acids of the same class as D.

3. Draw the structure of cysteine at pH 1.

4. Match the amino acids in the left column with the appropriate side chain types in the right column.

(a) Lys		(1)	nonpolar aliphatic
(b) Glu		(2)	nonpolar aromatic
(c) Leu		(3)	basic
(d) Cys		(4)	acidic
(e) Trp		(5)	sulfur-containing
(f) Ser		(6)	hydroxyl-containing

5. Which of the following amino acids have side chains that are negatively charged under physiologic conditions (i.e., near pH 7)?

- (a) Asp
- (b) His
- (c) Trp
- (d) Glu
- (e) Cys

6. Why does histidine act as a buffer at pH 6.0? What can you say about the buffering capacity of histidine at pH 7.6?

Essential Amino Acids Must Be Obtained from the Diet

7. Which of these amino acids is essential?

- (a) Aspartate
- (b) Alanine
- (c) Asparagine
- (d) Arginine
- (e) Proline

8. Why would weaning lead to malnutrition in some children in Africa and elsewhere?

ANSWERS TO SELF-TEST

1. The amino acid shown is D-Alanine, you can see that the H and carboxyl have been swapped—in the Fischer projection this always inverts the configuration. Glycine, with no R group (only H) is neither D nor L (achiral).

2. (a) (a) C (b) D (c) B, D (d)D (e) B, D (f) A (g) D (h) B (i) C (j) B, D

(b) A is proline, B is tyrosine, C is leucine, and D is lysine.

(c) histidine and arginine (basic amino acids)

3. See the structure of cysteine. At pH 1, all the ionizable groups are protonated. Thus the carboxyl is uncharged (COOH), and the amino is positive (NH_3^+). The mercaptan side chain remains –SH.

$$
\begin{array}{c}
COOH \\
| \\
^+H_3N-C-H \\
| \\
CH_2 \\
| \\
SH
\end{array}
$$

Cysteine

4. (a) 3   (b) 4   (c) 1   (d) 5   (e) 2   (f) 6

5. a, d, the "acidic" amino acids.

6. Histidine acts as a buffer at pH 6.0 because this is the pK of the imidazole group (see Table 3.1). At pH 7.6, histidine is a poor buffer because no one ionizing group is partially protonated and therefore capable of donating or accepting protons without markedly changing the pH.

7. e. Proline is essential. (Arginine is essential in human infants but not in adults).

8. Mother's milk is nutritionally complete. If weaning leads to malnutrition then the other forms of "baby food" must be lacking in protein, or lacking in essential amino acids.

PROBLEMS

1. Where stereoisomers of biomolecules are possible, only one is usually found in most organisms; for example, only the L amino acids occur in proteins. What problems would occur if, for example, the amino acids in the body proteins of herbivores were in the L isomer form, whereas the amino acids in a large number of the plants they fed upon were in the D isomer form?

2. The charged form of the imidazole ring of histidine is believed to participate in a reaction catalyzed by an enzyme. At pH 7.0, what is the probability that the imidazole ring will be charged?

3. Calculate the pH at which a solution of cysteine would have no net charge.

4. Monosodium glutamate (MSG) is well-known as common ingredient in Chinese food, but it is also used as a flavor in many other food products. "Yeast protein" or "hydrolyzed vegetable protein" in fact means that MSG has been added. Which of the following represents glutamate at physiological pH?

A

$$
\begin{array}{c}
\quad\quad O \\
\quad\quad \| \\
^{\ominus}H_3N-CHC-O^{\ominus} \\
| \\
CH_2 \\
| \\
HC=O \\
| \\
OH
\end{array}
$$

B

$$
\begin{array}{c}
\quad\quad O \\
\quad\quad \| \\
^{\ominus}H_3N-CHC-O^{\ominus} \\
| \\
CH_2 \\
| \\
CH_2 \\
| \\
C=O \\
| \\
OH
\end{array}
$$

C

$$
\begin{array}{c}
\quad\quad O \\
\quad\quad \| \\
^{\oplus}H_3N-CHC-O^{\ominus} \\
| \\
CH_2 \\
| \\
CH_2 \\
| \\
C=O \\
| \\
O^{\ominus}
\end{array}
$$

D

$$
\begin{array}{c}
\quad\quad O \\
\quad\quad \| \\
^+H_3N-CHC-O^- \\
| \\
CH_2 \\
| \\
CH_2 \\
| \\
C=O \\
| \\
NH_2
\end{array}
$$

5. The essential amino acids are the amino acids that are too difficult for us to synthesize. Thus they include most of the aromatic amino acids, but not tyrosine. Why do you think tyrosine is not on the list?

ANSWERS TO PROBLEMS

1. All metabolic reactions in an organism are catalyzed by enzymes that are generally specific for either the D or the L isomeric form of a substrate. If an animal (an herbivore in this case) is to be able to digest the protein from a plant and build its own protein from the resulting amino acids, both the animal and the plant must make their proteins from amino acids having the same configuration. In this hypothetical case the L-amino acid animal would be poisoned by its D-amino acid food.

2.   Use the Henderson-Hasselbalch equation to calculate the concentration of histidine, whose imidazole ring is ionized at neutral pH. The value of pK for the ring is 6.0 for a histidine residue in a protein (see Table 3.1).

$$pH = pK + \log \frac{[His]}{[His^+]}$$

$$7.0 = 6.0 + \log \frac{[His]}{[His^+]}$$

$$\log \frac{[His]}{[His^+]} = 1.0$$

$$\frac{[His]}{[His^+]} = 10$$

At pH 7.0, the ratio of uncharged histidine to charged histidine is 10:1, making the probability that the side chain is charged only 9%.

3. To see which form of cysteine has no net charge, examine all the possible forms, beginning with the one that is most protonated:

Net charge	+1	0	−1	−2

The pH of the cysteine solution at which the amino acid has no net charge will be that point at which there are equal amounts of the compound with a single positive charge and a single negative charge. This is, in effect, the average of the two corresponding pK values, one for the α-carboxyl group and the other for the side chain sulfhydryl group. Thus, (1.8 + 8.3)/2 = 5.05. This value is also known as the *isoelectric point*.

4. (c) At physiological pH, the pK_as of both carboxylic acid groups have been exceeded, so these are predominantly ionized/deprotonated. The amino group has a pK_a below that of physiological pH, so it remains protonated.

5. Tyrosine is very close in structure to phenylalanine, which humans cannot synthesize. The only difference is a para-hydroxy group on the benzene ring (making it a phenol). It happens that we do have an enzyme that can hydroxylate phenylalanine in that position, making the rest of the synthesis irrelevant as long as we have phe in the diet.

Protein Three-Dimensional Structure

Proteins are macromolecules that play central roles in all the processes of life. Chapter 4 begins with a discussion of key properties of proteins. Following the discussion of amino acids in Chapter 3, this chapter turns to peptides and to the linear sequences of amino acid residues in proteins. Next, it describes the folding of these linear polymers into the specific three-dimensional structures of proteins. The primary structure (or sequence of amino acids) dictates the higher orders of structure including secondary (α, β, etc.), tertiary (often globular), and quaternary (with multiple chains). You should note that the majority of functional proteins exist in water and that their structures are stabilized by the weak forces and interactions you learned about in Chapter 2. Hydrophobic groups are folded into the interior of most globular proteins. Some diseases are caused by prions, including mad cow disease and Creutzfeldt-Jakob disease. These are diseases of protein folding—wrongly folded proteins precipitate and form damaging plaque in the brain. The chapter concludes with a discussion of the theory of how proteins fold, including attempts to predict protein folding from amino acid sequences.

LEARNING OBJECTIVES

When you have mastered this chapter, you should be able to accomplish the following objectives.

Primary Structure: Amino Acids Are Linked by Peptide Bonds to Form Polypeptide Chains (Text Section 4.1)

1. List the key properties of proteins.

2. Explain how proteins relate one-dimensional gene structure to three-dimensional structure in the cell, and their complex interactions with each other and various substrates.

3. Draw a *peptide bond* and describe its *conformation* and its role in *polypeptide* sequences. Indicate the *N-* and *C-terminal residues* in *peptides*.

4. Define *main chain, side chains,* and *disulfide bonds* in polypeptides. Give the range of *molecular weights* of proteins.

5. Explain the origin and significance of the unique *amino acid sequences* of proteins.

6. State four reasons why knowing the amino acid sequence of a protein is important.

7. Understand why nearly all peptide bonds are *trans.*

8. Define the ϕ and ψ angles used to describe a peptide bond, and be able to read a *Ramachandran plot.*

Secondary Structure: Polypeptide Chains Can Fold into Regular Structures (Text Section 4.2)

9. Differentiate between two major *periodic structures* of proteins: the α helix and the β-pleated sheet. Describe the patterns of hydrogen bonding, the shapes, and the dimensions of these structures.

10. List the types of interactions among amino acid side chains that stabilize the *three-dimensional structures* of proteins. Give examples of *hydrogen bond donors* and *acceptors.*

11. Describe the role and structure of β *turns* or *hairpin turns* and *omega loops* in the structure of common proteins.

12. Understand the structures of fibrous proteins including α-*keratin,* made of α *helical coiled coils,* and *collagen,* which has a tight triple helix.

Tertiary Structure: Water-Soluble Proteins Fold into Compact Structures (Text Section 4.3)

13. Using *myoglobin* and *porin* as examples, describe the main characteristics of native folded protein structures.

14. Rationalize the conformational preferences of different amino acids in proteins and polypeptides.

15. Explain what is understood about the role of protein folding in *mad cow disease* and *Alzheimer's disease.*

16. Describe the *nucleation-condensation* model of protein folding.

17. Give evidence that protein folding appears to be a cooperative transition, and explain why that means it is an "all-or-none" process.

18. Explain how *protein folding* proceeds through stabilization of *intermediate states* rather than through a sampling of all possible conformations.

19. Distinguish between *motifs* and *domains* in protein structure.

Quaternary Structure: Multiple Polypeptide Chains Can Assemble into a Single Protein (Text Section 4.4)

20. Describe the *primary, secondary, tertiary,* and *quaternary structures* of proteins.

The Amino Acid Sequence of a Protein Determines Its Three-Dimensional Structure (Text Section 4.5)

21. Using *ribonuclease* as an example, describe the evidence for the hypothesis that all of the information needed to specify the three-dimensional structure of a protein is contained in its amino acid sequence.

22. Discuss the methods and advances in the prediction of three-dimensional structures of proteins.

23. List examples of the *modification* and *cleavage* of proteins that expand their functional roles.

SELF-TEST

Primary Structure: Amino Acids Are Linked by Peptide Bonds to Form Polypeptide Chains

1. How many different dipeptides can be made from the 20 L amino acids? What are the minimum and the maximum number of pK_a values for any dipeptide? 2^{2b}

2. For the pentapeptide Glu-Met-Arg-Thr-Gly,
   (a) name the carboxyl-terminal residue.
   (b) give the number of charged groups at pH 7.
   (c) give the net charge at pH 1.
   (d) write the sequence using one-letter symbols.
   (e) draw the peptide bond between the Thr and Gly residues, including both side chains.

3. If a polypeptide has 400 amino acid residues, what is its approximate mass?
   (a) 11,000 daltons   (c) 44,000 daltons
   (b) 22,000 daltons   (d) 88,000 daltons

4. Which amino acid can stabilize protein structures by forming covalent cross-links between polypeptide chains?
   (a) Met   (d) Gly
   (b) Ser   (e) Cys
   (c) Gln

Secondary Structure: Polypeptide Chains Can Fold into Regular Structures

5. Discuss the significance of *Ramachandran diagram.* Contrast the conformational states of Gly and Pro in proteins compared with other amino acid residues.

6. Which of the following statements about the peptide bond are true?
   (a) The peptide bond is planar because of the partial double-bond character of the bond between the carbonyl carbon and the nitrogen.
   (b) There is relative freedom of rotation of the bond between the carbonyl carbon and the nitrogen.

(c) The hydrogen that is bonded to the nitrogen atom is *trans* to the oxygen of the carbonyl group.

(d) There is no freedom of rotation around the bond between the α carbon and the carbonyl carbon.

7. Which of the following statements about the α helix structure of proteins is correct?

(a) It is maintained by hydrogen bonding between amino acid side chains.

(b) It makes up about the same percentage of all proteins.

(c) It can serve a mechanical role by forming stiff bundles of fibers in some proteins.

(d) It is stabilized by hydrogen bonds between amide hydrogens and amide oxygens in polypeptide chains.

(e) It includes all 20 amino acids at equal frequencies.

8. Which of the following properties are common to α-helical and β pleated sheet structures in proteins?

(a) rod shape

(b) hydrogen bonds between main-chain CO and NH groups

(c) axial distance between adjacent amino acids of 3.5 Å

(d) variable numbers of participating amino acid residues

9. Explain why α helix and β pleated sheet structures are often found in the interior of water-soluble proteins.

Tertiary Structure: Water-Soluble Proteins Fold into Compact Structures

10. Which of the following amino acid residues are likely to be found on the inside of a water-soluble protein?

(a) Val   (d) Arg

(b) His   (e) Asp

(c) Ile

11. Which of the following statements about the structures of water-soluble proteins, exemplified by myoglobin, are NOT true?

(a) They contain tightly packed amino acids in their interior.

(b) Most of their nonpolar residues face the aqueous solvent.

(c) The main-chain NH and CO groups are often involved in H-bonded secondary structures in the interior of these proteins.

(d) Polar residues such as His may be found in the interior of these proteins if the residues have specific functional roles.

(e) All of these proteins contain β sheet structural motifs.

12. Which one of the following amino acids interrupts α helices, and also disrupts β sheets?

(a) Phe   (d) His

(b) Cys   (e) Pro

(c) Trp

13. Mad cow disease, Creutzfeldt-Jakob disease, and Alzheimer's disease are caused by

(a) Viruses

(b) Bacteria

(c) Misfolded proteins

14. If we know that a solution of protein is half-folded, what will we find in solution?

    (a) 100% half-folded protein
    (b) 50% fully folded, 50% unfolded
    (c) 33% fully folded, 34% half-folded, and 33% unfolded

Quaternary Structure: Multiple Polypeptide Chains Can Assemble into a Single Protein

15. Match the levels of protein structures in the left column with the appropriate descriptions in the right column.

    (a) primary
    (b) secondary
    (c) tertiary
    (d) quaternary

    (1) association of protein subunits
    (2) overall folding of a single chain, can include α-helical and β sheet structures
    (3) linear amino acid sequence
    (4) repetitive arrangement of amino acids that are near each other in the linear sequence

16. Hemoglobin has the structure $\alpha_2\beta_2$. Hemoglobin is a protein. What are α and β called?

The Amino Acid Sequence of a Protein Determines Its Three-Dimensional Structure

17. Which of the following statements are true?

    (a) Ribonuclease (RNase) can be treated with urea and reducing agents to produce a random coil.
    (b) If one oxidizes random-coil RNase in urea, it quickly regains its enzymatic activity.
    (c) If one removes the urea and oxidizes RNase slowly, it will renature and regain its enzymatic activity.
    (d) Although renatured RNase has enzymatic activity, it can be readily distinguished from native RNase.

18. When most proteins are exposed to acidic pH (e.g., pH 2), they lose biological activity. Explain why.

19. Several amino acids can be modified after the synthesis of a polypeptide chain to enhance the functional capabilities of the protein. Match the type of modifying group in the left column with the appropriate amino acid residues in the right column.

    (a) phosphate
    (b) hydroxyl
    (c) γ-carboxyl
    (d) acetyl

    (1) Glu
    (2) Thr
    (3) Pro
    (4) Ser
    (5) N-terminal
    (6) Tyr

20. How can a protein be modified to make it more hydrophobic?

ANSWERS TO SELF-TEST

1. The 20 L amino acids can form 20 × 400 dipeptides. The minimum number of pK_a values for any dipeptide is two; the maximum is four.

2. (a) glycine
    (b) 4, namely the 2 carboxyl groups of glutamate, the R group of arginine, and the alpha amino group of glycine
    (c) +2, contributed by the N-terminal amino group and the arginine residue
    (d) E-M-R-T-G
    (e) See the structure of the peptide bond below.

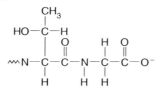

Peptide bond

3. c

4. e

5. A Ramachandran plot gives the possible ϕ and ψ angles for the main polypeptide chain containing different amino acid residues. The fact that <u>glycine lacks an R group means that it is much less constrained than other residues</u>. In Figure 4.10, the left-handed helix region, which occurs rarely, generally includes several Gly residues. This is the top right quadrant of the graph. In contrast to glycine, proline is more highly constrained than most residues because the R group is tied to the amino group. This fixes ϕ at about − 65°. In Figure 4.8, the rare *cis* form of the peptide bond is shown as occurring about half of the time in X-Pro peptide bonds.

6. a, c

7. c, d

8. b, d

9. In both α-helical and β sheet structures, the polar peptide bonds of the main chain are involved in internal hydrogen bonding, thereby eliminating potential hydrogen bond formation with water. Overall the secondary structures are less polar than the corresponding linear amino acid sequences.

10. a, c. Specific charged and polar amino acid residues may be found inside some proteins, in active sites, but most polar and charged residues are located on the surface of proteins.

11. b, e. Statement (b) is incorrect because globular, water-soluble proteins have most of their nonpolar residues buried in the interior of the protein. Statement (e) is incorrect because not all water-soluble proteins contain β sheet secondary structures. For example, myoglobin is mostly α-helical and lacks β sheet structures.

12. e

13. c

14. b

15. (a) 3   (b) 4   (c) 2   (d) 1

16. Hemoglobin is a protein, α is a protein, β is a protein. A protein is a macromolecule composed of amino acids whether it is one chain or many. α and β are also called subunits.

17. a, c

18. A low pH (pH 2) will cause the protonation of all ionizable side chains and will change the charge distribution on the protein; furthermore, it will impart a large net

positive charge to the protein. The resulting repulsion of adjacent positive charges and the disruption of salt bridges often cause unfolding of the protein and loss of biological activity.

19. (a) 2, 4, 6   (b) 3   (c) 1   (d) 5

20. The attachment of a fatty acid chain to a protein can increase its hydrophobicity and promote binding to lipid membranes. Acetylation of surface groups would also work.

PROBLEMS

1. The net charge of a polypeptide at a particular pH can be determined by considering the pK_a value for each ionizable group in the protein. For a linear polypeptide composed of 10 amino acids, how many α-carboxyl and α-amino groups must be considered?

2. For the formation of a polypeptide composed of 20 amino acids, how many water molecules must be removed when the peptide bonds are formed? Although the hydrolysis of a peptide bond is energetically favored, the bond is very stable in solution. Why?

3. Each amino acid in a run of several amino acid residues in a polypeptide chain has ϕ values of approximately $-140°$ and ψ values of approximately $+147$. What kind of structure is it likely to be?

4. A survey of the location of reverse turns in soluble proteins shows that most reverse turns are located at the surface of the protein, rather than within the hydrophobic core of the folded protein. Can you suggest a reason for this observation?

5. Wool and hair are elastic; both are α-keratins, which contain long polypeptide chains composed of α helices twisted about each other to form cablelike assemblies with cross-links involving Cys residues. Silk, on the other hand, is rigid and resists stretching; it is composed primarily of antiparallel β pleated sheets, which are often stacked and interlocked. Briefly explain these observations in terms of the characteristics of the secondary structures of these proteins.

6. In a particular enzyme, an alanine residue is located in a cleft where the substrate binds. A mutation that changes this residue to a glycine has no effect on activity; however, another mutation, which changes the alanine to a glutamate residue, leads to a complete loss of activity. Provide a brief explanation for these observations.

7. Glycophorin A is a glycoprotein that extends across the red blood cell membrane. The portion of the polypeptide that extends across the membrane bilayer contains 19 amino acid residues and is folded into a helix. What is the width of the bilayer that could be spanned by this helix? The interior of the bilayer includes long acyl chains that are nonpolar. Which of the 20 L amino acids would you expect to find among those in the portion of the polypeptide that traverses the bilayer?

8. (a) Early experiments on the problem of protein folding (notably Anfinsen's experiments on ribonuclease, described in Section 4.5 of the text) suggested that the native three-dimensional structure of a protein was an automatic consequence of its primary structure. Cite experimental evidence that shows that this is the case.
   (b) Later, the discovery that proteins are synthesized directionally on ribosomes, from the amino to the carboxy terminus, complicated the earlier view of protein folding. Explain what the complicating circumstance might be.
   (c) The discovery of chaperone proteins allows both earlier views to be reconciled. Explain how that might be the case.

9. Suppose you are studying the conformation of a monomeric protein that has an un-usually high proportion of aromatic amino acid residues throughout the length of the polypeptide chain. Compared with a monomeric protein containing many aliphatic residues, what might you observe for the relative α-helical content for each of the two types of proteins? Would you expect to find aromatic residues on the outside or the inside of a globular protein? What about aliphatic residues?

10. As more and more protein sequences and three-dimensional structures become known, there is a proliferation of computer algorithms for the prediction of folding based on sequence. How might it be possible to winnow through the possibilities and find the best computer programs? Bear in mind that if the sequence and the structure are avail-able, it is too easy to "reverse engineer" a routine that will produce the correct answer.

11. In its discussion of protein modification and cleavage, the text refers to the synthesis and cleavage of a large polyprotein precursor of virus proteins, as well as to the syn-thesis of multiple polypeptide hormones from a single polypeptide chain. Is there an advantage to synthesizing a large precursor chain and then cleaving it to create a num-ber of products?

12. When diseases such as mad cow disease and scrapie (a similar disease in sheep) were first discovered, many people thought that they were caused by "slow viruses." On the one hand it seemed clear that the diseases were transmissible, but on the other it could take ten years after "infection" for the disease to manifest itself clinically. Carleton Gajdusek visited Papua New Guinea in the 1950's and described a similar human brain disease called kuru. The Fore tribe had customs which brought the liv-ing into contact with recently deceased relatives, and somehow kuru was being passed from the dead to the living. How would you show that the disease is caused by in-fection and not by some sort of genetic transmission? How would you prove that the agent of infection is not a tiny bacterium or a "slow virus"?

13. Jello (or "jelly" if you're from Britain or a British tradition) is composed of collagen derived from animal bones, hides, and inedible connective tissue. Why is jello not a particularly useful source of dietary protein?

14. Humalog is an analog of fast-acting human insulin that is also known as Lispro. The difference between Humalog/Lispro and normal human insulin is that two amino acids are switched on the B-chain at positions 28 and 29. The result is an insulin that is absorbed faster under the skin and has a shorter duration of action. Which of the following would you expect to be true about Lispro? (The name is a big clue.)

   (a) L and P on the A chain are reversed.
   (b) K and P on the B chain are reversed.
   (c) L and P on the B chain are reversed.
   (d) L and R on the B chain are reversed.
   (e) The B chain becomes kinked.

ANSWERS TO PROBLEMS

1. Only the N-terminal α-amino group and the C-terminal α-carboxyl group will un-dergo ionization. The internal groups will be joined by peptide bonds and are not ion-izable. Naturally ionizable R-groups will also contribute but this question focuses on the beginning and the end of the chain.

2. For a peptide of *n* residues, (*n* − 1) water molecules must be removed (19 in this case). A significant activation energy barrier makes peptide bonds kinetically stable.

3. From the Ramachandran plot in Figure 4.10 of the text, we see that β conformation is accommodated by φ values of approximately −140° and ψ values of approximately +147°. The structure is most likely a β sheet. In fact, the "low" numbers here imply that it is an antiparallel beta sheet. The parallel β sheet would have higher numbers, more like φ = −160° and ψ = +160°.

4. Figure 4.20 in the text shows that in a reverse turn the CO group of residue 1 is hydrogen-bonded to the NH group of residue 4. However, there are no adjacent amino acid residues available to form intrachain hydrogen bonds with the CO and NH groups of residues 2 and 3. These groups cannot form hydrogen bonds in the hydrophobic environment found in the interior portion of a folded protein. They are more likely to hydrogen bond with water on the surface of the protein.

5. When the α helices in wool are stretched, intrahelix hydrogen bonds are broken as are some of the interhelix disulfide bridges; maximum stretching yields an extended β sheet structure. The Cys cross-links provide some resistance to stretch and help pull the α helices back to their original positions. In silk, the β sheets are already maximally stretched to form hydrogen bonds. Each β pleated sheet resists stretching, but since the contacts between the sheets primarily involve van der Waals forces, the sheets are somewhat flexible.

6. Both alanine and glycine are neutral nonpolar residues with small side chains, whereas the side chain of glutamate is acidic and bulkier than that of alanine. Either feature of the glutamate R group could lead to the loss of activity by altering the protein conformation or by interfering with the binding of the substrate.

7. Since each residue in the α helix is 1.5 Å from its neighbor, the length of the chain that spans the membrane bilayer is 19 × 1.5 Å = 28.5 Å, which is also the width of the membrane. One would expect to find nonpolar amino acid residues in the polypeptide portion associated with the membrane bilayer. These would include Phe, Ile, Leu, Val, Met, and Ala (FILMV + A). The actual sequence of the buried chain is

I-T-L-I-I-F-G-V-M-A-G-V-I-G-T-I-L-L-I

8. (a) In Anfinsen's experiment, native ribonuclease is treated with mercaptoethanol to disrupt disulfide bonds and with urea as a denaturant, it unfolds, as indicated by the fact that it becomes enzymically inactive. When urea is removed by dialysis and disulfide bonds reform by oxidation, it regains enzymic activity, suggesting that its native structure has been restored. Note that the refolding occurs in the absence of any cellular proteins or other biosynthetic machinery.

    (b) The discovery that proteins are synthesized directionally on ribosomes beginning at the amino terminus complicates matters somewhat because folding of the amino end of the polypeptide chain could begin before the carboxyl end had been synthesized. Such folding could represent the most stable conformation over a short range, but there would be no guarantee that it would be part of the energy minimum for the entire molecule.

    (c) Chaperone proteins could bind to an initially synthesized polypeptide and prevent it from undergoing final folding until the entire molecule was synthesized. Note that the final fold of the protein is still specified by the primary structure.

9. The higher the proportion of aromatic side chains (such as those of phenylalanine) in the protein, the more likely that steric hindrance among closely located residues could interfere with the establishment of the regular repeating structure of the α helix. Smaller aliphatic side chains like those of leucine, isoleucine, and valine would be less likely to in-

terfere. Structural studies on many proteins reveal that the number of aromatic residues in α-helical segments is relatively low, while the content of aliphatic side chains in such segments is unremarkable, compared to that of other nonhelical regions of a folded protein. Both aliphatic and aromatic side chains (especially that of phenylalanine) are hydrophobic, so that many of them are buried inside a globular protein, away from water molecules.

10. Protein scientists have devised a competition called CASP, or Critical Assessment of Techniques for Protein Structure Prediction, which is held every other year. Laboratories that are working on determination of three-dimensional structure by x-ray crystallography (or nmr) announce that they expect to release the structure in a few months. They give a description of the sequence of the protein and its use in the cell, and withhold the actual structural coordinates until a certain date. In the meantime, laboratories with predictive algorithms publicly post the structure they think the protein will have. The success or failure of the prediction takes place in a public arena, and the better predictors have bragging rights. CASP-4 in 2000 showed that there are several effective programs available, notably ROSETTA, used by David Baker of the University of Washington (sometimes on a server known as ROBETTA). Results of the competition are published in the journal *Protein* and online (in technical language) at the website http://predictioncenter.org/. CASP-6 in 2004 was won by Krzysztof Ginalski of the University of Texas, using ROSETTA along with 3D-Jury and Meta-BASIC.

11. The primary advantage of precursor chain synthesis is that the production of related proteins can be coordinated. This could be important in viral infection, and it may also be important for coordinated synthesis of hormones with related activities. It is worth noting that there are other reasons for the synthesis of polyprotein precursors. For example, the genome of the poliovirus consists of a single RNA molecule that acts as a messenger on entering the cytoplasm of the host. In eukaryotic cells a messenger RNA molecule can be translated into only one polypeptide chain. Therefore the poliovirus can reproduce only by synthesizing its proteins by sequential cleavages.

12. The genetic hypothesis was ruled out by injecting material from Kuru-infected brains into chimpanzees. After a period of time, they came down with the disease. It was known that the incubation time was quite long. In fact it took decades to rule out the nanobacteria and "slow virus" hypotheses. Probably there are still a few scientists clinging to those ideas. Stanley Prusiner devoted his career to proving that diseases could be caused by infectious proteins (which he called prions). As he was able to purify the infectious agent (not an easy task—how do you assay during purification?) he reached a point where he could demonstrate that there were no nucleotides present in the solution. As you saw in Chapter 1 of the text, all cells and viruses contain DNA or RNA, which is made up of nucleotides. Adenine and guanine have to be present, and both are built on the bicyclic purine ring. Purines absorb ultraviolet light at certain characteristic frequencies but there is nothing in proteins that absorbs light at those frequencies.

13. Collagen is highly enriched in Glycine (1/3 of all residues) and Proline (or Hydroxyproline; 1/6 of all residues). Jello thus does not contain a sufficient variety of amino acids to be a rich nutritional source of amino acids.

14. (b) ("Lis" indicates Lysine, K; "Pro" indicates Proline, P)

Chapter 5

Techniques in Protein Biochemistry

hapter 5 extends Chapter 4 by introducing the most important methods used to investigate proteins. Many of these were essential in discovering the principles of protein structure and function presented in the previous chapter. These methods also constitute the armamentarium of modern biochemical research and underlie current developments in biotechnology. First, the authors define the concept of the proteome, the sum of functioning proteins in the cell and their interactions. Then they outline methodological principles for the analysis and purification of proteins. This is followed by a discussion of the use of immunology as a tool in the analysis and localization of proteins. Finally, the authors discuss the usefulness of knowing the sequence of amino acids in a protein, the primary structure, and important tools used in determination of protein sequence.

LEARNING OBJECTIVES

When you have mastered this chapter, you should be able to accomplish the following objectives.

The Proteome Is the Functional Representation of the Genome (Text Section 5.1)

1. Distinguish between the genome and the proteome, and define both terms.

The Purification of A Protein Is the First Step in Understanding Its Function (Text Section 5.2)

2. Describe how a quantitative enzyme assay can be used to calculate the specific activity during protein purification.

3. Define differential centrifugation, and describe how it would be used to produce a protein mixture from a cell homogenate.

4. List the properties of proteins that can be used to accomplish their separation and purification, and correlate them with the appropriate methods: gel-filtration chromatography, dialysis, salting out, ion-exchange chromatography, and affinity chromatography. Describe the basic principles of each of these methods.

5. Describe the principle of electrophoresis and its application in the separation of proteins.

6. Explain the determination of protein mass by SDS-PAGE: sodium dodecyl sulfate-polyacrylamide gel electrophoresis.

7. Define the isoelectric point (pI) of a protein and describe isoelectric focusing as a separation method.

8. Explain the quantitative evaluation of a protein purification scheme.

Immunology Provides Important Techniques with Which to Investigate Proteins (Text Section 5.3)

9. Define the terms antibody, antigen, antigenic determinant (epitope), and immunoglobin G.

10. Contrast polyclonal antibodies and monoclonal antibodies and describe their preparation.

11. Outline methods that use specific antibodies in the analysis or localization of proteins.

Determining Primary Structure Facilitates an Understanding of Protein Function (Text Section 5.4)

12. Give examples of the important information that amino acid sequences reveal. For example, comparison of sequences can reveal relationships in function, or evolutionary relationships.

13. Outline the steps in the determination of the amino acid composition and the amino-terminal residue of a peptide.

14. Describe the sequential Edman degradation method and the automated determination of the amino acid sequences of peptides.

15. List the most common reagents used for the specific cleavage of proteins. Explain the application of overlap peptides to protein sequencing.

SELF-TEST

The Proteome Is the Functional Representation of the Genome

1. The genome sequence tells us all of the proteins an organism can make. Are all of these proteins expressed?

The Purification of A Protein Is the First Step in Understanding Its Function

2. The following five proteins, which are listed with their molecular weights and isoelectric points, were separated by SDS-polyacrylamide gel electrophoresis. Give the order of their migration from the top (the point of sample application) to the bottom of the gel.

		Molecular weight (daltons)	pI
(a)	α-antitrypsin	45,000	5.4
(b)	cytochrome c	13,400	10.6
(c)	myoglobin	17,000	7.0
(d)	serum albumin	69,000	4.8
(e)	transferrin	90,000	5.9

Top ——————— Bottom

3. If the five proteins in Question 2 were separated in an isoelectric-focusing experiment, what would be their distribution between the positive (+) and negative (−) ends of the gel? Indicate the high and low pH ends.

Cathode (−) ——————— (+) Anode

4. Which of the following statements are NOT true?
   (a) The pI is the pH value at which a protein has no charges.
   (b) At a pH value equal to its pI, a protein will not move in the electric field of an electrophoresis experiment.
   (c) An acidic protein will have a pI greater than 7.
   (d) A basic protein will have a pI greater than 7.

5. SDS-polyacrylamide gel electrophoresis and the isoelectric-focusing method for the separation of proteins have which of the following characteristics in common? Both
   (a) separate native proteins.
   (b) make use of an electrical field.
   (c) separate proteins according to their mass.
   (d) require a pH gradient.
   (e) are carried out on supporting gel matrices.

6. Examine Table 5.1 in the text, evaluating a protein purification scheme. Does "total activity" go up or down as the protein is purified? Would it have been a good idea to try affinity chromatography at an earlier stage of purification?

Immunology Provides Important Techniques with Which to Investigate Proteins

7. Match the terms in the left column with the appropriate item or items from the right column.

   (a) antigens
   (b) antigenic determinants
   (c) polyclonal antibodies
   (d) monoclonal antibodies

   (1) immunoglobins
   (2) foreign proteins, polysaccharides, or nucleic acids
   (3) antibodies produced by hybridoma cells
   (4) groups recognized by antibodies
   (5) heterogeneous antibodies
   (6) homogeneous antibodies
   (7) antibodies produced by injecting an animal with a foreign substance
   (8) epitopes

8. Explain why immunoassays are especially useful for detecting and quantifying small amounts of a substance in a complex mixture.

Determining Primary Structure Facilitates an Understanding of Protein Function

9. Treating a protein with 6 M HCl at 110° for 24 hours will have what effect?

   (a) The protein will unfold (denature)
   (b) All peptide bonds will be destroyed, releasing the amino acids
   (c) All amino acids will be destroyed

10. Which of the following statements concerning the Edman degradation method are true?

    (a) Phenyl isothiocyanate is coupled to the amino-terminal residue.
    (b) Under mildly acidic conditions, the modified peptide is cleaved into a cyclic derivative of the terminal amino acids and a shortened peptide (minus the first amino acid).
    (c) Once the PTH amino acid is separated from the original peptide, a new cycle of sequential degradation can begin.
    (d) If a protein has a blocked amino-terminal residue (as does N-formyl methionine, for example), it cannot react with phenyl isothiocyanate.

11. When sequencing proteins, one tries to generate overlapping peptides by using cleavages at specific sites. Which of the following statements about the cleavages caused by particular chemicals or enzymes are true?

    (a) Cyanogen bromide cleaves at the carboxyl side of threonine.
    (b) Trypsin cleaves at the carboxyl side of Lys and Arg.
    (c) Chymotrypsin cleaves at the carboxyl side of aromatic and bulky amino acids.
    (d) 2-Nitro-5-thiocyanobenzoate cleaves on the amino side of cysteine residues.
    (e) Chymotrypsin cleaves at the carboxyl side of aspartate and glutamate.

12. What treatments could you apply to the following hemoglobin fragment to determine the amino-terminal residue and to obtain two sets of peptides with overlaps so that the complete amino acid sequence can be established? Give the sequences of the peptides obtained.

    Val-Leu-Ser-Pro-Ala-Lys-Thr-Asn-Val-Lys-Ala-Ala-Trp-Gly-Lys-Val-Gly-Ala-His-Ala-Gly-Glu-Tyr-Gly-Ala-Glu-Ala-Thr-Glu

13. Which of the following are important reasons for determining the amino acid sequences of proteins?

(a) Knowledge of amino acid sequences helps elucidate the molecular basis of biological activity.

(b) Alteration of an amino acid sequence may cause abnormal functioning and disease.

(c) Amino acid sequences provide insights into evolutionary pathways and protein structures.

(d) The three-dimensional structure of a protein can be predicted from its amino acid sequence.

(e) Amino acid sequences provide information about the destination and processing of some proteins.

(f) Amino acid sequences allow prediction of the DNA sequences encoding them and thereby facilitate the preparation of DNA probes specific for the regions of their genes.

ANSWERS TO SELF-TEST

1. In any given cell, at any given time, it is quite likely that many genes capable of producing protein are not being expressed. Single-celled organisms tend to respond to their environment, producing enzymes to deal with the nutrients and conditions in the area. Multicellular organisms need different proteins for different parts of the body. Humans have very different needs in the retina, the liver, and muscle cells. This is why the proteome is a useful concept, it is a description of the proteins actually present in a functioning cell.

2. Top $\dfrac{\text{e d a c b}}{}$ Bottom

3. High pH (–) $\dfrac{\text{b c e a d}}{}$ Low pH (+)

4. a, c. Regardless of the pH, a protein is never devoid of charges; at the pI, the sum of all the charges is zero.

5. b, e

6. Total activity drops as material is lost in each step of purification. In a good purification, total protein drops much faster, so that specific activity goes up dramatically. Not all proteins can be purified with affinity chromatography. When a protein has a unique substrate and works this well with affinity chromatography, it may be a good idea to leave out the ion exchange and molecular exclusion steps, and go straight to the "home run" technique. A standard source on protein purification states that "One-step purifications of 1,000-fold with nearly 100% recovery have been reported" with this technique. (R. K. Scopes. [1994]. *Protein purification, principles and practice,* 3rd ed. New York: Springer-Verlag.)

7. (a) 2   (b) 4, 8   (c) 1, 5, 7   (d) 1, 3, 6

8. Because the interaction of an antibody with its antigen is highly specific, recognition and binding can occur in the presence of many other substances. If the antibody is coupled to a radioactive or fluorescent group or an enzyme whose activity can be detected in situ, then a sensitive method is available for the detection and quantitation of the antigen-antibody complex.

9   b. Students encountering amino acid analysis may underestimate the violence of the procedure. Water boils at 100° so you need a sealed glass vial (or pressure cooker) just to achieve that temperature. And 6M HCl is dangerous even at room temperature. Plus 24 hours is a long reaction time. Besides destroying all peptide bonds, the technique actually destroys three of the amino acids in the protein, glutamine, asparagine, and tryptophan.

10. a, b, c, d

11. b, c, d

12. The amino-terminal residue of the hemoglobin fragment can be determined by analyzing the intact fragment by the Edman degradation method; this shows that the amino-terminal residue is Val. Trypsin digestion, separation of peptides, and Edman degradation give

Val-Leu-Ser-Pro-Ala-Lys
Thr-Asn-Val-Lys
Ala-Ala-Trp-Gly-Lys
Val-Gly-Ala-His-Ala-Gly-Glu-Tyr-Gly-Ala-Glu-Ala-Thr-Glu
Chymotrypsin digestion, separation of peptides, and Edman degradation give
Val-Leu-Ser-Pro-Ala-Lys-Thr-Asn-Val-Lys-Ala-Ala-Trp
Gly-Lys-Val-Gly-Ala-His-Ala-Gly-Glu-Tyr
Gly-Ala-Glu-Ala-Thr-Glu

13. a, b, c, e, f. Answer (d) may be correct in some cases where homologous proteins are compared in terms of amino acid sequences and known three-dimensional structures.

PROBLEMS

1. How can a protein be assayed if it is not an enzyme?

2. Many of the methods described in Chapter 5 are used to purify enzymes in their native state. Why would the use of SDS-polyacrylamide gel electrophoresis be unlikely to lead to the successful purification of an active enzyme? What experiments would you conduct to determine whether salting out with ammonium sulfate would be useful in enzyme purification?

3. Of the techniques for analyzing proteins discussed in Chapter 5 of the text, which one would be the easiest to use for accurately determining the molecular weight of a small monomeric protein? Comment on the standards you would wish to use in this technique. What types of proteins might not be analyzed accurately by your suggested method?

4. A hexapeptide that is part of a mouse polypeptide hormone is analyzed by a number of chemical and enzymatic methods. When the hexapeptide is hydrolyzed and analyzed by ion-exchange chromatography, the following amino acids are detected:

Tyr Cys Glu

Ile Lys Met

Two cycles of Edman degradation of the intact hexapeptide released the following PTH-amino acids (see Figure 5.1):

FIGURE 5.1

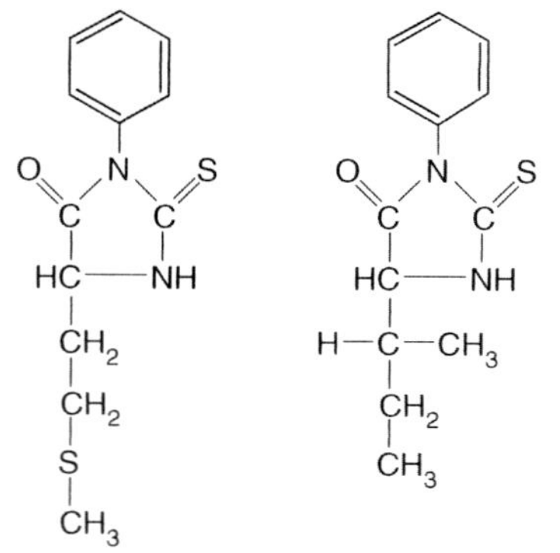

Cleavage of the intact protein with cyanogen bromide yields methionine and a pentapeptide. Treating the intact hexapeptide with trypsin yields a dipeptide, which contains tyrosine and glutamate, and a tetrapeptide. When the intact hexapeptide is treated with carboxypeptidase A, a tyrosine residue and a pentapeptide are produced. Bearing in mind that the hexapeptide is isolated from a mouse, write its amino acid sequence, using both three-letter and one-letter abbreviations.

5. The production of a small acidic protein, HCG or human chorionic gonadotropin, during pregnancy is the basis of most pregnancy test kits. What method makes the most sense for detecting a known protein like this?

ANSWERS TO PROBLEMS

1. This is a rather serious problem. Some proteins have a slight catalytic activity that can be utilized in an assay although they are not enzymes. Or perhaps the protein will serve as a substrate for a reaction. If a protein has no enzyme activity, but the molecular weight and/or pI is known, it can be detected by gel electrophoresis by looking for protein concentration at the right spot on the gel. Some proteins actually fluoresce, like the GFP (green fluorescent protein) produced by jellyfish. In these cases, the intensity of the fluorescence could serve as the basis for an assay.

   If the gene is known, then there are ways to "fish" out the protein in very high yield by modifying the sequence. This bypasses the need for an assay. One common procedure is "his-tagging" in which six tandem histidines are added to the sequence of the gene. The protein expressed can then be purified in one step on a nickel-containing column, and eluted with imidazole. This method is mentioned in the text as a special case of affinity chromatography. (A good review of various "Affinity Fusion Strategies" [Nilsson et al., *Prot. Exp. Purif.* 11(1997):1].)

2. SDS disrupts nearly all noncovalent interactions in a native protein, so the renaturation of a purified protein, which is necessary to restore enzyme activity, could be difficult or impossible. You should therefore conduct small-scale pilot tests to determine whether enzyme activity would be lost upon SDS denaturation. Similarly, when salting out with ammonium sulfate is considered, pilot experiments should be conducted. In many instances, concentrations of ammonium sulfate can be chosen such that the active enzyme remains in solution while other proteins are precipitated, thereby affording easy and rapid purification.

3. SDS-polyacrylamide gel electrophoresis, a sensitive and rapid technique which takes only a few hours and which has a high degree of resolution, is probably the easiest and most rapid method for providing an estimate of molecular weight. Small samples (as low as 0.02 mg) can be detected on the gel. For standards or markers on the gel, you should use two or more proteins whose molecular weights are higher than that of the protein to be analyzed, as well as two or more whose molecular weights are lower. The relative mobilities of these markers on the gel can then be plotted against the logarithms of their respective molecular weights, providing a straight line that can be used to establish the molecular weight of the protein to be analyzed. Proteins that have carbohydrate molecules covalently attached, or those that are embedded in membranes, often do not migrate according to the logarithm of their mass. The reasons for these anomalies are not clear; in the case of glycoproteins, or those with carbohydrate residues, the large heterocyclic rings of the carbohydrates may retard the movement of the proteins through the polyacrylamide gel. Membrane proteins often contain a high proportion of hydrophobic amino acid residues and may not be fully soluble in the gel system.

Modern variations of mass spectrometry can yield highly accurate MW values very quickly.

4. The sequence of the mouse hexapeptide is Met-Ile-Cys-Lys-Glu-Tyr, or MICKEY. Cyanogen bromide treatment cleaves methionine from one end, and the PTH-Met derivative places Met at the N-terminal end, with Ile next in the sequence. Trypsin treatment cleaves on the carboxyl side of Lys, so that Lys is on the C-terminal end of the tetrapeptide, next to Cys. Tyrosine is located on the C-terminal end, as shown by the observation that it is released as a single amino acid when the intact hexapeptide is treated with carboxypeptidase A. Glutamate must therefore be located between Lys and Tyr.

5. Most blood proteins do not show up in the urine, but HCG does. And it is produced very soon after the egg is fertilized, and then in increasing amounts as the pregnancy progresses. Sandwich ELISA (see Figure 5.22 in the text) is the ideal method for complex biological fluids, and it is relatively easy to produce two different monoclonal antibodies to epitopes on opposite sides of the protein. All home pregnancy test kits are based on variations of this method.

For a better understanding of the use of ELISA in home pregnancy tests, view the Animated Technique: Elisa Method for Detecting HCG at www.whfreeman.com/biochem5.

Chapter 6

Basic Concepts of Enzyme Action

Enzymes catalyze almost all chemical reactions in a cell and are also involved in the transformations of one form of energy into another. Most enzymes are proteins, but RNA also catalyzes physiologically important reactions. The authors begin this chapter with a brief overview of the catalytic power and specificity of enzymes. They point out that many enzymes require small molecule partners (cofactors) to effect catalysis. They then explain how the thermodynamic concepts of free energy change and free energy of activation are used to determine whether or not chemical reactions can occur and the rate at which they will occur, respectively. They explain how enzyme binding to the transition state of a reaction provides the chemical basis for catalysis. They explain how the velocity of enzyme-catalyzed reactions is analyzed, and they describe enzyme inhibitors and their analysis. This chapter draws on your knowledge of protein structure (Chapter 4) and the interactions between biomolecules (Chapter 2). It sets the stage for the majority of the remaining chapters of the text that deal with biochemical reactions.

LEARNING OBJECTIVES

When you have mastered this chapter, you should be able to accomplish the following objectives.

Enzymes Are Powerful and Highly Specific Catalysts (Text Section 6.1)

1. Explain why *enzymes* are versatile *biological catalysts*.

2. Appreciate that *catalytic power* and *specificity* are critical characteristics of enzymes. Give examples of the rate enhancements of enzymes and the substrate selectivity they display.

3. Realize that both *protein* and *RNA molecules* are enzymes.

4. Provide examples of *proteases* with diverse *substrate specificity*, and explain how substrate specificity arises from precise interactions of the enzyme with the substrate.

5. Provide examples of enzymes that transduce one form of energy into another.

Many Enzymes Require Cofactors for Activity (Text Section 6.2)

6. Define the terms *substrate, prosthetic group, apoenzyme,* and *holoenzyme*. Relate *vitamins* to cofactors.

Free Energy Is a Useful Thermodynamic Function for Understanding Enzymes (Text Section 6.3)

7. Describe how ΔG can be used to predict whether a reaction can occur spontaneously.

8. Write the equation for the ΔG of a chemical reaction. Define the *standard free-energy change* ($\Delta G°$); define $\Delta G'$ and $\Delta G°'$. Interconvert *kilojoules* and *kilocalories*.

9. Derive the relationship between $\Delta G°'$ and the *equilibrium constant* (K'_{eq}) of a reaction. Relate each tenfold change in K'_{eq} to the change in $\Delta G°'$ in kilojoules per mole (kJ/mol) or kcal/mol.

10. Relate the concentrations of reactants and products to $\Delta G'$. Define *endergonic* and *exergonic*.

11. Explain why enzymes do not alter the *equilibrium* of chemical reactions but change only their *rates*.

Enzymes Accelerate Reactions by Facilitating the Formation of the Transition State (Text Section 6.4)

12. Define the *transition state* and the *free energy of activation* ($\Delta G^{\ddagger}$), and describe the effect of enzymes on $\Delta G^{\ddagger}$.

13. Describe the formation of *enzyme-substrate (ES) complexes* and discuss their properties.

14. Summarize the common features of the *active sites* of enzymes, and relate them to the specificity of binding of the substrate.

15. Define the *binding energy* for the association of an enzyme and its substrate in terms of free energy change and describe the chemical bases for the interaction.

16. Explain why enzyme-catalyzed reaction rates reach a maximum value.

SELF-TEST

Enzymes Are Powerful and Highly Specific Catalysts

1. Which of the following are NOT true of enzymes?
   (a) Enzymes are proteins.
   (b) Enzymes have great catalytic power.
   (c) Enzymes bind substrates with high specificity.
   (d) Enzymes use hydrophobic interactions exclusively in binding substrates.
   (e) The catalytic activity of enzymes is often regulated.

2. Enzymes catalyze reactions by
   (a) binding regulatory proteins.
   (b) covalently modifying active-site residues.
   (c) binding substrates with great affinity.
   (d) selectively binding the transition state of a reaction with high affinity.

3. The combination of an apoenzyme with a cofactor forms what? What are the two types of cofactors? What distinguishes a prosthetic group from a cosubstrate?

4. Name a process that converts the energy of light into the energy of chemical bonds.

Many Enzymes Require Cofactors for Activity

5. Can any metal ions be considered as cofactors? Which ones?

Free Energy Is a Useful Thermodynamic Function for Understanding Enzymes

6. Which of the following statements is correct? The free energy change of a reaction
   (a) if negative, enables the reaction to occur spontaneously.
   (b) if positive, enables the reaction to occur spontaneously.
   (c) is greater than zero when the reaction is at equilibrium.
   (d) determines the rate at which a reaction will attain equilibrium.

7. Explain why the thermodynamic parameter ΔS cannot be used to predict the direction in which a reaction will proceed.

8. If the standard free-energy change ($\Delta G°$) for a reaction is zero, which of the following statements about the reaction are true?
   (a) The entropy ($\Delta S°$) of the reaction is zero.
   (b) The enthalpy ($\Delta H°$) of the reaction is zero.
   (c) The equilibrium constant for the reaction is 1.0.
   (d) The reaction is at equilibrium.
   (e) The concentrations of the reactants and products are all 1 M at equilibrium.

9. The enzyme triose phosphate isomerase catalyzes the following reaction:

   $$\text{dihydroxyacetone phosphate} \underset{k_{-1}}{\overset{k_1}{\rightleftharpoons}} \text{glyceraldehyde 3-phosphate}$$

   The $\Delta G°'$ for this reaction is 7.66 kJ/mol (1.83 kcal/mol). In light of this information, which of the following statements are correct?
   (a) The reaction would proceed spontaneously from left to right under standard conditions.

(b) The rate of the reaction in the reverse direction is higher than the rate in the forward direction at equilibrium.

(c) The equilibrium constant under standard conditions favors the synthesis of the compound on the left, dihydroxyacetone phosphate.

(d) The data given are sufficient to calculate the equilibrium constant of the reaction.

(e) The data given are sufficient to calculate the left-to-right rate constant (k_1).

10. Glycogen phosphorylase, an enzyme involved in the metabolism of the carbohydrate polymer glycogen, catalyzes the reaction:

$$\text{Glycogen}_n + \text{phosphate} \rightleftharpoons \text{glucose 1-phosphate} + \text{glycogen}_{n-1}$$

$$K'_{eq} = \frac{[\text{glucose 1} - \text{phosphate}][\text{glycogen}_{n-1}]}{[\text{phosphate}][\text{glycogen}_n]} = 0.088$$

Based on these data, which of the following statements are correct?

(a) Because glycogen phosphorylase normally *degrades* glycogen in cellular metabolism, there is a paradox in that the equilibrium constant favors synthesis.

(b) The $\Delta G^{o\prime}$ for this reaction at 25°C is 5.98 kJ/mol (1.43 kcal/mol).

(c) The phosphorolytic cleavage of glycogen consumes energy, that is, it is endergonic.

(d) If the ratio of phosphate to glucose 1-phosphate in cells is high enough, phosphorylase will degrade glycogen.

11. The reaction of the hydrolysis of glucose 6-phosphate to give glucose and phosphate has a $\Delta G^{o\prime} = -13.8$ kJ/mol (−3.3 kcal/mol). The reaction takes place at 25°C. Initially, the concentration of glucose 6-phosphate is 10^{-5} M, that of glucose is 10^{-1} M, and that of phosphate is 10^{-1} M. Which of the following statements pertaining to this reaction are correct?

(a) The equilibrium constant for the reaction is 260.

(b) The equilibrium constant cannot be calculated because standard conditions do not prevail initially.

(c) The $\Delta G'$ for this reaction under the initial conditions is −3.26 kJ/mol (−0.78 kcal/mol).

(d) Under the initial conditions, the synthesis of glucose 6-phosphate will take place rather than hydrolysis.

(e) Under standard conditions, the hydrolysis of glucose 6-phosphate will proceed spontaneously.

Enzymes Accelerate Reactions by Facilitating the Formation of the Transition State

12. The transition state of an enzyme-catalyzed reaction that converts a substrate to a product

(a) is a transient intermediate formed along the reaction coordinate of the reaction.

(b) has higher free energy than either the substrates or products.

(c) is the most populated species along the reaction coordinate.

(d) is increased in concentration because the enzyme binds tightly to it.

(e) determines the velocity of the reaction.

13. Explain briefly how enzymes accelerate the rate of reactions.

14. Which of the following statements is true? Enzyme catalysis of a chemical reaction
    (a) decreases $\Delta G'$ so that the reaction can proceed spontaneously.
    (b) increases the energy of the transition state.
    (c) does not change $\Delta G^{o'}$, but rather changes the ratio of products to reactants at equilibrium.
    (d) decreases the entropy of the reaction.
    (e) increases the forward and reverse reaction rates.

15. Which of the following statements regarding an enzyme-substrate complex (ES) is true?
    (a) The heat stability of an enzyme frequently changes upon the binding of a substrate.
    (b) At sufficiently high concentrations of substrate, the catalytic sites of the enzyme become filled and the reaction rate reaches a maximum.
    (c) An enzyme-substrate complex can usually be isolated.
    (d) Enzyme-substrate complexes can usually be visualized by x-ray crystallography.
    (e) Spectroscopic changes in the substrate or the enzyme can be used to detect the formation of an enzyme-substrate complex.

16. Why is there a high degree of stereospecificity in the interaction of enzymes with their substrates?

17. Explain why the forces that bind a substrate at the active site of an enzyme are usually weak.

ANSWERS TO SELF-TEST

1. d. (a) is incorrect because some enzymes are RNA.

2. d. (c) is incorrect because, although tight binding to the substrates helps confer specificity on the reaction, it increases the activation barrier to reaction. Tight substrate binding makes binding to the transition state of the reaction more energetically costly, that is, it increases the free energy of activation of the reaction.

3. Holoenzyme. Cofactors may be metal ions or low molecular weight organic molecules. A prosthetic group is a tightly bound cofactor that seldom dissociates from the enzyme. Cofactors that are loosely bound behave like cosubstrates; they are easily bound and released from the enzyme.

4. Photosynthesis. The sun provides light energy that photosynthesis converts into chemical bond energy in the form of ATP. Other examples of energy transduction include the use of an ion gradient in mitochondria to drive the synthesis of chemical bonds, and the use of the energy in ATP to cause the movement of muscles.

5. See Table 6.2—Zinc, Magnesium, Nickel, Molybdenum, Selenium, Manganese, and Potassium.

6. a

7. The thermodynamic parameter ΔS for a chemical reaction is not easily measured. Even if it were easily determined, its value depends on changes that occur not only in the system under study but also in the surroundings (see Chapter 2). Intrinsically unfavorable reactions ($\Delta G^{o'} > 0$) can take place if a change in the surroundings compensates for a decrease in the entropy (negative ΔS) of the reaction.

8. c, e. $\Delta G^{o} = -RT \ln K_{eq}$. When $K_{eq} = 1$, $\Delta G^{o} = 0$ because the natural log of $1 = 0$. (e) is correct by definition.

9. c, d

10. All of the statements are correct.

(a) The paradox is that although glycogen normally degrades glycogen to form glucose 1-phosphate, the standard free energy change of the reaction is positive, that is, the reaction is endergonic. See the answer to (d) for a resolution of the paradox.

(b) Using K'_{eq}, one can calculate the $\Delta G^{\circ\prime}$ for the phosphorylase reaction:

$$\Delta G^{\circ\prime} = -RT \ln K'_{eq}$$

$$= -8.31 \frac{J}{mol^{\circ}K} \times 298 \ {}^{\circ}K \times \ln (0.088)$$

$$= -2476 \ J/mol \times -2.43$$

$$= 6017 \ J/mol = 6.02 \ kJ/mol \ (1.44 \ kcal/mol)$$

(c) In part (b) the $\Delta G^{\circ\prime}$ for the phosphorylase reaction of 6.02 kJ/mol was calculated; therefore, energy is consumed rather than released by this reaction.

(d) In cells, the ratio of phosphate to glucose 1-phosphate is so large that phosphorylase is mainly involved with glycogen degradation.

11. a, d, e

(a)
$$\Delta G^{\circ\prime} = -RT \ln K'_{eq}$$

$$-13.8 \ kJ/mol = -8.31 \frac{J}{mol \ {}^{\circ}K} \times 298 \ {}^{\circ}K \times \ln K'_{eq}$$

$$\ln K'_{eq} = 5.56$$

$$K'_{eq} = 260$$

(b) Incorrect. K'_{eq} is a constant; it is independent of the initial concentrations.

(c) Incorrect.

$$\Delta G' = \Delta G^{\circ\prime} + RT \ \ln \frac{[glucose][phosphate]}{[glucose \ 6\text{-}phosphate]}$$

$$= -13.8 \ kJ/mol + \left(2.48 \ kJ/mol \times \ln \frac{10^{-1} \times 10^{-1}}{10^{-5}} \right)$$

$$= -13.8 \ kJ/mol + \left(2.48 \ kJ/mol \times \ln 1000 \right)$$

$$= -13.8 \ kJ/mol + (2.48 \ kJ/mol \times 6.91)$$

$$= +3.3 \ kJ/mol \ (+0.79 \ kcal/mol)$$

(d) Correct. Under the initial conditions, $\Delta G'$ is positive; therefore, the reaction will proceed toward the formation of glucose 6-phosphate.

(e) Correct. The negative $\Delta G^{\circ\prime}$ value (at standard conditions) indicates that the reaction will proceed spontaneously toward the hydrolysis of glucose 6-phosphate.

12. a, b, d, e. (c) is incorrect because it has the most energy and is therefore hardest to form. The velocity of the reaction is directly proportional to the concentration of the transition state.

13. Enzymes have evolved to bind tightly the transition state of the reaction they catalyze. By binding the transition state with high affinity, they facilitate its formation. Hydrogen bonds and ionic and hydrophobic interactions can be involved in binding the transition state. The more transition state formed, the faster the reaction.

14. e. The enzyme speeds up the rate of attainment of equilibrium.

15. a, b, e. Turnover of ES to form P usually makes isolating ES difficult. In reactions requiring two substrates, an enzyme-substrate complex of one of the substrates can be isolated in the absence of the other substrate if the complex is very stable. The absence of the cosubstrate precludes turnover of ES. The same consideration applies to ES complexes formed for x-ray crystallography.

16. The formation of an enzyme-substrate complex involves a close, complementary fitting of the atoms of the amino-acid-residue side chains that make up the active site of the enzyme with the atoms of the substrate. Since stereoisomers have different spatial arrangements of their atoms, only a single stereoisomer of the substrate usually fits into the active site in a form capable of being acted upon by the enzyme.

17. The enzyme-substrate and enzyme-product complexes must be reversible for catalysis to proceed; therefore, weak forces are involved in the binding of substrates to enzymes.

PROBLEMS

1. Calculate the values for $\Delta G^{\circ\prime}$ that correspond to the following values of K'_{eq}. Assume that the temperature is 25°C.
   (a) 1.5×10^4
   (b) 1.5
   (c) 0.15
   (d) 1.5×10^{-4}

2. Calculate the values for K'_{eq} that correspond to the following values of $\Delta G^{\circ\prime}$. Assume that the temperature is 25°C.
   (a) −41.84 kJ/mol (−10 kcal/mol)
   (b) −4.18 kJ/mol (−1 kcal/mol)
   (c) +4.18 kJ/mol (+1 kcal/mol)
   (d) +41.84 kJ/mol (+10 kcal/mol)

3. The enzyme aldolase catalyzes the following reaction:

$$\text{Fructose 1,6-bisphosphate} \rightleftharpoons$$

dihydroxyacetone phosphate + glyceraldehyde 3-phosphate

For this reaction, $\Delta G^{\circ\prime} = +23.8$ kJ/mol (+ 5.7 kcal/mol).

   (a) Calculate the change in free energy $\Delta G'$ for this reaction under typical intracellular conditions using the following concentrations: fructose 1,6-bisphosphate,

0.15 mM; dihydroxyacetone phosphate, 4.3×10^{-6} M; and glyceraldehyde 3-phosphate, 9.6×10^{-5} M. Assume that the temperature is 25°C.

(b) Explain why the aldolase reaction occurs in cells in the direction written despite the fact that it has a positive free-energy change under standard conditions.

4. The text states (Table 6.3) that a decrease of 5.69 kJ/mol (1.36 kcal/mol) in the free energy of activation of an enzyme-catalyzed reaction has the effect of increasing the rate of conversion of substrate to product by a factor of 10. What effect would this decrease of 5.69 kJ/mol in the free energy of activation have on the reverse reaction, the conversion of product to substrate? Explain.

ANSWERS TO PROBLEMS

1. The values for $\Delta G^{\circ\prime}$ are found by substituting the values for K'_{eq} into equation 5 in Section 6.3 of the text.

   (a) $\quad \Delta G^{\circ\prime} = -RT \ln K'_{eq}$

   $$= -8.31 \times 298 \ln (1.5 \times 10^4)$$

   $$= -20.4 \text{ kJ} / \text{mol} (-5.7 \text{ kcal} / \text{mol})$$

   (b) -1.00 kJ/mol (-0.24 kcal/mol)

   (c) $+4.60$ kJ/mol ($+1.1$ kcal/mol)

   (d) $+21.76$ kJ/mol($+5.2$ kcal/mol)

2. Equation 6 in Section 6.3 is used to find the answers.

   (a)
   $$K'_e = e^{\frac{-\Delta G^{\circ\prime}}{RT}} = e^{\frac{-\Delta G^{\circ\prime}}{2.48}}$$

   $$= e^{\frac{41.84}{2.48}} = e^{16.87}$$

   $$= 2.12$$

   (b) 5.42

   (c) 0.18

   (d) 4.71×10^{-8}

3. (a) The applicable relationship is equation 2 in Section 6.3:

   $$\Delta G' = \Delta G^{\circ\prime} + RT \ln \frac{[C][D]}{[A][B]}$$

   $$= \Delta G^{\circ\prime} + RT \ln \frac{[DHAP][G3P]}{[FBP]}$$

   $$= +2.38 \text{ kJ} / \text{mol} + \left(248\right)$$

   $$\times \ln \frac{\left(4.3 \times 10^{-6}\right) \times \left(9.6 \times 10^{-5}\right)}{0.15 \times 10^{-3}}$$

   $$= +23.8 \text{ kJ} / \text{mol} - 31.7 \text{ kJ} / \text{mol}$$

   $$= -7.9 \text{ kJ} / \text{mol} (-1.9 \text{ kcal} / \text{mol})$$

(b) The reaction occurs in the direction written because of the effects of the concentrations on the free-energy change. The concentration term in the equation is much smaller than 1.0, which is its value under standard conditions. Removal of G3P by a subsequent reaction keeps its concentration low.

4. The rate of the reverse reaction must also increase by a factor of 10. Enzymes do not alter the equilibria of processes; they affect the rate at which equilibrium is attained. Since the equilibrium constant K_{eq} is the quotient of the rate constants for the forward and reverse reactions, both rate constants must be altered by the same factor. If the rate of the forward reaction is increased by a factor of 10, the rate of the reverse reaction must also increase by the same factor.

Kinetics and Regulation

Chapter 7 continues the discussion of enzymes from the previous chapter, but focuses on a mathematical approach to the consideration of reaction rates. The study of rates is kinetics, and there are two main models. The simpler enzymes can be described by the Michaelis-Menten Equation, while more complex enzymes tend to have allosteric kinetics. The chapter shows how the Michaelis-Menten Equation is derived, and how it can be used. The significance of the K_m and V_{max} are discussed, and then the authors describe models for enzymes with multiple substrates. Finally there is an important discussion of allosteric kinetics, with models of cooperativity showing transitions from tense (T) to relaxed (R) conformations.

LEARNING OBJECTIVES

When you have mastered this chapter, you should be able to accomplish the following objectives.

Kinetics Is the Study of Reaction Rates (Text Section 7.1)

1. Review the fundamental terms and equations of the kinetics of chemical reactions. Define *first-order*, *second-order*, and *zero-order* reactions.

The Michaelis-Menten Model Describes the Kinetics of Many Enzymes (Text Section 7.2)

2. Outline the *Michaelis-Menten model of enzyme kinetics* and describe the molecular nature of each of its components.

3. Reproduce the derivation of the *Michaelis-Menten equation* in the text. Relate the Michaelis-Menten equation to experimentally derived plots of *velocity* (V) versus *substrate concentration* [S]. List the assumptions underlying the derivation.

4. Define V_{max} and K_M, and explain how these parameters can be obtained from a plot of V versus [S] or a plot of 1/V versus 1/[S] (a *Lineweaver-Burk plot*).

5. Explain the significance of V_{max}, K_M, k_2, k_{cat}, and k_{cat}/K_M. Define *kinetic perfection* as it pertains to enzyme catalysis.

6. Distinguish *sequential displacement* and *double displacement* in reactions involving multiple substrates. Provide examples of enzymes using each mechanism.

Allosteric Enzymes Are Catalysts and Information Sensors (Text Section 7.3)

7. Contrast the *kinetics of allosteric enzymes* with those displaying simple Michaelis-Menten kinetics. Describe the molecular basis of allostery.

8. Understand that allosteric enzymes provide controls to biochemical pathways via mechanisms such as *feedback inhibition*.

9. Compare and contrast the MWC *concerted* model and the Koshland *sequential* model for the mechanism behind allosteric kinetics.

10. Explain how loss of allosteric control can lead to disease.

Enzymes Can Be Studied One Molecule At a Time (Text Section 7.4)

11. Explain why it would be desirable to study enzymes as single molecules instead of the populations of millions of molecules.
12. Name two methods that allow study of single molecules.

SELF-TEST

Kinetics Is the Study of Reaction Rates

1. One of the fundamental laws of chemistry is the principle of mass action, written for a first order reaction as V = k[A]. If V has units of moles per liter second, and A is

$$\frac{m}{L \cdot s} = k \cdot \frac{m}{L} \qquad k = \frac{1}{s}$$

in moles per liter, what are the dimensions of the rate constant k? What are the units of k for a second order reaction?

2. Explain what is meant by a pseudo-first-order reaction.

The Michaelis-Menten Model Describes the Kinetics of Many Enzymes

3. Which of the following statements regarding simple Michaelis-Menten enzyme kinetics are correct?
   (a) The maximal velocity V_{max} is related to the maximal number of substrate molecules that can be "turned over" in unit time by a molecule of enzyme.
   (b) K_M is expressed in terms of a reaction velocity (e.g., mol s^{-1}).
   (c) K_M is the dissociation constant of the enzyme-substrate complex.
   (d) K_M is the concentration of substrate required to achieve half of V_{max}.
   (e) K_M is the concentration of substrate required to convert half the total enzyme into the enzyme-substrate complex.

4. Explain the relationship between K_M and the dissociation constant of the enzyme-substrate complex K_{ES}.

5. From the plot of velocity versus substrate concentration shown in Figure 7.1, obtain the following parameters. (The amount of enzyme in the reaction mixture is 10^{-3} mmol.)
   (a) K_M
   (b) V_{max}
   (c) k_2/K_M
   (d) Turnover number

FIGURE 7.1   Plot of reaction velocity versus substrate concentration.

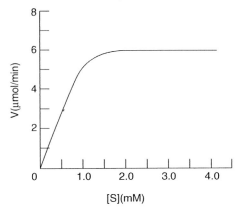

6. What is the significance of k_{cat}/K_M?

7. Which of the following statements is correct? The turnover number for chymotrypsin is 100 s^{-1}, and for DNA polymerase it is 15 s^{-1}. This means that
   (a) chymotrypsin binds its substrate with higher affinity than does DNA polymerase.
   (b) the velocity of the chymotrypsin reaction is always greater than that of the DNA polymerase reaction.
   (c) the velocity of the chymotrypsin reaction at a particular enzyme concentration and saturating substrate levels is lower than that of the DNA polymerase reaction under the same concentration conditions.
   (d) the velocities of the reactions catalyzed by both enzymes at saturating substrate levels could be made equal if 6.7 times more DNA polymerase than chymotrypsin were used.

Allosteric Enzymes Are Catalysts and Information Sensors

8. Allosteric enzymes do not obey the Michaelis-Menten Equation, and so they do not have a K_m. Do they have a V_{max}?

9. Signal molecules modulate the R = T equilibrium. What is a signal molecule?

Enzymes Can Be Studied One At a Time

10. Does the chapter reveal modern techniques that allow reactions to be observed kinetically using a single enzyme model?

ANSWERS TO SELF-TEST

1. First order k is 1/sec. Second order k is liters per mole second. The text expresses this as $M^{-1} s^{-1}$.

2. Some second-order reactions have two substrates, say A and B. If the concentrations are mismatched, for example much more A than B, then the reaction will appear to be first order, and only dependent on the concentration of A.

3. a, d. Answer (e) is correct only when $K_M = K_{ES}$. See Question 4.

4. K_M can be equal to K_{ES} when the rate constant $k_2 \ll k_{-1}$. Since $K_M = (k_2 + k_{-1})/k_1$, when k_2 is negligible relative to k_{-1}, K_M becomes equal to k_{-1}/k_1, which is the dissociation constant of the enzyme-substrate complex.

5. (a) $K_M = 5 \times 10^{-4}$ M. The value of the asymptote in Figure 7.1 is 6.0 µmol/min. K_M is equal to [S] at 1/2 V_{max}. Note that the units of [S] are mM.

   (b) $V_{max} = 6$ µmol/min. V_{max} is obtained from Figure 7.1; it is the maximum velocity.

   (c) $k_2/K_M = 2 \times 10^5 s^{-1} M^{-1}$. In order to calculate this ratio, k_2 must be known. Since $V_{max} = k_2[E_T]$, $k_2 = V_{max}/[E_T]$. Thus

$$k_2 = \frac{6\,\mu mol\,/\,min}{10^{-3}\,\mu mol}$$

$$= 6 \times 10^3\,min^{-1}$$

$$= 100\,s^{-1}$$

   Using K_M from part (a),

$$\frac{k_2}{K_M} = \frac{100\,s^{-1}}{5 \times 10^{-4}\,M} = 2 \times 10^5\,s^{-1}\,M^{-1}$$

   (d) The turnover number is $100\,s^{-1}$, equal to k_2, which was calculated in part (c).

6. Since $V_0 = (k_{cat}/K_M)$ [ET] [S], k_{cat}/K_M represents the second-order rate constant for the encounter of S with E. The ratio k_{cat}/K_M thus allows one to estimate the catalytic efficiency of an enzyme. The upper limit for k_{cat}/K_M, 10^8 to $10^9\,M^{-1}\,s^{-1}$, is set by the rate of diffusion of the substrate in the solution, which limits the rate at which it encounters the enzyme. If an enzyme has a k_{cat}/K_M in this range, its catalytic velocity is restricted only by the rate at which the substrate can reach the enzyme, which means that the enzymatic catalysis has attained kinetic perfection.

Understanding Concepts

7. d. $V_{max} = k_2[E_T]$; thus, if 6.7 times more DNA polymerase than chymotrypsin is used, V_{max} for both enzymes is the same:

$$100 \text{ s}^{-1} = 6.7 \times 15 \text{ s}^{-1}$$

Answer (a) is incorrect because the affinity of substrate for the enzyme is given by $K_{ES} = k_{-1}/k_1$. Answer (b) is incorrect because the velocity of the enzymatic reactions is a function of K_M, V_{max}, and substrate concentration. Answer (c) is incorrect because for the same enzyme concentration, $V_{max} = k_2[E_T]$ is greater for chymotrypsin than for DNA polymerase.

8. All enzymes have a maximum rate. This allows derivation of a useful number to replace the K_m. If you find the V_{max} and then look at how much substrate is required to produce a rate that is one half V_{max}, you can call that the $K_{0.5}$, and that is a useful thing to know.

9. This topic will be discussed in detail in future chapters. Here the point is that the world "allo-steric" is Greek for "another place." In other words the reaction rate is partly determined by the substrate bound to the active site, and partly determined by other molecules bound to "another place." Sometimes these are substrate molecules bound to other subunits, and sometimes they are entirely different molecules that serve as "allosteric modulators" changing T to R and altering the kinetics of the enzyme.

10. Not really. The two methods mentioned are patch-clamp recording, which is only useful for ion channels (not enzymes) and single molecule fluorescence, which does not have an obvious connection to determination of kinetics of enzymes.

PROBLEMS

1. What is the ratio of [S] to K_M when the velocity of an enzyme-catalyzed reaction is 80% of V_{max}?

2. The simple Michaelis-Menten model, $V = V_{max}$ [S]/([S] + K_M), applies only to the initial velocity of an enzyme-catalyzed reaction, that is, to the velocity when no appreciable amount of product has accumulated. What feature of the model is consistent with this constraint? Explain.

3. Two first-order rate constants, k_{-1} and k_2, and one second-order rate constant, k_1, define K_M by the relationship

$$K_M = \frac{k_{-1} + k_2}{k_1}$$

By substituting the appropriate units for the rate constants in this expression, show that K_M must be expressed in terms of concentration.

4. Suppose that two tissues, tissue A and tissue B, are assayed for the activity of enzyme X. The activity of enzyme X, expressed as the number of moles of substrate converted to product per gram of tissue, is found to be five times greater in tissue A than in tissue B under a variety of circumstances. What is the simplest explanation for this observation?

5. Sketch the appropriate plots on the following axes. Assume that simple Michaelis-Menten kinetics apply, and that the pre-steady state occurs so rapidly that it need not be considered (see Section 7.2).

FIGURE 7.2

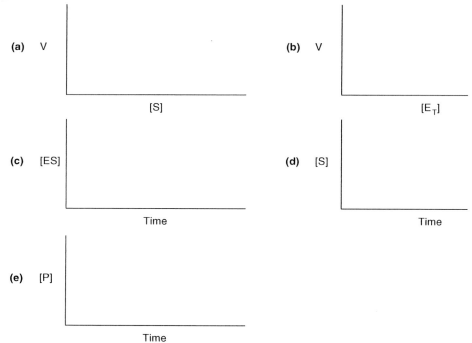

6. Suppose that the data shown below are obtained for an enzyme-catalyzed reaction.

[S](mM)	V (mmol ml^{-1} min^{-1})
0.1	3.33
0.2	5.00
0.5	7.14
0.8	8.00
1.0	8.33
2.0	9.09

(a) From a double-reciprocal plot of the data, determine K_M and V_{max}.

(b) Assuming that the enzyme present in the system had a concentration of 10^{-6} M, calculate its turnover number.

7. Suppose that the data shown below are obtained for an enzyme-catalyzed reaction in the presence and absence of inhibitor X.

[S](mM)	V (mmol ml^{-1} min^{-1}) Without X	With X
0.2	5.0	3.0
0.4	7.5	5.0
0.8	10.0	7.5
1.0	10.7	8.3
2.0	12.5	10.7
4.0	13.6	12.5

(a) Using double-reciprocal plots of the data, determine the type of inhibition that has occurred.

(b) Does inhibitor X combine with E, with ES, or with both? Explain.

(c) Calculate the inhibitor constant K_i for substance X, assuming that the final concentration of X in the reaction mixture was 0.2 mM.

8. Proteins such as cell surface receptors are often described by a value called $K_{0.5}$. This value is analogous to a K_m in that it reflects tightness of binding. It is defined as the concentration of ligand required to reach 50% saturation. Brain cells have glucose-binding proteins called GLUT 3 receptors on their membranes. Muscle and fat cells have similar receptors called GLUT 4 receptors. Will the $K_{0.5}$ of brain GLUT 3 receptors be higher or lower than the $K_{0.5}$ of muscle/fat GLUT 4 receptors? What is the physiological significance of this difference?

9. Although the double-reciprocal plot is the most widely used plotting form for enzyme kinetic data, it suffers from a major disadvantage. If linear increments of substrate concentration are used, thereby minimizing measurement errors in the laboratory, data points will be obtained that cluster near the vertical axis. Thus the intercept on the ordinate can be determined with great accuracy, but the slope of the line will be subject to considerable error, because the least reliable data points, those obtained at low substrate concentrations, have greater weight in establishing the slope. (Remember that many enzymes are protected against denaturation by the presence of their substrates at high concentrations.)

Because of the limitation of double-reciprocal plots described above, other linear plotting forms have been devised. One of these, the Eadie plot, graphs V versus V/[S]. Another, the Hanes-Woolf plot, ([S]/V versus [S]) is perhaps the most useful in minimizing the difficulties of the double-reciprocal plot.

(a) Rearrange the Michaelis-Menten equation to give [S]/V as a function of [S].

(b) What is the significance of the slope, the vertical intercept, and the horizontal intercept in a plot of [S]/V versus [S]?

(c) Data shown below were obtained for the hydrolysis of o-nitrophenyl-β-D-galactoside (ONPG) by E. coli β-galactosidase. Use both double-reciprocal and Hanes-Woolf plots to analyze these data, and calculate values for K_M and V_{max} from both plots. (We suggest that you use a graphing program to generate a scatterplot, and then fit the data using a linear curve-fitting algorithm.)

[S](mM)	V (μmol ml^{-1} min^{-1})
0.5	8.93
1.0	14.29
1.5	16.52
2.0	19.20
2.5	19.64

(d) Make a sketch of a plot [S]/V versus [S] in the absence of an inhibitor as in the presence of a competitive inhibitor and in the presence of a noncompetitive inhibitor.

10. The enzyme DNA ligase catalyzes the formation of a phosphodiester bond at a break (nick) in the phosphodiester backbone of a duplex DNA molecule. The enzyme from

bacteriophage T4 uses the free energy of hydrolysis ATP as the energy source for the formation of the phosphodiester bond. A covalently modified form of the enzyme in which AMP is bound to a lysine side chain is an intermediate in the reaction. The intermediate is formed by the reaction of E + ATP to form E-AMP + PP$_i$. In the next step, the AMP is transferred from the enzyme to a phosphate on the DNA to form a pyrophosphate-linked DNA-AMP. In the last step of the reaction, the phosphodiester bond is formed by the free enzyme to seal the nick in the DNA and AMP is released.

(a) Write chemical equations that show the individual steps that occur over the course of the overall reaction.

(b) Does this enzyme catalyze a double-displacement reaction?

(c) Do you think that if DNA were omitted from the reaction mixture, the enzyme would catalyze a partial reaction? If so, what reaction might it catalyze?

11. If you were studying an enzyme that catalyzed the reaction of ATP and fructose 1-phosphate to form fructose 1,6-bisphosphate and ADP and discovered that a plot of the initial velocity of formation of fructose 1,6-bisphosphate versus ATP concentration was not hyperbolic, but rather sigmoid, what would you suspect?

12. Converting between calories and joules is a skill that scientists frequently need. A rule of thumb is to remember that a calorie is about one-fourth of a joule. Specifically, 0.239 cal = 1 J. The following problem puts this conversion in context. In Europe, food energy content is expressed in kJ rather than kcal. (Food "calories" are really kcal.) If a cup of yogurt has 1370 kJ of energy and you are trying to keep your lunch to a maximum of 350 kcal (food calories), could you eat the entire container of yogurt? How many kcal are represented by 1370 kJ?

ANSWERS TO PROBLEMS

1. Start with the Michaelis-Menten equation, equation 7 in Section 7.2 of the text:

$$V = V_{max} \frac{[S]}{[S] + K_M}$$

Substituting 0.8 V_{max} for V yields

$$0.8\,V_{max} = V_{max} \frac{[S]}{[S] + K_M}$$

$$0.8[S] + 0.8K_M = [S]$$

$$0.8K_M = 0.2[S]$$

$$[S] = 4K_M$$

$$\frac{[S]}{K_M} = 4$$

Thus, a substrate concentration four times greater than the Michaelis constant yields a velocity that is 80% of maximal velocity.

2. Equation 6 in Section 7.2 of the text shows the k_2 step as being irreversible. This is true in practice at the initial stage of the reaction because P and E cannot recombine to give ES at an appreciable rate if negligible P is present. Note that the equation

reveals nothing about the relative magnitudes of k_2 and the reverse rate constant for this step, k_{-2}:

$$E + S \overset{k_1}{\underset{k_{-1}}{\leftrightarrow}} ES \overset{k_2}{\underset{k_{-2}}{\leftrightarrow}} E + P$$

The reverse constant k_{-2} may actually be quite large compared with k_2; nevertheless, the reverse reaction will not occur when little product is present, since the rate of the k_{-2} step depends on the concentrations of P and E as well as on the magnitude of its rate constant.

3. The first-order rate constants have the dimensions t^{-1} (one over time), whereas the second-order constant has the dimension $conc^{-1}$ $time^{-1}$ (one over concentration times one over time). Thus, we can carry out the following dimensional analysis:

$$K_M = \frac{k_{-1} + k_2}{k_1}$$

$$= \frac{t^{-1} + t^{-1}}{conc^{-1}t^{-1}}$$

$$= conc$$

4. For the activity of enzyme X to be five times greater in tissue A than in tissue B, tissue A must have five times the amount of enzyme X as does tissue B. Enzyme activity is directly proportional to enzyme concentration.

5. The sketches should resemble the following:

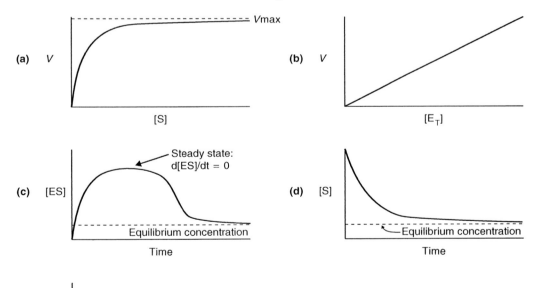

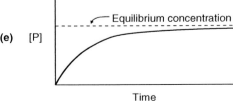

6. (a) See the graph, Figure 7.3. $V_{max} = 1/0.1 = 10$ mmol ml^{-1} min^{-1}.

$$\text{Slope} = \frac{0.3 - 0.1}{10} = 0.02$$

$$\text{Slope} = \frac{K_M}{V_{max}}$$

$K_M = 0.02 \times 10 = 0.2$ mM

FIGURE 7.3   A double-reciprocal plot of data for problem 11.

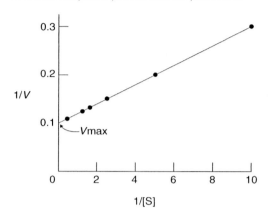

(b) The turnover number is equal to the rate constant k_2 in equation 11, Section 7.2 of the text. Rearrangement of the equation gives

$$k_2 = \frac{V_{max}}{[E_T]}$$

$$= \frac{10 \text{ mmol ml}^{-1} \text{ min}^{-1}}{10^{-6} \text{ mol liter}^{-1}}$$

$$= \frac{10 \text{ mol liter}^{-1} \text{ min}^{-1}}{10^{-6} \text{ mol liter}^{-1}}$$

$$= 10^7 \text{ min}^{-1} \quad \text{or} \quad 1.7 \times 10^5 \text{ s}^{-1}$$

7. Hexokinase binds more strongly to glucose. It takes less substrate to reach half the V_{max}, so the K_m is lower and the binding is tighter. On the other hand, a higher concentration of fructose is required to reach half the V_{max}, so fructose shows more dissociation from the enzyme. Remember that the K_m can be thought of like a K_d.

8. The $K_{0.5}$ of brain cell GLUT 3 will be lower. This means that GLUT 3 will bind glucose more tightly and will reach saturation at a lower concentration of glucose than is seen with the muscle/fat GLUT 4 receptors. This lower affinity of the GLUT 4 receptors for glucose helps to ensure that the organ that most needs glucose, that is, the brain, receives it preferentially. In conditions of low blood sugar, brain glucose receptors will still be available to bind glucose.

9. (a) We start with the Michaelis-Menten equation:

$$V = V_{max} [S]/(K_M + [S])$$

Cross multiplying yields

$$V(K_M + [S]) = V_{max}[S]$$

Division of both sides by V/V_{max} gives

$$[S]/V = (K_M + [S])/V_{max}$$

$$[S]/V = K_M/V_{max} + [S]/V_{max}$$

$$[S]/V = (1/V_{max})[S] + K_M/V_{max}$$

(b) The linear equation above is in the form, $y = mx + b$, where m is the slope, and b the y-intercept. Therefore, the slope of a Hanes-Woolf plot is $(1/V_{max})$, and the intercept on the y-axis is K_M/V_{max}. The plot will intercept the x-axis when $[S]/V$ is zero. Then

$$0 = (1/V_{max})[S] + K_M/V_{max}$$

$$-K_M/V_{max} = (1/V_{max})[S]$$

$$[S] = -K_M$$

(c) See Figure 7.4. The y-intercept of the double-reciprocal plot is $1/V_{max}$. Therefore $V_{max} = 1/0.034 = 29.4$ µmol l^{-1} min^{-1}. The slope of the double-reciprocal plot is K_M/V_{max}. Therefore,

$$0.039 = K_M/29.4$$

$$K_M = 1.15 \text{ mM}$$

FIGURE 7.4   A double-reciprocal plot of data for problem 9.

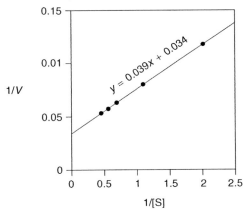

See Figure 7.5. The slope of the Hanes-Woolf plot is $1/V_{max}$. Therefore $V_{max} = 1/0.035 = 28.6$ mmol l^{-1} min^{-1}. The y-intercept of the Hanes-Woolf plot is K_M/V_{max}. Therefore,

$$0.037 = K_M/28.6$$

$$K_M = 1.06 \text{ mM.}$$

FIGURE 7.5 Hanes-Woolf plot of data for problem 9.

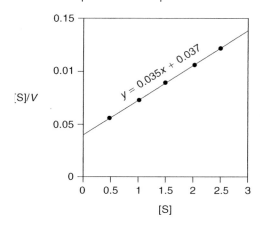

In this instance, both plots give good fits of the data, and the values derived from each for K_M and V_{max} do not differ significantly. We can conclude that the measurements at low substrate concentration are reliable.

(d) See Figure 7.6.

FIGURE 7.6 Hanes-Woolf plots depicting effects of competitive and noncompetitive inhibitors.

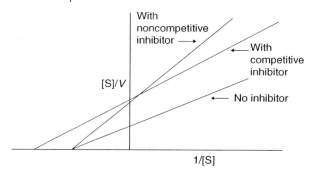

10. (a) The overall reaction proceeds as follows:

$$(1)\ E + ATP \longleftrightarrow E\text{-}AMP + PP_i$$
$$(2)\ E\text{-}AMP + \text{nicked DNA} \longleftrightarrow \text{nicked DNA-AMP} + E$$
$$\underline{(3)\ \text{nicked DNA-AMP} + E \longleftrightarrow \text{sealed DNA} + E}$$
$$\Sigma\ \ ATP + \text{nicked DNA} \longleftrightarrow \text{sealed DNA} + AMP + PP_i$$

(b) Yes, a substituted enzyme intermediate (E-AMP) is formed.

(c) In the absence of DNA, the enzyme catalyzes the partial reaction of the formation of the E-AMP with the release of PP_i. DNA is not involved in the first part of the double-displacement reaction. (This problem is derived from B. Weiss, and C. C. Richardson. Enzymatic breakage and joining of deoxyribonucleic acid. 3. An enzyme-adenylate intermediate in the polynucleotide ligase reaction. *J. Biol. Chem.* 243[1964]:4556–4563. See also I. R. Lehman. DNA ligase: Structure, mechanism, and function. *Science* 186[1974]:790–797, for a complete review.)

11. In the absence of additional information, you would suspect that the enzyme had allosteric properties; its initial velocity was being influenced by binding of one of the substrates to a site different from the active site.

12. $1370\ \text{kJ}\left(\dfrac{0.239\ \text{kcal}}{\text{kJ}}\right)$ = 327 kcal or 327 food calories Yes, you could eat the entire container of yogurt and keep your food calories under 350.

Chapter 8

Mechanisms and Inhibitors

This chapter is the third in a series of enzyme chapters, continuing the discussion of enzyme kinetics to include various sorts of inhibition. The chapter begins by outlining four catalytic strategies, including *covalent catalysis, general acid-base catalysis,* and *metal ion catalysis.* Then there is a discussion of how reaction rates can be affected by environmental variables including *temperature, pH,* and *inhibitors.* Types of inhibitors are described including *competitive, non-competitive,* and *uncompetitive.* Each of these produces recognizable changes in the Michaelis-Menten graphs, especially when the data is viewed using a *double reciprocal plot.* The authors then discuss the uses of irreversible inhibitors, and go into detail about the mechanism of action of penicillin. Finally, the mechanism of chymotrypsin action is also described in detail.

LEARNING OBJECTIVES

When you have mastered this chapter, you should be able to accomplish the following objectives.

A Few Basic Catalytic Strategies Are Used by Many Enzymes (Text Section 8.1)

1. Define *binding energy* as it relates to enzyme–substrate interactions and explain how it can be used in *enzyme catalysis*.

2. List four strategies commonly employed by enzymes to effect catalysis.

Enzyme Activity Can Be Modulated by Temperature, pH, and Inhibitory Molecules (Text Section 8.2)

3. List environmental factors that affect enzyme activity, and describe how those factors exert their effects on enzymes.

4. Understand that most enzymes show a maximum rate at close to the pH of the normal environment for each enzyme.

5. Know that in general, heating a reaction makes it speed up, but very high heat can ruin the structure of an enzyme by denaturing it.

6. Describe the functions and uses of *enzyme inhibitors*. Contrast *reversible* and *irreversible* inhibitors.

7. Describe the effects of *competitive, uncompetitive,* and *noncompetitive inhibitors* on the kinetics of enzyme reactions. Apply kinetic measurements and analysis to determine the nature of an inhibitor. Know how inhibitors change double-reciprocal plots.

8. Explain how irreversible inhibitors are used to learn about the active sites of enzymes. Provide examples of *group-specific, reactive substrate-analog, suicide,* and *transition-state* inhibitors. Know how DIPF reacts with chymotrypsin.

9. Contrast the properties of substrates and *transition-state analogs*.

10. Describe the formation of *catalytic antibodies* and recognize their uses.

11. Outline the mechanism of action of the antibiotic *penicillin*.

Chymotrypsin Illustrates Basic Principles of Catalysis and Inhibition (Text Section 8.3)

12. Define *proteolysis*. Draw the reaction for peptide-bond hydrolysis, and explain why peptide bonds are resistant to spontaneous hydrolysis.

13. List the evidence that indicates that a *serine* hydroxyl serves as a nucleophile in the reaction catalyzed by chymotrypsin.

14. Explain why Ser195 is especially reactive in chymotrypsin.

15. Explain why a *burst* of product appears when chymotrypsin reacts with a *chromogenic ester* substrate, and relate this phenomenon to *covalent catalysis*.

16. Summarize the roles of the *catalytic triad* in the mechanism of chymotrypsin and the relationship of the *oxyanion hole* to the tetrahedral intermediate of the reaction. Appreciate that these features are present in other *proteases, esterases,* and *lipases*.

17. Indicate the amino acid sequence specificity of the cleavage catalyzed by *chymotrypsin* and explain its molecular basis.

SELF-TEST

A Few Basic Catalytic Strategies Are Used by Many Enzymes

1. The free energy released when an enzyme binds a substrate
    (a) arises from many weak intermolecular interactions.
    (b) contributes to the catalytic efficiency of the enzyme.
    (c) is more negative when an incorrect substrate is bound.
    (d) becomes more positive as the transition state of the reaction develops.
    (e) becomes more negative the more tightly the enzyme binds the substrate.

2. Which of the following are used by enzymes to catalyze specific reactions?
    (a) metal ions   (d) general acid–base reactions
    (b) temperature changes   (e) covalent enzyme-substrate complexes
    (c) proximity between substrates

Enzyme Activity Can Be Modulated by Temperature, pH, and Inhibitory Molecules

3. Are most enzymes most active near neutral pH (pH = 7)?

4. What sort of organisms produce enzymes that are active at very high temperatures?

5. Which of the following statements about the different types of enzyme inhibition are correct?
    (a) Competitive inhibition occurs when a substrate competes with an enzyme for binding to an inhibitor protein.
    (b) Competitive inhibition occurs when the substrate and the inhibitor compete for the same active site on the enzyme.
    (c) Uncompetitive inhibition of an enzyme cannot be overcome by adding large amounts of substrate.
    (d) Competitive inhibitors are often similar in chemical structure to the substrates of the inhibited enzyme.
    (e) Noncompetitive inhibitors often bind to the enzyme irreversibly.

6. If the K_M of an enzyme for its substrate remains constant as the concentration of the inhibitor increases, what can be said about the mode of inhibition?

7. The kinetic data for an enzymatic reaction in the presence and absence of inhibitors are plotted in Figure 8.1. Identify the curve that corresponds to each of the following:
    (a) no inhibitor
    (b) noncompetitive inhibitor
    (c) competitive inhibitor
    (d) mixed inhibitor

FIGURE 8.1 Effects of inhibitors on a plot of V versus [S].

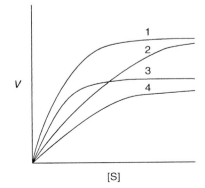

8. Draw approximate double reciprocal plots for each of the inhibitor types in the previous question.

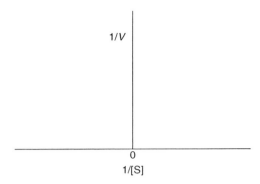

9. Which statements are NOT true about a transition state analog?

   (a) It fits better in the active site than the substrate.
   (b) It increases the rate of product formation.
   (c) It can be used as a hapten to produce catalytic antibodies.
   (d) It is usually a distorted or strained molecule.
   (e) It is a potent inhibitor of the enzyme.

10. The inhibition of bacterial cell wall synthesis by penicillin is a classic example of a medically significant inhibition of an enzymatic reaction. Which of the following statements about the inhibition of glycopeptide transpeptidase by penicillin is true?

    (a) The inhibition is noncompetitive.
    (b) Penicillin binds irreversibly to an allosteric site of the enzyme.
    (c) Penicillin inhibits bacterial cell wall synthesis by incorrectly cross-linking the peptides of the proteoglycan.
    (d) The penicilloyl-enzyme intermediate may be dissociated by high concentrations of D-alanine.
    (e) Penicillin resembles acyl-D-Ala-D-Ala, one of the substrates of the transpeptidase.

Chymotrypsin Illustrates Basic Principles of Catalysis and Inhibition

11. Why is the peptide bond, which is thermodynamically unstable, resistant to spontaneous hydrolysis?

12. The alkoxide group on chymotrypsin that attacks the carbonyl oxygen of the peptide bond of the substrate arises from which amino acid side chain?

    (a) aspartate
    (b) histidine
    (c) serine
    (d) threonine
    (e) tyrosine

13. Which of the following experimental observations provide evidence for the formation of an acyl-enzyme intermediate during the chymotrypsin reaction?

    (a) A biphasic release of p-nitrophenol occurs during the hydrolysis of the p-nitrophenyl ester of N-acetyl-phenylalanine.
    (b) The active serine can be specifically labeled with organic fluorophosphates.
    (c) The pH dependence of the catalytic rate is bell shaped, with a maximum at pH 8.
    (d) A deep pocket on the enzyme can accommodate a large hydrophobic side chain of the recognized substrate.

14. Three essential amino acid residues in the active site of chymotrypsin form a catalytic triad. Which of the following are roles for these residues in catalysis?
    (a) The histidine residue facilitates the reaction by acting as an acid–base catalyst.
    (b) The aspartate residue orients the histine properly for reaction.
    (c) The serine residue acts as a nucleophile during the reaction with the substrate.
    (d) The aspartate residue acts as an electrophile during the reaction with the substrate.
    (e) The aspartate residue initiates the deacylation step by a nucleophilic attack on the carbonyl carbon of the acyl intermediate.
    (f) They make up the oxyanion hole.

ANSWERS TO SELF-TEST

1. a, b, e. The $\Delta G^{o'}$ of the reaction becomes more negative as the binding affinity of the enzyme for the substrate increases. Interactions between the substrate and the enzyme promote the reaction when they are fully formed during the development of the transition state of the reaction. Favorable interactions between the enzyme and the substrate in its ground state before development of the transition state can hinder the reaction by lowering the valley preceding the activation barrier in the reaction coordinate diagram if they do not also contribute to binding the transition state. For instance a substrate analog that is a good competitive inhibitor forms strong interactions with the enzyme, but cannot develop a transition state.

2. a, c, d, e

3. Enzymes tend to be most active near the pH of their normal environment. So many enzymes are most active near neutral pH but many enzymes have other maxima. The two examples shown in the text are pepsin, with pH maximum between pH 1 and 2, and chymotrypsin, with a pH maximum near 8.

4. Thermophiles and hyperthermophiles live in the hottest environments. The organisms that can tolerate the highest temperatures are the Archaea, which are prokaryotic like the Bacteria (no nucleus) but are more closely related to the Eukarya.

5. b, c, d

6. The inhibition is noncompetitive because the proportion of bound substrate remains the same as the concentration of the inhibitor increases.

7. (a) 1 (b) 3 (c) 2 (d) 4

8. See Figure 8.2. Plots 1 and 2 have the same 1/V intercept; plots 1 and 3 have the same 1/[S] intercept; and plots 1 and 4 have different 1/V and 1/[S] intercepts.

FIGURE 8.2 Double-reciprocal plots for competitive (2), noncompetitive (3), and mixed (4) inhibition, relative to the enzymatic reaction in the absence of inhibitors (1).

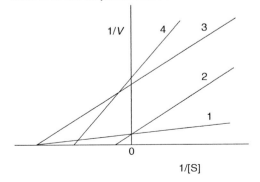

9. b, d. Answer (b) is incorrect because transition state analogs are inhibitors of the corresponding enzymes. Therefore, they decrease rather than increase enzyme reaction rates. Answer (d) is incorrect because transition-state analogs are not necessarily strained or distorted; rather, they mimic the shape of the transition state, which may itself be strained or distorted.

10. e

11. A peptide bond is stabilized by resonance, which gives the carbonyl–carbon-to-amide–nitrogen link partial double-bond character, making it more stable to hydrolysis. In addition, the carbonyl carbon of the peptide bond is linked to a partially negatively charged carbonyl oxygen that decreases the susceptibility of the carbon atom to nucleophilic attack by a hydroxyl ion.

12. c

13. a, b. The pH versus activity curve indicates only that some step in the mechanism is sensitive to the state of dissociation of a proton donor on the protein.

14. a, b, c. (d) is incorrect because the aspartic acid carboxylate is ionized, and bearing a negative charge, it is not an electrophile.

PROBLEMS

1. Why is histidine a particularly versatile amino acid residue in its involvement in enzymatic reaction mechanisms?

2. Suppose that the data shown below are obtained for an enzyme-catalyzed reaction in the presence and absence of inhibitor X.

[S](mM)	V (mmol ml^{-1} min^{-1})	
	Without X	With X
0.2	5.0	3.0
0.4	7.5	5.0
0.8	10.0	7.5
1.0	10.7	8.3
2.0	12.5	10.7
4.0	13.6	12.5

(a) Using double-reciprocal plots of the data, determine the type of inhibition that has occurred.
(b) Does inhibitor X combine with E, with ES, or with both? Explain.
(c) Calculate the inhibitor constant K_i for substance X, assuming that the final concentration of X in the reaction mixture was 0.2 mM.

3. Suppose that the data shown below are obtained for an enzyme-catalyzed reaction in the presence and absence of inhibitor Y.

[S](mM)	V (mmol ml^{-1} min^{-1})	
	Without Y	With Y
0.2	5.0	2.0
0.4	7.5	3.0
0.8	10.0	4.0
1.0	10.7	4.3
2.0	12.5	5.0
4.0	13.6	5.5

(a) Using double-reciprocal plots of the data, determine the type of inhibition that has occurred.

(b) Does inhibitor Y combine with E, with ES, or with both? Explain.

(c) Calculate the inhibitor constant K_i for substance Y, assuming that the final concentration of Y in the reaction mixture was 0.3 mM.

4. Suppose that a modifier Q is added to an enzyme-catalyzed reaction with the results depicted in Figure 8.3. What role does Q have? Does it combine with E, with ES, or with both E and ES?

FIGURE 8.3 Effects of modifier Q on a plot of 1/V versus 1/[S].

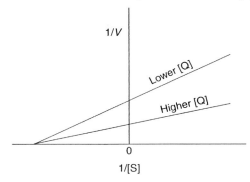

5. Although chymotrypsin is a proteolytic enzyme, it is quite resistant to digesting itself. How would you explain its resistance to self-proteolysis?

6. A pH-enzyme activity curve is shown in Figure 8.4. Which of the following pairs of amino acids would be likely candidates as catalytic groups? (See Table 3.1 in the text for the pK_a values of amino acid residues.)

(a) glutamic acid and lysine

(b) aspartic acid and histidine

(c) histidine and cysteine

(d) histidine and histidine

(e) histidine and lysine

FIGURE 8.4

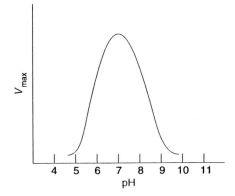

7. Trypsin, chymotrypsin, and carboxypeptidase A fail to cleave peptide bonds involving proline. Trypsin, for example, will not cleave a peptide at a Lys-Pro junction. Why do you think this is the case?

8. Place slash marks at the sites where you would expect chymotrypsin to cleave the following peptide:

Lys-Gly-Phe-Thr-Tyr-Pro-Asn-Trp-Ser-Tyr-Phe

9. Many enzymes can be protected against thermal denaturation during purification procedures by the addition of substrate. Propose an explanation for this phenomenon.

10. What are the main structural features of an enzyme that determine its substrate specificity?

11. Acetylcholinesterase is a serine protease found at the synapses between nerve cells. It cleaves the neurotransmitter acetylcholine. Organic fluorophosphates such as DIPF (Diisopropylphosphofluoridate, shown below) inhibit acetylcholinesterase. Suggest how this enzyme might be inhibited by DIPF.

$$
\begin{array}{ccccc}
CH_3 & & O & & CH_3 \\
| & & || & & | \\
H-C-O- & \!\!\!\!P\!\!\!\! & -O-C-H \\
| & & | & & | \\
CH_3 & & F & & CH_3
\end{array}
$$

ANSWERS TO PROBLEMS

1. The imidazole ring of histidine can act as an acid–base catalyst, a nucleophile, or a chelator (coordinator) of metal ions. The first and third functions were illustrated by chymotrypsin and carbonic anhydrase, respectively.

2. (a) See Figure 8.5. The double-reciprocal plots intersect on the y-axis, so the inhibition is competitive.

FIGURE 8.5 A double-reciprocal plot of data for problem 12 showing the effects of an inhibitor X.

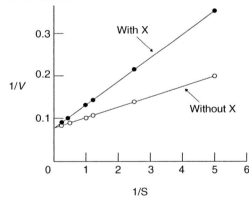

(b) The inhibitor combines only with E, the free enzyme. A competitive inhibitor cannot combine with ES because the inhibitor and the substrate compete for the same binding site on the enzyme.

(c) An inhibitor increases the slope of a double-reciprocal plot by a factor of $1 + [I]/K_i$:

$$
Slope_{inhib} = slope_{uninhib}\left(1 + \frac{[I]}{K_i}\right)
$$

The slope with X is

$$
Slope_{inhib} = \frac{0.333 - 0.067}{5} = 0.0532
$$

The slope without X is

$$Slope_{uninhib} = \frac{0.200 - 0.067}{5} = 0.0266$$

Substituting in these values yields

$$0.0532 = 0.0266 \left(1 + \frac{0.2 \text{ mM}}{K_i}\right)$$

$$K_i = 0.2 \text{ mM}$$

3. (a) See Figure 8.6. The inhibition was noncompetitive, as indicated by the fact that the double-reciprocal plots intersect to the left of the y-axis.

FIGURE 8.6 A double-reciprocal plot of data for problem 13 showing the effects of an inhibitor Y.

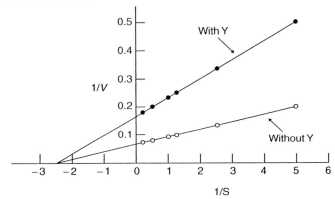

(b) A noncompetitive inhibitor combines at a site other than the substrate binding site. Thus, it may combine with both E and ES. In the case illustrated, the inhibitor has equal affinity for E and ES, which is shown by the fact that the plots intersect on the x-axis.

(c) Again, the slope increases by a factor of $1 + [I]/K_i$ in the presence of an inhibitor.

$$Slope_{inhib} = Slope_{uninhib}\left(1 + \frac{[I]}{K_i}\right)$$

4. Q increases the rate of reaction, so it is an activator, or perhaps a second substrate. It combines with both E and ES.

5. Chymotrypsin specifically cleaves peptide bonds whose C-terminal amino acid is adjacent to nonpolar aromatic amino acid residues or the bulky, hydrophobic methionine. Because these residues are often buried in the interior of proteins, including chymotrypsin, the self-hydrolysis of native, folded chymotrypsin is very inefficient. In fact, during digestion, chymotrypsin acts most effectively on partially degraded and denatured (unfolded) proteins.

6. c

7. Because of its ring structure, the imino acid proline cannot be accommodated in the substrate binding sites of trypsin, chymotrypsin, or carboxypeptidase A. Therefore these proteases fail to cleave peptide bonds involving proline.

8. Chymotrypsin would produce the following four fragments:

Lys-Gly-Phe, Thr-Tyr-Pro-Asn-Trp, Ser-Tyr, and Phe

9. When the substrate occupies the active site in the enzyme, the weak bonds that it forms with groups on the enzyme help to stabilize the tertiary structure of the enzyme and protect it against thermal denaturation.

10. The enzyme must have functional groups in the active site that can interact specifically with the substrate to distinguish it from other similar molecules and position it properly for a productive reaction. Usually, the enzyme must also have catalytic residues that react with a specific chemical bond of the substrate during the development of the transition state. Both ground-state interactions with the substrate by specific binding and the ability to catalyze the chemistry of the reaction determine the ability of an enzyme to convert a substrate to a product.

11. DIPF is an affinity label. The serine O^- attacks the phosphate group and displaces the F^-. But there is no leaving group for any additional chemistry, so the DIPF stays bound and prevents acetylcholine from entering the active site.

Hemoglobin:
An Allosteric Protein

Chapter 9

A t this point in the text, students should have enough information to understand what proteins are and how they are investigated in the laboratory. Homologous proteins should also be a familiar concept. In this chapter, the authors describe the structure and function relationships of two very important, well-studied proteins: hemoglobin and myoglobin. These homologous proteins have the important jobs of carrying oxygen in the blood and storing oxygen in the muscles. They also provide a clear example of the difference between allosteric (sigmoidal) binding and simpler (hyperbolic) single-ligand binding. The cooperative binding of oxygen to hemoglobin is critical to its ability to transport oxygen efficiently in blood and release it to myoglobin in tissues. Because it is also regulated by H^+, CO_2, and 2,3 BPG, hemoglobin also provides an excellent example of allosteric regulation of proteins. Finally the chapter describes the genetic diseases sickle-cell anemia and thalassemia, which are caused by abnormal hemoglobin genes.

LEARNING OBJECTIVES

When you have mastered this chapter, you should be able to accomplish the following objectives.

Hemoglobin Displays Cooperative Behavior (Text Section 9.1)

1. Describe the physiologic roles of *myoglobin* and *hemoglobin* in vertebrates.

2. Compare myoglobin and hemoglobin, and explain how they can have such similar structural folding and such different properties.

3. Summarize the general properties of an allosteric protein, as exemplified by hemoglobin.

4. Explain the significance of the differences in *oxygen dissociation curves*, in which the *fractional saturation* (Y) of the oxygen-binding sites is plotted for myoglobin and hemoglobin as a function of the *partial pressure of oxygen* (pO_2).

Myoglobin and Hemoglobin Bind Oxygen in Heme Groups (Text Section 9.2)

5. Describe the structure of the *heme prosthetic group* and its properties when free and when bound to the *globins*.

6. Describe how the distal histidine in myoglobin prevents release of superoxide anion and formation of metmyoglobin.

7. Define fMRI, and know it uses changes in hemoglobin to allow noninvasive imaging of the brain.

Hemoglobin Binds Oxygen Cooperatively (Text Section 9.3)

8. Contrast the *oxygen-binding* properties of myoglobin and hemoglobin. Define the *cooperative binding* of oxygen by hemoglobin and summarize how it makes hemoglobin a better oxygen transporter.

9. Discuss the three-dimensional structures of myoglobin and hemoglobin and how the heme groups attach to each one.

10. State the major structural differences between the *oxygenated* and *deoxygenated* forms of hemoglobin.

11. Distinguish between the *sequential model* and the *concerted model* for cooperative interactions between the subunits of proteins.

An Allosteric Regulator Determines the Oxygen Affinity of Hemoglobin (Text Section 9.4)

12. Explain the effect of *2,3-bisphosphoglycerate (BPG)* (also known as 2,3-diphosphoglycerate) on the affinity of hemoglobin for oxygen.

13. Rationalize the existence of *fetal hemoglobin*.

14. Describe *sickle-cell anemia* as a genetically transmitted *molecular disease*.

15. Contrast the biochemical and structural properties of deoxygenated *sickle-cell hemoglobin (HbS)* with those of *hemoglobin A (HbA)*.

16. Correlate the clinical observations of patients with *sickle-cell anemia* and the *sickle-cell trait* to their hemoglobins.

17. Explain how deoxyhemoglobin S forms *fibrous precipitates*.

18. Outline the possible functional consequences of *amino acid substitutions* in *mutant hemoglobins*.

Hydrogen Ions and Carbon Dioxide Promote the Release of Oxygen
(Text Section 9.5)

19. Explain the effects of CO_2 and H^+ (the *Bohr effect*) and 2,3-bisphosphoglycerate (BPG) on the binding of oxygen by hemoglobin. Describe the structural bases for the effects of these molecules on the binding of oxygen by hemoglobin. Explain the consequences of the metabolic production of CO_2 and H^+ on the oxygen affinity of hemoglobin.

SELF-TEST

Hemoglobin Displays Cooperative Behavior

1. Where are hemoglobin and myoglobin located in the body?

2. Which of the following statements are false?
   (a) The oxygen dissociation curve of myoglobin is sigmoidal, whereas that of hemoglobin is hyperbolic.
   (b) The affinity of hemoglobin for O_2 is regulated by organic phosphates, whereas the affinity of myoglobin for O_2 is not.
   (c) Hemoglobin has a higher affinity for O_2 than does myoglobin.
   (d) The affinity of both myoglobin and hemoglobin for O_2 is independent of pH.

Myoglobin and Hemoglobin Bind Oxygen at Iron Atoms in Heme Groups

3. Which of the following statements about heme structure is true?
   (a) Heme contains a tetrapyrrole ring with four methyl, four vinyl, and four propionate side chains.
   (b) The iron atom in heme may be present in the ferrous or the ferric state.
   (c) The iron atom is coplanar with the tetrapyrrole ring in deoxymyoglobin.
   (d) The axial coordination positions of heme are occupied by tyrosine residues in myoglobin.

Hemoglobin Binds Oxygen Cooperatively

4. Hemoglobin differs from myoglobin in that it has four binding sites for oxygen (compared to myoglobin's single binding site) and is cooperative. Are all molecules with multiple binding sites cooperative?

5. Hemoglobin is a tetrameric protein consisting of two α and two β polypeptide subunits. The structures of the α and β subunits are remarkably similar to that of myoglobin. However, at a number of positions, hydrophilic residues in myoglobin have been replaced by hydrophobic residues in hemoglobin.
   (a) How can this observation be reconciled with the generalization that hydrophobic residues fold into the interior of proteins?
   (b) In this regard, what can you say about the nature of the interactions that determine the quaternary structure of hemoglobin?

6. One effect of carbon monoxide binding to hemoglobin is that it increases hemoglobin's affinity for oxygen. Why isn't that a good thing?

An Allosteric Regulator Determines the Oxygen Affinity of Hemoglobin

7. Which of the following answers completes the sentence *incorrectly*? Hemoglobin differs from myoglobin in that
   (a) hemoglobin is multimeric whereas myoglobin is monomeric.
   (b) myoglobin binds O_2 more tightly than does hemoglobin at any given O_2 concentration.
   (c) hemoglobin binds CO_2 more effectively than does myoglobin.
   (d) myoglobin is more sensitive to allosteric modulators than hemoglobin.
   (e) the binding of O_2 by hemoglobin depends on the concentrations of CO_2, H^+, and BPG, whereas the binding of O_2 by myoglobin does not.

8. The book describes one structural difference between fetal hemoglobin (HbF) and adult hemoglobin (HbA). What is it?

9. Explain why fetal hemoglobin has a higher affinity for oxygen than does maternal hemoglobin and why this is a necessary adaptation.

10. Which of the following answers are true? Hemoglobin S forms fibrous precipitates
    (a) because the valine at position 6 of the β chain forms a sticky hydrophobic patch on the surface of the protein.
    (b) that are reversible upon oxygenation.
    (c) that distort the shape of cells.
    (d) only in the deoxy form.
    (e) only in homozygotes.

Hydrogen Ions and Carbon Dioxide Promote the Release of Oxygen

11. The oxygen dissociation curve for hemoglobin reflects allosteric effects that result from the interaction of hemoglobin with O_2, CO_2, H^+, and BPG. Which of the following structural changes occur in the hemoglobin molecule when O_2, CO_2, H^+, or BPG bind?
    (a) The binding of O_2 pulls the iron into the plane of the heme and causes a change in the interaction of all four globin subunits, mediated through the proximal His.
    (b) BPG binds at a single site between the four globin subunits in deoxyhemoglobin and stabilizes the deoxyhemoglobin form by cross-linking the β subunits.
    (c) The deoxy form of hemoglobin has a greater affinity for H^+ because the molecular environment of His and the α-NH_2 groups of the a chains changes, rendering these groups less acidic when O_2 is released.

12. Several oxygen dissociation curves are shown in Figure 9.1. Assuming that curve 3 corresponds to isolated hemoglobin placed in a solution containing physiologic concentrations of CO_2 and BPG at a pH of 7.0, indicate which of the curves reflects the following changes in conditions:
    (a) decreased CO_2 concentration
    (b) increased BPG concentration
    (c) increased pH
    (d) dissociation of hemoglobin into subunits

FIGURE 9.1   Oxygen dissociation curves.

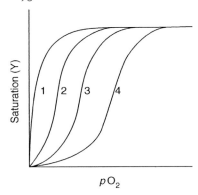

13. Which of the following statements concerning the Bohr effect are true?

   (a) Lowering the pH shifts the oxygen dissociation curve of hemoglobin to the right.
   (b) The acidic environment of an exercising muscle allows hemoglobin to bind O_2 more strongly.
   (c) The affinity of hemoglobin for O_2 is diminished by high concentrations of CO_2.
   (d) In the lung, the presence of higher concentrations of H^+ and CO_2 allows hemoglobin to become oxygenated.
   (e) In the lung, the presence of higher concentrations of O_2 promotes the release of CO_2 and H^+.

14. In the transition of hemoglobin from the oxy to the deoxy form, an aspartate residue is brought to the vicinity of His 146. This increases the affinity of this histidine for protons. Explain why.

ANSWERS TO SELF-TEST

1. Hemoglobin is found in red blood cells and myoglobin in muscles. "Haem" is a Greek prefix meaning blood, and "myo" is a Greek prefix meaning muscle.

2. a, c, d

3. b

4. No. A simple example would be the phosphate molecule, PO_3^{-3} which can bind one, two, or three protons. The binding of one proton does not change the affinity of the molecule for a second or third proton. Hence the whole population of phosphate molecules will have one, two, or three protons depending on the pH. In contrast, binding one oxygen molecule "opens" hemoglobin to binding a second, third, and fourth molecule (because of its cooperative nature) so that only the deoxy and tetra-oxy forms can be observed. The mono-, di-, and tri-oxy forms are essentially transition states.

5. (a) Hydrophobic patches occur on the surface of the hemoglobin subunits where the α and β chains fit together. As a result, these patches are not on the surface of the multimeric protein.
   (b) Hydrophobic interactions play an important role in stabilizing the tetrameric subunit structure of hemoglobin.

6. The higher hemoglobin's affinity for oxygen is, the closer its loading curve is to the loading curve of myoglobin. The amount of oxygen released to tissues is represented

by the space between those two curves. See text Figure 9.1. Both carbon monoxide's tight binding to hemoglobin, and the change it causes in the affinity for oxygen, lead to oxygen starvation of the tissues.

7. (d)

8. Fetal hemoglobin has a serine residue replacing a histidine residue in its γ chains (there are 2 γ and 2 α chains in HbF). This makes the central cavity where 2,3 BPG binds have less of a positive charge, and thus it binds less and has slightly more affinity for oxygen than HbA. See text Figure 9.11.

9. Fetal hemoglobin is composed of different subunits than adult hemoglobin and binds BPG less strongly. As a result, the affinity of fetal hemoglobin for oxygen is higher, and the fetus can extract the O_2 that is transported in maternal blood.

10. a, b, c, d

11. a, b, c

12. (a) 2   (b) 4   (c) 2   (d) 1

13. a, c, e

14. The pK values of ionizable groups are sensitive to their environment. The change in the environment of His 146 in deoxyhemoglobin increases its affinity for protons as a result of the electrostatic attraction between the negative charge of the aspartate and the proton.

PROBLEMS

1. The dense, rich color of human blood tells us that there are very many erythrocytes in every drop of blood. About how many red blood cells are in the adult human body? About what percent of human cells would this be? Considering that red blood cells have a half-life of only about 120 days, the supply of erythrocytes must be replaced about every 4 months.

2. Glutathione is a tripeptide consisting of glutamic acid, cysteine, and glycine; it is abundant in human erythrocytes as well as in many types of tissue. Reduced glutathione (GSH) acts as a reducing agent in tissues because its side-chain —SH group can be readily oxidized to form disulfide bonds. Unless glutathione is maintained substantially in its reduced form as opposed to its oxidized form in erythrocytes, they lose their ability to transport oxygen effectively. Why do you think this is so?

3. The heme prosthetic group found in hemoglobin and myoglobin is also found in cytochromes b and c, which are proteins that transfer electrons in the electron transport chain. How can the same prosthetic group serve such different functions as oxygen binding and electron transport?

4. The iron in hemoglobin must be in the ferrous (+2) state to bind oxygen. If the iron of hemoglobin becomes oxidized to the ferric (+3) state, the corresponding hemoglobin, called methemoglobin, cannot bind oxygen. To maintain iron in the ferrous state, red blood cells contain a reducing system to convert any methemoglobin back to hemoglobin. Some variant forms of hemoglobin, such as hemoglobin M, cannot be reduced by that system. What would be the expected clinical presentation of a patient having HbM?

5. If fMRI shows what is happening inside someone's brain, do you think it would provide the basis of the best possible lie detector? What other uses might there be for fMRI?

6. An effective respiratory carrier must be able to pick up oxygen from the lungs and deliver it to peripheral tissues. Oxygen dissociation curves for substances A and B are shown in Figure 9.2. What would be the disadvantage of each of these substances as a respiratory carrier? Where would the curve for an effective carrier appear in the figure?

FIGURE 9.2   Oxygen dissociation curves for substances A and B.

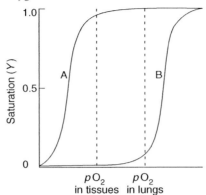

7. A portion of the lungs of patients suffering from pneumonia are filled with fluid, and therefore the lung surface area available for oxygen exchange is reduced. Standard hospital treatment of these patients involves placing them on a ventilating machine set to deliver enough oxygen to keep their hemoglobin approximately 92% saturated. Why is this value selected rather than one lower or higher?

8. What major differences exist between the sequential and concerted models for allostery in accounting for hemoglobin that is partially saturated with oxygen?

9. Predict whether each of the following manipulations will increase or decrease the tendency of HbS molecules to polymerize in vitro. Give a brief rationale for each answer.

   (a) increase in temperature
   (b) increase in the partial pressure of oxygen
   (c) stripping the HbS molecules of BPG
   (d) increase in the pH

10. One avenue of approach to therapy for sickle-cell anemia involves finding a way of turning on the synthesis of HbF in afflicted adults. Briefly explain why such a manipulation might be beneficial.

11. One approach to the management of sickle-cell anemia involves a search for osmotically active agents that would expand the volume of erythrocytes.

    (a) Give a brief rationale for this approach.
    (b) Suppose that the volume of an erythrocyte is increased by 10%. Calculate the rate of HbS polymer formation in the enlarged cell as a fraction of its rate in a normal-sized cell.

12. Prenatal diagnosis of sickle-cell anemia can be carried out by the treatment of fetal DNA with the restriction endonuclease MSTII, which recognizes the sequence CCTNAGG, where N is any nucleotide. Digestion of the β^S gene with MSTII yields a 1.3-kb fragment, whereas digestion of the β^A gene yields a 1.1-kb fragment.

    (a) Using your knowledge of the amino acid substitution that occurs in HbS, give the identity of nucleotide N on both the β^A and β^S genes. Also identify the mutational change at the DNA level that leads to the amino acid substitution.

Explain your answer. (Refer to the genetic code in your text.) Note that the (+) strand of DNA is given so you need to look for the complementary antiparallel RNA sequence.

(b) Give the identity of the amino acid at position 5 in the β chain using the information provided here and the genetic code.

13. The cooperative nature of hemoglobin can be understood using either the sequential model, in which each of the four subunits changes from T to R individually upon binding oxygen, or the MWC symmetry model, in which the whole tetramer shifts at once from T to R. What structural features of hemoglobin support each model?

14. Why is endemic malaria such a powerful selective force for the sickle-cell trait? Why can't malaria be treated with antibiotic drugs?

ANSWERS TO PROBLEMS

1. According to this Web site, written for a popular audience—
   http://www.madsci.org/posts/archives/feb2001/981770369.An.r.html
   —there are about 30 trillion RBC (red blood cells) in the adult human body, or 3×10^{13} cells (a trillion = 10^{12}). Of the roughly 90 trillion cells in the average human body, about 40 trillion are bacteria in the gut and other places. So the RBC make up about half of the "human" cells in the body.

2. Reduced glutathione helps keep the iron of hemoglobin in the ferrous (+2) valence state. When the iron of heme is oxidized to the ferric (+3) state to form methemoglobin, it can no longer combine reversibly with oxygen.

3. The oxidation state and the binding properties of heme vary markedly with its environment; therefore, the different environments caused by the different amino acids in these two classes of proteins change the functions of the heme.

4. An individual with HbM would have a bluish appearance, a condition called *cyanosis*, because of the lower concentration of ferrous hemoglobin ++ and thus less O_2 in RBC's.

5. Use of fMRI as a lie detector occurred to several people around the world, and there are some who claim to have systems that work. The central problem appears to be that the method works too well, in a sense. Some people will consider lying before they actually tell the truth. The same area of your brain "lights up" if you actually lie, or if you just think about lying. Still the research potential of fMRI seems limitless, and one could study decision making, or what part of the brain is active during religious meditation or prayer, and other things which are otherwise almost impossible to visualize.

6. Substance A would never unload oxygen to peripheral tissues. Substance B would never load oxygen in the lungs. An effective carrier would have an oxygen dissociation curve between the curves depicted for substance A and substance B. It would be relatively saturated with oxygen in the lungs and relatively unsaturated in the peripheral tissues.

7. Administering enough oxygen to give saturation levels greater than approximately 92% would be wasteful of oxygen, because one reaches the point of diminishing returns. Administering oxygen in amounts less than that required for 92% saturation runs the risk of compromising oxygen delivery to the tissues.

8. According to the concerted model, hemoglobin partially saturated with oxygen is composed of a mixture of fully oxygenated molecules, with all subunits in the R form, and fully deoxygenated molecules, with all subunits in the T form. According to the sequential model, individual molecules would have some subunits that are oxygenated (in the R form) and some that are deoxygenated (in the T form).

9. (a) An increase in temperature will favor the polymerization of HbS. The interaction between Hb molecules in polymer formation is hydrophobic in nature. Hydrophobic interactions have negative temperature coefficients; that is, they become more stable with increasing temperature.

   (b) An increase in the partial pressure of oxygen will inhibit polymerization because only deoxyhemoglobin S polymerizes.

   (c) BPG stabilizes deoxyhemoglobin S. Since only the deoxy form polymerizes, the removal of BPG from HbS would inhibit polymer formation.

   (d) Increasing the pH (decreasing the acidity) stabilizes oxyhemoglobin S. Since only the deoxy form polymerizes, this would inhibit formation.

10. HbF is devoid of β chains, having γ chains instead, so it does not polymerize. If adults with sickle-cell anemia could synthesize HbF, each erythrocyte would contain a mixture of HbS and HbF, which would reduce the degree of polymerization of HbS.

11. (a) The rate of polymerization of HbS is proportional to the tenth power of its concentration. Therefore, increasing the cell volume would decrease the HbS concentration, which would slow the rate of HbS polymerization.

   (b) If the cell has been expanded by 10%, the HbS concentration has been decreased to 10/11 or 90.9% of its original value. The rate of polymerization under these conditions is $(0.909)^{10} = 0.386$ of the rate in an unexpanded cell.

12. (a) Nucleotide N must be C on both the β^A and β^S genes. In HbA, Glu is present at position 6; it is encoded by GAG (on mRNA). Therefore, the sequence CTC must be present on the informational strand of β^A DNA. The mutation that leads to the substitution of Val for Glu at position 6 is T ->A.

   (b) The amino acid at position 5 in the β chain is Pro, which is encoded by CCU on RNA (or AGG on DNA).

13. The sequential model is supported by the fact that as each globin subunit binds oxygen, the iron moves into the heme plane pulling on the proximal histidine. This alters the position of the attached alpha helix and directly produces a conformational change. The MWC symmetry model is supported by the fact that each tetramer contains only one molecule of 2,3-BPG. The fact that 2,3-BPG must be either present or absent supports the concept that the tetramer should either be tense (in the presence of BPG) or relaxed (in its absence). In fact both models produce the same sigmoidal curve and both are useful ways of looking at hemoglobin.

14. Even though people who are heterozygotic for sickle cell (and have both HbS and HbA in every erythrocyte) are unlikely to have serious sickling attacks, there is still some formation of HbS fibers. This is enough to shorten the life of erythrocytes, which normally have a half-life in the body of 120 days. When the cells break down, the *Plasmodium falciparum* (malaria) parasites inside are exposed to the body's immune system and destroyed. So individuals with the sickle-cell trait survive while many with normal HbA die from the disease. Antibiotics are generally effective only against prokaryotes (bacteria). Malaria and several other tropical diseases are caused by eukaryotes.

Carbohydrates

Carbohydrates are one of the four major classes of biomolecules; the others are proteins, nucleic acids, and lipids. In Chapter 10, the authors describe the chemical nature of carbohydrates and summarize their principal biological roles. First, they introduce monosaccharides, the simplest carbohydrates, and describe their chemical properties. Since these sections assume familiarity with the properties of aldehydes, ketones, alcohols, and stereoisomers, students with a limited background in organic chemistry should review these topics in any standard organic chemistry text. Next, the chapter discusses simple derivatives of monosaccharides, including sugar phosphates and disaccharides. *Sugar* is the common name for monosaccharides and their derivatives. Then the text discusses poly-saccharides and oligosaccharides as storage and structural polymers and as components of proteoglycans and glycoproteins.

Glycoproteins are proteins with carbohydrates attached, generally as oligosaccharides. The attachment of sugars takes place either in the lumen of the endoplasmic reticulum or in the Golgi complex. One reason for attachment of sugars is the targeting of specific proteins to specific sites. For example, attachment of mannose 6-phosphate sends proteins from the Golgi complex to the lysosomes. A eukaryotic cell has many different subcellular compartments, each of which has to have a certain array of enzymes and proteins. The Golgi complex functions as the "post office" for the cell, and the attached oligosaccharides function as the "ZIP codes." Attached sugars can also function as signals for proper folding, or as sites of interaction between cells. Lectins and selectins are proteins that bind specific oligosaccharide clusters on the cell surface. The A, B, and O blood group antigens are examples of cell-surface oligosaccharides. Hemagglutinin allows the influenza virus to bind to sialic acid and thus attach to cells before invading them.

LEARNING OBJECTIVES

When you have mastered this chapter, you should be able to accomplish the following objectives.

Monosaccharides Are the Simplest Carbohydrates (Text Section 10.1)

1. List the main roles of *carbohydrates* in nature.

2. Define *carbohydrate* and *monosaccharide* in chemical terms.

3. Relate the absolute configuration of monosaccharide D or L *stereoisomers* to those of *glyceraldehyde*.

4. Associate the following monosaccharide class names with their corresponding structures: *aldose* and *ketose*; *triose, tetrose, pentose, hexose*, and *heptose*; *pyranose* and *furanose*.

5. Distinguish among *enantiomers, diastereoisomers*, and *epimers* of monosaccharides.

6. Draw the *Fischer* (open-chain) *structures* and the most common *Haworth* (ring) *structures* of D-*glucose*, D-*fructose*, D-*galactose*, and D-*ribose*.

7. Explain how ring structures arise through the formation of *hemiacetal* and *hemiketal* bonds. Draw a ring structure, given a Fischer formula.

8. Distinguish between α and β *anomers* of monosaccharides.

9. Compare the *chair* and *boat conformations* of monosaccharides.

10. Define *O-glycosidic* and *N-glycosidic* bonds in terms of *acetal* and *ketal* bonds. Draw the bonds indicated by such symbols as α-1,6 or β-1,4.

11. Explain what makes a sugar a reducing sugar.

12. Explain how Advanced Glycation End-Products (AGEs) arise.

Monosaccharides Are Linked to Form Complex Carbohydrates (Text Section 10.2)

13. Explain the role of O-glycosidic bonds in the formation of monosaccharide derivatives, *disaccharides*, and *polysaccharides*.

14. Draw the structures of *sucrose, lactose*, and *maltose*. Give the natural sources of these common disaccharides.

15. Describe the structures and biological roles of *glycogen, starch, amylose, amylopectin*, and *cellulose*.

16. Give examples of enzymes involved in the digestion of carbohydrates in humans.

17. List the major kinds of *glycosaminoglycans* and name their sugar components.

18. Describe *proteoglycans* and explain their importance in cartilage.

19. Explain the differences between the oligosaccharide antigens for A, B, and O blood types.

Carbohydrates Are Attached to Proteins to Form Glycoproteins (Text Section 10.3)

20. Name the amino acid residues that are used for attachment of carbohydrates to glycoproteins.

21. Discuss *erythropoietin* (EPO) structure and function.

22. State the molecular basis of *I-cell disease*. Explain how this disorder revealed the molecular signal that directs hydrolytic enzymes to the lysosome.

Lectins Are Specific Carbohydrate-Binding Proteins (Text Section 10.4)

23. Give examples of *lectins* and outline their functions and uses.

24. Describe the functions of *selectins* in the human body.

25. Explain why the influenza virus would have two proteins, hemagglutinin and neuraminidase, which perform diametrically opposite tasks.

SELF-TEST

1. Which of the following are roles of carbohydrates in nature? Carbohydrates

    (a) serve as energy stores in plants and animals.
    (b) are major structural components of mammalian tissues.
    (c) are constituents of nucleic acids.
    (d) are conjugated to many proteins and lipids.
    (e) are found in the structures of all the coenzymes.

2. In the human diet, carbohydrates constitute approximately half the total caloric intake, yet only 1% of tissue weight is carbohydrate. Explain this fact.

Monosaccharides Are the Simplest Carbohydrates

3. Examine the five sugar structures in Figure 10.1:

FIGURE 10.1

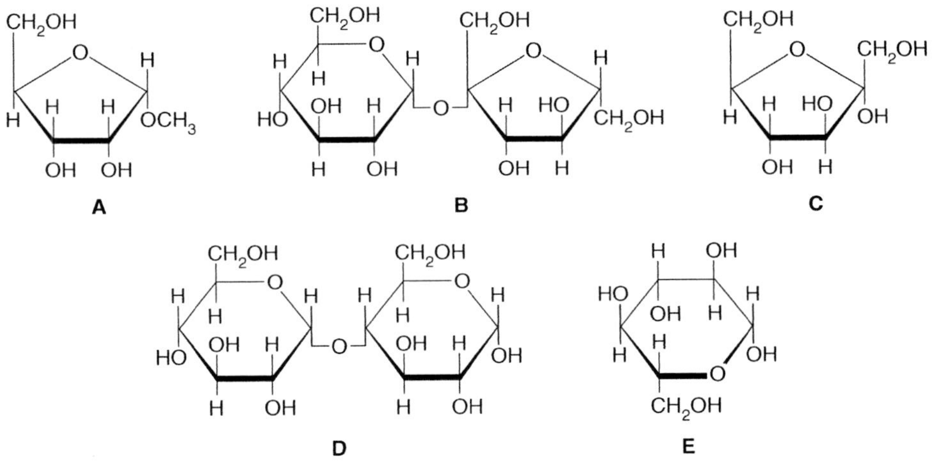

Which of these sugars

    (a) contain or are pentoses?
    (b) contain or are ketoses?
    (c) contain the same monosaccharides? Name the monosaccharides.
    (d) will yield different sugars after chemical or enzymatic hydrolysis of glycosidic bonds?
    (e) are reducing sugars?
    (f) contain a β-anomeric carbon?
    (g) is sucrose?
    (h) are released upon the digestion of starch?

4. Consider the aldopentoses in Figure 10.2.

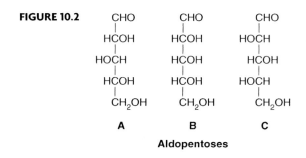

FIGURE 10.2

Aldopentoses

   A   B   C

(a) Name the types of stereoisomers represented by each pair.
   A and B are
   B and C are
   A and C are
(b) Name sugar B.
(c) Draw the α-anomeric form of the furanose Haworth ring structure for sugar A.

5. Identify the properties common to D-glucose and D-ribose. Both monosaccharides
(a) are reducing sugars.
(b) form intramolecular hemiacetal bonds.
(c) have functional groups that can form glycosidic linkages.
(d) occur in hexose form.
(e) are major constituents of glycoproteins.

6. Referring to the structure of ATP in Figure 10.3, which of the statements are true?

FIGURE 10.3

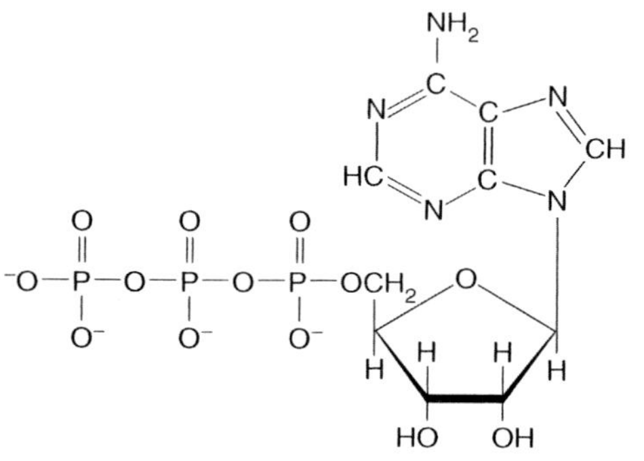

Adenosine triphosphate (ATP)

The structure of ATP
(a) contains a β-N-glycosidic linkage.
(b) contains a pyranose ring.
(c) exists in equilibrium with the open Fischer structure of the sugar.
(d) preferentially adopts a chair conformation.
(e) contains a ketose sugar.

Monosaccharides Are Linked to Form Complex Carbohydrates

7. Draw the structure of the disaccharide glucosyl α-1,6-galactose in the β-anomeric form.

8. If one carries out the partial mild acid hydrolysis of glycogen or starch and then isolates from the product oligosaccharides all the trisaccharides present, how many different kinds of trisaccharides would one expect to find? Disregard α or β anomers.

   (a) 1
   (b) 2
   (c) 3
   (d) 4
   (e) 5

9. A sample of bread gives a faint positive color with Nelson's reagent for reducing sugars. After an equivalent bread sample has been chewed, the test becomes markedly positive. Explain this result.

10. Why does cellulose form dense linear fibrils, whereas amylose forms open helices?

11. For the polysaccharides in the left column, indicate all the descriptions in the right column that are appropriate.

   (a) amylose
   (b) cellulose
   (c) dextran
   (d) glycogen
   (e) starch

   (1) contains α-1,6 glucosidic bonds
   (2) is a storage polysaccharide in yeasts and bacteria
   (3) can be effectively digested by humans
   (4) contains β-1,4 glucosidic bonds
   (5) is a branched polysaccharide
   (6) is a storage polysaccharide in humans
   (7) is a component of starch

12. α-Amylase
   (a) removes glucose residues sequentially from the reducing end of starch.
   (b) breaks the internal α-1,6 glycosidic bonds of starch.
   (c) breaks the internal α-1,4 glycosidic bonds of starch.
   (d) cleaves the α-1,4 glycosidic bond of lactose.
   (e) can hydrolyze cellulose in the presence of an isomerase.

13. Which of the following statements about glycosaminoglycans are true?
   (a) They contain derivatives of either glucosamine or galactosamine.
   (b) They constitute 5% of the weight of proteoglycans.
   (c) They contain positively charged substituent groups.
   (d) They include heparin, chondroitin sulfate, and keratan sulfate.
   (e) They have repeating units of four sugar groups.

14. Look at Figure 10.24 in the text, which shows the structures of the A, B, and O blood antigens. Based on the structures of the three antigens, can you suggest why type O blood is the "universal donor" and can be transfused into people with type A or type B without provoking an immune response?

Carbohydrates Are Attached to Proteins to Form Glycoproteins

15. Glycoproteins
   (a) contain oligosaccharides linked to the side chain of lysine or histidine residues.
   (b) contain oligosaccharides linked to the side chain of asparagine, serine, or threonine residues.
   (c) contain linear oligosaccharides with a terminal glucose residue.
   (d) bind to liver cell-surface receptors that recognize sialic acid residues.
   (e) are mostly cytoplasmic proteins.

16. Which of the following statements about I-cell disease are correct?

    (a) It results from the inability of lysosomes to hydrolyze glycosaminoglycans and gly-colipids.
    (b) It results from a chromosomal deletion of the genes specifying at least eight acid hydrolases ordinarily found in the lysosomes.
    (c) It arises from a deficiency in an enzyme that transfers mannose 6-phosphate onto a core oligosaccharide that is normally found on lysosomal enzymes.
    (d) It arises from the absence of a mannose 6-phosphate receptor in the *trans* Golgi complex.

Lectins Are Specific Carbohydrate-Binding Proteins

17. Which of the following statements are true? Lectins

    (a) are produced by plants and bacteria.
    (b) contain only a single binding site for carbohydrate.
    (c) are glycosaminoglycans.
    (d) recognize specific oligosaccharide patterns.
    (e) mediate cell-to-cell recognition.

18. Which of the following statements are true? Selectins

    (a) circulate in blood as free proteins.
    (b) are cell-surface receptor proteins.
    (c) are carbohydrate-binding adhesive proteins.
    (d) recognize and bind collagen in the extracellular matrix.
    (e) mediate the binding of immune cells to sites of injury during the inflammation process.

ANSWERS TO SELF-TEST

1. a, c, d

2. Most of the carbohydrates in the human diet are used as fuel to supply the energy re-quirements of the organism. Although some carbohydrate is stored in the form of glyco-gen, the mass stored is relatively small compared with adipose tissue and muscle mass. The carbohydrate present in nucleic acids, glycoproteins, glycolipids, and cofactors, al-though functionally essential, contributes relatively little to the weight of the body.

3. (a) A
   (b) B, C
   (c) B and C contain fructose; B, D, and E contain or are glucose. Note that glucose is in the α-anomer form in sugars B and D and is in the β-anomer form in sugar E.
   (d) A, B, D
   (e) C, D, E
   (f) B and E. In structure B, the fructose ring is flipped over, and E is D-glucose filpped over.
   (g) B
   (h) D and E. Although E is in the β-anomer form, recall that in solution it can "mu-tarotate" or change back to the α-anomer.

4. (a) A and B are 3-epimers. B and C are diastereoisomers. A and C are enantiomers.
   (b) D-ribose
   (c) See Figure 10.4.

FIGURE 10.4

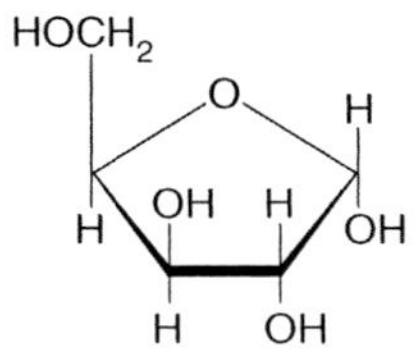

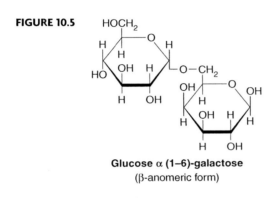

Sugar A
(α-anomeric form)

5. a, b, c. Note that *glycosidic* refers to bonds involving any sugars; however, *glucosidic* and *galactosidic* refer specifically to bonds involving the anomeric (reducing) carbons of glucose and galactose, respectively.

6. a

7. See Figure 10.5.

FIGURE 10.5

Glucose α (1–6)-galactose
(β-anomeric form)

8. Both c and d are correct. Since there are two glucosidic bonds in each trisaccharide and each bond can be α-1,4 or α-1,6, the total number of possible kinds of trisaccharides is four. However, two consecutive α-1,6 bonds would be very rare in glycogen or starch; therefore, one would be more likely to find three kinds.

9. The carbohydrate in bread is mostly starch, which is a polysaccharide mixture containing D-glucose residues linked by glucosidic bonds. All the aldehyde groups in each polysaccharide, except one at the free end, are involved in acetal bonds and do not react with Nelson's reagent. During mastication (chewing), α-amylase in saliva breaks many of the internal α-1,4 glucosidic bonds and exposes reactive aldehyde groups (reducing groups). Note: Nelson's reagent consists of copper sulfate in a hot alkaline solution; a reducing sugar, such as glucose, reduces the copper, which in turn reduces the arsenomolybdate in the reagent, producing a blue complex.

10. Both cellulose and amylose are linear polymers of D-glucose, but the glucosidic linkages of cellulose are β-1,4 whereas those of amylose are α-1,4. The different configuration at the anomeric carbons determines a different spatial orientation of consecutive glucose residues. Thus, cellulose is capable of forming a linear, hydrogen-bonded structure, whereas amylose forms an open helical structure (see Figure 10.14 in the text).

11. (a) 3, 7   (b) 4   (c) 1, 2, 5   (d) 1, 3, 5, 6   (e) 1, 3, 5, and, if you wish, 7.

12. c

13. a, d

14. The O antigen lacks the extra galactose or N-acetylgalactosamine that the other antigens have. Antibodies will react to the presence of an unfamiliar "bump" in the shape

of an oligosaccharide but will evidently not react to the lack of a sugar. It is also possible that individuals with Type A or Type B blood have a small amount of O antigen because of inefficient transfer of the final galactose or perhaps hydrolysis of the galactose. This would prevent the immune system from seeing the O antigen as "foreign."

15. b

16. c. The disease results from a deficiency in a sugar phosphotransferase that initiates a two-step sequence leading to the formation of a mannose 6-phosphate terminus on an oligosaccharide substituent of the eight or more affected lysosomal hydrolases. The phosphotransferase attaches a GlcNAc phosphate to a mannose residue of the oligosaccharide. Removal of the GlcNAc leaves the phosphate on the mannose. The enzymes lacking this mannose 6-phosphate "address" label are erroneously exported from the cell rather than being directed to the lysosomes. (See Figure 10.25 of the text.)

17. a, d, e

18. b, c, e. Collagen is a fibrous protein that is bound by proteins called "integrins."

PROBLEMS

1. Glucose and other dietary monosaccharides like fructose and galactose are very soluble in water at neutral pH. For example, over 150 g of glucose can be dissolved in 100 ml g water at 25°C.

   (a) What features of the chemical structure of glucose make it so soluble in water?
   (b) What features of the proteoglycans found in cartilage make them so highly hydrated and contribute to their ability to spring back after deformation?

2. Indicate whether the following pairs of molecules are enantiomers, epimers, diastereoisomers, or anomers.

   (a) D-xylose and D-lyxose
   (b) α-D-galactose and β-D-galactose
   (c) D-allose and D-talose
   (d) L-arabinose and D-arabinose

3. What is the name of the compound that is the mirror image of α-D-glucose?

4. Compound X, an aldose, is enzymatically reduced using NADPH as an electron donor, yielding D-sorbitol (Figure 10.6). This sugar alcohol is then oxidized at the C-2 position with NAD^+ as the electron acceptor; the products are NADH and a ketose, compound Y.

FIGURE 10.6

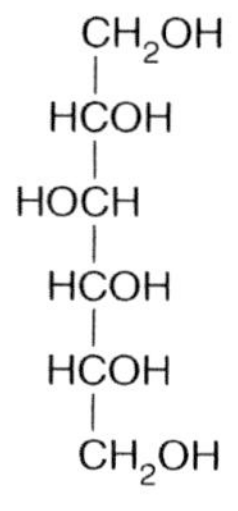

$$CH_2OH$$
$$HCOH$$
$$HOCH$$
$$HCOH$$
$$HCOH$$
$$CH_2OH$$

D-Sorbitol

   (a) Name compound X and write its structure.
   (b) Will sorbitol form a furanose or pyranose ring? Why?
   (c) Name compound Y and write its structure.

5. In Section 10.1 of the text, reducing sugars are defined as those with a free aldehyde or keto group that can reduce cupric ion to the cuprous form. The reactive species in the reducing sugar reaction is the open-chain form of the aldose or ketose. The reaction can be used to estimate the total amount of glucose in a solution such as blood plasma. An aqueous solution of glucose contains only a small amount of the open-chain form. How can the reaction be used to provide a *quantitative* estimate of glucose concentration?

6. Compare the number of dimers that can be prepared from a pair of alanine molecules and from a pair of D-galactose molecules, each of which is present as a pyranose ring. For the galactose molecules, pairs may be made using the α or β anomers.

7. Storage polysaccharides, like starch and glycogen, often contain over a million glucose units. The energetic cost of synthesizing polysaccharides is high (about one high-energy phosphate bond per sugar residue added). Suppose that in a liver cell, the glucosyl residues in large numbers of glycogen molecules were replaced with an equivalent number of molecules of free glucose. What problems would this cause for the liver cell?

8. You have a sample of glycogen that you wish to analyze using exhaustive methylation and acid hydrolysis. You incubate a sample of 0.4 g glycogen with methyl iodide, which methylates all *free* primary or secondary alcohol groups on sugars. Then you subject the sample to acid hydrolysis, which cleaves glycosidic linkages between adjacent glucose residues. You then determine the yield of 2,3-dimethylglucose in your sample.

    (a) Why is a 2,3-dimethylglucose residue produced from a branch point in glycogen?
    (b) The yield of 2,3-dimethylglucose is 0.247 mmol. What fraction of the total residues in each sample are branch points? The molecular weight of a glucosyl residue in glycogen is 162.
    (c) Could you use this technique to determine the anomeric nature of the glycogen branch? Why?

9. Shown in Figure 10.7 is one example of the storage oligosaccharides that account in part for the flatulence caused by eating beans, peas, and other legumes. These oligosaccharides cannot be digested by enzymes in the small intestine, but they can be metabolized by anaerobic microorganisms in the large intestine. There, they undergo oxidation, with the production of large quantities of carbon dioxide, hydrogen sulfide, and other gases. Solutions are now on the market containing one or more enzymes that, when ingested with the offending legumes at mealtime, convert the oligosaccharides to digestible products.

FIGURE 10.7

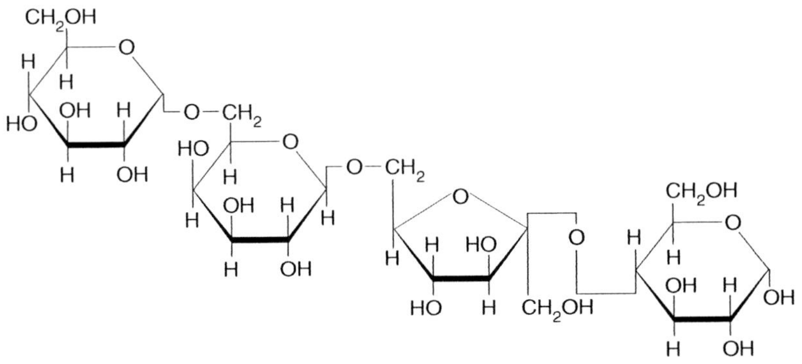

(a) Name the oligosaccharide shown in the figure.

(b) Given that free hexoses can pass easily through intestinal cells into the blood, what types of enzymes do you think are included in the commercial products that aid in legume oligosaccharide digestion?

(c) The concentration of oligosaccharides in beans can be reduced by cooking or by sprouting. What happens to the oligosaccharides in cooking? When the beans sprout before cooking or eating?

(d) When small amounts of cellulose are ingested purposely or accidentally (for example, by pets or young children), there is usually no gas production. In fact, the primary concern about paper ingestion by pets or small children is intestinal blockage. Why?

10. Why is the structural analysis of an oligosaccharide containing eight monosaccharide residues more complicated than a similar analysis for an octanucleotide or an octapeptide? This is not a quantitative question; a qualitative description will do.

11. In the 1950s, Morgan and Watkins showed that N-acetylgalactosamine and its α-methylglycoside inhibit the agglutination of type A erythrocytes by type A-specific lectins, whereas other sugars had little effect. What did this information reveal about the structure of the glycoprotein on the surface of type A cells?

12. Because red blood cells (RBC) carry oxygen, athletes have long been interested in finding ways to increase the numbers of RBC in their bodies. Honest athletes go through physical training, which increases their blood volume. Thirty years ago, some dishonest athletes hit on the idea of "donating" blood that could be centrifuged so that their own RBC could be reinjected before an athletic event (blood doping). More recently some athletes in endurance events (like cycling) have been caught using EPO, a hormone that stimulates production of RBC. As described in the text, EPO is a protein that is rather easy to produce by modern techniques. In the year 2000 tests were developed that could reveal the presence of EPO based on differences in glycosylation. These differences were there because human genes had been expressed in hamster cells. In 2004, a new form of EPO called dynEPO was produced using human cell lines. The glycosylation appears to be identical because this is a human protein expressed by human cells. Can you think of any way to detect athletes who cheat using this highly engineered product?

13. Exercise is fueled primarily by the oxidation of glucose (glycolysis) and fat (a process called β-oxidation). A typical runner might oxidize carbohydrate at the rate of 4 g/min and fat at the rate of 0.5 g/minute. The glucose that is being oxidized can come from the breakdown of liver and muscle glycogen. What advantages does the structure of glycogen provide for a runner?

14. Blood glucose is carefully regulated so that its normal concentration (the level between meals) is approximately 4.4–6.1 mM (82–110 mg/dL). This concentration represents about four teaspoons of dissolved glucose. Many mechanisms exist for blood glucose homeostasis (keeping blood glucose levels as constant as possible). Why is glucose homeostasis so important? (That is, what are the negative effects of high blood glucose levels?)

15. If you have ever ripped a piece of newspaper, then you may have noticed that if you tear the paper in one direction, you get a smooth tear. If you tear it in the perpendicular direction, the paper is more difficult to tear smoothly and you get a jagged edge. Given that newsprint is made from cellulose, explain this phenomenon.

16. Alcoholic beverages are made from the fermentation of glucose. A source of glucose can be the amylose and amylopectin of potatoes (for vodka), barley (for beer), or rice

(for sake). The starch is treated with amylases that are similar to the α-amylase secreted by the salivary glands and pancreas. Malted barley (barley that has begun to germinate) is a source of these enzymes. This treatment hydrolyzes amylose to glucose and maltose and a few short oligosaccharides. The same products appear from amylopectin but with the addition of a class of products called "limit dextrins." What would you expect would be the structure of these limit dextrins?

ANSWERS TO PROBLEMS

1. (a) Glucose and other hexose monosaccharides have five hydroxyl groups and an oxygen in the heterocyclic ring that can all form hydrogen bonds with water. The ability to form these hydrogen bonds with water and other polar molecules enables hexoses and other carbohydrates to dissolve easily in aqueous solution.

   (b) In addition to hydrogen bonding of water to hydroxyl groups and oxygen atoms in the repeating disaccharide units of cartilaginous proteoglycans like keratan sulfate and chondroitin sulfate, these molecules also contain charged sulfate and carboxylate groups that can also interact with water. Compression of these large hydrated polyanions can drive some water out of the cavities between them, but the high degree of hydration of the molecules, as well as charge repulsion between the sulfate and carboxylate groups, contributes to the tendency of these compounds to resume their normal conformations after deformation.

2. (a) D-Xylose and D-lyxose differ in configuration at a single asymmetric center; they are epimers.

   (b) α-D-Galactose and β-D-galactose have differing configurations at the C-1, or anomeric, carbon; they are anomers.

   (c) D-Allose and D-talose are diastereoisomers because they have opposite configurations at one or more chiral centers, but they are not complete mirror images.

   (d) L-arabinose and D-arabinose are mirror images of each other and are therefore enantiomers.

3. Although the mirror image of a D compound is an L compound, the mirror image of an α compound is an α compound. (An α compound has a 1-hydroxyl group in the α position.) Thus, α-L-glucose is the compound that is the mirror image, or enantiomer, of α-D-glucose.

4. (a) Compound X is D-glucose; it is the only D-aldose whose reduction will yield a hexitol with the same conformation as that of D-sorbitol. The less common sugar L-glucose would also yield the same result. L-sorbitol is commonly used for applications like sweetening toothpaste (without promoting decay). With sugar alcohols, there is no most-oxidized carbon, so it is hard to define which end is "carbon one," but the use of an enzyme greatly favors D-aldose as the starting material. L-Sorbitol probably originates from D-glucose. Turn the molecule upside down to see the relationship.

   (b) Sorbitol cannot form a hemiacetal because it has no aldehyde or ketone group. Therefore, neither type of ring can be formed by sorbitol.

   (c) Compound Y is D-fructose, a ketose that is produced by the oxidation of sorbitol. Enzymes would be very unlikely to produce an L-ketose, so this is the only expected result.

5. In water, an equilibrium exists among three forms of glucose. Two-thirds is present as the β anomer, one-third as the α anomer, and less than 1% as the open-chain

form. When excess cupric ion reacts with the open-chain form, glucose is oxidized to gluconic acid. Through the law of mass action, the α and β anomers of glucose are then converted to the open-chain aldose form. Continued production of gluconic acid from the open-chain form leads to the ultimate conversion of all glucopyranoses to the open-chain form, which reacts quantitatively with cupric ion. Thus the total amount of glucose in a known volume of blood plasma or other solution can be determined.

6. Only one dimer, alanylalanine, can be made from two alanine molecules linked via a peptide bond. However, the presence of several hydroxyl groups and the aldehydic function at the C-1 position of each D-galactose molecule provides an opportunity to make a larger number of dimers. Both the α and β forms of one molecule can form glycosidic linkages with the C-2, C-3, C-4, or C-6 hydroxyl groups of the other. Recall that the C-5 position is not available, because it participates in the formation of the pyranose ring. To these eight dimers can be added dimers formed through glycosidic linkages involving the αα, αβ, or ββ configurations. Thus, 11 possible dimers exist. If one is allowed to use L forms, then the number of possible dimers increases greatly. This variety of linkages makes the sugars very versatile molecules and yields many different structures that may be useful in biology. However, this variety has also made the systematic study of the chemistry of polysaccharides very difficult.

7. The primary consequence of a high concentration of free glucose molecules in the cell would be a dramatic and probably catastrophic increase in osmotic pressure. In aqueous solutions, colligative properties like boiling and freezing points, vapor pressure, and osmotic pressure depend primarily on the number of molecules in the solution. Thus a glycogen molecule containing a million glucose residues exerts one-millionth the osmotic pressure of a million molecules of free glucose. Osmotic pressure exerted by high glucose concentration would induce entry of water into the cell in an attempt to equalize pressure inside and outside the cell. Unlike bacterial or plant cells which have a rigid cell wall that can help resist high pressures, animal cells have a comparatively fragile plasma membrane, which will burst when osmotic pressures are too high.

8. (a) A glucosyl residue at a branch point has three of its five carbons linked to other glucose residues; these are carbons 1, 4, and 6. Only C-2 and C-3 of a branch point residue will have alcohol or hydroxyl groups that are free and therefore available for methylation. Thus residues at a branch point are converted to 2,3-dimethylglucose after methylation and hydrolysis. The glucosyl residues not at a branch point would be converted to 2,3,6-trimethylglucose by the same procedure, except for the single residue at the reducing end, which could be converted to 1,2,3,6-tetramethylglucose.

   (b) The original sample of 0.4 g corresponds to 0.4 g ÷ 162 g/mole, or 2.47×10^{-3} mole, or 2.47 mmol glucose residues, which is 10% of the total sample. Thus 10% of the glucosyl residues are at branch points.

   (c) The analysis using methylation and acid hydrolysis does not allow determination of the anomeric linkage. Acid hydrolysis cleaves both α- and β-anomeric linkages and does not allow distinctions between them.

9. (a) Glu α-1,6 Gal α-1,6 Fru β-1,4 Glu.

   (b) The solution must contain enzymes that hydrolyze the glycosidic linkages between the monosaccharides. For example, an activity that would be required for the oligosaccharide shown would be a type of α-1,6-glycosidase, which would cleave the α-1,6 linkage between glucose and galactose. Another would be the β-1,4-fructosidase, a different glycosidase. The glycosidases are needed to convert the oligosaccharides to free hexoses, which then pass easily into the circulation. The three common sugars found in the oligosaccharide shown in this problem are easily metabolized by the liver and other cells.

(c) Cooking by heating in water probably hydrolyzes some of the glycosidic linkages found in the oligosaccharides. Sprouting or germinating beans undergo a reduction in oligosaccharide concentration because hydrolase proteins induced during germination produce free hexoses, which can be used in the developing plant tissues as a source of carbon for biosynthesis.

(d) Because cellulose is an unbranched polymer of glucose residues joined by β-1,4 linkages, the molecule is resistant to hydrolysis even by anaerobic bacteria in the human intestine. Small amounts of cellulose and other indigestible complex carbohydrates are virtually unaltered as they pass through the digestive system. Thus no gases from carbohydrate breakdown are generated in the large intestine. Intestinal blockage may result from ingestion of large quantities of cellulose because there are no enzymes available to cleave the glycosidic linkages. Organisms that use cellulose as an energy source (for example, cows and termites) have gut flora that make cellulase and can provide the service of breaking these β-1,4 bonds.

10. In oligosaccharides, there are a number of different types of potential glycosidic linkages that can be formed among eight residues, because each free hydroxyl group as well as the anomeric carbon on a particular monosaccharide could be linked to similar groups on adjacent residues. An octo-oligosaccharide could be linear or branched and could be composed of as many as eight different monosaccharides, each of which could require additional steps to analyze completely. Analysis of an oligonucleotide is somewhat less complicated, because usually only four different bases are found during the analysis, and the linkage between adjacent nucleotides is almost always 3' ⟶ 5'; in addition, the oligonucleotide molecule is not likely to be branched. Although there may be as many as eight different amino acid residues in an octapeptide, all 20 different amino acids found in most proteins are relatively easy to characterize and the octapeptide is unlikely to be branched.

11. The observations of Morgan and Watkins suggested that the sugar N-acetylgalactosamine in a linkage is the determinant of blood group A specificity. The galactose derivative binds to type A lectins, occupying the sites that would otherwise bind to glycoproteins having N-acetylgalactosamine end groups on the surfaces of type A cells. The papers establishing the structures of the blood group oligosaccharides were among the first of Winifred M. Watkins's long and distinguished career. The fields of biochemistry and molecular biology have provided several early female role models including such important scientists as Maud Menten (who collaborated with L. Michaelis to study enzymology) and Rosalind Franklin (who determined the structure of the A-form and worked on the B-form of double-helical DNA). Dr. Watkins was elected as a Fellow of the Royal Society in 1998. [W. M. Watkins & W. T. J. Morgan, *Nature* 178[1956]:1289, and other papers.]

12. Assuming that dynEPO is identical to normal human EPO, it could be impossible to detect as a "foreign substance" because it is not "foreign." It should be possible to have some indication that a person is using illegal drugs by following their hematocrit (which shows levels of RBC in the blood) and other secondary effects. In other words, if you can't see the drug, you still should be able to see the effect of the drug. Here is an article about the difficulties of testing:

http://hum-molgen.org/NewsGen/08-2004/msg19.html

and an article about dynEPO and the sport of cycling:
http://www.bike-zone.com/features/?id=EPOv2

13. Glycogen consists of a homopolymer of glucose molecules linked via α1→4 linkages with branches of the same attached via α1→6 linkages every 10 residues or so. Glycogen is broken down into monomers of glucose-1-phosphate by the enzyme glycogen phosphorylase. One advantage of the glycogen structure lies in its branches. Each branch has a non-reducing end and because glycogen is broken down from these ends, the branches simply increase the number of ends that are accessible to glycogen phosphorylase. The branches thus enable glucose 1-phosphate to be released at a faster rate than it would be without these branches. The process provides the body with more glucose to meet its energy demands.

14. Glucose homeostasis is important because glucose is so reactive in its linear form. It will react with the primary amines found in proteins (N-termini, Lys residues, etc.) to form Advanced Glycation Endproducts (AGEs). Many enzymes and proteins do not work as well when they are glycosylated. Second, as you will learn later in this course, elevated blood glucose levels can result in increased insulin secretion, and insulin is a hormone that directs biochemical processes toward fat storage and away from fat oxidation. Elevated insulin levels are associated with obesity and type 2 diabetes.

15. Cellulose is made of glucose monomers with β1→4 linkages. These linkages result in a rather straight chain. Thus, these chains are able to line up side-by-side as well as above and below, and they hydrogen bond with each other. When you rip the newsprint between these hydrogen-bonded chains, the newsprint rips smoothly. When you rip the newsprint in the perpendicular direction, you are ripping it at natural breaks in the cellulose chain. That is, you are ripping it where there is no β(1→4) covalent bond. The jagged-edged tear shows the random distribution of these breaks in the cellulose polymers.

16. Limit dextrins are the branched structures that remain when only the α1→4 linkages of amylopectin are hydrolyzed. Unlike amylose, which is made entirely of α(1→4) linkages, amylopectin has branches that are attached via α(1→6) linkages. These linkages are not hydrolyzed by the α-amylase enzymes. What remains after amylase treatment are short oligosaccharides with branches. Additional enzymes (sometimes from mold) must be added to hydrolyze the α(1→6) bonds at these branches.

Lipids

This short chapter introduces the student to the world of *lipids*. All lipids are hydrophobic, and thus more soluble in organic solvents than in water. But they come in a variety of shapes and sizes, which leads to different uses in the cell. *Fatty acids* are a basic building block for some lipids, and are used as fuel in the cell. Each molecule of *triacylglycerol* contains three fatty acid molecules. Triacylglycerols are the main component of stored fat tissue. *Phosphoglycerides* are a form of *phospholipid*, which is like a triacylglycerol with one of the fatty acids replaced with a polar head group. This makes a difference in the behavior and use, so that these lipids are used in membranes and not as fat storage. Other phospholipids are also used in membranes, including *sphingolipids* and *glycolipids*. *Steroids* such as *cholesterol* can be found in membranes but have various other important roles in the cell. The *archaea* live in extreme environments such as very hot water, or acidic water, or high salt concentration. They have unusual membrane lipids with long methyl-branched alcohols instead of fatty acids. The alcohols connect to glycerol via an *ether linkage*, which leads to greater chemical stability.

LEARNING OBJECTIVES

When you have mastered this chapter, you should be able to accomplish the following objectives.

Fatty Acids Are a Main Source of Fuel (Text Section 11.1)

1. Draw the general chemical formula of a *fatty acid* and be able to use standard notation for representing the number of carbons and double bonds in a fatty acid chain.
2. Distinguish between *saturated* and *unsaturated* fatty acids.
3. Explain the relationship between fatty acid *chain length* and *degree of saturation* and the physical property of *melting point*.
4. Understand the significance of the ω-*carbon atom* in fatty acids.

Triacylglycerols Are the Storage Form of Fatty Acids (Text Section 11.2)

5. Describe the functions of *adipose tissue* in fuel storage and thermal insulation.
6. Understand that *triacylglycerols* are a highly concentrated energy source.

There Are Three Common Types of Membrane Lipids (Text Section 11.3)

7. Define *lipid* and list the major kinds of *membrane lipids*.
8. Recognize the structures and the constituent parts of *phospholipids* (*phosphoglycerides* and *sphingomyelin*), *glycolipids*, and *cholesterol*.
9. Describe the general properties of the *fatty acid chains* found in phospholipids and glycolipids.
10. Draw the general chemical formula of a phosphoglyceride, and recognize the most common *alcohol moieties* of phosphoglycerides (e.g., *choline*, *ethanolamine*, and *glycerol*).
11. Distinguish between membranes of *archaea* and those of eukaryotes and bacteria.
12. Describe the composition of *glycolipids*. Note the location of the carbohydrate components of membranes.
13. Recognize the structure of *cholesterol*.
14. Describe the properties of an *amphipathic molecule*.

SELF-TEST

Fatty Acids Are a Main Source of Fuel

1. Which of the following fatty acids is polyunsaturated?
   (a) arachidate
   (b) arachidonate
   (c) oleate
   (d) palmitate
   (e) stearate

2. True or False The double bonds in naturally occurring fatty acids tend to be *cis*.

3. When a fatty acid has more than one double bond, they tend to be how many carbons apart?
   (a) adjacent: one carbon apart
   (b) conjugated: two carbons apart
   (c) unconjugated: three carbons apart

Triacylglycerols Are the Storage Form of Fatty Acids

4. Soaps are produced by treating biological fats and oils with strong bases like sodium hydroxide (NaOH). Sodium linolenate would be a soap. Draw sodium linolenate.

5. Besides insulation and energy storage, can you think of other uses for adipose tissue in humans?

There Are Three Common Types of Membrane Lipids

6 . Which of the following substances are membrane lipids?
   (a) cholesterol
   (b) glycerol
   (c) phosphoglycerides
   (d) choline
   (e) cerebrosides

7. The phosphoinositol portion of the phosphatidyl inositol molecule is called the
   (a) amphipathic moiety.
   (b) hydrophobic moiety.
   (c) hydrophilic moiety.
   (d) micelle.
   (e) polar head group.

8. Acid hydrolysis will break all ester, amide, and acetal chemical linkages. Which of the following statements about the acid hydrolysis of various lipids is NOT correct?
   (a) A cerebroside releases two fatty acids and one monosaccharide per mole of cerebroside.
   (b) Phosphatidylcholine releases two fatty acids and one glycerol molecule per mole of phosphatidylcholine.
   (c) Sphingomyelin and phosphatidylcholine releases equivalent molar amounts of choline and phosphoric acid.
   (d) Cerebrosides and sphingomyelin each release one mole of sphingosine.

9. After examining the structural formulas of the four lipids in Figure 11.1, answer the following questions:
   (a) Which formulas are phosphoglycerides?
   (b) Which is a glycolipid?
   (c) Which contain sphingosine?
   (e) Which contain glycerol?
   (d) Which contain choline?
   (f) Name the lipids.

FIGURE 11.1 Membrane lipids R₁ and R₂ represent hydrocarbon chains.

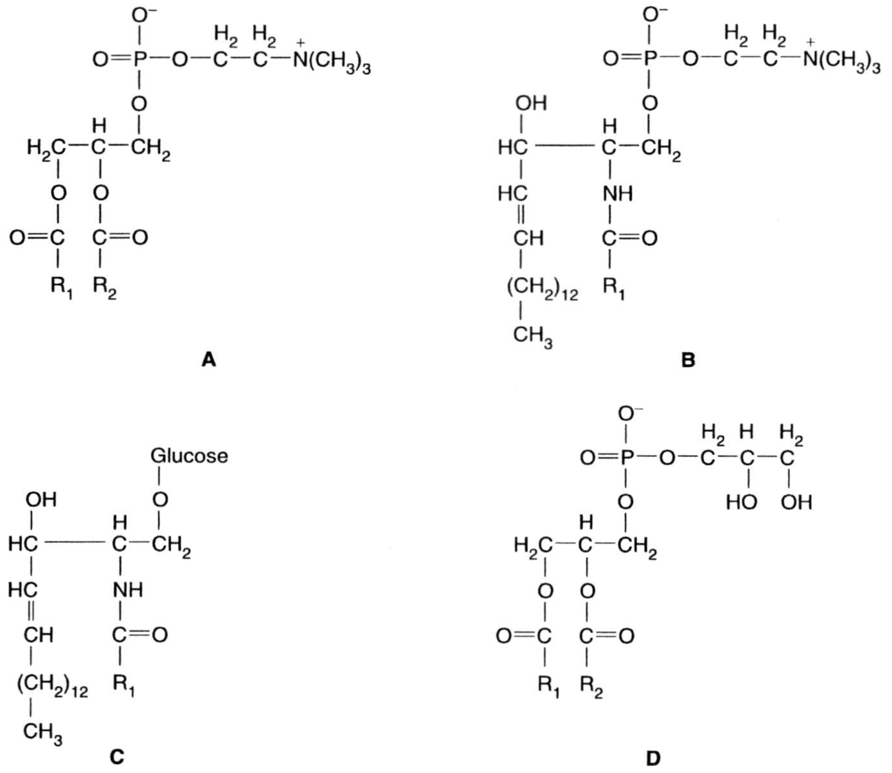

A

B

C

D

ANSWERS TO SELF-TEST

1. b. In this list, only arachidonic acid is polyunsaturated.

2. True. Trans-fatty acids sometimes found in processed foods are bad for cholesterol levels and are considered unnatural and unhealthy.

3. c. Unconjugated. Immediately adjacent double bonds (as in allene) are very rare. Double bonds one carbon apart are conjugated, and so they behave as a single system. Having two carbons separating double bonds allows them to be treated individually.

4. Saponification—mixing animal fats with lye—produces soap.

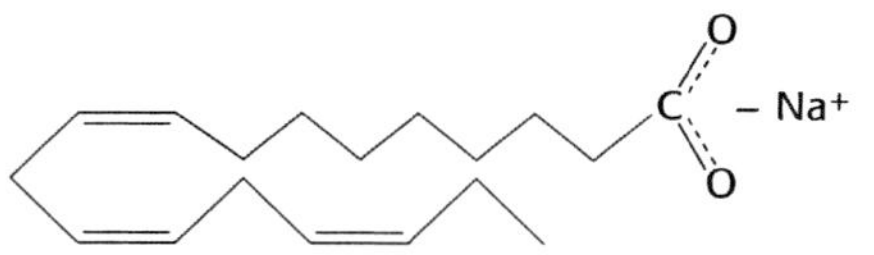

α-Linolenate

5. Fat is found where the human body needs cushioning, for example, when sitting down. Fat often is important in human perception of attractiveness—whether it is present as a pot belly or "pretty" curves.

6. a, c, e

7. c, e

8. a

9. (a) A, D (b) C   (c) B, C   (d) A, B   (e) A, D   (f) A is phosphatidyl choline, B is sphingomyelin, C is cerebroside, and D is phosphatidyl glycerol.

PROBLEMS

1. Bacteria and eukaryotic cells have membranes that contain fatty acids esterified to glycerol-3-phosphate. Archaea have no fatty acids, no esters between glycerol and hydrophobic groups, and glycerol-1-phosphate. Why are the archaea so different?

2. One sphingolipid shown in the text chapter is named sphingomyelin. Another sphingolipid mentioned is known a cerebroside. What sort of tissues are implied by these names?

3. Do you think it is possible for the body to discriminate between the different fatty acids we ingest? For example, while it is not mentioned in the chapter, seafood contains a small percentage of 17 carbon fatty acids. If you eat seafood will your own fat storage also have 17 carbon fatty acids?

4. Biochemistry labs that work with proteins often have a bottle on the shelf labeled "Sodium Lauryl Sulfate." Look at Table 11.1 and decode "Lauryl" into systematic nomenclature. What is this compound used for?

ANSWERS TO PROBLEMS

1. The differences between archaea and other cells must be very ancient. Archaea tend to live in extreme environments—hot, salty, acidic, etc. These environments would easily hydrolyze the fatty acid esters found in "normal" cells. Having phytyl ethers instead (see structure on page 187 of the textbook) makes for a much stabler compound under difficult conditions. Nobody really knows why archaeal lipids have a "backward" glycerol phosphate structure.

2. Sphingomyelin makes us think of the myelin sheath around nerve cells. Cerebroside makes us think of the cerebrum, a part of the brain, also neural tissue. Sphingomyelin is found in all sorts of tissues, but it is particularly abundant in the myelin sheath, which explains the origin of the name. Other sphingolipids not mentioned in this chapter also suggest neural tissue; for example, gangliosides make us think of ganglia, nerve clusters. The name sphingosine refers to the sphinx, or the riddle of the sphinx. When first discovered the compound was considered mysterious and contradictory (by the German biochemist Thudichum) because it contains both alcohol groups and an amine but it is insoluble in water.

3. There is no "screening" of ingested fats, so especially in the case of lipids, "you are what you eat." And eating seafood can give you as much as 5% odd chain fatty acids (these are discussed in Chapter 27 of the textbook). Odd chain fatty acids are not unhealthy, but trans fatty acids are, so one should try to avoid eating food known to contain those. It is also a good idea never to use cooking oil or salad oil that smells "a little off" because rancid fats will also go right into your body and become part of your tissues.

4. Sodium lauryl sulfate is SDS, sodium dodecyl sulfate, used as the denaturing detergent in SDS-PAGE, polyacrylamide gel electrophoresis. This technique was described in Chapter 5 of the textbook.

Membrane Structure and Function

In this chapter, the authors describe the composition, structural organization, and general functions of biological membranes and their ability to organize into vesicles and bilayers in water are then described. An important functional feature of membranes is their selective permeability to molecules, in particular the inability of ions and most polar molecules to cross membrane bilayers. This aspect of membrane function is discussed next and will be revisited when the mechanisms for transport of ions and polar molecules across membranes are discussed in Chapter 13.

Next, the authors turn to membrane proteins, the major functional constituents of biological membranes. The arrangement of proteins and lipids in membranes is described and the asymmetric, fluid nature of membranes is stressed. The important differentiation between integral and peripheral membrane proteins is discussed as well as the chemical forces that bind them to the membrane. The high-resolution analyses of the structures of selected membrane proteins are discussed, including structure prediction of membrane-spanning proteins. The chapter concludes with a discussion of internal membranes within eukaryotic cells and the mechanisms by which proteins are targeted to specific compartments within cells.

LEARNING OBJECTIVES

When you have mastered this chapter, you should be able to accomplish the following objectives.

Phospholipids and Glycolipids Form Bimolecular Sheets (Text Section 12.1)

1. List the functions of *biological membranes*.
2. Describe the common features of biological membranes.
3. Distinguish among *oriented monolayers, micelles,* and *lipid bilayers.*
4. Describe the *self-assembly process* for the formation of lipid bilayers. Note the stabilizing intermolecular forces.
5. Outline the methods used to prepare *lipid vesicles (liposomes)* and *planar bilayer membranes.* Point out some applications of these systems.
6. Explain the relationship between the *permeability coefficients* of small molecules and ions and their *solubility* in a nonpolar solvent relative to their solubility in water.

Membrane Fluidity Is Controlled by Fatty Acid Composition and Cholesterol Content (Text Section 12.2)

7. Know that a *cis double bond* in a fatty acid produces lipids that have a lower melting temperature, and hence are more fluid.
8. Understand that *cholesterol* enhances fluidity by forming specific complexes with membrane lipids, especially *sphingolipids.*
9. Define *lipid rafts* or *membrane rafts.*

Proteins Carry Out Most Membrane Processes (Text Section 12.3)

10. Distinguish between *peripheral* and *integral membrane proteins.*
11. Give an example of α-helical and β-sheet membrane-bound proteins.

Lipids and Many Membrane Proteins Diffuse Laterally in the Membrane (Text Section 12.4)

12. Describe the evidence for the *lateral diffusion* of membrane lipids and proteins. Contrast the rates for *lateral diffusion* with those for *transverse diffusion.*
13. Describe the features of the *fluid mosaic model* of biological membranes.
14. Explain the roles of the fatty acid chains of membrane lipids and cholesterol in controlling the *fluidity of membranes.*
15. Describe the components of lipid rafts and discuss their effect on *membrane fluidity.*
16. Discuss the origin and the significance of membrane asymmetry.

SELF-TEST

Phospholipids and Glycolipids Form Bimolecular Sheets

1. Which of the following statements about biological membranes are true?
    (a) They constitute selectively permeable boundaries between cells and their environment and between intracellular compartments.
    (b) They are formed primarily of lipid and carbohydrate.
    (c) They are involved in information transduction.
    (d) Targeting across them requires specific systems.
    (e) They are dynamic structures.

2. Which of the following statements about biological membranes is NOT true?

   (a) They contain carbohydrates that are covalently bound to proteins and lipids.
   (b) They are very large, sheetlike structures with closed boundaries.
   (c) They are symmetric because of the symmetric nature of lipid bilayers.
   (d) They can be regarded as two-dimensional solutions of oriented proteins and lipids.
   (e) They contain specific proteins that mediate their distinctive functions.

3. Which of the following statements about a micelle and a lipid bilayer are NOT true?

   (a) Both assemble spontaneously in water.
   (b) Both are made up of amphipathic molecules.
   (c) Both are very large, sheetlike structures.
   (d) Both have the thickness of two constituent molecules in one of their dimensions.
   (e) Both are stabilized by hydrophobic interactions, van der Waals forces, hydrogen bonds, and electrostatic interactions.

4. A triglyceride (triacylglycerol) is a glycerol derivative that is similar to a phosphoglyceride except that all three of its glycerol hydroxyl groups are esterified to fatty acid chains. Would you expect a triglyceride to form a lipid bilayer? Explain.

5. What is the volume of the inner water compartment of a liposome that has a diameter of 500 Å and a bilayer that is 40 Å thick?

   (a) 5.6×10^5 Å^3
   (b) 7.3×10^6 Å^3
   (c) 3.9×10^7 Å^3
   (d) 7.3×10^7 Å^3
   (e) 3.9×10^8 Å^3

6. Arrange the following substances in the order of decreasing permeability through a lipid bilayer.

   (a) urea
   (b) tryptophan
   (c) H_2O
   (d) Na^+
   (e) glucose

Membrane Fluidity Is Controlled by Fatty Acid Composition and Cholesterol Content

7. Would a trans double bond produce the same sort of disruption in packing of fatty acid chains as a cis double bond?

8. Cholesterol is an enhancer of membrane fluidity. Why would cholesterol be particularly common in animal cell membranes and rare in plant cell membranes?

Proteins Carry Out Most Membrane Processes

9. Why is an α-helix the preferred structure for transmembrane protein segments?

10. Show which of the properties listed at the right are characteristics of peripheral membrane proteins and which are characteristics of integral membrane proteins.

    (a) peripheral
    (b) integral

    (1) require detergents or organic solvent treatment for dissociation from the membrane
    (2) require mild salt or pH treatment for dissociation from the membrane
    (3) bind to the surface of membranes
    (4) have transmembrane domains

Lipids and Many Membrane Proteins Diffuse Laterally in the Membrane

11. Which of the following statements about the diffusion of lipids and proteins in membranes is NOT true?

    (a) Many membrane proteins can diffuse rapidly in the plane of the membrane.
    (b) In general, lipids show a faster lateral diffusion than do proteins.
    (c) Membrane proteins do not diffuse across membranes at measurable rates.
    (d) Lipids diffuse across and in the plane of the membrane at equal rates.

12. Which of the following statements about the asymmetry of membranes are true?

    (a) It is absolute for glycoproteins.
    (b) It is absolute for phospholipids, but only partial for glycolipids.
    (c) It arises during biosynthesis.
    (d) It is structural but not functional.

13. If phosphoglyceride A has a higher T_m than phosphoglyceride B, which of the following differences between A and B may exist? (In each case only one parameter—either chain length or double bonds—is compared.)

    (a) A has shorter fatty acid chains than B.
    (b) A has longer fatty acid chains than B.
    (c) A has more unsaturated fatty acid chains than B.
    (d) A has more saturated fatty acid chains than B.
    (e) A has trans unsaturated fatty acid chains, whereas B has cis unsaturated fatty acid chains.

14. Explain how the presence of lipid rafts modifies the original fluid mosaic model for biological membranes.

ANSWERS TO SELF-TEST

1. a, c, d, e

2. c

3. c

4. No. Although a triglyceride has hydrophobic fatty acyl chains attached to a glycerol backbone, it lacks a polar head group; therefore, it is not an amphipathic molecule and is incapable of forming a bilayer.

5. The correct answer is (c). The volume of a sphere is $4/3 \, \pi \, r^3$, so we just need the radius of the inner compartment to do the calculation. Using Figure 12.1 to represent the liposome, we can calculate the diameter of the inner water compartment by subtracting the width of the bilayer from the left and right sides of the liposome from the diameter of the outer compartment.

FIGURE 12.1

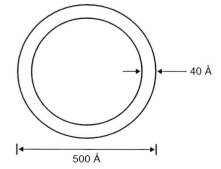

40 Å

500 Å

Diameter of inner water compartment = 500 Å − (2 × 40 Å) = 420 Å

Since the radius of a circle is half the diameter, the radius of the inner compartment $r = 1/2(420$ Å$) = 210$ Å.

Therefore the volume of inner water compartment in the liposome 4/3 π (210 Å)³ = 3.9 × 10⁷ Å³.

6. c, a, b, e, d

7. No, a trans double bond in a fatty acid allows the fatty acid to be very nearly linear, so the stacking would be about the same as with entirely saturated fatty acids.

8. Plant cells tend to be surrounded by cell walls and to have an unchanging shape. Animal cells have an irregular flowing membrane, like that of an amoeba, and the changes from convex to concave require a lot of fluidity. Thus, in the grocery store plant products like peanut butter and corn oil can always say "cholesterol free!" on the label.

9. Transmembrane protein segments usually consist of nonpolar amino acids. The main-chain peptide CO and NH groups, however, are polar and tend to form hydrogen bonds with water. In an α helix, these groups hydrogen-bond to each other, thereby decreasing their overall polarity and facilitating the insertion of the protein segment into the lipid bilayer.

10. (a) 2, 3   (b) 1, 4

11. d

12. a, c

13. b, d, e. Trans unsaturated fatty acid chains have a straighter conformation than do cis unsaturated chains; the packing of trans chains in bilayers is therefore more highly ordered, so they require higher temperatures to melt.

14. Lipid rafts are formed from cholesterol in specific complexes with lipids that contain the sphingosine backbone and with GPI-anchored proteins. Lipid rafts moderate membrane fluidity (making them less fluid) and at the same time make them less subject to phase transitions. The fluid mosaic model says that membrane fluidity is controlled by fatty acid composition and cholesterol content. Normally the addition of cholesterol will increase membrane fluidity by disrupting packing between fatty acid chains, but when in a lipid raft complex, may actually decrease membrane fluidity.

PROBLEMS

1. Phytol, a long-chain alcohol, appears as an ester in plant chlorophyll. When consumed as part of the diet, phytol is converted to phytanic acid (see Figure 12.2).

FIGURE 12.2

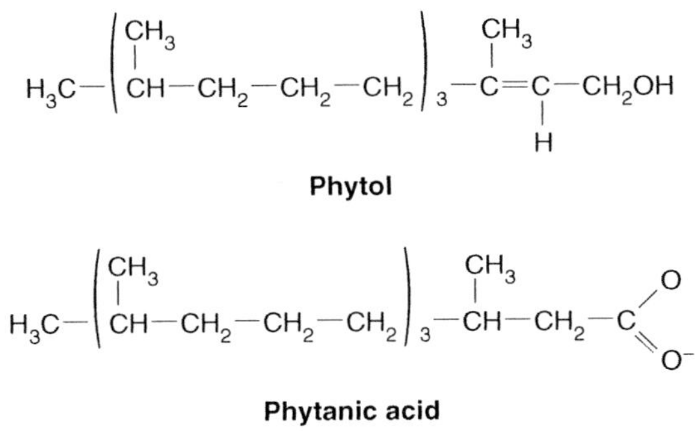

Phytol

Phytanic acid

People who cannot oxidize phytanic acid suffer from a number of neurological disorders that together are known as *Refsum's disease*. The symptoms may be related to the fact that phytanic acid accumulates in the membranes of nerve cells. What general effects of phytanic acid on these membranes would be observed?

2. Bacterial mutants that are unable to synthesize fatty acids will incorporate them into their membranes when fatty acids are supplied in their growth medium. Suppose that each of two cultures contains a mixture of several types of straight-chain fatty acids, some saturated and some unsaturated, ranging in chain length from 10 to 20 carbon atoms. If one culture is maintained at 18°C and the other is maintained at 40°C over several generations, what differences in the composition of the cell membranes of the two cultures would you expect to observe?

3. Given two bilayer systems, one composed of phospholipids having saturated acyl chains 20 carbons in length and the other having acyl chains of the same length but with cis double bonds at C-5, C-8, C-11, and C-14, compare the effect of the acyl chains on T_m for each system.

4. Hopanoids are pentacyclic molecules that are found in bacteria and in some plants. A typical bacterial hopanoid, bacteriohopanetetrol, is shown in Figure 12.3. Compare the structure of this compound with that of cholesterol. What effect would you expect a hopanoid to have on a bacterial membrane?

FIGURE 12.3

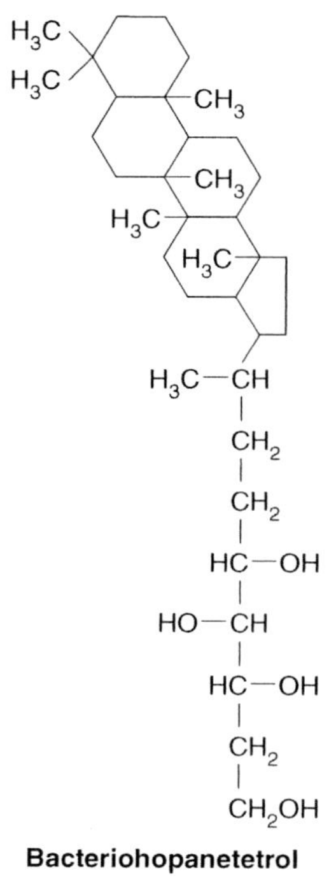

Bacteriohopanetetrol

5. As early as 1972, it was known that many biological membranes are asymmetric in the distribution of phospholipids between the inner and outer leaflets of the bilayer. Once such asymmetry is established, what factors act to preserve it?

6. As discussed in the text, the length and degree of saturation of the fatty acyl chains in membrane bilayers can affect the melting temperature T_m.

   (a) The value of T_m for a pure sample of phosphatidyl choline that contains two 12-carbon fatty acyl chains is −1°C. Values for phosphatidyl choline species with longer acyl chains increase by about 20°C for each two-carbon unit added. Why?

   (b) Suppose you have a phosphatidyl choline species that has one palmitoyl group esterified to C-1 of the glycerol moiety, as well as an oleoyl group esterified at

C-2 of glycerol. How would T_m for this species compare with that of dipalmitoylphosphatidyl choline, which contains two esterified palmitoyl groups?

(c) Suppose you have a sample of sphingomyelin that has palmitate esterified to the sphingosine backbone. Compare the T_m for this phospholipid with that of dipalmitoylphosphatidyl choline.

(d) The transition temperature for dipalmitoylphosphatidyl ethanolamine is 63°C. Suppose you have a sample of this phospholipid in excess water at 50°C, and you add cholesterol until it constitutes about 50% of the total lipid, by weight, in the sample. What would you expect when you attempt to determine the transition temperature for the mixture?

7. At least two segments of the polypeptide chain of a particular glycoprotein span the membrane of an erythrocyte. All the sugars in the glycoprotein are *O*-linked.

(a) Which amino acids might be found in the portion of the chain that is buried in the lipid bilayer?

(b) Why would you expect to find serine or threonine residues in the glycoprotein?

8. (a) Many integral membrane proteins are composed of a number of membrane-spanning segments, which form bundles of α helices packed closely together, often forming a membrane channel or pore. Each membrane-spanning sequence of most integral membrane proteins is an α helix composed of 18 to 20 amino acids. What is the width of the hydrocarbon core of the membrane?

(b) The sequence of one of the α helices in a particular integral membrane protein is shown in Figure 12.4, and the 19 residues in this helix are plotted in a helical wheel plot. Such a plot projects the side chains of the amino acid residues along the axis of the α helix (z-axis) onto an x-y plane. In an α helix, a full turn occurs every 3.6 residues, so each successive residue is 100° apart on the helix wheel. Compare the location of hydrophobic side chains on the helix surface with those that are polar or hydrophilic. Where are the hydrophobic side chains, and how are they accommodated in the membrane? Where are the polar side chains? How are they accommodated in the protein-membrane complex?

Helix sequence:

Ser Val Tyr Asp Ile Leu Glu Arg Phe Asn Glu Thr Met Asn His Ala Val Ser Gly

FIGURE 12.4

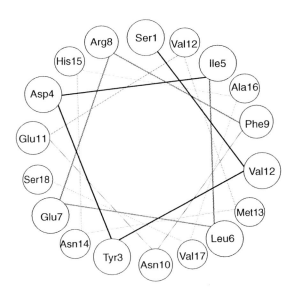

9. A series of experiments that shed some light on the movement of lipids in membranes was conducted by Rothman and Kennedy, using a gram-positive bacterium. They used 2,4,6-trinitrobenzenesulfonic acid (TNBS), which reacts with amino groups in phosphoethanolamine residues. Note that TNBS, shown in Figure 12.5, is charged at physiologic pH and cannot penetrate intact membrane vesicles. Incubation of TNBS with intact bacterial cells and with disrupted cells revealed that about two-thirds of the phosphoethanolamine molecules are located on the outside of the membrane, with the remaining residues on the inside. Rothman and Kennedy then incubated growing cells with a pulse of radioactive inorganic phosphate to label newly synthesized phosphoethanolamine molecules in the membrane. Using TNBS once again to distinguish between residues on the two sides of the membrane, they determined that immediately after the radioactive pulse, all newly synthesized phosphoethanolamine residues were located on the inner face of the membrane. After 30 minutes, however, the original distribution of phosphoethanolamine residues on the inner and outer faces of the bacterial cell membrane was restored. What do these observations suggest about the movement of phospholipids in membranes?

FIGURE 12.5

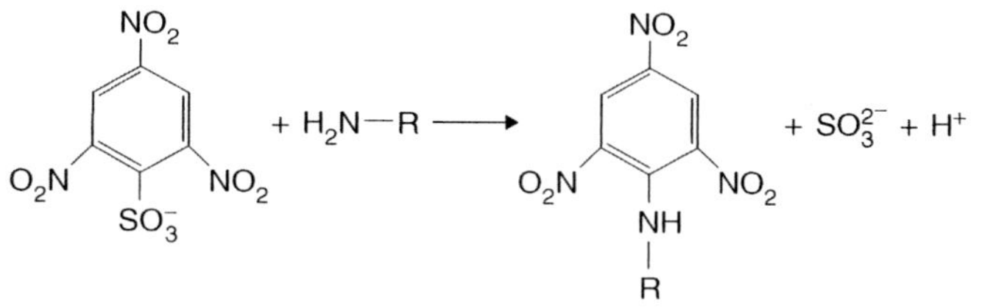

2,4,6-Trinitrobenzenesulfonic acid (TNBS)

10. Mycoplasma cells can be grown under conditions such that their plasma membrane contains one type of glycolipid, such as mono- or diglucosylated sphingosine molecules.

   (a) Membranes prepared from mycoplasma cells undergo a phase transition when heated. Suppose that sample A is isolated from cells whose glycolipids contain a very high percentage of unsaturated fatty acyl chains, whereas sample B is isolated from cells whose glycolipids contain a high percentage of saturated fatty acyl chains of the same length. When heated, which sample will exhibit a higher melting temperature? Why?

   (b) Glycolipids from samples A and B are analyzed for the carbohydrate content of their polar head groups. Those from sample A have a higher percentage of diglucosyl residues than those from sample B, which have mostly monoglucosyl residues. Explain how this observation is consistent with the lipid content of the two samples.

11. In mammals, lysophosphoglycerides (1-monoacylglycerol-3-phosphates) are generated in small quantities to trigger physiologic responses. Hydrolysis of a fatty acyl group from the C-2 position of a glycerophospholipid yields a lysophosphoglyceride. The reaction is catalyzed by phospholipase A_2, whose activity is strictly regulated. However, large quantities of phospholipase A_2 are found in snake venom, and the active venom enzyme can generate high concentrations of lysophosphoglycerides from membranes of snakebite victims. Lysophosphoglycerides are so named because in high concentrations they can disrupt membrane structure. Why?

12. What features of liposomes make them potentially useful as a delivery system for transporting water-soluble drugs to target cells? Suggest how one could prepare a liposome that is specific for a particular type of cell.

13. Explain the role of cholesterol in cell membranes.

14. During the solubilization of membranes, the purification of integral membrane proteins, and the reconstitution of membranes, gentler detergents, such as octyl glucoside, are used in preference to sodium dodecyl sulfate (SDS). Explain why.

15. Why do membrane proteins not diffuse, that is, flip-flop, across membranes?

16. In a membrane, an integral membrane protein diffuses laterally an average distance of 4×10^{-6} m in 1 minute, whereas a phospholipid molecule diffuses an average distance of 2 μm in 1 second.

   (a) Calculate the ratio of the diffusion rates for these two membrane components in meters per second.

   (b) Provide reasons for the difference between the two rates.

ANSWERS TO PROBLEMS

1. The four methyl side chains of each phytanic acid molecule interfere with the ordered association of fatty acyl chains; thus, they increase the fluidity of nerve cell membranes. This increase in fluidity could interfere with myelin function or ion transport, but the actual molecular basis for the symptoms is not yet known. Many of the symptoms of Refsum's disease can be eliminated by adopting diets that are free of phytol. The primary source of phytol in the human diet is from dairy products and other fats from ruminants. Cows, for example, consume large quantities of chlorophyll as they ingest grasses and plant materials. The symbiotic bacteria that inhabit the bovine rumen readily degrade chlorophyll, releasing free phytol, which is then converted to phytanic acid. Up to 10% of the fatty acids in bovine blood plasma are found as phytanic acid, which can then be incorporated into cell membranes and milk. For those who have Refsum's disease, it is therefore necessary to restrict consumption of beef as well as dairy products like milk and butter. Because humans do not degrade chlorophyll extensively during digestion, restriction of green plants in the diet is usually unnecessary.

2. You would expect to find that the bacteria grown at the higher temperature has incorporated a higher number of the longer fatty acids and a greater proportion of the saturated fatty acids. The membranes of bacteria grown at 18°C have more short-chain fatty acids and more that are unsaturated. These cells select fatty acids that will remain fluid at a lower temperature in order to prevent their membranes from becoming too rigid. The cells grown at the higher temperatures can select fatty acids that pack more closely. Cells in both cultures thus employ strategies designed to achieve optimal membrane fluidity.

3. The higher the number of cis double bonds, the less ordered the bilayer structure and the more fluid the membrane system. You would therefore expect T_m for the bilayer system containing the acyl chains with four unsaturated bonds to be much lower than that for the system containing the saturated fatty acid chains.

4. Like cholesterol, bacteriohopanetetrol is a pentacyclic molecule with a rigid, plate-like, hydrophobic ring structure; it has a hydrophilic region as well, although that region is on the opposite end of the molecule when compared with cholesterol. In bacterial membranes, hopanoids may have a function similar to that of cholesterol in mammalian membranes; that is, they may moderate bacterial membrane fluidity by blocking the motion of fatty acyl chains and by preventing their crystallization.

5. Phospholipids have polar head groups, so their transfer across the hydrophobic interior of the bilayer as well as their dissociation from water at the bilayer surface would require a positive change in free energy. Without the input of free energy to make the process a spontaneous one, the transfer of the polar head group is very unlikely, so the asymmetric distribution of the phospholipids is preserved.

6. (a) The longer the acyl groups, the larger the number of noncovalent interactions that can form among the hydrocarbon chains. Higher temperatures are therefore required to disrupt the interactions of phospholipid species that have longer fatty acyl groups.

   (b) The cis double bond in oleate produces a bend in the hydrocarbon chain, interfering with the formation of noncovalent bonds between the acyl chains. Less heat energy is therefore required to cause a phase transition; in fact, the melting temperature for phosphatidyl choline with a palmitoyl and an oleoyl unit is $-5°C$, and T_m for dipalmitoylphosphatidyl choline is 41°C.

   (c) The structures of phosphatidyl choline and of sphingomyelin are very similar to each other; both contain phosphoryl choline and both have a pair of hydrocarbon chains. Given similar chain lengths in palmitoylspingomyelin and in dipalmitoylphosphatidyl choline, you would expect that values of T_m for the two molecules are similar. Both species in fact exhibit a phase transition at 43°C.

   (d) At 50°C, you should expect cholesterol to diminish or even to abolish the transition, by preventing the close packing of the fatty acyl chains that impart rigidity to the molecular assembly. At higher temperatures, cholesterol in the mixture also prevents larger motions of fatty acyl chains, making the assembly less fluid. Studies show that in mixtures containing 30 to 35 mol % cholesterol, phase transitions are extinguished.

7. (a) You should expect to find nonpolar amino acid residues in the portions of the glycoprotein chain that are buried in the membrane. Because the core portion of the membrane is 30 Å wide, up to 20 amino acids could be included in the buried segments, assuming that the amino acids are part of an α helix, in which the translation distance for each amino acid is 1.5 Å.

   (b) The glycoprotein has O-linked carbohydrate residues, and in most such proteins the sugars are attached to the side chains of serine or threonine residues. Were the sugars N-linked instead, you would expect to find one or more asparagine residues in the glycoprotein.

8. (a) In an α helix, each amino acid residue extends 1.5 Å (1.5×10^{-1} nm) along the helix axis. Therefore a span of 20 amino acids in an α helix will be about 30 Å in length, corresponding to the width of the hydrophobic core of the membrane.

   (b) The plot clearly shows that hydrophobic amino acids are concentrated along one side of the surface of the helix. The side chains of those residues are likely to face the hydrophobic core of the membrane. Polar side chains are located on the opposite side of the helical surface; they are likely to be on the side of the chain that faces other α-helical bundles. They could form hydrogen or ionic bonds with polar residues in other bundles.

9. In model membrane systems, the transfer of phospholipid head groups from one side of the bilayer to the other is very slow, presumably because of the energy required to move the polar head group through the hydrophobic bilayer. The experiments carried out by

Rothman and Kennedy indicate that a process that mediates the flip-flop of membrane lipids is operating in bacterial cells. Phospholipid synthesis takes place on the cytosolic face (the inner leaflet) of the membrane, and some of the newly synthesized lipids are moved through the bilayer to the outside surface of the membrane bilayer. While aminophospholipid translocases that can move polar lipids across membranes have been found in eukaryotes, it is not yet known how such a process occurs in bacteria.

10. (a) You would expect sample B, with a higher percentage of saturated fatty acids, to have a higher melting point. The saturated chains will aggregate more closely with each other, requiring more thermal energy to disrupt that aggregation. The acyl chains of unsaturated fatty acids are kinked and therefore cannot aggregate in regular arrays like saturated acyl chains of the same length. They are therefore disrupted at a lower temperature.

    (b) In the membrane, the cross-sectional area occupied by unsaturated fatty acids is larger than that occupied by saturated chains because of kinks in the hydrocarbon chains due to double bonds. A diglucosyl head group is larger (has a larger cross-section size) than that of a monoglucosyl derivative, so the larger head group would match the increase in cross-sectional area in the interior of the bilayer composed of unsaturated fatty acyl chains.

11. Glycerophospholipids contain two fatty acyl groups esterified to glycerol, to which a polar head group is also attached at the C-3 carbon. When phospholipase A_2 removes one of the fatty acyl chains, the polar head group is too large in relation to the single hydrocarbon chain to allow optimal packing in the bilayer. The regular association of the hydrocarbon tails is disrupted, and the plasma membrane dissolves.

12. Liposomes are essentially impermeable to water-soluble molecules. Therefore, water-soluble drugs could be trapped inside the liposomes and then be delivered into the target cells by fusing the liposomes with the cell membrane. To make a liposome specific for a particular type of cell, antibodies that have been prepared against a surface protein of the target cell could be attached to the liposome via a covalent bond with a bilayer lipid, for example, phosphatidyl ethanolamine. This would enable the liposome to recognize the target cells. Of course, strategies would also have to be devised to prevent the premature, nonspecific fusion of the liposome with other cells.

13. Cholesterol modulates the fluidity of membranes. By inserting itself between the fatty acid chains, cholesterol prevents their "crystallization" at temperatures below T_m and sterically blocks large motions of the fatty acid chains at temperatures above T_m. In fact, high concentrations of cholesterol abolish phase transitions of bilayers. This modulating effect of cholesterol maintains the fluidity of membranes in the range required for biological function.

14. Although sodium dodecyl sulfate (SDS) is a very effective detergent for solubilizing membrane components, the strong electrostatic interactions of its polar head groups with charged groups on the membrane proteins disrupt protein structure. A detergent such as octyl glucoside, which has an uncharged head group, allows the proteins to retain their three-dimensional structures while it interacts with their hydrophobic domains.

15. Membrane proteins are very bulky molecules that contain numerous charged amino acid residues and polar sugar groups (in the case of glycoproteins) that are highly hydrated. Such molecules do not diffuse through the hydrophobic interior of the lipid bilayer.

16. (a) Rate of protein diffusion:

$$4 \times 10^{-6} \text{ m/min} = \frac{1 \text{ min}}{60 \text{ s}} = 6.7 \times 10^{-8} \text{ m/s}$$

Rate of phospholipid diffusion: 2 μm/s $= 2 \times 10^{-6}$ m/s

Ratio of phospholipid diffusion rate to protein diffusion rate:

$$\frac{2 \times 10^{-6} \text{ m/s}}{6.7 \times 10^{-8} \text{ m/s}} = 30$$

(b) The difference in diffusion rates is due primarily to the difference in mass between phospholipids, which have a molecular weight of approximately 800, and proteins, which have a molecular weight greater than 10,000. In addition, integral membrane proteins may associate with peripheral proteins, which would further decrease their lateral diffusion.

Signal-Transduction Pathways

In Chapter 11 you learned how biological membranes serve as semipermeable boundaries that isolate the cell from its surroundings and separate intracellular compartments from one another. Chapter 12 also described how selective, controlled breaching of the membrane barrier generates ion gradients across the bilayer, thereby producing electrical signals. In this chapter you will learn how molecules external to the cell bind to integral membrane protein receptors to initiate specific responses within the cell. The text describes how these binding and transmission mechanisms lead to an amplification of the initial signal and to specific effects that adapt the cell to its environment through effects on intracellular enzymes and regulatory proteins. The text also describes how disorders in these pathways of information flow can lead to diseases.

The authors use three examples of signal transduction pathways as examples. The first is the epinephrine-initiated pathway, the next is the pathway activated by insulin, and the last is the pathway activated by the epidermal growth factor. After a brief overview of signal transduction, the text describes the structure of the seven-helix transmembrane β-adrenergic receptor and indicates how it transmits to the intracellular side of the plasma membrane a signal arising from binding the hormone epinephrine on the extracellular surface of the cell. The common features of the G proteins are presented next. The description of the information-transmission pathway from hormone stimulus to G proteins to adenylate cyclase is completed by a discussion of how cAMP activates specific protein kinases to modulate the activities of the phosphorylated target proteins. A small number of hormone molecules outside the cell results in an amplified response because each activated enzyme in the triggered cascade forms numerous products. There are many distinct seven-helix transmembrane hormone receptors.

The text next describes an analogous hormone-stimulated system—the phospho-ionositide cascade. In this system, the hormone activates, by means of G proteins, a specific phospholipase (phospholipase C) that cleaves a plasma membrane phospholipid, phosphatidyl inositol 4,5-bisphosphate (PIP_2), to form two second messengers. The inositol phosphate derivative, inositol 1,4,5-trisphosphate (IP_3), which is short-lived, triggers the opening of ion channels so that the Ca^{+2} concentration in the cytosol is increased. The remnant of the PIP_2 molecule, diacylglycerol (DAG), is also a second messenger that activates protein kinase C. The increased Ca^{+2} levels and the activated protein kinase C affect a variety of biochemical reactions. The authors then describe the structure of Ca^{+2}-binding proteins, focusing on calmodulin, and explain how the binding of the ion is highly specific and leads to a large conformational change in the protein—qualities desirable in molecules serving as Ca^{2+} sensors and signal transducers.

The text then introduces another class of receptors, the transmembrane receptor tyrosine kinases that are often activated by a ligand-induced dimerization. The activated dimers phosphorylate some of their own tyrosine residues to provide docking sites for effector proteins on the cytosolic side of the membrane. Once bound, these effector enzymes are themselves phosphorylated and thereby activated by the tyrosine receptor kinase. The insulin and EGF receptors are used to discuss this class of receptors. A description of the susceptibility of signal transduction pathways to malfunctions that produce cancer follows, and the roles of oncogenes and their normal cellular counterparts (proto-oncogenes) in cell growth and differentiation are presented last.

LEARNING OBJECTIVES

When you have mastered this chapter, you should be able to accomplish the following objectives.

Signal Transduction Depends on Molecular Circuits (Text Section 13.1)

1. Identify the basic components of signal transduction pathways.

2. Draw a generalized *molecular circuit* based on a signal-transduction cascade. Outline the roles of *membrane receptors, ligands, primary messengers, second messengers, effectors,* and *cross talk* in the process.

3. Explain how a small number of *hormone* molecules outside the cell can effect a change involving many molecules within the cell, and consider that the cascade must be curtailed after being initiated.

Receptor Proteins Transmit Information Into the Cell (Text Section 13.2)

4. Describe the structure of the *seven-transmembrane-helix (7TM)* class of cell surface receptors. List some of the functions of members of this family and recognize their importance as drug targets.

5. Compare the structure of human *β-adrenergic receptor* ($β_2$-AR), which binds epinephrine, with that of *rhodopsin*.

6. Identify the cellular localization of *guanyl nucleotide-binding proteins* (*G proteins*) and describe their structures, catalytic characteristics, and molecular mechanisms of

activation and inactivation. Describe the roles of G proteins in coupling a *hormone-receptor complex* to *adenylate cyclase* and in amplifying the stimulus.

7. Understand that families of G proteins enable diverse hormones to effect a variety of physiologic functions.

8. Recognize the structure of *cAMP*, and write the reaction catalyzed by *Adenylate Cyclase* that forms it.

9. State the role of the hormone bound receptor in activation of *heterotrimeric G proteins* and describe the structural changes involved in the activation.

10. Describe the mechanism by which cAMP modulates the activity of *protein kinase A* *(PKA)*.

11. Explain the molecular mechanisms causing *cholera* and *pertussis*.

12. Write the reaction catalyzed by *phospholipase C* to produce the second messengers *inositol 1,4,5-trisphosphate* (IP_3) and *diacylglycerol* (DAG).

13. Describe the effects of IP_3 on the *IP_3-gated channel*. Describe the effects of Ca^{2+} released from endoplasmic reticulum of smooth muscle, and list some biochemical processes affected by an increased intracellular Ca^{2+} concentration.

Some Receptors Dimerize in Response to Ligand Binding and Recruit Tyrosine Kinases (Text Section 13.3)

14. Describe how the quaternary structure (*monomer-dimer equilibrium*) of the *human growth hormone receptor* changes on binding *human growth hormone*.

15. Discuss how the structure of the *epidermal growth factor receptor* (*EGFR*) provides evidence for why it is a monomer in the absence of the *epidermal growth factor* (*EGF*), but dimerizes in its presence. Explain how the structure and activity of the Her2 receptor supports this model.

16. Explain the role of *adaptor proteins* in signal transduction and give examples of their use.

17. Name some members of the *small G protein* family, and distinguish their structures from those of the heterotrimeric G proteins.

18. Appreciate the essential roles of the receptor tyrosine kinases and small G proteins in controlling cell growth and differentiation.

19. Outline the EGF signaling pathway including the mechanism for signal transmission between steps.

Metabolism in Context: Insulin Signaling Regulates Metabolism
(Text Section 13.4)

20. Describe the structure of the *insulin receptor* (*IR*) including the location of the insulin-binding site. Recognize the significance of the insulin-dependent dimerization of the receptor.

21. Describe the general structures of the *receptor tyrosine kinases* and outline the process that converts them from inactive proteins to active enzymes. List some of the hormones that activate tyrosine kinases.

22. Summarize the series of events that occur after binding of insulin to the IR.

23. Describe the mechanism of termination of the insulin signal transduction cascade.

Calcium is a Ubiquitous Cytoplasmic Messenger (Text Section 13.5)

24. Outline the features that suit Ca^{2+} in its role as a eukaryotic signaling ion.

25. Describe the structure of *calmodulin* and its biochemical function. Relate calmodulin to the *calmodulin-dependent protein kinase (CaM Kinase)*.

26. Describe the *EF hand structural motif* of *calcium-binding proteins*, explain how it binds Ca^{2+}, and describe how ion binding affects its structure.

27. Understand the opposing roles of Calmodulin and the Ca^{2+}–ATPase Pump in calcium signaling.

Defects in Signal-Transduction Pathways Can Lead to Diseases (Text Section 13.6)

28. Define *cancer* in terms of cell growth.

29. Appreciate that proto-oncogenes, which provide normal, essential functions in cell growth and proliferation, can give rise to cancer on mutation to oncogenes.

30. Outline the biochemical mechanism of *v-ras protein*–induced cancer and note the role of the normal (noncarcinogenic) *c-ras* protein in cellular growth. Appreciate that a diminished GTPase activity, in this case, leads to cancer.

31. Explain how an inhibitor of a specific protein kinase might be an effective anticancer drug. Compare it with the mechanism of *monoclonal antibodies* in treatment of cancer.

SELF-TEST

Signal Transduction Depends on Molecular Circuits

1. Signal transduction cascades are produced by molecular assemblies of which of the following components?
   - (a) enzymes
   - (b) regulatory proteins
   - (c) receptors
   - (d) transmembrane channels
   - (e) nuclear pores

2. Match the process in the left column with the function it performs in the right column.
   - (a) second messenger
   - (b) effectors
   - (c) membrane receptors
   - (d) signal terminator

   - (1) carries a signal outside the cell across the membrane into the cell
   - (2) returns the signal-transduction system to its original state
   - (3) Directly alter the physiological response
   - (4) relays information from the membrane receptor

Receptor Proteins Transmit Information Into the Cell

3. Describe an essential structural property of seven-transmembrane helix receptors (7TM) that allows them to respond to stimuli.

4. Guanyl nucleotide-binding proteins (G proteins) have which of the following properties?

   (a) bind GMP in their inactivated state
   (b) act as intermediates in 7TM receptor-initiated signal transductions
   (c) are heterodimers
   (d) have an intrinsic GTPase activity
   (e) can be activated in large numbers by a single activated membrane receptor

5. The β-adrenergic receptor is a member of which of the following receptor families?

   (a) G-protein coupled receptors (GPCR)
   (b) seven-transmembrane receptors (7TM)
   (c) serpentine receptors
   (d) all of the above
   (5) none of the above

6. Which nucleotides are bound to G proteins in their unactivated state and activated state, respectively? How does the 7TM activate a G protein? How is the activated state of a G protein returned to the unactivated form?

7. Which of the following statements about GTP and its role in the cAMP-mediated hormone response system are correct?

   (a) GTP is associated with the α subunit of a guanyl nucleotide–binding protein (G protein).
   (b) GTP reduces the magnitude of the hormone response because it is converted to cGMP—a compound that antagonizes the effects of cAMP.
   (c) GTP maintains the steady-state level of cAMP by rephosphorylating AMP to ATP in a nucleotide kinase-catalyzed reaction.
   (d) GTP activates G protein so that its G_α−GTP subunit interacts with adenylate cyclase.
   (e) GTP couples the stimulus from a hormone-receptor complex or an activated receptor to a system that produces an allosteric effector.
   (f) The effect of GTP on hormone response is antagonized by the GTPase activity of the G_α subunit of the G protein.
   (g) A single GTP-binding event with a stimulatory G protein leads to the formation of one cAMP molecule.

8. Which of the following are correct statements about G proteins and their functioning in cAMP-mediated hormonal systems?

   (a) G proteins bind hormones.
   (b) G proteins are integral membrane proteins.
   (c) G proteins are heterotrimers.
   (d) G proteins bind adenylate cyclase.
   (e) In their GDP form and in the absence of hormone, G proteins bind to hormone receptors and are converted to their GTP forms.
   (f) When G protein in the GDP form binds to a hormone-receptor complex, GTP exchanges with GDP.
   (g) The α subunit of G proteins is a GTPase.

9. If cells with β-adrenergic receptors are exposed for extended times to epinephrine, a hormone that causes activation of adenylate cyclase, the G protein fails to carry out efficiently the GDP–GTP exchange reaction and adenylate cyclase is no longer activated. What is the biological function of this phenomenon, and how does it occur?

10. Both cAMP and AMP contain one adenine base, one ribose, and one phosphorus atom. How are they different?

11. Which of the following statements about cAMP and its functioning in hormone action are correct?

    (a) Most effects of cAMP in eukaryotic cells are exerted through the activation of protein kinase A (PKA).

    (b) Cyclic AMP binds the catalytic subunits of PKA and activates the enzyme allosterically.

    (c) Cyclic AMP binds the regulatory subunits of PKA and activates the enzyme by releasing the catalytic subunits.

    (d) Cyclic AMP is bound by the activated hormone receptor and PKA simultaneously to convey the hormonal signal in order to activate the kinase.

12. Which of the following statements about cAMP and the second-messenger mechanism of hormone function are correct?

    (a) The hormonal stimulus leads to increased amounts of adenylate cyclase.

    (b) The formation of a hormone-receptor complex leads to the activation of adenylate cyclase.

    (c) Cyclic AMP acts as an allosteric modulator to affect the activities of specific protein kinases.

    (d) Cyclic AMP interacts with a hormone-receptor complex to dissociate the hormone.

    (e) The hormone-receptor complex enters the cell and affects the activities of target enzymes.

13. Why do you think the cells of one kind of tissue respond to a given hormone, whereas cells of another tissue may NOT do so?

14. Suppose a patient is suffering from a disorder in which adenylate cyclase is impaired and, as a result, cAMP levels are not readily increased by hormones. Explain why the infusion of cAMP probably will not remedy the problem.

15. Cholera toxin (choleragen)

    (a) inactivates a G protein by locking it in the off state (inactivates the GTPase).

    (b) A subunit enters the cell and ADP-ribosylates the $G_{\alpha S}$ subunit of a G protein.

    (c) B subunit interacts with a GM_1 ganglioside on the target-cell surface.

    (d) causes the activation of protein kinase A, which opens a membrane channel and inhibits a Na^+–H^+ exchanger.

    (e) causes the retention of Cl^- in the cell.

Some Receptors Dimerize in Response to Ligand Binding and Recruit Tyrosine Kinases

16. Which of the following statements about the phosphoinositide cascade are correct?

    (a) The phosphoinositide cascade depends on the hydrolysis of a phospholipid component of the plasma membrane.

    (b) A polypeptide hormone interacts with a G_{M1} ganglioside on the cell surface to trigger the phosphoinositide cascade.

    (c) In some cases, a G-protein system acts to transduce the stimulus from the receptor to the phosphoinositidase.

    (d) At least four kinds of phospholipase C play a crucial role in the phosphoinositide cascade.

    (e) The phosphoinositide cascade directly produces a unique second-messenger molecule.

17. Which of the following are the second messengers that are produced by the phosphoinositide cascade?

    (a) phosphatidyl inositol 4,5-bisphosphate (PIP_2)
    (b) inositol 1,4,5-trisphosphate (IP_3)
    (c) inositol 4-phosphate
    (d) inositol 1,3,4,5-tetrakisphosphate
    (e) inositol 1,3,4-trisphosphate
    (f) diacylglycerol (DAG)

18. Which of the following statements about inositol 1,4,5-trisphosphate (IP_3) are correct?

    (a) IP_3 leads to the uptake of Ca^{2+} by the endoplasmic reticulum and the sarcoplasmic reticulum.
    (b) IP_3 may be rapidly inactivated by either a phosphatase or a kinase.
    (c) IP_3 opens calcium ion channels in the membranes of the endoplasmic reticulum and the sarcoplasmic reticulum.
    (d) IP_3 reacts with CTP to form CDP-inositol phosphate, a precursor of PIP_2.
    (e) IP_3 acts by altering the intracellular-to-extracellular Na^+-to-K^+ ratio, thereby altering the transmembrane potential.

19. Which of the following statements about the actions or targets of the second messengers of the phosphoinositide cascade are correct?

    (a) Diacylglycerol (DAG) activates protein kinase C (PKC).
    (b) Most of the effects of IP_3 and DAG are antagonistic.
    (c) DAG increases the affinity of PKC for Ca^{2+}.
    (d) PKC requires Ca^{2+} for its activity.

20. Which of the following statements about the tyrosine kinases or hormones that affect them are correct?

    (a) Epidermal growth factor (EGF) stimulates epidermal and epithelial cells to divide.
    (b) EGF is a protein kinase that phosphorylates tyrosine residues.
    (c) EGF and insulin share the common mechanism of dimerization for signal transduction across the plasma membrane.
    (d) Receptors for EGF and insulin are integral membrane proteins.
    (e) Some oncogenes encode tyrosine kinases.
    (f) Specialized adaptor proteins link the phosphorylation of the EGF receptor to the stimulation of cell growth.

Metabolism in Context: Insulin Signaling Regulates Metabolism

21. Which of the following statements about the protein kinase domain of the insulin receptor are true?

    (a) It is a tyrosine kinase.
    (b) The kinase domain is inactive when covalently modified.
    (c) The protein kinase domain is a dual-specificity kinase in that is it phosphorylates Ser, Thr, and Tyr.
    (d) An activation loop is responsible for inactivation of the kinase domain in the IR.
    (e) The kinase recognizes the sequence Tyr-X-X-Met in substrates.

22. Place the following events in the insulin signal transduction domain in order of occurrence.

    (a) activation of Akt
    (b) phosphorylation of IRS
    (c) dimerization of the insulin receptor
    (d) binding of IRS to the insulin receptor
    (e) phosphorylation of the insulin receptor

(f) binding of IRS to Phosphatidyl-inositol-3 kinase

(g) activation of PDK1

23. Which of the following answers complete the sentence correctly? Receptor tyrosine kinases

(a) are seven-transmembrane-helix receptors.

(b) are integral membrane enzymes.

(c) activate their targets via the G-protein cascade.

(d) are often activated by ligand-induced dimerization.

(e) can phosphorylate themselves on their cytoplasmic domains when activated.

(f) that have been activated by hormone binding are recognized by target proteins having SH2 (src protein homology region 2) sequences.

(g) are so named because they contain extraordinarily high amounts of tyrosine.

Calcium is a Ubiquitous Cytoplasmic Messenger

24. Which of the following statements about Ca^{2+} and its roles in the regulation of cellular metabolism are correct?

(a) The solubility product of calcium phosphate is small; therefore, low Ca^{2+} levels must be maintained in the cell to avoid its precipitation.

(b) Intracellular Ca^{2+} is maintained at concentrations that are several orders of magnitude smaller than the extracellular concentration by ATP-dependent Ca^{2+} pumps.

(c) The transient opening of ion channels in the plasma membrane or endoplasmic reticulum can rapidly raise cytosolic Ca^{2+} levels.

(d) The binding of Ca^{2+} by a protein can induce a large conformational change because the ion simultaneously coordinates to several anionic groups within the protein.

(e) Ca^{2+} is bound by a family of regulatory proteins that have a characteristic EF hand, helix-loop-helix structure.

(f) When calmodulin binds Ca^{2+} at its low-affinity site, it undergoes a conformational change that allows the complex to interact with target proteins.

25. Explain how a Ca^{2+} ionophore could mimic the effects of a hormone.

26. If it were incubated with cells *in vitro*, why would EGTA prevent either a Ca^{2+}-triggering hormone or a Ca^{2+} ionophore from acting?

27. Which of the following answers complete the sentence correctly? Calmodulin

(a) is a member of the EF hand family of calcium-binding proteins.

(b) activates target molecules by recognizing negatively charged β sheets.

(c) serves as a calcium sensor in most eukaryotic cells.

(d) is activated when intracellular Ca^{2+} concentrations rise above 0.5 μM.

(e) activates CAM kinase II, which then phosphorylates many different proteins.

(f) undergoes a large conformational change on binding Ca^{2+} ions.

28. Match each compound in the left column with its characteristic in the right column.

(a) cyclic AMP	(1)	is cleaved by phospholipase C
(b) GTP	(2)	binds the regulatory subunits of specific protein kinases
(c) G proteins		
(d) adenylate cyclase	(3)	exchanges with GDP on G_α subunits
(e) PIP_2	(4)	is a downstream hormone product of PIP_2 catabolism
(f) Ca^{2+}		
(g) IP_3	(5)	binds epinephrine

(h) DAG
(i) insulin receptor
(j) Ras
(k) β-Adrenergic receptor
(l) arachidonic acid

(6) is a second messenger arising from PIP_2
(7) is a small G protein GTPase
(8) transduces hormone stimulus from an activated 7TM membrane receptor to adenylate cyclase
(9) has inducible tyrosine kinase activity.
(10) is activated by G_α-GTP
(11) has its intracellular concentration increased by IP_3
(12) activates protein kinase C

Defects in Signaling Pathways Can Lead to Diseases

29. Which of the following answers complete the sentence correctly? A mammalian protein, src,
    (a) has a viral counterpart, v-src, that is oncogenic.
    (b) is a proto-oncogene.
    (c) is a component of a signaling pathway for cell growth and differentiation.
    (d) can be converted to an oncogene by the alteration of some of its C-terminal amino acids.
    (e) is a protein tyrosine kinase.

30. Which of the following statements about hormones in mammals are correct?
    (a) Hormones are enzymes.
    (b) Hormones are synthesized in specific tissues.
    (c) Hormones are secreted into the blood.
    (d) Hormones alter one or more activities in the cells to which they are targeted.
    (e) Hormones display specificity toward the tissues with which they interact.

    (f) Hormones are involved in biochemical amplification systems.

ANSWERS TO SELF-TEST

1. a, b, c, d
2. (a) 4   (b) 3   (c) 1   (d) 2
3. A signal, in the form of a molecule or a photon interacts with a part of a 7TM on the outside surface of the cell. This interaction causes a conformational change in the protein that is transmitted to the inside of the cell.
4. b, d, e. G proteins are heterotrimers and alternate between states in which GTP or GDP is bound.
5. d.
6. GDP is bound to G proteins when they are inactive and GTP when they are activated. The 7TM receptor, when activated by binding its cognate signaling molecule outside the cell, catalyzes the exchange on a G protein of GDP by GTP inside the cell to activate the G protein. An intrinsic GTPase of the G protein converts GTP to GDP to cause inactivation.
7. a, d, e, f. Answer (g) is incorrect because the GTP form of the G protein activates adenylate cyclase and it forms many cAMP molecules; that is, an amplification occurs.

8. c, d, f, g. Answers (a) and (b) are incorrect because G proteins are peripheral membrane proteins inside cells. They do bind not the hormone but rather the activated hormone-receptor complex, and they carry the signal to adenylate cyclase. Answer (e) is incorrect because the hormone receptor must have the hormone bound to it or it must have been activated by hormone binding before the G protein will bind.

9. The phenomenon is called *desensitization* or *adaptation*. It allows the system to adapt to a given level of hormone so that it can respond to changes in hormone concentrations rather than to absolute amounts. Desensitization is effected by phosphorylation by β-adrenergic receptor kinase at multiple seine and threonine sites on the carboxyl-terminal region of the β-adrenergic receptor when it has epinephrine bound to it. These covalent modifications of the hormone-receptor complex allow β-arrestin to bind it and further inhibit but not completely prevent the GDP–GTP exchange. These events thereby decrease the activation of adenylate cyclase. However, the desensitized receptor can still respond to an increase in epinephrine concentrations. Ultimately, a phosphatase reverses the effects of the modification and resensitizes the receptor.

10. AMP has a single phosphomonoester attached to the 5′-hydroxyl of the adenosine moiety. cAMP has its single phosphate group attached to both the 5′ and 3′ hydroxyls of its adenosine to form a phosphodiester bond.

11. a, c

12. b, c. Answer (a) is incorrect because the hormone leads to an increase in the activity of adenylate cyclase, not an increase in the amount of the enzyme. Answer (e) is incorrect because the hormone need not enter the cell to carry out its action.

13. The simplest explanation for the tissue specificity of hormones is the presence or absence of receptors for particular hormones on the extracellular surfaces of the tissues. Whether or not a given cell type has a given hormone receptor depends upon which genes have been expressed within it.

14. Aside from the likelihood that serum phosphodiesterases might destroy it, cAMP is a polar molecule that does not readily traverse the plasma membrane. Even if a more hydrophobic derivative, such as dibutyryl-cAMP, were used to overcome the permeability problem, there would be no tissue specificity, and all cells would have increased cAMP levels, leading to a massive, nonspecific response.

15. b, c, d. Choleragen stabilizes the GTP form of the G protein to keep it in the activated state, resulting in a loss of Cl^- and H_2O from the cell.

16. a, c, d. Answer (e) is incorrect because two messengers are formed.

17. b, f. Answer (a) is incorrect because PIP_2 is the precursor of the second messengers. The other incorrect choices are all downstream products of IP_3 metabolism.

18. b, c. Answer (a) is incorrect because IP_3 causes the release, not the uptake, of Ca^{2+}. Answer (b) is correct because not only does a phosphatase act on IP_3 but a specific kinase phosphorylates it to form the inactive tetrakisphosphate derivative. Answer (d) is incorrect because free inositol reacts with CDP-diacylglycerol to form phosphatidyl inositol, which is then phosphorylated to form PIP_2.

19. a, c, d. Answer (b) is incorrect because most of the effects of IP_3 and Ca^{2+} are synergistic, not antagonistic.

20. a, d, e, f. Answer (b) is incorrect because the hormone itself does not have tyrosine kinase activity; only the activated receptor is an active tyrosine kinase. Answer (c) is incorrect because the insulin receptor exists as a dimer and merely requires binding insulin to activate its intrinsic tyrosine kinase activity.

21. The correct order is c, e, d, b, f, g, a.

22. a, c, d, e, f. Answer (b) is incorrect because activated calmodulin recognizes complementary positively charged amphipathic α helices on target proteins. Complementary hydrophobic interactions also contribute to the recognition.

23. b, d, e, f. Answer (g) is incorrect because the name arises from the amino acid that they phosphorylate in their target proteins.

24. a, b, c, d, e, f

25. The ionophore allows Ca^{2+} to enter cells by rendering the membrane permeable to the ion. Since the extracellular Ca^{2+} concentration is higher than the intracellular concentration, the ion enters the cell and the cytosolic level increases. Because some hormones act to raise intracellular Ca^{2+} levels to carry out their physiological roles, the ionophore could lead to the same response.

26. EGTA is a specific Ca^{2+} chelator. It would bind tightly to the ion and markedly lower Ca^{2+} concentration in the extracellular medium. Consequently, when a hormone or a Ca^{2+} ionophore acted to allow Ca^{2+} influx, none could occur because the concentration gradient of Ca^{2+} would be insufficient.

27. a, d, e. Phosphorylation (covalent modification) of the activation loop leads to activation of the receptor kinase. So b is incorrect and d is correct. The specificity is for Tyr residues so a is correct and c is incorrect.

28. (a) 2 (b) 3 (c) 8 (d) 10 (e) 1 (f) 11 (g) 6 (h) 12 (i) 9 (j) 7 (k) 5 (l) 4

29. a, b, c, d, e

30. b, c, d, e, f

PROBLEMS

1. Based on the material so far covered in the text and your general understanding of regulation and signal transduction, list properties that a substance should have for it to be classified as a hormone.

2. Bee venom is particularly rich in phospholipase A_2, an enzyme that hydrolytically removes the fatty acyl residue at position 2 of phospholipids. The action of phospholipase A_2 on phosphatidyl choline is shown in Figure 13.1. One of the mediators of the inflammatory response following a bee sting (swelling, redness, pain, heat, and loss of function) is lysophosphatidyl choline, the remainder of the phospholipid following the hydrolysis of the fatty acyl residue at position 2. Lysophosphatidyl choline stimulates mast cells to release histamine, which triggers the inflammatory response.

FIGURE 13.1 Action of phospholipase A2 on phosphatidyl choline.

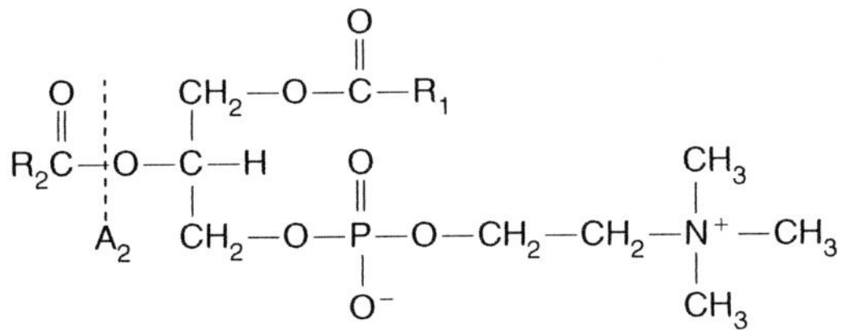

(a) Explain the major point of similarity between the system described here and one (phospholipase C hydrolysis of PIP_2) described in Section 13.1 in the text.

(b) Suppose that the hydrolysis product of phosphatidyl choline that is important as a mediator of the inflammatory response were unknown. Suggest an experiment that might help establish the identity of the active agent.

3. Suppose that epinephrine stimulates the conversion of compound A to compound B in liver cells by means of a regulatory cascade involving a G protein, cAMP, protein kinase A, and enzymes E_1 and E_2, as shown in Figure 13.2. Assume that each catalytically active enzyme subunit in the regulatory cascade has a turnover number of 1000 s^{-1}. Assume further that 10 G-GTP are formed for each molecule of epinephrine bound to receptor. Calculate the theoretical number of molecules of A that would be converted to molecules of B per second as a result of the interaction of one molecule of epinephrine with its receptor on a liver cell membrane.

FIGURE 13.2   Hypothetical regulatory cascade for problem 3.

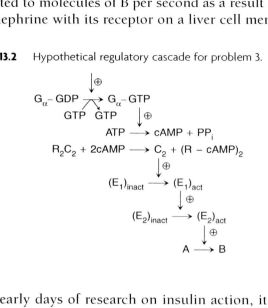

4. In the early days of research on insulin action, it was not known whether insulin might enter cells and directly mediate intracellular effects or whether it might act through a second messenger. In a classic experiment, Pedro Cuatrecasas attached insulin covalently to Sepharose beads many times the size of fat cells and showed that the addition of the insulin-Sepharose complexes to isolated fat cells gave the same stimulation of glucose oxidation as did addition of insulin alone.

   (a)   What conclusion might follow from this experiment? Explain.
   (b)   What assumptions have you made about the effects of adding sepharose without attached insulin to fat cells and about the attachment of the insulin to the Sepharose bead?

5. In kinetic studies on the interaction of human growth hormone with its receptor, each functional receptor dimer was found to bind one hormone molecule, and the monomer receptors needed to dimerize in order to transduce the signal from the hormone. Explain how this occurs.

6. To be effective, intracellular signals must be readily inactivated when their effects are no longer needed. Give a method of inactivation for each of the following classes of intracellular messengers;

   (a)   G proteins   (d)   calcium ion
   (b)   cyclic nucleotides   (e)   inositol 1,4,5-trisphosphate (IP_3)
   (c)   phosphoproteins   (f)   diacylglycerol

7. A tissue is known to increase cyclic AMP production on stimulation by a certain hormone. Addition of an analog of GTP in which the terminal phosphate group is replaced by a sulfate to a homogenate of the tissue results in sustained production of cyclic AMP. Propose an explanation for this observation.

8. What properties of Ca^{2+} render it so useful as a messenger in cells? What protein is often used in cells to "sense" Ca^{2+}? How does the cell overcome the problem of the low-solubility product of Ca^{2+} with P_i, phosphorylated compounds, and carboxyl groups?

9. What signal-transduction functions do SH2 domains in proteins serve?

10. After the insulin–insulin-receptor complex autophosphorylates itself, a series of down-stream events carries the signal to molecules directly involved in promoting, among other things, the entry of glucose into muscle and adipose cells. Insulin thus promotes a lowering of the blood glucose (hypoglycemia). When both copies of the gene (*Akt2*) for a particular serine–threonine kinase (a protein kinase B isoform) were ablated in a strain of mice, the "knockout" mice could no longer lower their blood glucose by taking it into muscle cells upon administration of insulin. (Isoenzymes are sometimes called isoforms.) What conclusions can you draw about the role of the Akt2 isoform of protein kinase B in glucose homeostasis? Can you think of alternative explanations for the observation with the knockout mice?

11. List three characteristics of many signaling pathways and give an example of each.

ANSWERS TO PROBLEMS

1. The major criteria for classifying a substance as a hormone are:
   (1) In order to carry messages from one tissue to another, it should be produced by one type of cell and have effects on another type of cell.
   (2) Its effects should involve the chemical amplification of the original signal.
   (3) It should be produced in response to a stimulus, and its production should cease upon cessation of the stimulus.
   (4) It should be selectively destroyed following cessation of the stimulus.
   (5) The addition of the purified substance to tissues should mimic physiologic responses produced in vivo.
   (6) Specific inhibitors of the physiologic response should also abolish the response elicited by the addition of the purified substance to tissues.
   (7) Specific receptors for the hormone should exist and should be more abundant in tissues that are more sensitive to the hormone.

2. (a) The bee venom system resembles the phosphoinositide cascade discussed in section 13.2 of the text. In that system, a membrane phospholipid is also converted into an active mediator of the response of several hormones.

   (b) One could inject each of the hydrolysis products—lysophosphatidyl choline and the fatty acid—into tissues separately to see which might elicit the inflammatory response.

3. The theoretical number of molecules of A converted to B per second would be 10^{13}. One molecule of epinephrine would result in the production of 10 G-GTP. Each activated α subunit would stimulate adenylate cyclase to produce 1000 cAMP molecules for a total of 10,000 molecules of cAMP. Each of these cAMP molecules would activate one catalytic subunit of protein kinase. (Remember that a molecule of protein kinase exists as an R_2C_2 complex. Two cAMP molecules combine with two R subunits to give two catalytically active C subunits.) Each of the 10,000 active C subunits would result in the production of 1000 molecules of active E_1 for a total of 10^7 molecules of active E_1. Each molecule of active E_1 would in turn activate 1000 molecules of E_2 for

a total of 10^{10} molecules of active E_2. Since each molecule of active E_2 would convert 1000 molecules of A to B per second, the total would be $1000 \times 10^{10} = 10^{13}$ per second. (*Note:* This is a greatly oversimplified example, but it illustrates the profound chemical amplification that can occur in systems under hormonal control.)

4. (a) A reasonable conclusion is that insulin need not enter the cell to have an effect. The results are consistent with the notion that insulin affects cells by combining with a membrane receptor site outside the cell thereby causing some second messenger to be formed within the cell that mediates the effects. Note that the experiment does not prove that insulin fails to enter cells.

   (b) You probably assumed that the addition of Sepharose alone gave no stimulation of glucose oxidation. You also have to assume that the covalent attachment of the insulin to the Sepharose is stable so that free insulin is not formed during the course of the experiment.

5. A given molecule of growth hormone contains two domains, each of which binds a receptor monomer. Thus, a single molecule of growth hormone could be bound by two receptors, bringing them together to form the activated hormone-receptor dimer complex.

6. (a) G proteins are active while GTP is bound, but they become inactive as GTP is hydrolyzed to GDP and phosphate.

   (b) Cyclic nucleotides are converted by phosphodiesterases to 5'-mononucleotides.

   (c) Phosphates are cleaved from phosphoproteins by protein phosphatases.

   (d) Calcium ions are pumped from the cell interior into the extracellular fluid or intracellular storage organelles, for example, the endoplasmic reticulum.

   (e) Inositol 1,4,5-trisphosphate can be degraded to inositol and inorganic phosphate by the sequential action of phosphatases or it can be phosphorylated by a kinase to form inositol 1,3,4,5-tetrakisphosphate.

   (f) Diacylglycerol may be converted to phosphatidate or hydrolyzed to glycerol and fatty acids.

7. The observation could be explained if the sulfate-containing analog of GTP bound to G protein, stimulating cyclic AMP production, could not be hydrolyzed to GDP and sulfate by the GTPase activity of G. Thus the production of cyclic AMP would persist.

8. Energy-requiring molecular pumps maintain a steep concentration gradient of Ca^{2+} across the plasma membrane between the outside and inside of the cell and across the membrane between intracellular organelles and the cytoplasm. When the membrane, for instance, is rendered permeable to Ca^{2+} as a result of the opening of a Ca^{2+} channel, a flux of ions passes through the membrane raising the cytoplasmic Ca^{2+} concentration. Such a sudden increase in Ca^{2+} can act as a signal to Ca^{2+}-sensing proteins within the cell. Calmodulin binds Ca^{2+} and interacts with several proteins and enzymes as a consequence of the binding. Because Ca^{2+} can interact simultaneously with several anionic amino acid side chains, the carbonyls of the peptide backbone, or the carbonyls of Gln and Asn, it can cause large conformational changes in the protein to which it binds. Conformational changes in response to binding a ligand are the hallmarks of a molecular switch. Thus, the ability to rapidly change its concentration and to effect large conformational changes renders Ca^{2+} an effective intracellular messenger. The cell avoids precipitating the Ca^{2+} salts of its intracellular components by maintaining the Ca^{2+} concentration below the solubility product for various compounds. Endergonic pumps and exchangers maintain the low intracellular Ca^{2+} concentrations.

9. SH2 domains bind to peptides or sections of proteins that contain phosphotyrosine residues in particular sequence contexts. The formation of phosphorylated tyrosine residues in a receptor often results from hormone activation of the receptor. The phosphorylated tyrosine-containing peptides in the receptor can be recognized and bound by other proteins that have SH2 domains. The SH2 domain allows different proteins to respond to and be affected by the phosphorylated tyrosines that arise in proteins as a result of a signal transduction event.

10. The simplest interpretation of the observation is that this particular protein kinase B isoform is directly involved in mediating the ability of insulin to lower blood glucose concentrations by facilitating its entry into muscle cells. The kinase presumably acts by phosphorylating a target molecule that, in turn, facilitates the movement of a glucose transporter (GLUT4) to the surface of the cell. An alternative explanation could be that the lack of the Akt2 kinase during the growth of the knockout mouse led to the failure to synthesize a molecule that was, itself, the active component in the insulin-signaling pathway. The mutation-induced lack of the protein in some other tissue could also have caused the effect if that tissue normally supplied a compound needed in the muscle cells for the insulin response. For instance, adipose tissue is known to affect glucose uptake by muscle cells. The gene deletion could have affected the ability of adipose tissue to make that compound. Further experiments would be required to verify the simplest conclusion. (This problem is based on H. Cho, J. Mu, J. K. Kim, J. L. Thorvaldsen *et al.* Insulin resistance and a diabetes mellitus-like syndrome in mice lacking the protein kinase Akt2 (PKBβ). *Science* 292[2001]:1728–1731.)

11. The text lists three common themes in signal transduction. The first is that protein kinases are central to many pathways. The kinases can be either part of receptors or cytoplasmic. Although not discussed in the text, kinases with a specificity for serine and threonine phosphyorylation are actually more common than tyrosine kinases. All three signal-transduction pathways discussed in the text contain protein kinases, either as tyrosine-kinase receptors (IR, EGFR) or as cytoplasmic kinases (PKA, Raf, MEK, ERK). The second theme is that second messengers participate in many signal-transduction pathways. The text discusses several, including cAMP, Ca^{2+}, IP_3, and DAG. These messengers are mobile so they can move between signaling components and can be either soluble (cAMP, Ca^{2+}, and IP_3) or membrane-associated (DAG). The last theme is that specialized domains that mediate specific interactions are present in many signaling proteins. Protein-protein interactions lie at the heart of cellular signaling. These are mediated in large part through protein domains which repeat in a large number of signaling components and may even be present in multiple copies within a particular protein. Some examples given in the text are SH2 and SH3 domains, which bind phosphotryosines and polyprolines respectively and PH which interact with the lipid PIP_3.

Chapter 14

Digestion: Turning a Meal into Cellular Biochemicals

Just as the process of digestion prepares food for metabolism, this chapter on digestion provides preparation for the chapters on metabolism of food molecules. Macroscopic food items (the chapter uses the example of a pizza) must be ground up, moistened, and the large molecules of starch and protein must be broken down by enzymes into smaller units—the sugars and amino acids. The authors point out that the process (in humans) begins in the mouth with chewing and salivary enzymes. Then further chemical breakdown occurs with acid and enzymes in the stomach, followed by more intense enzyme digestion in the small intestine with the aid of the pancreas and the gall bladder. The pancreas is protected from its own enzymes because they are produced as inactive zymogens, which must be cleaved by digestive enzymes to become active. α-Amylase in the saliva starts the breakdown of starch and glycogen. Fats and oils are lipids that require some special treatment because they are not very water soluble. The authors describe the digestion process in poisonous snakes, which inject digestive enzymes as part of their venom, and then swallow the prey whole. Finally the chapter is linked to the previous chapter with a description of a cell signaling circuit involving G proteins to connect the hormone CCK to release of zymogens from the pancreas.

LEARNING OBJECTIVES

When you have mastered this chapter, you should be able to accomplish the following objectives:

Digestion Prepares Large Biomolecules for Use in Metabolism (Text Section 14.1)

1. Describe the three stages of catabolism.
2. Understand how the stomach prepares proteins for degradation.

Proteases Digest Proteins into Amino Acids and Peptides (Text Section 14.2)

3. List the enzymes and other substances released by the pancreas during digestion.
4. Explain the concept of *zymogen activation*.

Dietary Carbohydrates Are Digested by α-Amylase (Text Section 14.3)

5. Diagram the digestion of starch by *α-amylase*.
6. Define the term *limit dextrin*.
7. Outline the digestion of common *disaccharides*.

The Digestion of Lipids Is Complicated by Their Hydrophobicity (Text Section 14.4)

8. Understand how forming an *emulsion* aids in digestion of fats.
9. Describe the reaction catalyzed by *lipase* enzymes.
10. Define *micelle*, *steatorrhea*, and *chylomicrons*.

Metabolism in Context: Cell Signaling Facilitates Caloric Homeostasis (Text Section 14.5)

11. Compare signaling by the hormone *cholecystokinin* (CCK) and glucagon-like peptide 1 (GLP-1) to signaling by epinephrine (described in the previous chapter).

SELF-TEST

Digestion Prepares Large Biomolecules for Use in Metabolism

1. Which stage of metabolism produces the most ATP? Which stage produces no ATP at all?
2. What does the stomach do, specifically, to start breaking down proteins?
3. Digestion begins in the mouth. Explain how this is true? Is it also true for snakes, which eat their prey whole?

Proteases Digest Proteins into Amino Acids and Peptides

4. During digestion, intestinal cells release the hormones secretin and CCK. Specifically what effect does each hormone have?

5. Which of the following would not be an active enzyme?

   A. Trypsin
   B. Pepsinogen
   C. Chymotrypsin
   D. Elastase
   E. Lipase

6. What job does enteropeptidase do?

Dietary Carbohydrates Are Digested by α-Amylase

7. Which of the following is not a disaccharide?

   A. lactase
   B. maltose
   C. sucrose
   D. maltotriose
   E. lactose

8. What sort of sugar linkages can α-Amylase break down? What is an example of a bond that it cannot hydrolyze?

The Digestion of Lipids Is Complicated by Their Hydrophobicity

9. Which would be the most water soluble: triacylglycerol, diacylglycerol, or monoacylglycerol?

10. What does it mean that glycocholate and other molecules are amphipathic? What structural features make it amphipathic?

11. Define chylomicrons and tell how they are used.

12. Roughly how many proteins and peptides are present in a typical snake venom? What sort of enzymes are found in venom?

Metabolism in Context: Cell Signaling Facilitates Caloric Homeostasis

13. What specific effects do CCK and GLP-1 produce in the body? Would they make you feel hungry or full?

ANSWERS TO SELF-TEST

1. The diagram in Figure 14.1 (originated by Sir Hans Krebs) shows that Stage 1 of catabolism—the digestive stage—yields no useable ATP energy. And most of the processes in Stage 1 occur outside the cells, so it would be hard to trap any energy that might be released. Stage 3 has the highest ATP yield.

2. The stomach has a very low pH due to a high concentration of HCl, hydrochloric acid. Some protein breakdown occurs simply because of the acidic environment, but the stomach also releases the enzyme pepsin, which efficiently breaks down peptide bonds in proteins despite the ambient pH of 1 or 2. The peptides produced by the initial breakdown in the stomach stimulate the release of secretin and CCK by the small intestine.

3. Chewing provides a mechanical breakdown of food components, which are also mixed with saliva to make a wet slurry which is easier for enzymes to attack. And saliva contains amylase which begins the digestion of starch. If we swallowed a whole chunk of meat or potato, the enzymes would have to start working on the surface, and further digestion would be quite slow. For snakes, it is true in a way, because

while the prey is not contained in the snake's mouth, the venom for digestion comes from the snake's mouth, injected via the fangs.

4. Secretin stimulates the pancreas to release enough sodium bicarbonate ($NaHCO_3$) to neutralize the stomach acid that arrives in the small intestine with the food from the stomach. As shown in the chapter, CCK stimulates the release of various zymogens from the pancreas, and these are then activated to become the most important enzymes for protein digestion—trypsin, chymotrypsin, elastase, and carboxypeptidase.

5. B. Pepsinogen. The -ogen ending tells us that this is a zymogen, and zymogens are inactive.

6. Zymogens are proteins, and they must be cut in order to be activated. And when they are activated, they are protease enzymes, which means that they cut other proteins. So there is a sort of cascade of protease enzymes cutting zymogens which become protease enzymes and cut other zymogens. See Figure 14.4. Enteropeptidase is at the very top of this cascade, and its job is to cut trypsinogen forming trypsin, which then cuts several other zymogens as well as food proteins.

7. There are two answers, A and D. Lactase is an enzyme and therefore a protein and not a sugar at all. Maltotriose is a sugar, but a trisaccharide and not a disaccharide.

8. α-Amylase can only cut α-1,4 linkages between glucose molecules. Thus there are many linkages that it cannot cut. The one mentioned in the chapter is α-1,6, which occurs in glycogen. Another example of a bond it can't cut would be β-1,4.

9. See Figure 14.8, which shows the actions of pancreatic lipase enzymes. The fewer fatty acids, the more soluble a molecule will be, so the monoacylglycerol will be the most water soluble.

10. Amphipathic molecules have both a hydrophobic part and a hydrophilic part. Soaps and detergents are good examples of this. In glycocholate (Figure 14.7) the most hydrophilic part would be the carboxylate anion, but the hydroxyls also contribute to water solubility. The hydrophobic part would be the steroid ring system.

11. To understand chylomicrons, it is best to take a peek at a much later chapter in the book. The lipid chapter, Chapter 29, has a table of "plasma lipoproteins" (Table 29.1) and a picture of a lipoprotein (Figure 29.14). Lipids are light and proteins are heavy, so the larger lipoproteins, with the most lipid in the center and less protein in proportion, have the lowest density. Small lipoproteins have proportionately more protein in their outer "shell" and are much denser. Chylomicrons are simply the largest and lowest density lipoproteins. They are also the first lipoproteins formed, arising from the digestive processes and carrying lipids through the lymph and blood. Lipids need to be "carried" by external proteins because they will not dissolve and can't travel through water based systems on their own.

12. The chapter states that snake venoms contain "50 to 60" different proteins and peptides. The enzymes are very effective at destroying tissues, and include phospholipases, collagenase, hyaluronidase, and a variety of proteases. In some cases the venom includes both enzymes that produce blood clots and enzymes that break down blood clots.

13. See Figure 14.12. CCK and GLP-1 would make you feel full—that is what "satiety" means. So you eat less and your weight goes down. Also, insulin and β-cells increase.

PROBLEMS

1. Living cells contain many different proteins which do important jobs to keep the cells alive. What would happen if pancreatic cells synthesized a digestive enzyme like Trypsin right in their own cytoplasm? How does the use of zymogens solve this problem?

2. Some "health food stores" sell expensive enzyme pills. Most enzymes are proteins. Looking at the diagram showing the digestion and absorption of proteins, does it make sense to buy enzyme pills? Can your body tell ingested enzymes from ingested hamburgers?

3. The text gives an explanation of emulsions, which are enhanced by amphipathic molecules like bile salts. Other amphipathic molecules are used in everyday life as cleaning agents. Can you suggest a couple, and describe how the formation of emulsions helps with the cleaning process?

4. In Figure 14.1 of the textbook we see that stage 3 of catabolism requires oxygen. What can we deduce about metabolism in obligate anaerobes? Many prokaryotes (Eubacteria and Archaea) are anaerobic.

SOLUTIONS TO PROBLEMS

1. A protease enzyme like trypsin or chymotrypsin would be a real "bull in a china shop" if released in the cytoplasm. Many vital cellular proteins would be destroyed and the cell would probably die as a result. Obviously this cannot be allowed to happen. So one line of defense is to make the enzyme as an inactive zymogen, that is, trypsinogen. A second line of defense is that even the zymogen is not made in the cytoplasm but rather, during protein synthesis, the zymogen is extruded through a membrane so it never exists in the cytoplasmic compartment. There are forms of pancreatitis caused by digestive proteases backing up in the pancreatic duct and damaging the tissues there.

2. If ingested proteins routinely showed up in the blood, there would be large problems because they would trigger allergies and antibodies would form to attack any nonhuman proteins. So no, your digestive processes do not really distinguish between hamburger and expensive enzyme tablets, and both are chopped up into peptides and amino acids before being absorbed into the blood. Hamburger is much cheaper. Note that some enzymes are not intended to be absorbed; for example, lactase is sold in tablets which can either be put into milk or eaten by those with lactose intolerance. This enzyme is intended to work during digestion, in the glass or in the stomach, and it does not matter that it is subsequently broken down and digested.

3. Soaps and detergents are amphipathic molecules used in cleaning. Whether you want to get a film of butter off a plate, or a smear of grease off your hands, you need a molecule that has a hydrophobic moiety that will "attach" itself to the grease, and a second moiety that will "pull" the grease into aqueous solution. Look at Figure 11.1 in the lipid chapter, which shows ionized fatty acids. If you write Na^+ next to one and K^+ next to the other, then you are showing them as sodium and potassium salts, and those would be examples of soaps. Soaps take hand grease or food grease and emulsify it so that water can wash it away.

4. Anaerobic organisms cannot perform "stage 3" of catabolism as shown in Figure 14.1. As a result, they obtain much less energy from each molecule of glucose ingested or synthesized. They utilize fuel very inefficiently compared to aerobic organisms. One molecule of glucose metabolized anaerobically yields only 2 ATP, whereas aerobic catabolism of glucose yields about 30 ATP. Obviously this disadvantage doesn't slow down the "germs"—they simply eat more food to stay alive.

Chapter 15

Metabolism: Basic Concepts and Design

This chapter is an introduction to the next two parts of the text, which are devoted to metabolism. Metabolism is the interconnected, integrated ensemble of chemical reactions cells use to extract energy and reducing power from their environments, synthesize the building blocks of their macromolecules, and carry out all the other processes that are required to sustain life. Basic thermodynamic postulates were presented in Chapter 6 and should now be reviewed for a better understanding of the principles of metabolism presented in this chapter. Because energy is an essential concept in understanding metabolism, the authors begin this chapter with a review of free-energy changes in the context of a description of coupled reactions. They explain how an energetically unfavorable reaction can occur if it is coupled to one that occurs spontaneously. The most important molecules for storing and carrying energy in metabolic processes, including ATP, the universal currency of energy in biological systems, are described next. The role of creatine phosphate, the specialized energy storage molecule of vertebrate muscle, is also given.

The authors present a broad outline of energy metabolism. The energy for ATP synthesis comes from the oxidation of carbon compounds, and the pathways that perform these oxidations can be classified into three stages. All living cells draw on a spectrum of a few activated carriers to help run these reactions, including the electron carriers NAD^+ and FAD, plus CoA, thiamine, biotin, and several others. Most metabolic reactions fall into a handful of predictable types of reactions. The student would do well to pay particular attention to this discussion because these reactions form a major part of the subsequent part of the text, and learning them now can save time and energy later. The chapter concludes with a cogent discussion of regulation of metabolic pathways, followed by speculation about the origin of nucleotide-containing cofactors.

LEARNING OBJECTIVES

When you have mastered this chapter, you should be able to accomplish the following objectives.

Metabolism Is Composed of Many Interconnecting Reactions (Text Section 15.1)

1. Define *metabolism*.

2. Define *catabolism* and *anabolism*.

3. State the significance of the *free-energy change* (ΔG) of reactions and the relationship of ΔG to $\Delta G^{o\prime}$, the *equilibrium constant*, and the *concentrations of reactants* and *products* of the reaction.

4. Describe the *additivity* of ΔG values for *coupled reactions* and explain the ability of a thermodynamically favorable (exergonic) reaction to drive an energetically unfavorable (endergonic) one.

ATP Is the Universal Currency of Free Energy (Text Section 15.2)

5. Give the structure of *adenosine triphosphate*. Describe the role of ATP as the major energy-coupling agent (*energy currency*) in metabolism.

6. Explain how coupling a reaction with the hydrolysis of ATP can change the equilibrium ratio of the concentrations of the products to the concentrations of the reactants by a factor of 10^8. Know the ΔG for ATP hydrolysis under typical celllular conditions.

7. Describe the structural and electronic bases for the *high-phosphoryl group-transfer potential* of ATP, and give the free energy liberated by the hydrolysis of ATP under standard and cellular conditions.

8. Recognize that compounds that have a *high group-transfer potential*, that is, compounds that release large amounts of free energy on hydrolysis or oxidation.

9. Describe how *creatine phosphate* serves as a "high-energy" buffer in vertebrate muscle.

The Oxidation of Carbon Fuels Is an Important Source of Cellular Energy (Text Section 15.3)

10. Describe the *ATP–ADP cycle* of energy exchange in biological systems.

11. Explain in general terms how oxidation of carbon compounds can drive the formation of ATP.

12. Define *proton gradient*, and explain how a proton gradient can couple unfavorable reactions to favorable ones.

Metabolic Pathways Contain Many Recurring Motifs (Text Section 15.4)

13. Recognize the structures of *nicotinamide adenine dinucleotide* (NAD^+) and *flavin adenine dinucleotide* (FAD), describe their reduction to NADH and $FADH_2$, and explain their roles in metabolism.

14. Contrast the metabolic roles of *NADPH* and *NADH*.

15. Explain the fact that most *high-energy compounds* and *reduced electron carriers* are kinetically stable, despite their high-energy status, and that they require enzymes for their reactions.

16. Describe the structure of *coenzyme A (CoA)* and its role as a *carrier of acetyl* or *acyl groups*.

17. List the major *activated carriers*, both of electrons and activated groups, in metabolic reactions.

Metabolic Processes Are Regulated in Three Principal Ways (Text Section 15.5)

18. Discuss the three major mechanisms for the *regulation of metabolism.*

19. Define *energy charge* and compare it with the *phosphorylation potential.*

20. Describe the common structural features of NAD, FAD, and ATP.

SELF-TEST

Metabolism Is Composed of Many Interconnecting Reactions

1. Which of the following functions is not a purpose of metabolism?
   (a) extract chemical energy from substances obtained from the external environment
   (b) form and degrade the biomolecules of the cell
   (c) convert exogenous foodstuffs into building blocks and precursors of macromolecules
   (d) equilibrate extracellular substances and the biomolecules of the cell
   (e) assemble the building-block molecules into macromolecules

2. If the ΔG of the reaction A $\longrightarrow$ B is -12.5 kJ/mol (-3.0 kcal/mol), which of the following statements are correct?
   (a) The reaction will proceed spontaneously from left to right at the given conditions.
   (b) The reaction will proceed spontaneously from right to left at standard conditions.
   (c) The equilibrium constant favors the formation of B over the formation of A.
   (d) The equilibrium constant could be calculated if the initial concentrations of A and B were known.
   (e) The value of $\Delta G^{\circ\prime}$ is also negative.

ATP Is the Universal Currency of Free Energy

3. The text compares ATP to currency. How is ATP similar to money?

4. Glucose 1-phosphate is converted to fructose 6-phosphate in two successive reactions:

   Glucose-1-phosphate $\longrightarrow$ glucose-6-P $\Delta G' = -7.1$ kJ/mol (-1.7 kcal/mol)

   Glucose-6-phosphate $\longrightarrow$ fructose-6-P $\Delta G^{\circ\prime} = -1.7$ kJ/mol (-0.4 kcal/mol)

   What is the $\Delta G^{\circ\prime}$ for the overall reaction?
   (a) -8.8 kJ/mol (-2.1 kcal/mol)   (d) 5.4 kJ/mol (1.3 kcal/mol)
   (b) -7.1 kJ/mol (-1.7 kcal/mol)   (e) 8.8 kJ/mol (2.1 kcal/mol)
   (c) -5.4 kJ/mol (-1.3 kcal/mol)

5. The reaction

$$\text{phosphoenolpyruvate} + \text{ADP} + \text{H}^+ \longrightarrow \text{pyruvate} + \text{ATP}$$

has a $\Delta G^{o\prime} = -31.4$ kJ/mol (-7.5 kcal/mol). Calculate $\Delta G^{o\prime}$ for the hydrolysis of PEP.

6. Inside cells, the ΔG value for the hydrolysis of ATP to ADP + P_i is approximately -50 kJ/mol (-12 kcal/mol). Calculate the approximate ratio of [ATP] to [ADP][P_i] found in cells at 37°C.

   (a) 5000/1
   (b) 4000/1
   (c) 2000/1
   (d) 1000/1
   (e) 200/1

7. Which of the following processes are ways by which two reactions can be coupled energetically to each other?

   (a) As common intracellular components of a compartment, two reactions become automatically coupled.
   (b) An ionic gradient across a membrane that is formed by one reaction can drive another reaction that uses the gradient to render it exergonic.
   (c) A shared, common intermediate can couple two reactions.
   (d) A protein that is activated by binding another molecule or by being covalently modified can provide energy to drive another reaction.

8. Which of the following statements about the structure of ATP are correct?

   (a) It contains three phosphoanhydride bonds.
   (b) It contains two phosphate ester bonds.
   (c) The sugar moiety is linked to the triphosphate by a phosphate ester bond.
   (d) The nitrogenous base is called *adenosine*.
   (e) The active form is usually in a complex with Mg^{2+} or Mn^{2+}.

9. Which of the following factors contributes to the high-phosphate group-transfer potential of ATP?

   (a) greater resonance stabilization of ADP and P_i than of ATP
   (b) increase in the electrostatic repulsion of oxygens on hydrolysis of ATP
   (c) interaction of the terminal phosphoryl group with the ribose group in ADP
   (d) formation of a salt bridge between the base amino group and the negative charges of the phosphate oxygens in ATP

10. Which of the following are high-energy compounds?

    (a) glycerol 3-phosphate
    (b) adenosine diphosphate
    (c) glucose 1-phosphate
    (d) 1,3-bisphosphoglycerate
    (e) fructose 6-phosphate

11. ATP falls in the middle of the list of compounds having high phosphate group-transfer potentials. Explain why this is advantageous for energy coupling during metabolism.

12. Which of the following statements about the phosphoryl transfer potential of skeletal muscle are correct?

    (a) The ATP of muscle can sustain contraction for less than a second.
    (b) Creatine phosphate serves as a phosphoryl reservoir that replenishes the ATP pool.
    (c) Creatine phosphate can support contraction for up to 4 minutes.
    (d) The phosphoguanidino group of creatine phosphate has a large negative standard free energy of hydrolysis.
    (e) Creatine phosphate is formed by a reaction between creatine and ATP.

The Oxidation of Carbon Fuels Is an Important Source of Cellular Energy

13. Which of the following features are part of the ATP–ADP cycle in biological systems?
    (a) ATP hydrolysis is used to drive reactions that require an input of free energy.
    (b) The oxidation of fuel molecules forms $ADP + P_i$ from ATP.
    (c) The oxidation of fuel molecules forms ATP from $ADP + P_i$.
    (d) Light energy drives ATP hydrolysis.
    (e) A transmembrane proton-motive force drives ATP synthesis.

14. Which of the following statements about the third of the three stages of metabolism that generate energy from foodstuffs are correct?
    (a) It is common to the oxidation of all fuel molecules.
    (b) It involves the breakdown of the macromolecular components of food into smaller units, such as amino acids, sugars, and fatty acids.
    (c) It releases relatively little energy compared with the second stage.
    (d) It involves the conversion of sugars, fatty acids, and amino acids into a few common metabolites.
    (e) It produces most of the ATP and CO_2 in cells.

Metabolic Pathways Contain Many Recurring Motifs

15. Which of the following answers complete the sentence correctly? NAD^+
    (a) is a flavin nucleotide.
    (b) is the major electron acceptor used in fuel metabolism.
    (c) contains a nicotinamide ring that accepts a hydride ion during reduction.
    (d) loses a plus charge upon reduction.
    (e) contains ATP as a part of its structure.

16. Which of the following answers complete the sentence correctly? During the reduction of FAD,
    (a) a flavin group is transferred.
    (b) an equivalent of a hydride ion is transferred.
    (c) the isoalloxazine ring becomes charged.
    (d) two hydrogen atoms are added to the isoalloxazine ring.
    (e) the adenine ring opens.

17. Match the four cofactors in the left column with the appropriate structural features and properties from the right column.
(a) ATP	(1) nicotinamide ring
(b) FAD	(2) adenine group
(c) NAD^+	(3) phosphoanydride bond
(d) CoA	(4) sulfur atom
	(5) isoalloxazine ring
	(6) ribose group
	(7) acyl group transfer
	(8) electron transfer
	(9) phosphate transfer

18. ATP and NADH release large amounts of free energy on the transfer of the phosphate group to H_2O and electrons to O_2, respectively. However, both molecules are relatively stable in the presence of H_2O or O_2. Explain why.

19. Which of the following pairs correctly matches a coenzyme with the group transferred by the coenzyme?

    (a) CoA, electrons
    (b) biotin, CO_2
    (c) ATP, one-carbon unit
    (d) NADPH, phosphoryl group
    (e) thiamine pyrophosphate, acyl group

20. Which of the following water-soluble vitamins forms part of the structure of CoA?

    (a) pantothenate
    (b) thiamine
    (c) riboflavin
    (d) pyridoxine
    (e) folate

21. Which of the following statements are reasons the biochemical pathway for the catabolism of a molecule is almost never the same as the pathway for the biosynthesis of that molecule?

    (a) It would be extremely difficult to regulate the pathway if it served both functions.
    (b) The free-energy change would be unfavorable in one direction.
    (c) The reactions never take place in the same type of cell.
    (d) Enzyme-catalyzed reactions are irreversible.
    (e) Biochemical systems are usually at equilibrium.

Metabolic Processes Are Regulated in Three Principal Ways

22. Which of the following phrases are ways by which metabolism is regulated?

    (a) accessibility of substrates
    (b) pressure fluxes
    (c) amounts of enzymes
    (d) control of enzyme activities
    (e) temperature cycles

23. Which of the following statements about the energy charge are correct?

    (a) It can have a value between 0 and 1.
    (b) It is around 0.1 in energy-consuming cells, such as the muscle cells.
    (c) It can regulate the rates of reactions in energy-consuming and energy-producing pathways.
    (d) It is also called the *phosphorylation potential.*
    (e) It is buffered in the sense that its value is maintained within narrow limits.

ANSWERS TO SELF-TEST

1. d. The intracellular and extracellular concentrations of most substances are not at equilibrium, and one of the functions of metabolism is to maintain these nonequilibrium concentrations.

2. a, d. The expression for ΔG contains two variables: $\Delta G^{o\prime}$ (a derivative of K_{eq}) and the ratio of the product concentrations to the reactant concentrations. Therefore, ΔG alone cannot provide information about $\Delta G^{o\prime}$ or K_{eq}. Answer (d) is correct because $\Delta G^{o\prime}$ and K_{eq} can be calculated when ΔG and the reactant and product concentrations are known.

3. The way ATP is used in the cell is remarkably similar to the way money is used in society. The ATP is "earned" by oxidizing food molecules and "spent" to build "expensive" molecules. It is useful to put energetic calculations into these terms—"I am spending $30.50 worth of ATP to buy $9.20 worth of glycerol-3-phosphate, so my

change will be $21.30." In other words, there will be -21.3 kJ/mol left over to drive the reaction far to the right.

4. a

5. The answer is -61.9 kJ/mol (-14.8 kcal/mol).

The overall reaction can be separated into two steps:

(1) PEP $\longrightarrow$ Pyruvate + P_i unknown $\Delta G^{o\prime}$
(2) ADP + $P_i \longrightarrow$ ATP $\Delta G^{o\prime} = -30.5$ kJ/mol ($+7.3$ kcal/mol)

The sum of standard free energies for the two steps is -31.4 kJ/mol (-7.5 kcal/mol). Combining what we know,

$$\Delta G^{o\prime} = -31.4 \text{ kJ/mol} - (+30.5 \text{ kJ/mol}) = -61.9 \text{ kJ/mol}$$

or in kcal: $-7.5 \text{ kcal/mol} - (+7.3 \text{ kcal/mol}) = -14.8 \text{ kcal/mol}$

6. (c) ATP $\longrightarrow$ ADP + P_i $\Delta G^{o\prime} = -30.5$ kJ/mol (-7.3 kcal/mol)

$$\text{Using } \Delta G = \Delta G^{\circ\prime} + RT \ln \frac{[ADP][P_i]}{[ATP]}$$

$$-50 \text{ kJ/mol} = -30.5 \text{ kJ.mol} + 0.0083 \text{ kJ/mol K} \times 310 \text{ K} \times \ln \frac{[ADP][P_i]}{[ATP]}$$

$$-50 + 30.5 = -19.5 \text{ kJ/mol}$$

$$0.0083 \text{ kJ/mol K} \times 310 \text{ K} = 2.57 \text{ kJ/mol}$$

$$-19.5 = 2.57 \ln \frac{[ADP][P_i]}{[ATP]}$$

$$\frac{[ADP]}{[ATP][P_i]} = \text{anti ln } (-7.6) = e^{-7.6} = 5 \times 10^{-4}$$

$$\text{so} \frac{[ATP]}{[ADP][P_i]} = \frac{1}{5 \times 10^{-4}} = 2000$$

Alternatively, in calories,

$$-12 \text{ kcal/mol} = -7.3 \text{ kcal/mol} + 2.303 \times 1.98 \text{ cal/mol K} \times 310 \text{ K} \times \log_{10} \frac{[ADP][P_i]}{[ATP]}$$

$$-12 + 7.3 = -4.7 \text{ kcal/mol}$$

$$2.30 \times 0.00198 \text{ kcal/mol K} \times 310 \text{ K} = 1.41 \text{ kcal/mol}$$

$$-4.7 = 1.414 \log_{10} \frac{[ADP][P_i]}{[ATP]}$$

$$\frac{[ADP][P_i]}{[ATP]} = \text{antilog } (-3.32) = 10^{-3.32} = 4.79 \times 10^{-4}$$

$$\text{so} \frac{[ATP][P_i]}{[ADP]} = \frac{1}{4.79 \times 10^{-4}} = 2089$$

Answers slightly different due to approximation. 12 kcal/mol is more like 50.15 kJ/mol.

7. b, c, d. Being in the same compartment does not necessarily couple two reactions.

8. c, e

9. a

10. b, d

11. The intermediate phosphate group-transfer potential of ATP means that, although ATP hydrolysis can drive a very large number of thermodynamically unfavorable biochemical reactions in metabolic pathways, it can itself be regenerated by coupling with other reactions that release more free energy than -30.5 kJ/mol (-7.3 kcal/mol). Thus, ATP can act as an effective carrier, since it both accepts and donates phosphoryl groups.

12. a, b, d, e. Answer (c) is incorrect because the amount of creatine phosphate is sufficient to maintain only a few seconds of intense contraction. The ATP for the creatine kinase-catalyzed reaction given in (d) is generated by glycolysis in anaerobic muscle or by respiration in muscle with sufficient oxygen.

13. a, c, e

14. a, e

15. b, c, d. Answer (e) is incorrect because ADP, not ATP, forms a part of the structure of NAD^+.

16. d

17. (a) 2, 3, 6, 9   (b) 2, 3, 5, 6, 8   (c) 1, 2, 3, 6, 8   (d) 2, 3, 4, 6, 7

18. Although the transfer reactions of the cofactors ATP and NADH have large negative free-energy changes, there are high activation-energy barriers that greatly slow spontaneous reactions with H_2O or O_2, respectively. In other words, cofactors with high group-transfer potentials and fuel molecules are thermodynamically unstable yet kinetically stable. Consequently, specific enzymes are required to catalyze their reactions.

19. b

20. a

21. a, b

22. a, c, d

23. a, c, e

PROBLEMS

1. Under standard conditions, the free energy of hydrolysis of L-glycerol phosphate is -9.2 kJ/mol (-2.2 kcal/mol), and for ATP hydrolysis it is -30.5 kJ/mol (-7.3 kcal/mol). Show that when ATP is used as a phosphoryl donor for the formation of L-glycerol phosphate, the value of the equilibrium constant is altered by a factor of over 10^5.

2. When a hexose phosphate is hydrolyzed to free hexose and inorganic phosphate, the ratio of the concentration of hexose to the concentration of hexose phosphate at equilibrium is 99 to 1. What is the free-energy change for the reaction under standard conditions?

3. Sucrose phosphorylase catalyzes the phosphorolytic cleavage of sucrose in certain microorganisms.

$$\text{sucrose} + P_i \longrightarrow \text{glucose-1-phosphate} + \text{fructose}$$

(a) Use the following information to calculate the standard free-energy change for the phosphorolysis of sucrose.

$$\text{sucrose} + H_2O \longrightarrow \text{glucose} + \text{fructose} \qquad \Delta G^{o\prime} = -29.3 \text{ kJ/mol } (-7.0 \text{ kcal/mol})$$

$$\text{glucose 1-phosphate} + H_2O \longrightarrow \text{glucose} + P_i \qquad \Delta G^{o\prime} = -20.9 \text{ kJ/mol } (-5.0 \text{ kcal/mol})$$

(b) Calculate the equilibrium constant for the phosphorolysis of glucose at 25°C.

4. Phosphocreatine can be used as a phosphoryl donor for the synthesis of ATP in a reaction catalyzed by creatine kinase. Refer to Section 15.2 of the text for free energies of hydrolysis of ATP and creatine phosphate.

   (a) What effect does creatine kinase have on the value of $\Delta G°'$ for the reaction?
   (b) From the typical concentrations of ATP, ADP, creatine phosphate, and creatine cited in Section 15.2 of the text, calculate ΔG for the reaction in a resting muscle cell at 25°C.
   (c) Suppose that during muscle contraction the concentration of creatine phosphate drops to 1 mM, and ATP concentration drops to 3.9 mM. At these concentrations, will creatine phosphate serve as a donor of phosphoryl groups to ADP at 25°C?

5. Chemotrophs derive free energy from the oxidation of fuel molecules, such as glucose and fatty acids. Which compound, glucose or a saturated fatty acid containing 18 carbons, would yield more free energy per carbon atom when subjected to oxidation in the cell? See Figure 15.10 in the text for a comparison.

6. The process of catabolism releases free energy, some of which is stored as ATP and some of which is lost as heat to the surroundings. Explain how these observations are consistent with the fact that catabolic pathways are essentially irreversible.

7. It is well known that putting sugar in the gas tank of an internal combustion engine will disable the engine. But sugar is mostly carbon, and a sugar cube burns readily. Explain why it causes a problem on a molecular level, and relate the problem to this chapter.

8. In a typical cell, the concentrations of pyridine nucleotides ($NAD^+/NADP^+$) and flavins (FAD/FMN) are relatively low compared with the number of substrate molecules that must be oxidized. What does this observation suggest about the rate of oxidation and reduction of these electron carriers?

9. The flavins FAD and FMN (flavin mononucleotide) are both bright yellow compounds; in fact, the name *flavin* was taken from *flavus*, the Latin word for "yellow." The corresponding reduced compounds, $FADH_2$ and $FMNH_2$, are nearly colorless. What portion of a flavin molecule accounts for these color changes? The enzyme glucose oxidase, found in fungi, catalyzes the conversion of free glucose to gluconic acid. Glucose oxidase utilizes two molecules of FAD as cofactors. How could you use the light-absorbing properties of flavins as a means of monitoring glucose oxidase activity?

10. The flow of electrons from reduced pyridine nucleotides, such as NADH, provides energy that can drive the formation of ATP. Why must the reaction

$$NADH \rightarrow NAD^+ + H^+ + 2\,e^-$$

have a negative value for $\Delta G°'$?

11. Refer to problem 13 in the homework problems of the text. The formation of a number of other important compounds in biosynthetic reactions involves the generation of pyrophosphate and its subsequent hydrolysis to two molecules of P_i. For example, the formation of UDP-glucose from UTP and glucose 1-phosphate yields PP_i, which is then cleaved. What does this tell you about the group transfer potential of UDP-glucose?

12. Many important reactions are "driven to completion" by formation of pyrophosphate in the reaction ATP $\rightarrow$ AMP + PP_i followed by $PP_i \rightarrow 2\,P_i$. Examples would include DNA polymerase, attachment of amino acids to transfer RNA, synthesis of NAD^+, synthesis

of acyl CoA derivatives, and many other reactions. Yet in text Table 15.1, the standard free energy of hydrolysis of pyrophosphate is given as -19.3 kJ/mol (-4.6 kcal/mol), a rather low value. Why should a reaction with such a small standard free-energy change be utilized in such critically important processes?

13. In Table 15.2 in the text, pantothenate, part of coenzyme A, is listed as a vitamin precursor. Coenzyme A also contains AMP and mercaptoethylamine. Why do you think these components are not listed as vitamins?

14. The coenzyme biotin acts as a carrier of carbon dioxide molecules in carboxylase enzymes. During catalytic cycles biotin undergoes successive carboxylation and decarboxylation, but the coenzyme itself is not chemically altered at the end of each cycle. Yet a small amount of biotin is required on a daily basis in the diet. Why?

15. Look in the index of the textbook and find leucine catabolism. The degradation of the amino acid leucine produces isovaleryl CoA, which is then further catabolized. What features of this catabolism are familiar from Section 15.4?

16. Why is it desirable for a cell to regulate the *first* reaction in a biosynthetic pathway?

17. The text discusses the fact that many cofactors contain nucleotides as evidence for the former existence of an RNA world. Are there other "fossil" nucleotide-containing carriers not mentioned in Section 15.4? Do all of these "fossils" prove that RNA came before protein in living cells?

18. Approximately 4% of cellular enzymes use coenzyme A. Understanding the role of this cofactor is critical to understanding many metabolic processes such as glucose oxidation and fatty acid oxidation. What is coenzyme A? What is its role (or the role of Acetyl-CoA) in metabolism? What advantages does this cofactor impart?

19. It will be critical later on to know which forms of the nicotinamide adenine dinucleotides and mononucleotides are the reduced forms and which are the oxidized forms. The following exercises will help to reinforce this knowledge. Using the abbreviated structure below, fill in the blanks for the reactions for the reduction of NAD^+.

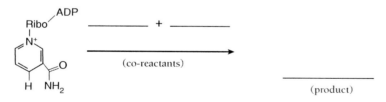

20. The sale of nutritional supplements has become an enormously profitable industry. The following are supplements that are available for over-the-counter purchase. Identify the role of these substances in metabolism.
   (a) Pantothenic acid (vitamin B_5)
   (b) Biotin
   (c) Niacin or Nicotinate
   (d) Creatine
   (e) Riboflavin (vitamin B_2)

21. NAD^+ and FAD are both oxidizing agents, but they participate in different types of reactions. What are these two reaction types?

ANSWERS TO PROBLEMS

1. For the synthesis of L-glycerol phosphate from glycerol and phosphate, the value of $\Delta G^{o\prime}$ is $+9.2$ kJ/mol ($+2.2$ kcal/mol). Under standard conditions,

$$\Delta G^{o\prime} = -RT \ \ln \ K_{eq}^{\prime}$$

$$+9.2 \ \text{kJ/mol} = (.0083 \ \text{kJ}/^{\circ}\text{Kmol})(298\text{K}) \ln K_{eq}^{\prime}$$

$$\ln \ K_{eq}^{\prime} = \frac{+9.2}{(-2.47)}$$

$$= -3.72$$

$$K_{eq}^{\prime} = \ e^{-3.72} = 0.024 = 2.40 \times 10^{-2}$$

[In Chapter 6 of the text, we saw that $RT\ln K_{eq}$ could be calculated using standard conditions ($T = 298$) and base 10 logs so that $RT*2.303 = 1.36$ assuming that R is in cal

$$\Delta G^{o\prime} = 1.36 \ log_{10} \ K_{eq}^{\prime} \ (using \ calories)$$

$$log_{10} \ K_{eq}^{\prime} = \frac{(+2.2)}{(-1.36)}$$

$$= -1.62$$

$$K_{eq}^{\prime} = anti \, log \ (-1.62)$$

$$= 2.40 \times 10^{-2} \ (the \ same \ answer.)]$$

The overall value of $\Delta G^{o\prime}$ for the formation of L-glycerol phosphate using ATP as a phosphoryl donor is equal to the sum of the free-energy values for the two individual reactions:

$$= (+9.2) + (-30.5) = -21.3 \ \text{kJ/mol}$$

The equilibrium constant for the overall reaction is

$$\ln K_{eq}^{\prime} = \frac{-21.3}{(-2.47)} \ (as \ in \ the \ calculations \ above)$$

$$= +8.62$$

$$K_{eq}^{\prime} = 5.6 \times 10^{3}$$

[Using calories, and 1.36 as described above, we get

$$= (+2.2) + (-7.3) = -5.1 \ kcal / mol$$

$$\log_{10} K'_{eq} = \frac{(-5.1)}{(-1.36)}$$

$$= +3.75$$

$$K'_{eq} = antilog \ 3.75$$

$$= 5.6 \times 10^3 \ (the \ same \ anwer.)]$$

The ratio of the two equilibrium constants is $5.6 \times 10^3 \div 2.4 \times 10^{-2} = 2.3 \times 10^5$.

2. The reaction is

hexose phosphate + $H_2O \longrightarrow$ hexose + P_i

The expression for the equilibrium constant is

$$K'_{eq} = \frac{[\text{hexose}][P_i]}{[\text{hexose phosphate}]} = \frac{99}{1}$$

Thus, $\log_{10} K'_{eq}$ is approximately equal to 2 (note that ln 99 = 4.6). Using the free-energy equation,

$$\Delta G^{\circ\prime} = RT \ln K'_{eq} = -(0.0083)(298) \ln 99 = -(2.47)(4.6) = -11.4 \ kJ / mol$$

$$[\Delta G^{\circ\prime} = -1.36 \times 2 \ (in \ calories)$$

$$= -2.72 \ kcal/mol$$

For the origin of the "1.36" term, see problem 1.]

3. (a) To calculate the standard free-energy change for the phosphorolysis of sucrose, add the standard free-energy changes of the two reactions written so that their sum yields the required net reaction:

H_2O + sucrose $\longrightarrow$ glucose + fructose $\qquad \Delta G^{\circ\prime} = -29.3$ kJ/mol

glucose + $P_i \longrightarrow$ glucose 1-phosphate + $H_2O \qquad \Delta G^{\circ\prime} = +20.9$ kJ/mol

Net:

sucrose + $P_i \longrightarrow$ glucose 1-phosphate + fructose $\qquad \Delta G^{\circ\prime} = -8.4$ kJ/mol

[H_2O + sucrose $\longrightarrow$ glucose + fructose $\qquad \Delta G^{\circ\prime} = -7.0$ kcal/mol

glucose + $P_i \longrightarrow$ glucose 1-phosphate + $H_2O \qquad \Delta G^{\circ\prime} = +5.0$ kcal/mol

Net:

sucrose + $P_i \longrightarrow$ glucose 1-phosphate + fructose $\qquad \Delta G^{\circ\prime} = -2.0$ kcal/mol]

(b) The equation that describes the relationship between the standard free energy and the equilibrium constant is

$$\Delta G^{o\prime} = -RT \ln K'_{eq} = -(0.0083)(298) \ln K'_{eq} = -2.47 \ln K'_{eq}$$

Solving for K'_{eq},

$$K'_{eq} = \text{antiln}(-\Delta G^{o\prime}/(2.47)) = \text{antiln}(-(-8.4)/(2.47)) = e^{+3.4} = 30$$

Alternatively,

$$[\Delta G^{o\prime} = -1.36 \log_{10} K'_{eq} \text{ at } 25°C \text{ in calories}).$$

Solving for K'_{eq},

$$\log_{10} K'_{eq} = -\Delta G^{o\prime}/1.36$$

$$= -(-2.0/1.36) = +1.47$$

$$K'_{eq} = \text{antilog } 1.47 = 30$$

For the origin of the "1.36" term see problem 1.]

4. (a) Although the enzyme controls the rate at which equilibrium is attained, it has no effect on the equilibrium constant, K'_{eq}. Because $\Delta G^{o\prime}$ is a function of the equilibrium constant, the action of the enzyme has no effect on its value.

(b) Under the conditions described in the text we know that

ADP + P_i + H^+ ⟶ ATP + H_2O $\Delta G^{o\prime} = +30.5$ kJ/mol

creatine phosphate + H_2O ⟶ creatine + P_i + H^+ + $\Delta G^o = -43.1$ kJ/mol

so adding these two reactions we know that

creatine phosphate + ADP ⟶ creatine + ATP $\Delta G^{o\prime} = -12.6$ kJ/mol

$$\text{So } \Delta G = -12.6 \text{ kJ/mol} + RT \ln \frac{[ATP][creatine]}{[ADP][creatine\ phosphate]}$$

$$\Delta G = -12.6 \text{ kJ/mol} + (0.0083) \times (298) \ln \frac{[4\ mM][13\ mM]}{[0.03\ mM][25\ mM]}$$

Note that the brackets imply molar concentrations. We can use millimolar concentrations because the expression has the form A × B / C × D and the concentrations cancel out. With expressions of the form A × B / C it is important to do the work in moles per liter and not mM.

$$\Delta G = -12.6 \text{ kJ/mol} + (2.47) \ln (160) = -12.6 + 12.5$$

$$\Delta G = -0.1 \text{ kJ/mol, practically zero}$$

At these concentrations, there is no free energy released in the reaction, and there is no net formation of ATP.

Alternatively,

[ADP + P_i + H^+ ⟶ ATP + H_2O $\Delta G^{o\prime} = +7.3$ kcal/mol

creatine phosphate + H_2O ⟶ creatine + P_i + H^+ + $\Delta G^o = -10.3$ kcal/mol

so adding these two reactions we know that

creatine phosphate + ADP ⟶ creatine + ATP $\Delta G^{o\prime} = -3.0$ kcal/mol

$$So\ \Delta G = -3.0 + RT\ 2.303\ log_{10} \frac{[ATP][creatine]}{[ADP][creatine\ phosphate]}$$

$$\Delta G = -3.0\ kcal/mol + 1.36\ log_{10} \frac{[4\ mM][13\ mM]}{[0.03\ mM][25\ mM]}$$

$$\Delta G = -3.0 + 1.36\ log_{10}\ (160) = -3.0 + 1.36\ (2.2)$$

$$\Delta G = -0.01\ kcal/mol,\ practically\ zero]$$

(c) Under these conditions, because the sum of (creatine + creatine phosphate) remains the same, the concentration of creatine is 37 mM, and by the same logic the concentration of ADP increases to about 0.113 mM. (AMP levels will be constant and low enough to ignore here.) Using the free-energy equation,

$$\Delta G = -12.6\ kJ/mol + (0.0083)(298)\ ln \frac{[3.9\ mM][37\ mM]}{[0.113\ mM][1\ mM]}$$

$$\Delta G = -12.6\ kJ/mol + 2.47\ ln\ (1277) = -12.6 + 2.47\ (7.15)$$

$$\Delta G = -12.6 + 17.7 = +5.1\ kJ/mol$$

Alternatively,

$$[\Delta G = -3.0\ kcal/mol + 1.36\ log_{10} \frac{[3.9\ mM][37\ mM]}{[0.113\ mM][1\ mM]}$$

$$\Delta G = -3.0\ kcal/mol + 1.36\ log_{10}\ (1277) = -3.0 + 1.36(3.105)$$

$$\Delta G = -3 + 4.2 = +1.2\ kcal/mol]$$

The positive value of ΔG shows that the reaction will not proceed toward the net formation of ATP, so that under these conditions, creatine phosphate does not serve as a donor of phosphoryl groups to ATP. Instead, the reaction proceeds toward the net formation of creatine phosphate, with phosphoryl groups donated from ATP.

5. Of the 18 carbon atoms in a saturated fatty acid, 17 are saturated (as $-CH_2-$groups) and are more reduced than the partially oxidized carbon atoms in glucose. In glucose, five of the six carbons are partially oxidized to the hydroxymethyl level, and the sixth is at the more oxidized aldehyde level. A greater number of electrons per carbon are available in the fatty acid, so more metabolic energy is available from it than from glucose.

6. The heat that is lost contributes to an increase in the entropy of the surroundings. A positive change in entropy means that the free energy for a catabolic process is more likely to be negative. Reactions with negative free-energy values are irreversible in that they require an input of energy to proceed in the opposite direction.

7. Look at Figure 15.11 in the text. Gasoline is largely composed of octane, which would be similar to the structure of the fatty acid shown—truncated to eight carbons and missing the carboxyl group on the left. "Sugar" could be thought of as the glucose structure shown. Octane is much more highly reduced than sugar, which has many hydroxyl groups. Sugar, or syrup, can't provide enough power to propel a vehicle. Octane also burns cleaner—sugars tend to form "caramel" when heated and oxidized, and this would mean that pistons would jam and valves would stick.

8. Pyridine nucleotides, such as NADH, serve as acceptors and donors of electrons in many metabolic reactions, including those that generate energy for the cell. Because the absolute number of pyridine nucleotides in the cell is low, the cycle of oxidation and reduction for these compounds must occur rapidly for the oxidation of fuel molecules to proceed at a sufficient rate.

9. The conjugated π system in the isoalloxazine ring of oxidized flavins like FAD and FMN accounts for their intense yellow color. The reduced molecules are partially saturated, and their remaining double bonds are not conjugated, making them nearly colorless. To monitor glucose oxidase activity, one could use spectrophotometry to determine the wavelength of maximum absorption for FAD and then monitor the oxidation of the flavin in the enzyme by observing changes in absorption. As glucose is oxidized and FAD is reduced to $FADH_2$, one would observe a corresponding decrease in absorption.

10. For the synthesis of ATP to proceed spontaneously, the overall value of $\Delta G^{o\prime}$ must be negative. The value of $\Delta G^{o\prime}$ for ATP synthesis is positive, so a negative value would be expected for the oxidation of NADH to NAD^+.

11. The text's answer to this problem shows that the cleavage of pyrophosphate ensures that the coupled reactions will proceed toward the net formation of desired product; that is, the overall reaction will have a rather large negative free-energy value. The fact that PP_i is formed during the synthesis of UDP-glucose suggests that the free energy released by the coupled reactions for the formation of UDP-glucose and the hydrolysis of UTP is small. Therefore, the free energy of the hydrolysis of UDP-glucose would be similar to that of UTP. Thus, you should surmise that the group transfer potential of glucose from UDP-glucose would be high. This is the case, as UDP-glucose serves as a donor of glucose residues for the synthesis of glycogen.

12. If you look at older biochemistry textbooks, you will see that many of them list the $\Delta G^{o\prime}$ for pyrophosphate hydrolysis as a much more negative number, between -29 and -33 kJ/mol (-7 and -8 kcal/mol). A recent paper by Perry A. Frey (*Biochem.* 34[1995]:11307) shows that the real driving force in such reactions is the high energy of the α, β phosphoanhydride bond. In other words, it is the first reaction ATP $\longrightarrow$ AMP + PP_i with a $\Delta G^{o\prime}$ of about -64.9 kJ/mol (-15.5 kcal/mol), which provides the driving force for such reactions. The subsequent pyrophosphatase step $PP_i \longrightarrow 2P_i$ (-19.2 kJ/mol)(-4.6 kcal/mol) makes only a relatively minor contribution to functional irreversibility.

13. AMP and mercaptoethylamine are not listed as vitamins because they can be synthesized *de novo* from other precursors in cells. Pantothenate is required in the diet because one or more of the biochemical steps needed to synthesize it are deficient in higher organisms. All three components of coenzyme A can be put together by a cell to form the required cofactor.

14. In cells, there is constant synthesis and degradation of enzymes in response to the need for enzymatic activity. Enzyme degradation through proteolysis will often release coenzymes like biotin. Although some biotin molecules can be incorporated into newly synthesized proteins, others are carried by the blood to the kidney, where they are then excreted. Daily excretion of coenzymes leads to a requirement for their replenishment in the diet.

15. The point here is that most steps in this pathway fall into a familiar pattern. The oxidation of isovaleryl CoA produces a C=C bond, and the cofactor is FAD. The subsequent carboxylation with ATP as a cofactor resembles reaction 3. Browsing through the many chapters on metabolic pathways would reveal many similar examples.

16. Regulation of the first reaction in a biosynthetic pathway ensures that the intermediates in the pathway will be synthesized only when the ultimate product is required. In this way the cell can conserve energy as well as precursors of all intermediates. Such a regulatory scheme will be found when none of the intermediates are utilized in other pathways.

17. In Table 15.2 in the text, we also see uridine diphosphate glucose and cytidine diphosphate diacylglycerol. So besides the ADP in common redox cofactors and CoA, we also have CDP and UDP. These "fossils" make a convincing case that RNA played a greatly expanded role in the distant past. But just because we find dinosaur bones, and they resemble chicken bones, we can't conclude that dinosaurs (or chickens) were the first form of life on Earth. There is positive evidence for an RNA world, but there isn't really negative evidence showing a complete lack of protein during or before this phase of evolution.

18. Coenzyme A is a thiol that reacts with carboxylic acids (such as pyruvate from glycolysis and fatty acids, as we shall see) to form a thioester. It serves as a carrier of acyl groups and it activates carboxylic acids for further reaction. Commonly, this acyl group is an acetyl group and the molecule formed is Acetyl-CoA. Two important roles for Acetyl CoA that will emerge are its shuttling carbon atoms from glycolysis or from fatty acids from the cytoplasm to the mitochondria to be oxidized. One advantage of esterifying acyl groups to coenzyme A is that the hydrolysis of a thioester has a large negative $\Delta G^{\circ\prime}$ value (-31.4 kJ/mol or -7.5 kcal/mol). This exergonic reaction can then be used to drive other reactions forward.

19.

20. (a) Panthothenic acid (vitamin B_5)—part of coenzyme A. Coenzyme A is a cofactor that carries two-carbon acetyl groups, activating them as a thioester.
    (b) Biotin—used to carry CO_2 groups.
    (c) Niacin or Nicotinate—precursor to the nicotinamide ring that stores electrons in NADH and NADPH.
    (d) Creatine-used to create creatine phosphate, a molecule with a high phosphoryl potential that serves as a reservoir of phosphoryl groups to transfer to ADP in muscle during strenuous exercise.
    (e) Riboflavin (Vitamin B_2)—precursor to the isoalloxazine ring of Flavin Adenine Dinucleotides (FAD, $FADH_2$) and Flavine Mononucleotides (FMN, $FMNH_2$), used to carry electrons.

21. NAD^+ tends to participate in reactions in which it oxidizes alcohols to carboxylic acids, producing NADH and H^+. FAD participates in the oxidation of alkanes to alkenes, producing $FADH_2$.

Glycolysis

Chapters 16 and 17 examine some of the most well-studied metabolic pathways—the metabolism of carbohydrates via the glycolytic and gluconeogenic pathways. Glycolysis, discussed in this chapter, is a series of reactions that converts glucose into pyruvate with the concomitant trapping of a portion of the energy as ATP. Gluconeogenesis, discussed in Chapter 17, is a biosynthetic pathway that generates glucose from non-carbohydrate precursors. This chapter describes glycolysis, a classic metabolic pathway whose study ushered in biochemistry as a discipline separate from chemistry. The glycolytic pathway can be broken down into three distinct stages: (1) the conversion of glucose into fructose-1,6-bisphosphate; (2) cleavage of fructose-1,6-biphosphate into triose phosphate intermediates; and (3) the oxidation of the three-carbon fragments into pyruvate, leading to the formation of ATP. The authors discuss the individual reactions within each stage, along with some of the reaction mechanisms and enzyme structures of particular interest.

After summarizing the energetics of glycolysis, the authors discuss the various fates of pyruvate (conversion to ethanol, lactate or acetyl CoA), which differs depending on the organism, cell type, and metabolic state. In addition to glucose, fructose and galactose can also be oxidized by enzymes in the glycolytic pathway, and their mode of entry into glycolysis is described, as are the physiological results of defects in lactose and galactose metabolism. The regulation of glycolysis by the enzymes that catalyze the irreversible reactions in the pathway is discussed next. Phosphofructokinase, the most prominent regulatory enzyme in glycolysis, is examined in detail. Hexokinase and pyruvate kinase, two other important glycolytic regulatory enzymes, are also discussed. The discussion of glycolysis continues with a description of the family of glucose transporters as examples of the ability of isoforms of proteins to perform diverse and specialized functions. Finally there is a discussion of clinical topics—the relationship of glycolysis to cancer, and how glycolysis helps pancreatic beta cells to sense glucose.

LEARNING OBJECTIVES

When you have mastered this chapter, you should be able to accomplish the following objectives.

Glycolysis Is an Energy-Conversion Pathway (Text Section 16.1)

1. Define *glycolysis* and explain its role in the generation of *metabolic energy.*
2. List the alternative end points of the glycolytic degradation of *glucose.*
3. Outline the early work in delineating the glycolytic pathway.
4. Discuss reasons why glucose is such an important fuel for most organisms.
5. Outline the three stages of glycolysis.
6. Discuss the *induced-fit rearrangements* that occur in hexokinase upon glucose binding and list two important consequences of this step in glycolysis.
7. Describe the steps in the conversion of glucose to *fructose 1,6-bisphosphate,* including all the intermediates and enzymes. Note the steps where *ATP* is consumed.
8. List the reactions that convert fructose 1,6-bisphosphate, a hexose, into the triose *glyceraldehyde 3-phosphate.* Summarize the most important features of the catalytic mechanism of *triosephosphate isomerase I.*
9. Outline the steps in glycolysis between glyceraldehyde 3-phosphate and *pyruvate.* Recognize all the intermediates and enzymes and the cofactors that participate in the ATP-generating reactions. Summarize the most important features of the catalytic mechanism of *glyceraldehyde 3-phosphate dehydrogenase.*
10. Explain the role of 2,3-BPG in the interconversion of 3-phosphoglycerate and *2-phosphoglycerate.*
11. Explain the role of the *enol* to *ketone conversion* in the *phosphoryl transfer* catalyzed by *pyruvate kinase.*

NAD⁺ Is Regenerated from the Metabolism of Pyruvate (Text Section 16.2)

12. Write the net reaction for the transformation of glucose into pyruvate and enumerate the ATP and NADH molecules formed.
13. Outline the reactions for the conversion of pyruvate into *ethanol, lactate,* or *acetyl CoA.* Explain the role of *alcoholic fermentation* and lactate formation in the regeneration of NAD⁺.
14. Describe the structure of the NAD⁺-binding region common to many *NAD⁺-linked dehydrogenases.*

Fructose and Galactose Are Converted into Glycolytic Intermediates
(Text Section 16.3)

15. Outline the pathways for the conversion of *fructose* and *galactose* into *glyceraldehyde 3-phosphate* and *glucose-6-phosphate,* respectively. Note the role of *UDP-activated sugars.*
16. Describe the biochemical defects in *lactose intolerance* and *galactosemia.*

The Glycolytic Pathway Is Tightly Controlled (Text Section 16.4)

17. Identify the features of a regulated enzyme in a metabolic pathway and list the regulated enzymes in glycolysis.

18. Describe the allosteric regulation of *phosphofructokinase* including the reason AMP is used as a positive regulator rather than ADP. Explain the role of *fructose 2,6-bisphosphate* in its regulation.

19. Discuss the regulation of *hexokinase*. Contrast the properties and physiologic roles of hexokinase and *glucokinase*.

20. Describe the regulation of the isozymes of *pyruvate kinase*.

21. Compare the regulation of glycolysis in skeletal muscle cells to that in liver cells.

22. Describe the features of the five different isozymes of *glucose transporters*.

23. Define HIF-1 and describe the role it plays in some tumors and in physical exercise training.

Metabolism In Context: Glycolysis Helps Pancreatic β-Cells Sense Glucose
(Text Section 16.5)

24. Describe the origin and function of insulin.

25. Explain how changes in K^+ and Ca^{2+} levels lead to insulin release from the pancreas.

SELF-TEST

Glycolysis Is an Energy-Conversion Pathway

1. Which of the following are reasons why glucose is so prominent (relative to other monosaccharides) as a metabolic fuel?
   (a) It has a relatively low tendency to nonenzymatically glycosylate proteins.
   (b) It can be formed from formaldehyde under prebiotic conditions.
   (c) It has a strong tendency to stay in the ring formation.
   (d) Its oxidation yields more energy than other monosaccharides.

2. What are the three primary fates of pyruvate?

3. For each of the following types of chemical reactions, give one example of a glycolytic enzyme that carries out such a reaction.
   (a) aldol cleavage
   (b) dehydration
   (c) phosphoryl transfer
   (d) phosphoryl shift
   (e) isomerization
   (f) phosphorylation coupled to oxidation

4. Which of the following answers completes the sentence correctly? Hexokinase
   (a) catalyzes the conversion of glucose 6-phosphate into fructose 1,6-bisphosphate.
   (b) requires Ca^{2+} for activity.
   (c) uses inorganic phosphate to form glucose 6-phosphate.
   (d) catalyzes the transfer of a phosphoryl group to a variety of hexoses.
   (e) catalyzes a phosphoryl shift reaction.

5. During the phosphoglucose isomerase reaction, the pyranose structure of glucose 6-phosphate is converted into the furanose ring structure of fructose 6-phosphate. Does this conversion require an additional enzyme? Explain.

6. The steps of glycolysis between glyceraldehyde 3-phosphate and 3-phosphoglycerate involve all of the following except
   (a) ATP synthesis.
   (b) utilization of P_i.
   (c) oxidation of NADH to NAD^+.
   (d) formation of 1,3-bisphosphoglycerate.
   (e) catalysis by phosphoglycerate kinase.

7. In the mechanism of G3PDH, glyceraldehyde-3-phosphate forms a covalent bond with which amino acid residue of the enzyme?
   (a) lysine
   (b) serine
   (c) cysteine
   (d) glutamate
   (e) histidine

8. Why are there bubbles in beer and champagne? Why does bread "rise"?

9. Which of the following answers complete the sentence correctly? The phosphofructokinase and the pyruvate kinase reactions are similar in that
   (a) both generate ATP.
   (b) both involve a "high-energy" sugar derivative.
   (c) both involve three-carbon compounds.
   (d) both are essentially irreversible.
   (e) both enzymes undergo induced-fit rearrangements after binding of the substrate.

10. The reaction phosphoenolpyruvate + ADP + H^+ ⟶ pyruvate + ATP has a $\Delta G^{o\prime} = -31.4$ kJ/mol and a $\Delta G' = -16.7$ kJ/mol under physiologic conditions. Explain what these free-energy values reveal about this reaction.

11. If the C-1 carbon of glucose were labeled with ^{14}C, which of the carbon atoms in pyruvate would be labeled after glycolysis?
    (a) the carboxylate carbon
    (b) the carbonyl carbon
    (c) the methyl carbon

12. Starting with fructose 6-phosphate and proceeding to pyruvate, what is the net yield of ATP molecules?
    (a) 1   (d) 4
    (b) 2   (e) 5
    (c) 3

13. Which of the following statements about triosphosphate isomerase (TIM) is NOT true?
    (a) The mechanism of action of TIM involves a conformational change in the structure of the enzyme that prevents escape of an activated intermediate.
    (b) The rate-limiting step in the reaction catalyzed by TIM is the release of the product glyceraldehyde 3-phosphate.
    (c) The $kcat/K_M$ ratio for the reaction catalyzed by TIM is close to the diffusion-controlled limit for a bimolecular reaction.
    (d) The isomerization of a hydrogen atom from one carbon atom to another in the TIM-catalyzed reaction is assisted by a base (the γ -carboxyl of a glutamate residue) in the enzyme.
    (e) TIM catalyzes an intramolecular oxidation-reduction reaction.

NAD⁺ Is Regenerated From the Metabolism of Pyruvate

14. Since lactate is a "dead-end" product of metabolism in the sense that its sole fate is to be reconverted into pyruvate, what is the purpose of its formation?

Fructose and Galactose Are Converted into Glycolytic Intermediates

15. Galactose metabolism involves the following reactions: (1) galactose + ATP $\rightarrow$ galactose 1-phosphate + ADP + H⁺; (2) ?; (3) UDP-galactose $\rightarrow$ UDP-glucose.
    (a) Write the reaction for step 2.
    (b) Which step is defective in galactosemia?
    (c) Which enzymes catalyze steps 1, 2, and 3?

The Glycolytic Pathway Is Tightly Controlled

16. The essentially irreversible reactions that control the rate of glycolysis are catalyzed by which of the following enzymes?
    (a) pyruvate kinase
    (b) aldolase
    (c) glyceraldehyde 3-phosphate
    (d) phosphofructokinase
    (e) hexokinase
    (f) phosphoglycerate kinase dehydrogenase

17. Both phosphofructokinase and pyruvate kinase are inhibited by high levels of ATP. Why is this logical?

18. In which of the following is the enzyme correctly paired with its allosteric effector?
    (a) hexokinase: ATP
    (b) phosphofructokinase: glucose 6-phosphate
    (c) pyruvate kinase: alanine
    (d) phosphofructokinase: AMP
    (e) glucokinase: fructose 2,6-bisphosphate

19. Match hexokinase and glucokinase with the descriptions from the right column that are appropriate.
    (a) hexokinase
    (b) glucokinase

    (1) is found in the liver
    (2) is found in nonhepatic tissues
    (3) is specific for glucose
    (4) has a broad specificity for hexoses
    (5) requires ATP for reaction
    (6) has a high K_M for glucose.
    (7) is inhibited by glucose 6-phosphate

20. Which of the following statements about glucose transporters is NOT true?
    (a) They are transmembrane proteins.
    (b) They accomplish the movement of glucose across animal cell plasma membranes.
    (c) Their tissue distribution and concentration can depend on the tissue type and metabolic state of the organism.
    (d) Their glucose binding site is moved from one side of the membrane to the other by rotation of the entire protein.
    (e) They constitute a family of five isoforms of a protein.

Metabolism In Context: Glycolysis Helps Pancreatic β-Cells Sense Glucose

21. Glucose enters pancreatic β cells via which transporter?

    (a) GLUT1   (d) GLUT4

    (b) GLUT2   (e) GLUT5

    (c) GLUT3

22. Which conditions lead to release of insulin from the pancreas, according to the text?

    (a) high K^+ and high Ca^{2+}

    (a) low K^+ and high Ca^{2+}

    (a) high K^+ and low Ca^{2+}

    (a) low K^+ and low Ca^{2+}

ANSWERS TO SELF-TEST

1. a, b, c

2. ethanol, lactate, and CO_2/water

3. (a) aldolase

   (b) enolase

   (c) hexokinase, phosphofructokinase, phosphoglycerate kinase, or pyruvate kinase

   (d) phosphoglycerate mutase

   (e) phosphoglucose isomerase, triosephosphate isomerase

   (f) glyeraldehyde 3-phosphate dehydrogenase

4. d

5. No. The reaction catalyzed by phosphoglucose isomerase is a simple isomerization between an aldose and a ketose and involves the open-chain structures of both sugars. Since glucose 6-phosphate and fructose 6-phosphate are both reducing sugars, their Haworth ring structures are in equilibrium with their open-chain forms. This equilibration is very rapid and does not require an additional enzyme. Note that this isomerization reaction is of the same type as that catalyzed by triosephosphate isomerase.

6. c

7. (c) cysteine. The resulting thioester bond is important catalytically.

8. See text Figure 16.4. Anaerobic glycolysis in yeast produces ethanol and carbon dioxide gas. Louis Pasteur's studies on this alcoholic fermentation gave rise to the entire science of biochemistry. So capping a bottle before the fermentation is finished gives rise to carbonation, or bubbles. The bubbles in champagne are generally "real" carbonation produced directly by yeast. Beer is generally fermented to completion and then artificially carbonated, but the bubbles originated in the same way. In bread dough, the alcohol cooks off when the bread is baked but it is there and it gives a sweet smell to the rising dough. The bubbles that make the bread rise are CO_2, just as in beer and champagne.

9. d

10. The large negative $\Delta G^{o\prime}$ value indicates that equilibrium favors product formation by a very large margin. The -16.7 kJ/mol value for $\Delta G'$ means that under physiologic conditions the reaction will also proceed toward product formation essentially irreversibly. The fact that $\Delta G'$ has a smaller negative value than $\Delta G^{o\prime}$ indicates that under

physiologic conditions the ratio of the concentrations of products over reactants is considerably smaller than in the standard state.

11. c

12. c

13. b. The rate-limiting step of the reaction, which by definition can be no faster than the rate at which the product appears, is the diffusion-controlled encounter of the substrate with the enzyme, not the release of product.

14. The reduction of pyruvate to lactate converts NADH to NAD^+, which is required in the glyceraldehyde 3-phosphate dehydrogenase reaction. This prevents glycolysis from stopping owing to too low a concentration of NAD^+ and allows continued production of ATP.

15. (a) Galactose 1-phosphate + UDP-glucose $\longrightarrow$ glucose 1-phosphate + UDP-galactose
    (b) Step 2 is defective in galactosemia.
    (c) Galactokinase catalyzes step 1; galactose 1-phosphate uridyl transferase catalyzes step 2; and UDP-galactose 4-epimerase catalyzes step 3.

16. a, d, e

17. Control points are generally the irreversible steps in a pathway, and for glycolysis that means the kinase enzymes. Catabolic pathways produce ATP by breaking down food metabolites, so it is appropriate for any catabolic pathway to be inhibited by a high energy charge, or high ATP. If you have enough ATP you should stop "burning" your fuel supply; the concept is like a thermostat controlling the temperature in a house. If your house is at 80°F, turn off the furnace!

18. a, c, d

19. (a) 1, 2, 4, 5, 7   (b) 1, 3, 5, 6

20. d

21. (b) $Glut_2$

22. (a) both are high

PROBLEMS

1. The text states that lactose intolerance in adult humans is the "normal" state, and that the mutation that allows for lactose tolerance should not be older than 10,000 years because that is when the practice of dairying started. Can you think of a way that this can be proven, that a certain mutation is relatively "young"? Hint, it involves DNA and chromosomes.

2. Inorganic phosphate labeled with ^{32}P is added with glucose to a glycogen-free extract from liver, and the mixture is then incubated in the absence of oxygen. After a short time, 1,3-bisphosphoglycerate (1,3-BPG) is isolated from the mixture. On which carbons would you expect to find radioactive phosphate? If you allow the incubation to continue for a longer period, will you find any change in the labeling pattern? Why?

3. Mannose, the 2-epimer of glucose (Figure 10.2 in text), and mannitol, a sugar alcohol, are widely used as dietetic sweeteners. Both compounds are transported only slowly across plasma membranes, but they can be metabolized by the liver. Propose a scheme by which mannitol and mannose can be converted into intermediates of the glycolytic pathway. You may wish to take advantage of the fact that hexokinase is relatively nonspecific. Why should such sugars be brought into glycolysis as early in the sequence as possible?

4. The value of $\Delta G^{\circ\prime}$ for the hydrolysis of sucrose to glucose and fructose is -31.4 kJ/mol. You have a solution that is 0.10 M in glucose and that contains sufficient sucrase enzyme to bring the reaction rapidly to equilibrium.

   (a) What concentration of fructose would be required to yield sucrose at an equilibrium concentration of 0.01 M, at 25°C?

   (b) The solubility limit for fructose is about 3.0 M. How might this limit affect your experiment?

5. In 1905, Harden and Young, two English chemists, studied the fermentation of glucose using cell-free extracts of yeast. They monitored the conversion of glucose to ethanol by measuring the evolution of carbon dioxide from the reaction vessel. In one set of experiments, Harden and Young observed the evolution of CO_2 when inorganic phosphate (P_i) was added to a yeast extract containing glucose. In the graph in Figure 16.2, curve A shows what happens when no P_i is added. Curve B shows the effect of adding P_i in a separate experiment. As the evolution of CO_2 slows with time, more P_i is added to stimulate the reactions; this is shown in curve C.

   (a) Why is glucose fermentation dependent on P_i?

   (b) During fermentation, what is the ratio of P_i consumed to CO_2 evolved?

   (c) How does the formation of ethanol ensure that the fermentation process is in redox balance?

   (d) Harden and Young found that they could recover phosphate from the reaction mixture, but it was not precipitable by magnesium citrate, as is P_i. Name at least three organic compounds that would be phosphorylated when P_i is added to the fermenting mixture.

   (e) As the rate of CO_2 evolution decreased, Harden and Young found that an unusual compound accumulated in the reaction mixture. In 1907, Young identified the compound as a hexose bisphosphate. Name the compound and explain why it might accumulate when P_i becomes limiting.

   (f) Later, Meyerhof showed that the addition of adenosine triphosphatase (ATPase, an enzyme that hydrolyzes ATP to yield ADP and P_i) to the reaction mixture stimulates the evolution of CO_2. Explain this result.

FIGURE 16.2   Evolution of CO_2 in the Harden-Young experiment.

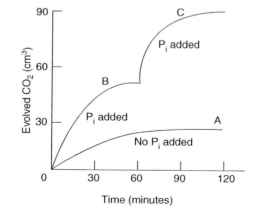

6. Ahlfors and Mansour studied the activity of purified sheep phosphofructokinase (PFK) as a function of the concentration of ATP in experiments that were carried out at a constant concentration of fructose 6-phosphate. Typical results are shown

in Figure 16.3. Explain these results, and relate them to the role of PFK in the glycolytic pathway.

FIGURE 16.3 The effects of ATP concentration on sheep PFK.

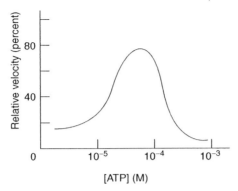

7. Hexokinase catalyzes the formation of glucose 6-phosphate at a maximum velocity of 2×10^{-5} mol/min, whereas V_{max} for the formation of fructose 6-phosphate is 3×10^{-5} mol/min. The value of K_M for glucose is 10^{-5} M, whereas K_M for fructose is 10^{-3} M. Suppose that in a particular cell the observed rates of phosphorylation are 1.0×10^{-8} mol/min for glucose and 1.5×10^{-5} mol/min for fructose.

   (a) Estimate the concentrations of glucose and fructose in the cell.
   (b) Which of these hexoses is more important in generating energy for this cell?

8. Galactose is an important component of glycoproteins. Explain why withholding galactose from the diet of galactosemic patients has no effect on their synthesis of glycoproteins.

9. For the glyceraldehyde 3-phosphate dehydrogenase reaction, explain how the oxidation of the aldehyde group ultimately gives rise to an acyl phosphate product.

10. Explain the high phosphoryl group-transfer potential of phosphoenolpyruvate as it is displayed in the pyruvate kinase reaction.

11. Glycerol can enter the glycolytic pathway through phosphorylation to glycerol 3-phosphate, catalyzed by glycerol kinase, and then by oxidation to dihydroxyacetone phosphate, catalyzed by glycerol 3-phosphate dehydrogenase. Glyceraldehyde is funneled into the glycolytic pathway through phosphorylation to glyceraldehyde 3-phosphate, catalyzed by triose kinase. Glycerate enters the glycolytic pathway when it is phosphorylated to 3-phosphoglycerate by glycerate kinase. Lactate-forming bacteria can metabolize glycerol, glyceraldehyde, or glycerate in the presence of oxygen, but only one of these substrates can be converted to lactate under anaerobic conditions. Which one, and why?

12. Hexokinase and glucokinase are isozymes, which is to say that they are related and they both catalyze the phosphorylation of glucose at carbon 6. Hexokinase is the first enzyme of glycolysis and is thus more or less universal in living cells. Why do we need a different isozyme, found only in certain organs (liver and pancreas)?

13. The textbook points out that both certain kinds of cancer and anaerobic exercise produce similar responses. Both result in *hypoxia-inducible transcription factor* (HIF-1). How does this make sense? Can you see a parallel logic for development of a tumor and development of stronger muscles?

ANSWERS TO PROBLEMS

1. Even students who have not studied DNA in detail might know that there is a steady level of recombination in chromosomes. A part of one chromosome is swapped for part of another chromosome. So in the very first generation with a helpful gene (like lactose tolerance in adults)—say a woman has this mutation, and several of her children have it. At that time, everyone with the gene will have the entire chromosome, the whole chromosome will be 100% the same. Over the centuries, bits of that chromosome will be swapped away, but the portion that contains the useful gene will often cause the survival of that individual (during a famine) and thus be passed on. The region passed on with the gene becomes smaller and smaller over time. What is interesting about the lactose tolerance mutation is that the northern European version of the gene is surrounded by a block of about a *million* base pairs. This is interpreted to imply that the mutation could have occurred as recently as 2000 years ago (Bersaglieri, T. et al., *Am. J. Hum. Genet.* 74 (2004) p. 1111). This matches the time frame mentioned in the text (less than 10,000 years) very nicely.

2. After a short incubation time, labeled phosphate will be found on C-1 of 1,3-BPG. Inorganic phosphate enters the glycolytic pathway at the step catalyzed by glyceraldehyde 3-phosphate dehydrogenase. However, after a longer incubation time, the radioactive label will be found on both C-1 and C-3 of 1,3-BPG because the step subsequent to the formation of 1,3-BPG involves the phosphorylation of ADP to form ATP, which will be radioactively labeled in the γ-phosphoryl group. In other glycolytic reactions, the radioactively labeled ATP can phosphorylate at C-1 of fructose 6-phosphate and C-6 of glucose, both of which are equivalent to C-3 in 1,3-BPG. Thus, after prolonged incubation, both labeled inorganic phosphate and labeled ATP will be present in the mixture, and 1,3-BPG with a radioactive label at both C-1 and C-3 will be present in the extract. One must assume that a small amount of unlabeled ATP is available at the start to initiate hexose phosphorylation.

3. The first step is the conversion of mannitol to mannose. This requires oxidation at the C-1 of mannitol, using a dehydrogenase enzyme with NAD^+ or $NADP^+$ as an electron acceptor. One could then propose a number of schemes, using nucleotide derivatives with isomerase or epimerase activities in combination with one or more phosphorylated intermediates. An established pathway uses hexokinase and ATP for the synthesis of mannose 6-phosphate; this is then converted by mannose phosphate isomerase to form fructose 6-phosphate, an intermediate of the glycolytic pathway. Bringing such sugars into the glycolytic pathway as soon as possible means that already existing enzymes can be used to process the intermediates derived from each of a number of different sugars. Otherwise, a separate battery of enzymes would be needed to obtain energy from each of the sugars found in the diet.

4. The reaction you are concerned with is glucose + fructose $\longrightarrow$ sucrose.

   (a) For the reaction in this direction, $\Delta G^{o\prime} = +31.4$ kJ/mol. The equilibrium constant K'_{eq} is

   $$K'_{eq} = \frac{[\text{sucrose}]}{[\text{glucose}][\text{fructose}]}$$

   At the start of the reaction, [sucrose] = 0, [glucose] = 0.10 M, and [fructose] = x. At equilibrium, [sucrose] = 0.01 M, [glucose] = 0.09 M, and [fructose] = $x - 0.01$ M. First, calculate K'_{eq} for the reaction at equilibrium:

$$\Delta G^{\circ\prime} = -RT \ln K_{eq}^{\prime} = (-8314 \, JK^{-1} mol^{-1})(298K) \ln K_{eq}^{\prime} = +31.4 \, kJ/mol$$

$$\ln K_{eq}^{\prime} = \frac{-31.4 \, kJ/mol}{(8.314 \, J \, K^{-1})(298K)} = -12.7$$

$$K_{eq}^{\prime} = 3.05 \times 10^{-6} \, M^{-1}$$

Then find the concentration of fructose that satisfies the conditions at equilibrium. Assume that the unknown concentration of fructose at equilibrium ($x - 0.01$ M) is approximately equal to x.

$$x = \frac{0.01 \, M}{(0.09 \, M)(3.05 \times 10^{-6} \, M^{-1})} = 3.64 \times 10^{4} \, M$$

(b) The concentration of fructose required to generate sucrose at a concentration of 0.01 M exceeds the solubility limit for fructose; it is therefore impossible to establish such conditions in solution.

5. Harden-Young Experiment

(a) Inorganic phosphate is required for one of the reactions of the glycolytic pathway: the phosphorylation by which glyceraldehyde 3-phosphate is converted to 1,3-bisphosphoglycerate.

(b) The P_i/CO_2 ratio is 1.0, with one P_i being consumed for each pyruvate that undergoes decarboxylation.

(c) In most cells, the absolute concentration of NAD^+ and NADH is low. Successive and continuous reduction and oxidation of NAD^+ and NADH, respectively, is necessary for them to continue to serve as donors and acceptors of electrons. In this case, NAD^+ must be constantly available for the continued activity of glyceraldehyde 3-phosphate dehydrogenase in the glycolytic pathway. The NADH generated during the oxidation of glyceraldehyde 3-phosphate is reoxidized to NAD^+ when acetaldehyde is reduced to ethanol.

(d) Initially, glyceraldehyde 3-phosphate is phosphorylated when P_i is added to the fermenting mixture. ADP is phosphorylated when 1,3-bisphosphoglycerate donates a phosphoryl group to the nucleotide and is itself converted to 3-phosphoglycerate. The ATP formed in this reaction can be used in two earlier reactions of glycolysis, the phosphorylations of glucose and of fructose 6-phosphate.

(e) The hexose bisphosphate is fructose 1,6-bisphosphate, the only such intermediate in the glycolytic pathway. This compound accumulates when glycolytic flux is blocked at the glyceraldehyde 3-phosphate dehydrogenase step by limited Pi availability. As the phosphorylation of glucose continues, intermediates from the steps preceding the formation of 1,3-bisphosphoglycerate build up.

(f) The hydrolysis of ATP to ADP and P_i makes more P_i available for the phosphorylation of glyceraldehyde 3-phosphate. Under such conditions, glycolytic activity and CO_2 production are stimulated.

6. See text Section 16.4. The rate of the reaction catalyzed by PFK initially increases with the ATP concentration because ATP is a substrate for the reaction; it binds at the active site of PFK with fructose 6-phosphate and serves as a phosphoryl donor. At higher concentrations, ATP binds not only at the active site but also at the allosteric site; this alters the conformation of the enzyme and decreases the level of its activity. The effects

of ATP on PFK are consistent with the role of PFK as a control element for the glycolytic pathway. When concentrations of ATP are relatively low, the activity of PFK is stimulated so that additional fructose 1,6-bisphosphate is made available for subsequent energy-generating reactions; when concentrations of ATP are higher and the demand of the cell for energy is lower, ATP inhibits PFK activity, thereby allowing glucose and other substrates to be utilized in other pathways. In many cells, ATP concentration is maintained at relatively high and constant levels, so that PFK is always subject to inhibition by ATP. Inhibition can be relieved by fructose 2,6-bisphosphate, which is synthesized when glucose is readily available. This allows cells to carry out glycolysis even when ATP levels are high, permitting the synthesis of building blocks from glucose.

7. Hexokinase kinetics

   (a) The values of V_{max}, K_M, and V, the measured velocity, are given for glucose and fructose. You can use the Michaelis-Menten equation by solving for [S], the substrate concentration:

   $$V = V_{max} \frac{[S]}{[S] + K_M}$$

   $$V_{max}[S] = V[S] + VK_M$$

   $$[S](V_{max} - V) = VK_M$$

   $$[S] = \frac{VK_M}{V_{max} - V}$$

   Then you can use the values provided to calculate the concentrations of the two sugars in the cell. For glucose, [S] = 5×10^{-9} M; whereas for fructose, [S] = 1×10^{-3} M.

   (b) The phosphorylation of a hexose such as glucose or fructose is the initial step in the oxidation of the sugar, a process in which energy in the form of ATP is generated. Fructose is more important in the provision of energy for the cell because V, the observed rate of formation, is 1500 times faster for fructose 6-phosphate than it is for glucose 6-phosphate.

8. Because their epimerase activity is normal, galactosemic patients are able to synthesize UDP-galactose from UDP-glucose. The UDP-galactose is then used in the synthesis of glycoproteins.

9. The oxidation of the aldehyde group by NAD^+ is an energetically favorable reaction that leads to the formation of a high-energy thioester bond between the substrate and the thiol group of a cysteine residue of the enzyme. Inorganic phosphate then attacks the thioester bond, which gives rise to an acyl phosphate product, 1,3-bisphosphoglycerate.

10. When pyruvate kinase transfers the phosphoryl group from phosphoenolpyruvate to ADP, the remaining enediol remnant, enolpyruvate, is much more unstable than its ketone tautomer, pyruvate. This enol-ketone tautomerization drives the overall reaction toward ATP formation by removing the enolpyruvate by converting it to pyruvate.

11. Only glyceraldehyde can be converted to lactate under anaerobic conditions. The pathway for glyceraldehyde to lactate produces net formation of one ATP with no net oxidation per molecule metabolized. Every glycerol molecule converted to lactate under

anaerobic conditions generates 2 NADH, one produced during the conversion of glycerol 3-phosphate into DHAP and another during the formation of 1,3-BPG from glyceraldehyde 3-phosphate. Because there is only one step, catalyzed by lactate dehydrogenase, that regenerates an NAD^+ molecule for every glyceraldehyde molecule metabolized, NADH accumulates. The glycolytic pathway is interrupted because there is no NAD^+ available to accept electrons from glycerol 3-phosphate or glyceraldehyde 3-phosphate. Glycerate cannot be metabolized under anaerobic conditions, because during its conversion to lactate there is no net formation of ATP. In addition, the pathway from glycerate to lactate has no pathway for generation of NADH, which would be required to balance the generation of NAD^+ during the reduction of pyruvate to form lactate.

12. Hexokinase phosphorylates glucose even at low concentrations. This is important in muscle and other tissues because phosphorylating newly absorbed glucose prevents it from leaving the cell. But remember that the liver must be able to export glucose, so allowing hexokinase to put a phosphate on right after the liver has gone to some trouble to allow glucose-6-phosphatase to take a phosphate *off* would make no sense. Thus both in liver and pancreas, glucokinase is used because it only works at high glucose concentrations. When glucose is particularly high it allows glycogen synthesis and helps to signal for secretion of the hormone insulin.

13. A malignant tumor is likely to grow. As new tissue is added, it won't have enough oxygen unless new blood vessels form. Thus it will be hypoxic, which will cause formation of HIF-1. This will stimulate a variety of responses (see Table 16.4 and textbook Figure 16.18) including growth of new blood vessels. Exercising enough to strengthen muscles also is likely to add new tissue as muscles get larger, producing the same situation. HIF-1 is produced and new blood vessels will form. As the text points out, one promising focus of chemotherapy is prevention of new blood vessel formation in tumors.

Chapter 17

Gluconeogenesis

This chapter amplifies the topic of glucose metabolism presented in the previous chapter by describing gluconeogenesis, or the synthesis of glucose from noncarbohydrate precursors such as lactate, amino acids, and glycerol. Gluconeogenesis is not simply a reversal of glycolysis, due to the fact that the equilibrium of glycolysis lies far on the side of pyruvate formation. The steps of glycolysis that lie near equilibrium are used in gluconeogenesis, and three new steps are substituted for those that are essentially irreversible. The authors discuss these three new steps in detail, in which (1) phosphoenolpyruvate is produced from pyruvate, in a two-step reaction with oxaloacetate as an intermediate; (2) fructose-6-phosphate is synthesized from fructose-1,6-biphosphate; and finally (3) glucose is produced from glucose-6-phosphate. The authors emphasize the reciprocal regulation of glycolysis and gluconeogenesis, ensuring that cells respond quickly to the need for energy.

LEARNING OBJECTIVES

When you have mastered this chapter, you should be able to accomplish the following objectives.

Glucose Can Be Synthesized from Noncarbohydrate Precursors (Text Section 17.1)

1. Describe the physiologic significance of *gluconeogenesis*. List the primary precursors of gluconeogenesis.

2. Describe the enzymatic steps in the conversion of *pyruvate* to *phosphoenolpyruvate*. Name the enzymes, intermediates, and cofactors involved in these reactions.

3. Name the major organs that carry out gluconeogenesis. Locate the various enzymes of gluconeogenesis in cell compartments.

4. Explain the role of *biotin* as a carrier for *activated CO_2* in the *pyruvate carboxylase* reaction. Describe the control of pyruvate carboxylase by *acetyl CoA* and its role in maintaining the level of citric acid cycle intermediates.

5. Calculate the number of high-energy phosphate bonds consumed during gluconeogenesis and compare it with the number formed during glycolysis.

Gluconeogenesis and Glycolysis Are Reciprocally Regulated (Text Section 17.2)

6. Describe the coordinated control of the enzymes in glycolysis and gluconeogenesis. Include a discussion of the effects of the hormones *insulin* and *glucagon*.

7. Describe the *fused-domain structure* of *phosphofructokinase 2 (PFK2)/fructose bisphosphatase 2* that forms and degrades fructose 2,6-bisphosphate. Describe the reciprocal regulation of the enzyme.

8. Explain how *substrate cycles* may *amplify metabolic signals* or *produce heat*.

9. Outline the *Cori cycle* and explain its biological significance.

10. Contrast the properties and roles of the *H* and *M isozymes* of *lactate dehydrogenase*.

SELF-TEST

Glucose Can Be Synthesized from Noncarbohydrate Precursors

1. Which of the following statements about gluconeogenesis are true?
   (a) It occurs actively in the muscle during periods of exercise.
   (b) It occurs actively in the liver during periods of exercise or fasting.
   (c) It occurs actively in adipose tissue during feeding.
   (d) It occurs actively in the kidney during periods of fasting.
   (e) It occurs actively in the brain during periods of fasting.

2. Glucose can be synthesized from which of the following noncarbohydrate precursors?
   (a) adenine   (d) palmitic acid
   (b) alanine   (e) glycerol
   (c) lactate

3. Which statement about glucose 6-phosphatase is true? Glucose 6-phosphatase

(a) is bound to the inner mitochondrial membrane.
(b) requires an associated Ca^{2+}-binding protein for activity.
(c) is directly associated with a glucose transporter.
(d) produces glucose and phosphate in a reaction that consumes energy.
(e) has an identical active site with hexokinase.

4. Figure 17.1 below shows the sequence of reactions of gluconeogenesis from pyruvate to phosphoenolpyruvate. Match the capital letters indicating the reactions of the gluoneogenic pathway with the following statements:

FIGURE 17.1 Reactions of gluconeogenesis from pyruvate to phosphoenolpyruvate.

Pyruvate $\longrightarrow$ oxaloacetate $\longrightarrow$ malate $\longrightarrow$ oxaloacetate $\longrightarrow$ phosphoenolpyruvate
           A   B   C   D

(a) occurs in the mitochondria
(b) occurs in the cytosol
(c) produces CO_2
(d) consumes CO_2

(e) requires ATP
(f) requires GTP
(g) is regulated by acetyl CoA
(h) requires a biotin cofactor

5. How many "high-energy" bonds are required to convert oxaloacetate to glucose?

(a) 2
(b) 3
(c) 4

(d) 5
(e) 6

Gluconeogenesis and Glycolysis Are Reciprocally Regulated

6. Which of the following statements correctly describe what happens when acetyl CoA is abundant?

(a) Pyruvate carboxylase is activated.
(b) Phosphoenolpyruvate carboxykinase is activated.
(c) Phosphofructokinase is activated.
(d) If ATP levels are high, oxaloacetate is diverted to gluconeogenesis.
(e) If ATP levels are low, oxaloacetate is diverted to gluconeogenesis.

7. When blood glucose levels are low, glucagon is secreted. Which of the following are the effects of increased glucagon levels on glycolysis and related reactions in liver?

(a) Phosphorylation of phosphofructokinase 2 and fructose bisphosphatase 2 occurs.
(b) Dephosphorylation of phosphofructokinase 2 and fructose bisphosphatase 2 occurs.
(c) Phosphofructokinase is activated.
(d) Phosphofructokinase is inhibited.
(e) Glycolysis is accelerated.
(f) Glycolysis is slowed down.

8. In the coordinated control of phosphofructokinase (PFK) and fructose 1,6-bisphosphatase (F-1,6-BPase),

(a) citrate inhibits PFK and stimulates F-1,6-BPase.
(b) fructose 2,6-bisphosphate inhibits PFK and stimulates F-1,6-BPase.
(c) acetyl-CoA inhibits PFK and stimulates F-1,6-BPase.
(d) AMP inhibits PFK and stimulates F-1,6-BPase.
(e) NADPH inhibits PFK and stimulates F-1,6-BPase.

9. Indicate which of the conditions listed in the right column *increase* the activity of the glycolysis or gluconeogenesis pathways.

   (a) glycolysis
   (b) gluconeogenesis

   (1) increase in ATP
   (2) increase in AMP
   (3) increase in F-2,6-BP
   (4) increase in citrate
   (5) increase in acetyl-CoA
   (6) increase in insulin
   (7) increase in glucagon
   (8) starvation
   (9) fed state

10. Which of the following statements about the Cori cycle and its physiologic consequences are true?

    (a) It involves the synthesis of glucose in muscle.
    (b) It involves the release of lactate by muscle.
    (c) It involves lactate synthesis in the liver.
    (d) It involves ATP synthesis in muscle.
    (e) It involves the release of glucose by the liver.

11. Which part of glycolysis appears to be evolutionarily "oldest": the hexose portion or the triose portion?

ANSWERS TO SELF-TEST

1. b, d

2. b, c, e

3. b. The other answers are incorrect because glucose 6-phosphatase is bound to the luminal side of the endoplasmic reticulum membrane. It is associated with the glucose 6-phosphate and phosphate transporters, but not with the glucose transporter. The hydrolysis of glucose 6-phosphate is an exergonic reaction. The active site of hexokinase is distinct from that of the phosphatase, since the hexokinase binds ATP.

4. (a) A, B (b) C, D (c) D (d) A (e) A (f) D (g) A (h) A

5. c. The two steps in gluconeogenesis that consume GTP or ATP are:

   Oxaloacetate + GTP $\rightarrow$ phosphoenolpyruvate + GDP + CO_2

   3-Phosphoglycerate + ATP $\rightarrow$ 1,3-bisphosphoglycerate + ADP

   Since two oxaloacetate molecules are required to synthesize one glucose molecule, a total of four "high-energy" bonds are required.

6. a, d

7. a, d, f

8. a

9. (a) 2, 3, 6, 9 (b) 1, 4, 5, 7, 8

10. b, d, e

11. According to the last paragraph of the textbook chapter, the triose portion of glycolysis is absolutely universal, unlike the hexose portion, which is missing in some

species, particularly among the archaea. The fact that the triose portion is universal means that it must have been present in LUCA, the Last Universal Common Ancestor, and hence it is probably at least 3 billion years old.

PROBLEMS

1. Aminotransferases are enzymes that catalyze the removal of amino groups from amino acids to yield α-keto acids. How could the action of such enzymes contribute to gluconeogenesis? Consider the utilization of alanine, aspartate, and glutamate in your answer.

2. Even if the concentration of lactate and other precursors were high, why is it unlikely that liver cells would be carrying out gluconeogenesis under anaerobic conditions?

3. Explain why a CO_2 is added to pyruvate in the pyruvate carboxylase reaction only to be subsequently removed by the phosphoenolpyruvate carboxykinase reaction. Identify the high-energy intermediate in the carboxylation reaction.

4. In liver, V_{max} for fructose bisphosphatase is three to four times higher than V_{max} for phosphofructokinase, whereas in muscle it is only about 10 percent of that of phosphofructokinase. Explain this difference.

5. In muscle, lactate dehydrogenase produces lactate from pyruvate, whereas in the heart it preferentially synthesizes pyruvate from lactate. Explain how this is possible.

6. Briefly explain what the purpose is of each of the following steps in glycolysis? In other words, why are these steps necessary or useful?

    a) Glucose $\longrightarrow$ Glucose-6-P
    b) Glucose-6-P $\longrightarrow$ Fructose-6-phosphate
    c) Dihydroxyacetone-phosphate $\longrightarrow$ Glyceraldehyde-3-phosphate
    d) 2-Phosphoglycerate $\longrightarrow$ Phosphoenolpyruvate

ANSWERS TO PROBLEMS

1. Examination of the structures of the α-keto acid analogs of alanine, aspartate, and glutamate shows that each can be used for gluconeogenesis. Specific amino transferases convert alanine to pyruvate, aspartate to oxaloacetate, and glutamate to α-ketoglutarate. These amino acids, along with others whose carbon skeletons can be used for the synthesis of glucose, are termed glucogenic amino acids.

2. Gluconeogenesis requires six high-energy phosphate bonds for every two molecules of pyruvate converted to glucose. These phosphate molecules come from ATP, most of which is generated in the liver by oxidative phosphorylation in the presence of oxygen. Under anaerobic conditions, the only source of ATP is glycolysis, but only two molecules of ATP are produced per glucose converted to pyruvate. The extra price of generating glucose from pyruvate would lead to a deficit in the supply of ATP. The balance between gluconeogenesis and glycolysis is stringently controlled; therefore, it seems unlikely that ATP generation via glycolysis would occur if cellular conditions favored gluconeogenesis.

3. The carboxylation reaction produces an activated carboxyl group in the form of a high-energy carboxybiotin intermediate. The cleavage of this bond and release of CO_2 in the

phosphoenolpyruvate carboxykinase reaction or the transfer of the CO_2 to acceptors in other reactions in which biotin participates allows endergonic reactions to proceed. Thus, the formation of phosphoenolpyruvate from oxaloacetate is driven by the release of CO_2 ($\Delta G^{o\prime} = -19.7$ kJ/mol) and the hydrolysis of GTP ($\Delta G^{o\prime} = -30.6$ kJ/mol).

4. In contrast to muscle tissue, which oxidizes glucose to yield energy, liver tissue generates glucose primarily for export to other tissues. Thus, one would expect the rate of gluconeogenesis in the liver to be greater than the rate of glycolysis. Therefore, the relative catalytic capacity (as measured by V_{max}) of fructose bisphosphatase, a key enzyme in gluconeogenesis, should be expected to exceed that of phosphofructokinase, which is a regulatory enzyme of the glycolytic pathway.

5. Muscle and heart have distinct lactate dehydrogenase isozymes. Heart lactate dehydrogenase contains mostly H-type subunits. This enzyme has higher affinity for substrates and is inhibited by high concentrations of pyruvate; that is, it is designed to form pyruvate from lactate. In contrast, muscle lactate dehydrogenase, which consists of M-type subunits, is more effective for forming lactate from pyruvate.

6. (a) The negatively charged phosphate keeps glucose from diffusing out of the cell.

   (b) The isomerization reaction sets up the sugar for a second phosphorylation at C-1 and symmetric cleavage by aldolase.

   (c) The isomerization allows both 3-C sugars to be oxidized by the same pathway.

   (d) The isomerization converts 2-phosphoglycerate (a low energy compound) into phosphoenolpyruvate whose hydrolysis can be coupled to ATP synthesis.

Chapter 18

Preparation for the Cycle

Glycolysis metabolizes glucose to produce pyruvate. In order for the carbons of pyruvate to enter the citric acid cycle, and stage III of catabolism, the pyruvate must be converted into acetyl CoA. That is the subject of this short chapter. The conversion process is complicated enough that it must be handled by an enzyme complex, which has three different enzyme activities. The complex is known as the pyruvate dehydrogenase complex, and in eukaryotic cells it is found in the mitochondrial matrix. The overall reaction includes a decarboxylation and is irreversible. The chapter discusses each of the three enzymes and how they work together in the cell, along with their five cofactors. The chapter then goes on to describe the two ways that pyruvate dehydrogenase is regulated—one by feedback inhibition, and one by addition of a phosphate (by a kinase enzyme) and removal of that phosphate (by a phosphatase enzyme). Finally, a clinical point is made—pyruvate dehydrogenase complex is so important that anything that makes it stop working will cause a disease. And thus the nutritional disease, Beri-Beri, which is caused by a deficiency of thiamine (one of the five cofactors) resembles certain types of heavy-metal poisoning, which remove lipoic acid (another of the five cofactors).

LEARNING OBJECTIVES

When you have mastered this chapter, you should be able to accomplish the following objectives.

Pyruvate Dehydrogenase Forms Acetyl Coenzyme A From Pyruvate
(Text Section 18.1)

1. Outline the role of the *citric acid cycle* in aerobic metabolism.
2. Locate the enzymes of the citric acid cycle in eukaryotic cells.
3. Account for the origins of *acetyl CoA* from various metabolic sources.
4. Describe *pyruvate dehydrogenase* as a *multienzyme complex*.
5. List the *cofactors* that participate in the pyruvate dehydrogenase complex reactions and discuss the roles they play in the overall reaction.

The Pyruvate Dehydrogenase Complex Is Regulated by Two Mechanisms
(Text Section 18.2)

6. Describe the two ways in which the activity of the pyruvate dehydrogenase complex is controlled in mitochondria.
7. Summarize the *regulation* of the pyruvate dehydrogenase complex through reversible *phosphorylation*. List the major *activators* and *inhibitors* of the kinase and the phosphatase.
8. Explain the role of calcium ion in the covalent activation of the pyruvate dehydrogenase complex.
9. Describe the consequences and the biochemical basis of *thiamine deficiency*. Compare the effects of heavy-metal poisoning with mercury or arsenite.

SELF-TEST

Pyruvate Dehydrogenase Forms Acetyl Coenzyme A From Pyruvate

1. If a eukaryotic cell were broken open and the subcellular organelles were separated by zonal ultracentrifugation on a sucrose gradient, in which of the following organs would the citric acid cycle enzymes be found?

    (a) nucleus
    (b) lysosomes
    (c) Golgi complex
    (d) mitochondria
    (e) endoplasmic reticulum

2. What are the potential advantages of a multienzyme complex with respect to the isolated enzyme components? Explain.

3. Match the cofactors of the pyruvate dehydrogenase complex in the left column with their corresponding enzyme components and with their roles in the enzymatic steps in the right column.

    (a) coenzyme A
    (b) NAD^+
    (c) thiamine pyrophosphate
    (d) FAD
    (e) lipoamide

    (1) pyruvate dehydrogenase component
    (2) dihydrolipoyl dehydrogenase
    (3) dihydrolipoyl transacetylase
    (4) oxidizes the hydroxyethyl group
    (5) decarboxylates pyruvate

(6) oxidizes dihydrolipoamide
(7) accepts the acetyl group from acetyl-lipoamide
(8) provides a long, flexible arm that conveys intermediates to different enzyme components
(9) oxidizes $FADH_2$

The Pyruvate Dehydrogenase Complex Is Regulated by Two Mechanisms

4. What are the allosteric inhibitors of the pyruvate dehydrogenase complex?

5. Does phosphorylating pyruvate dehydrogenase complex ("PDC") make it active or inactive? Is there a general rule that phosphorylating enzymes activates all of them (or inactivates all of them)?

6. In the liver, calcium activation of the PDC leads to "cross talk" with the phosphatidyl inositol pathway (see Chapter 13 of the text). How does this occur?

7. How do heavy metals inhibit the PDC?

8. Which of the following answers complete the sentence correctly? The pyruvate dehydrogenase complex is activated by:
   (a) phosphorylation of the pyruvate dehydrogenase component (E1).
   (b) stimulation of a specific phosphatase by Ca^{2+}.
   (c) inhibition of a specific kinase by pyruvate.
   (d) decrease of the $NADH/NAD^+$ ratio.
   (e) decreased levels of insulin.

ANSWERS TO SELF-TEST

1. d

2. A multienzyme complex can carry out the coordinated catalysis of a complex reaction. The intermediates in the reaction remain bound to the complex and are passed from one enzyme component to the next, which increases the overall reaction rate and minimizes side reactions. In the case of isolated enzymes, the reaction intermediates would have to diffuse randomly between enzymes.

3. (a) 3, 7   (b) 2, 9   (c) 1, 5   (d) 2, 6   (e) 3, 4, 8

4. It makes it easy to remember the inhibitors if you notice that they are the products of the reaction. Acetyl CoA and NADH are the immediate products, and high ATP is an eventual product. Normally "feedback inhibition" involves a product from several steps farther down a pathway, but this is a true allosteric inhibition and not a simple "product inhibition" based on the principle of mass action.

5. When a kinase enzyme phosphorylates the pyruvate dehydrogenase complex, it inactivates it. But there is no rule that phosphorylating enzymes causes them to become inactive; it seems almost random, some enzymes are turned on by a phosphate and others are turned off. You have to learn the individual cases.

6. Calcium ion is a second messenger in the activation of protein kinase C, and it also is a potent activator of PDC in the liver. So stimulation of one system also stimulates another system.

7. They complex with lipoic acid; see Figure 18.13.

8. b, c, d

PROBLEMS

1. In addition to its role in the action of pyruvate dehydrogenase, thiamine pyrophosphate (TPP) serves as a cofactor for other enzymes, such as pyruvate decarboxylase, which catalyzes the *nonoxidative* decarboxylation of pyruvate. Propose a mechanism for the reaction catalyzed by pyruvate decarboxylase. What product would you expect? Why, in contrast to pyruvate dehydrogenase, are lipoamide and FAD not needed as cofactors for pyruvate decarboxylase?

2. (a) A cell is deficient in pyruvate dehydrogenase phosphate phosphatase. How would such a deficiency affect cellular metabolism?

   (b) A cell has a metabolic defect in the citric acid cycle that causes inhibition of prolyl dehydrogenase kinase 2, and consequent activation of HIF-1, hypoxia-inducible factor 1. Compare the metabolic effects of this situation to part "a" of this problem.

3. ATP is an important source of energy for muscle contraction. Pyruvate dehydrogenase phosphate phosphatase is activated by calcium ion, which increases greatly in concentration during exercise. Why is activation of the phosphatase consistent with the metabolic requirements of muscle during contraction?

4. As the textbook points out, the symptoms of Beriberi are very similar to the symptoms of arsenite poisoning. At first glance this seems impossible because two very different cofactors are affected; Beriberi is a deficiency of thiamine, and arsenite inactivates lipoamide. Explain how the two are linked, and explain why the symptoms are neurological.

ANSWERS TO PROBLEMS

1. The mechanism is similar to that shown on page 320 of the text, in which the C-2 carbanion of TPP attacks the α-keto group of pyruvate. The subsequent decarboxylation of pyruvate is enhanced by the delocalization of electrons in the ring nitrogen of TPP. The initial product is hydroxyethyl-TPP, which is cleaved on protonation to yield acetaldehyde and TPP. In contrast to the reaction catalyzed by pyruvate dehydrogenase, no net oxidation occurs, so lipoamide and FAD, which serve as electron acceptors, are not needed.

2. (a) Pyruvate dehydrogenase phosphate phosphatase removes a phosphoryl group from pyruvate dehydrogenase, activating the enzyme complex and accelerating the rate of synthesis of acetyl CoA. Cells deficient in phosphatase activity cannot activate pyruvate dehydrogenase, so that the rate of entry of acetyl groups into the citric acid cycle will decrease, as will aerobic production of ATP. Under such conditions, stimulation of glycolytic activity and a subsequent increase in lactate production would be expected as the cell responds to a continued requirement for ATP synthesis. See the clinical note on page 324 of the text (*phosphatase deficiency*).

   (b) As described in the second clinical note on page 325 (*development of cancer*), the metabolic state of the cell is rather similar to the situation in part "a" of this problem. But instead of a deficiency in pyruvate dehydrogenase phosphatase, we see an increase in pyruvate dehydrogenase kinase. So in both cases the PDH is phosphorylated and hence "off" or inactive. But under the circumstances, with high HIF-1, just as described in the previous chapter of the textbook, aerobic glycolysis is favored so that the accumulating pyruvate will be channeled toward formation of lactate. This appears to contribute to the development of certain cancers.

3. As discussed in the previous problem, the phosphatase activates pyruvate dehydrogenase, stimulating the rate of both glycolysis and the citric acid cycle. Calcium-mediated activation of pyruvate dehydrogenase therefore promotes increased production of ATP, which is then available for muscle contraction.

4. Both thiamine and lipoamide are cofactors of the pyruvate dehydrogenase complex. So a deficiency of either cofactor will cause the complex to slow down or shut down. As described in the textbook, if this enzyme is not working then pyruvate will accumulate and glycolysis will be blocked, not for want of glucose, but through accumulation of product. Because nerve tissue is particularly dependent on glycolysis, this will have a deleterious effect on nerve functions.

Chapter 19

Harvesting Electrons from the Cycle

The citric acid cycle, also known as the *tricarboxylic acid cycle* or the *Krebs cycle,* is the final oxidative pathway for carbohydrates, lipids, and amino acids. It is also a source of precursors for biosynthesis. The previous chapter has a detailed discussion of the reaction mechanisms of the pyruvate dehydrogenase complex. This chapter begins with a description of the reactions of the citric acid cycle. This description includes details of mechanism and stereospecificity of some of the reactions. In the following sections, they describe the stoichiometry of the pathway including the energy yield (ATP and GTP) and then describe control mechanisms. They conclude the chapter with a summary of the biosynthetic roles of the citric acid cycle and its relationship to the glyoxylate cycle found in bacteria and plants.

LEARNING OBJECTIVES

When you have mastered this chapter, you should be able to accomplish the following objectives.

The Citric Acid Cycle Consists of Two Stages (Text Section 19.1)

1. Define the two stages of the citric acid cycle.
2. Define the two stages of cellular respiration.

Stage One Oxidizes Two Carbon Atoms to Gather Energy-Rich Electrons (Text Section 19.2)

3. Outline the enzymatic mechanism of *citrate synthase*.
4. Explain the importance of the *induced-fit* structural rearrangements in citrate synthase during catalysis.
5. Compare the reaction catalyzed by the *α-ketoglutarate dehydrogenase complex* to the reaction catalyzed by the *pyruvate dehydrogenase complex*.

Stage Two Regenerates Oxaloacetate and Harvests Energy-Rich Electrons (Text Section 19.3)

6. Describe the high energy intermediate in succinyl CoA synthetase.
7. Name all the *intermediates* of the citric acid cycle and draw their structures.
8. List the enzymatic reactions of the citric acid cycle in their appropriate sequence. Name all the enzymes.
9. Give examples of *condensation, dehydration, hydration, decarboxylation, oxidation,* and *substrate-level phosphorylation* reactions.
10. Indicate the steps of the cycle that yield CO_2, *NADH*, $FADH_2$, and *GTP*. Note the biological roles of GTP.
11. Calculate the *yield of ATP* from the complete oxidation of pyruvate or of acetyl CoA.

The Citric Acid Cycle Is Regulated (Text Section 19.4)

12. Summarize the *regulation* of the pyruvate dehydrogenase complex through reversible *phosphorylation*. List the major *activators* and *inhibitors* of the kinase and phosphatase.
13. Indicate the *control points* of the citric acid cycle and note the activators and inhibitors.
14. Understand how prolyl hydroxylase 2 and HIF-1 interact with certain enzymes of the citric acid cycle in some forms of cancer.
15. Explain how cancer could be considered a "metabolic disease"?
16. Indicate the citric acid cycle intermediates that may be used as *biosynthetic precursors*.
17. Describe the role of *anaplerotic reactions* and discuss the *pyruvate carboxylase* reaction.

The Glyoxylate Cycle Enables Plants and Bacteria to Convert Fats into Carbohydrates (Text Section 19.5)

18. Compare the reactions of the *glyoxylate cycle* and those of the citric acid cycle. List the reactions that are unique to the glyoxylate cycle.

SELF-TEST

The Citric Acid Cycle Consists of Two Stages

1. Between succinyl CoA and oxaloacetate all reactions are reversible. Which "stage" of the citric acid cycle is this? Is the other "stage" also reversible, as a whole?

Stage One Oxidizes Two Carbon Atoms to Gather Energy-Rich Electrons

2. Which of the following statements concerning the enzymatic mechanism of citrate synthase is correct?
   (a) Citrate synthase uses an NAD^+ cofactor.
   (b) Acetyl CoA binds to citrate synthase before oxaloacetate.
   (c) The histidine residues at the active site of citrate synthase participate in the hydrolysis of acetyl CoA.
   (d) After citryl CoA is formed, additional structural changes occur in the enzyme.
   (e) Each of the citrate synthase subunits binds one of the substrates and brings the substrates into close proximity to each other.

3. Citrate synthase binds acetyl CoA, condenses it with oxaloacetate to form citryl CoA, and then hydrolyzes the thioester bond of this intermediate. Why doesn't citrate synthase hydrolyze acetyl CoA?

Stage Two Regenerates Oxaloacetate and Harvests Energy-Rich Electrons

4. Which of the following answers complete the sentence correctly? Succinate dehydrogenase
   (a) transfers electrons directly to coenzyme Q.
   (b) contains FAD and NAD^+ cofactors like pyruvate dehydrogenase.
   (c) is an integral membrane protein unlike the other enzymes of the citric acid cycle.
   (d) carries out an oxidative decarboxylation like isocitrate dehydrogenase.

5. The conversion of malate to oxaloacetate has a $\Delta G^{o\prime} = +29.7$ kJ/mol (7.1 kcal/mol), yet in the citric acid cycle the reaction proceeds from malate to oxaloacetate. Explain how this is possible.

6. Given the biochemical intermediates of the pyruvate dehydrogenase reaction and the citric acid cycle (Figure 19.1), answer the following questions.
   (a) Name the intermediates **A** and **B**.
   (b) Draw the structure of isocitrate and show those atoms that come from acetyl CoA in bold letters.
   (c) Which reaction is catalyzed by α-ketoglutarate dehydrogenase?
   (d) Which enzyme catalyzes step 2?
   (e) Which reactions are oxidations? Name the enzyme that catalyzes each of them.
   (f) At which reaction does a substrate-level phosphorylation occur? Name the enzyme and the products of this reaction.
   (g) Which of the reactions require an FAD cofactor? Name the enzymes.
   (h) Indicate the decarboxylation reactions and name the enzymes.

FIGURE 19.1 Citric acid cycle and the pyruvate dehydrogenase reaction.

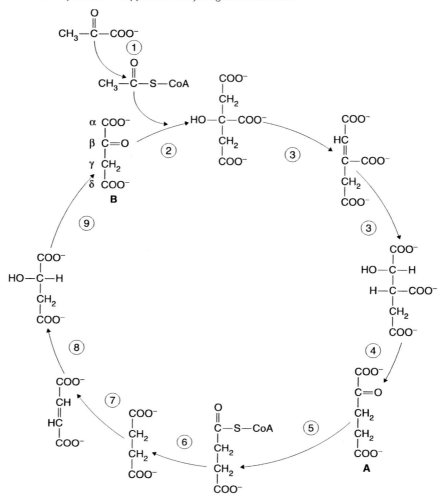

7. If the methyl carbon atom of pyruvate is labeled with ^{14}C, which of the carbon atoms of oxaloacetate would be labeled after one turn of the citric acid cycle? (See the lettering scheme for oxaloacetate in Figure 19.1 in this book.) Note that the "new" acetate carbons are the two shown at the bottom of the first few structures in the cycle, because aconitase reacts stereospecifically.

   (a) None. The label will be lost in CO_2.
   (b) α
   (c) β
   (d) γ
   (e) δ

8. Considering the citric acid cycle steps between α-ketoglutarate and malate, how many high-energy phosphate bonds, or net ATP molecules, can be generated?

   (a) 4   (d) 10
   (b) 5   (e) 12
   (c) 7

9. The standard free-energy change (in terms of net ATP production) when glucose is converted to 6 CO_2 and 6 H_2O is about how many times as great as the free-energy change when glucose is converted to two lactate molecules?

   (a) 2   (c) 15
   (b) 7   (d) 28

10. Although O_2 does not participate directly in the reactions of the citric acid cycle, the cycle operates only under aerobic conditions. Explain this fact.

The Citric Acid Cycle Is Regulated

11. First select the enzymes in the left column that regulate the citric acid cycle. Then match them with the appropriate control mechanisms in the right column.

(a) citrate synthase
(b) aconitase
(c) isocitrate dehydrogenase
(d) α-ketoglutarate dehydrogenase
(e) succinyl CoA synthetase
(f) succinate dehydrogenase
(g) fumarase
(h) malate dehydrogenase

(1) feedback inhibited by succinyl CoA
(2) allosterically activated by ADP
(3) inhibited by NADH
(4) regulated by the availability of acetyl CoA and oxaloacetate
(5) inhibited by ATP

12. Match the intermediates of the citric acid cycle in the left column with their biosynthetic products in mammals, in the right column.

(a) citrate
(b) α-ketoglutarate
(c) succinyl CoA
(d) cis-aconitate
(e) oxaloacetate

(1) aspartic acid
(2) glutamic acid
(3) cholesterol
(4) porphyrins
(5) none

13. Which of the following answers complete the sentence correctly? Pyruvate carboxylase

(a) catalyzes the reversible decarboxylation of oxaloacetate.
(b) requires thiamine pyrophosphate as a cofactor.
(c) is allosterically activated by NADH.
(d) requires ATP.
(e) is found in the cytoplasm of eukaryotic cells.

14. Although the ATP/ADP ratio and the availability of substrates and cycle intermediates are very important factors affecting the rate of the citric acid cycle, the $NADH/NAD^+$ ratio is of paramount importance. Explain why.

15. Prolyl hydroxylase 2 (PHD-2) regulates Hypoxia-Inducible Factor 1 (HIF-1). How does the regulation work? What is the cofactor for PHD-2? Have you seen a similar reaction with the same cofactor before?

16. Which specific enzymes of the citric acid cycle appear to be related to cancer, as described in the textbook?

The Glyoxylate Cycle Enables Plants and Bacteria to Convert Fats Into Carbohydrates

17. Malate synthase, an enzyme of the glyoxylate cycle, catalyzes the condensation of glyoxylate with acetyl CoA. Which enzyme of the citric acid cycle carries out a similar reaction? Would you expect the binding of glyoxylate and acetyl CoA to malate synthase to be sequential? Why?

18. All organisms require three- and four-carbon precursor molecules for biosynthesis, yet bacteria can grow on acetate whereas mammals cannot. Explain why this is so.

19. Starting with acetyl CoA, what is the approximate yield of high-energy phosphate bonds (net ATP formed) via the glyoxylate cycle?
    (a) 3
    (b) 6
    (c) 9
    (d) 12
    (e) 15

ANSWERS TO SELF-TEST

1. Succinyl CoA to osaloacetate is the second stage. The rest of the cycle is stage one, and it is irreversible (although it contains reversible steps) largely due to decarboxylations.

2. d

3. Citrate synthase binds acetyl CoA only after oxaloacetate has been bound and the enzyme structure is rearranged to create a binding site for acetyl CoA. After citryl CoA is formed, there are further structural changes that bring an aspartate residue and a water molecule into the vicinity of the thioester bond for the hydrolysis step. Thus, acetyl CoA is protected from hydrolysis.

4. a, c

5. Although this step is energetically unfavorable in standard conditions, in mitochondria the concentrations of malate and NAD^+ are relatively high and the concentrations of the products, oxaloacetate and NADH, are quite low, so the overall ΔG for this reaction is negative.

6. (a) **A**: α-ketoglutarate; **B**: oxaloacetate
   (b) See the structure of isocitrate in the margin. The text doesn't go into detail about the stereochemistry of the enzyme aconitase, but the enzyme always puts the double bond and then the hydroxyl on the side of the molecule away from the "new" carbons introduced from Acetyl CoA.

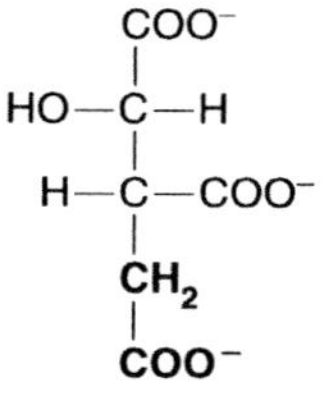

$$
\begin{array}{c}
COO^- \\
| \\
HO-C-H \\
| \\
H-C-COO^- \\
| \\
CH_2 \\
| \\
COO^-
\end{array}
$$

Isocitrate

   (c) reaction 5
   (d) citrate synthase
   (e) step 1, pyruvate dehydrogenase; step 4, isocitrate dehydrogenase; step 5, α-ketoglutarate dehydrogenase; step 7, succinate dehydrogenase; step 9, malate dehydrogenase
   (f) step 6; the enzyme is succinyl CoA synthetase; the products of the reaction are succinate, CoA, and GTP.
   (g) step 1, dihydrolipoyl dehydrogenase component of the pyruvate dehydrogenase complex; step 5, dihydrolipoyl dehydrogenase component of the α-ketoglutarate dehydrogenase complex; step 7, succinate dehydrogenase.
   (h) step 1, pyruvate dehydrogenase; step 4, isocitrate dehydrogenase; step 5, α-ketoglutarate dehydrogenase.

7. c and d. Both the middle carbons of oxaloacetate will be labeled because succinate is a symmetrical molecule.

8. b

9. c. From glucose to lactate, two ATP are formed; from glucose to CO_2 and H_2O, about 30 ATP are formed.

10. The citric acid cycle requires the oxidized cofactors NAD^+ and FAD for its oxidation–reduction reactions. The oxidized cofactors are regenerated by transfer of electrons through the electron transport chain to O_2 to give H_2O (see Chapter 18).

11. b, c, d

12. (a) 3   (b) 2   (c) 4   (d) 5   (e) 1

13. a, d

14. The oxidized cofactors NAD^+ and FAD are absolutely required as electron acceptors in the various dehydrogenation reactions of the citric acid cycle. When these oxidized cofactors are not available, as when their reoxidation stops in the absence of O_2 or respiration, the citric acid cycle also stops.

15. Normally PHD-2 hydroxylates proline residues on HIF-1, which causes it to be destroyed in the proteasome. The cofactor for the reaction is ascorbate, or vitamin C, although the enzyme also requires oxygen and α-ketoglutarate. Near the end of Chapter 2 in the textbook there is a discussion of the disease scurvy, which is caused by a lack of vitamin C. Specifically scurvy is a lack of mature collagen. One of the main differences between procollagen and collagen is that many of the proline residues have to be hydroxylated. So that is another prolyl hydroxylase that requires ascorbate as its cofactor.

16. The book mentions succinate dehydrogenase, fumarase, and pyruvate dehydrogenase kinase. The enzymes that are directly part of the citric acid cycle (succinate DH and fumarase) can be defective or lacking, in which case succinate and fumarate build up and spill out into the cytoplasm from the mitochondrial matrix. These are competitive inhibitors of PHD-2.

17. The condensation of glyoxylate and acetyl CoA carried out by malate synthase in the glyoxylate cycle is similar to the condensation of oxaloacetate and acetyl CoA carried out by citrate synthase in the citric acid cycle. The initial binding of glyoxylate, which induces structural changes in the enzyme that allow the subsequent binding of acetyl CoA, would be expected in order to prevent the premature hydrolysis of acetyl CoA. See Question 5.

18. Bacteria are capable, via the glyoxylate cycle, of synthesizing four-carbon precursor molecules for biosynthesis (for example, malate) from acetate or acetyl CoA. Mammals do not have an analogous mechanism; in the citric acid cycle, the carbon atoms from acetyl CoA are released as CO_2, and there is no net synthesis of four-carbon molecules.

19. a. One NADH is formed that can yield approximately 2.5 molecules of ATP.

PROBLEMS

1. Oysters and some other mollusks live their adult lives permanently cemented to a support on the seafloor. The local environment can occasionally become anaerobic. This means that these higher animals have to function as *facultative anaerobes*. When oysters are deprived of oxygen, they accumulate succinate. Even though the citric acid cycle cannot be run as a cycle in the absence of oxygen, the reactions can be exploited in a way that maintains redox balance. The "four-carbon" reactions are run

backward, from oxaloacetate to succinate, which produces reduced NAD^+ and FAD. Simultaneously, the cycle runs forward from citrate to succinate, which produces two molecules of NADH. Assuming that the oysters manage a steady supply of oxaloacetate to run these reactions, how much energy would they derive from this process?

2. Sodium fluoroacetate is a controversial poison also known as *compound 1080*. When an isolated rat heart is perfused with sodium fluoroacetate, the rate of glycolysis decreases and hexose monophosphates accumulate. In cardiac cells, fluoroacetate is condensed with oxaloacetate to give fluorocitrate. Under these conditions, cellular citrate concentrations increase while the levels of other citric acid cycle components decrease. What enzyme is inhibited by fluorocitrate? How can you account for the decrease in glycolysis and the buildup of hexose monophosphates?

3. The conversion of citrate to isocitrate in the citric acid cycle actually occurs by a dehydration-rehydration reaction with aconitate as an isolatable intermediate. A single enzyme, aconitase, catalyzes the conversion of citrate to aconitate and aconitate to isocitrate. An equilibrium mixture of citrate, aconitate, and isocitrate contains about 90%, 4%, and 6% of the three acids, respectively.

   (a) Why must citrate be converted to isocitrate before oxidation takes place in the citric acid cycle?
   (b) What are the respective equilibrium constants and standard free-energy changes for each of the two steps (citrate $\rightleftharpoons$ aconitate; aconitate $\rightleftharpoons$ isocitrate)? For the overall process at 25°C?
   (c) Could the citric acid cycle proceed under standard conditions? Why or why not?
   (d) Given the thermodynamic data you have gathered about the reactions catalyzed by aconitase, how can the citric acid cycle proceed under cellular conditions?

4. Lipoic acid and FAD serve as prosthetic groups in the enzyme isocitrate dehydrogenase. Describe their possible roles in the reaction catalyzed by the enzyme.

5. Malonate anion is a potent competitive inhibitor of succinate dehydrogenase, which catalyzes the conversion of succinate to fumarate.

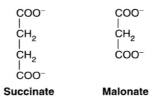

Succinate   **Malonate**

   (a) Why is malonate unreactive?
   (b) In work that led to the elucidation of the citric acid cycle, Hans Krebs employed malonate as an inhibitor of succinate dehydrogenase. Earlier studies by Martius and Knoop had shown that in animal tissues there is a pathway from citrate to succinate. Krebs had also noticed that citrate catalytically enhances respiration in minced muscle tissues. Knowing that malonate reduces the rate of respiration in animal cells, he then added citrate to malonate-poisoned muscle. In another experiment, Krebs added fumarate to malonate-poisoned muscle. What changes in succinate concentration did Krebs observe in each of the experiments with malonate-treated muscle, and what was the significance of each finding?
   (c) Krebs carried out a final set of crucial studies by showing that citrate can be formed in muscle suspensions if oxaloacetate is added. What is the significance of this experiment, and how did it provide a coherent scheme for terminal oxidation of carbon atoms?

6. Recent studies suggest that succinate dehydrogenase activity is affected by oxaloacetate. Would you expect the enzyme activity to be enhanced or inhibited by oxaloacetate?

7. Winemakers have to understand some biochemistry to know what is happening as crushed grapes turn to wine. The major pathway involved is glycolysis, leading to ethanol and CO_2. Early bottling can lead to sparkling wine as more CO_2 is produced. A secondary fermentation is allowed to take place in many wines, both red and white, called "malolactic fermentation." This fermentation is classically produced by bacteria that have an enzyme that binds L-malic acid and decarboxylates it to form L-lactate. This process alters the flavor, making the wine more complex and less acidic. The secondary fermentation is so desirable that biotechnologists inserted the gene for this enzyme into *Saccharomyces cerevisiae,* the yeast used to ferment wine or beer. Initial experiments failed to produce malolactic fermentation using only yeast, but after some thought, researchers inserted another gene into the yeast and the process succeeded.

   (a) Why does wine taste less acidic when malate is converted into lactate?

   (b) What was the second gene that researchers had to insert to make the process work?

8. The fermentation process for beer or Scotch whiskey begins with barley. The grains are moistened and allowed to swell and almost sprout (the process is called "malting") and then they are roasted in an oven (an "oast") before they are fermented. Why couldn't one simply grind up the grains, mix with water, and ferment without bothering with the malting process? What pathway is involved (one that humans do not have)?

9. In addition to the carboxylation of pyruvate, there are other anaplerotic reactions that help to maintain appropriate levels of oxaloacetate. For example, the respective amino groups of glutamate and aspartate can be removed to yield the corresponding α-keto acids. How can these α-keto acids be used to replenish oxaloacetate levels?

10. The oxidation of a fatty acid with an even number of carbon atoms yields a number of molecules of acetyl CoA, whereas the oxidation of an odd-numbered fatty acid yields molecules of not only acetyl CoA but also propionyl CoA, which then gives rise to succinyl CoA. Why does only the oxidation of odd-numbered fatty acids lead to the *net* synthesis of oxaloacetate?

ANSWERS TO PROBLEMS

1. Notice that the oysters (and other organisms) are running stage one forward and stage two backward, and accumulating succinate. This gives one GTP directly from succinyl CoA synthetase. The fact that stage one yields NADH by oxidizing substrate while stage two backwards is reducing substrates to yield NAD^+ and FAD actually leads to more energy, generated in the electron-transport chain (see next chapter). Some people think the citric acid cycle evolved from two linear pathways.

2. The accumulation of citrate and the decrease in the levels of other citric acid cycle intermediates suggest that aconitase is inhibited by fluorocitrate. Excess citrate inhibits phosphofructokinase, causing a decrease in the rate of glycolysis and an accumulation of hexose monophosphates such as glucose 6-phosphate and fructose 1,6-bisphosphate. The controversy over compound 1080 is between environmentalists, who want it banned from outdoor use, and farmers and ranchers, who find it useful against rodents and predators. Because of the way it acts on cells, there is no antidote and it produces a slow and painful death.

3. (a) The oxidation of isocitrate involves oxidation of a secondary alcohol. Citrate has an alcohol function, but it is a tertiary alcohol, which is much more difficult to oxidize. Isomerization of citrate to isocitrate provides an easier route to oxidative decarboxylation.

   (b) For the citrate–aconitate pair, the equilibrium constant is equal to the ratio of product and substrate concentration. Because $K_{eq} = (4/90) = 0.0444$, the value of the standard free-energy change for the citrate-aconitate pair would be

$$\Delta G^{o\prime} = -RT \ln K_{eq} = -0.0083 \, (298) \ln (4.44 \times 10^{-2})$$
$$= (-2.47) \times (-3.11) = +7.68 \text{ kJ/mol}$$

Similar calculations for the aconitate-isocitrate pair give $K_{eq} = 6/4 = 1.5$ and thus for the aconitate isocitrate pair we would have

$$= -0.0083(298) \ln (1.5) =$$
$$(-2.47) \times (0.405) = -1.00 \text{ kJ/mol}$$

Summing the two numbers, we get

$$= 7.68 - 1.00 = + 6.68 \text{ kJ/mol}$$

[In calories, $\Delta G^{o\prime}$ is $-1.36 \log_{10} (4.44 \times 10^{-2}) = -1.36(-1.35) = +1.84$ kcal/mol for the citrate–aconitate pair. Similar calculations for the aconitate–isocitrate pair give $K_{eq} = 6/4 = 1.5$ and of $\Delta G^{o\prime} = -0.24$ kcal/mol.

The overall standard free-energy value for the conversion of citrate to isocitrate is the sum of the two values for the individual reactions:

$$\Delta G^{o\prime} = 1.84 + (-0.24) = +1.60 \text{ kcal/mol.]}$$

(c) Under standard conditions, the citric acid cycle could not proceed because the positive free-energy value for the reaction indicates that it would proceed toward net formation of citrate. Note that under standard conditions, everything would be present at 1 molar concentration.

(d) The net conversion of citrate to isocitrate can occur in the mitochondrion if the isocitrate produced is then converted to α-ketoglutarate. This would lower the concentration of isocitrate, pulling the reaction toward net formation of that molecule. Concentrations of citrate could also be increased, driving the reaction once again toward the formation of isocitrate. Although accurate concentrations of metabolites in mitochondria are difficult to establish, it appears that both mechanisms may operate to ensure net isocitrate synthesis.

4. Lipoic acid contains a sulfhydryl group that could act as an acceptor for electrons from isocitrate. Those electrons could then be transferred to NAD$^+$ via FAD. The roles of the prosthetic groups would be similar to those they play in the reaction catalyzed by pyruvate dehydrogenase.

5. (a) Succinate, which has two methylene groups, loses two hydrogens during its oxidation by succinate dehydrogenase. Malonate, which has only one methylene group, cannot be dehydrogenated and is therefore unreactive.

(b) In both experiments, Krebs observed an increase in the concentration of succinate. We know now that both citrate and fumarate can be viewed as precursors of succinate or other components of the citric acid cycle. A malonate-induced block in the conversion of succinate to fumarate would cause an increase in succinate concentration. The first experiment, in which citrate addition caused an increase in succinate concentration, showed that the pathway from citrate to succinate is physiologically significant and is related to the process of respiration using carbohydrates as a fuel. The second experiment with fumarate suggested that a pathway from fumarate to succinate exists that is separate from the reaction catalyzed by succinate dehydrogenase. Krebs realized that a cyclic pathway could account for all these observations. The piece of the puzzle that was left was to learn how citrate might be generated from pyruvate or acetate. The results from those experiments are described in (c).

(c) The generation of citrate from oxaloacetate enabled Krebs to devise a scheme that incorporated two-carbon molecules from acetate or pyruvate into citrate, with oxaloacetate serving as an acceptor of the carbon atoms. He then was able to use the results of his experiments and those of others to show how a cyclic pathway could function to carry out oxidation of carbon molecules while regenerating oxaloacetate. Krebs was prepared for the development of the cyclic scheme because he had shown earlier that the ornithine cycle, which is used for urea synthesis, is also a cyclic metabolic pathway. Krebs's famous paper, which describes the entire cycle as well as the malonate inhibition study, appeared in *Enzymologia* 4(1937):148.

6. Oxaloacetate is derived from succinate by the sequential action of succinate dehydrogenase, fumarase, and malate dehydrogenase. When levels of oxaloacetate are high, one would expect the activity of the enzyme to be reduced. Low levels of oxaloacetate would call for an increase in succinate production.

7. (a) Malic acid has two carboxyl groups. Lactic acid has only one. The pH of the wine changes significantly as malate is converted into lactate and carbon dioxide.

   (b) The yeast cells with the extra gene for the malolactic enzyme were quite capable of running the reaction, but they had no transport system for malate. The researchers realized that they could also insert a gene for malate permease, which would allow malate to enter the yeast cells and be metabolized. With both genes, the system started working well. An example of a malate transporters is shown in the next chapter, see Figure 21.12 and Figure 21.4.

8. Fermentation starts with sugar. All that is inside un-malted barley (or many other grains) is starch and oil. The pathway involved here is the glyoxylate cycle, which allows many plants to convert stored supplies of oil into acetyl CoA, and then build the acetyl units up into molecules of glucose. By moistening the barley we convince the seeds that it is springtime and so they make a lot of glucose in preparation for turning it into cellulose for sprouts and leaves and roots. Roasting the malt kills the seeds and arrests the process at a stage where there is maximum sugar. At this point you have something that is easily fermented. As a side note, the smoke from the roasting process is what gives some Scotch whiskeys a smoky aroma.

9. Examination of the structures of the α-keto acid analogs of glutamate and aspartate shows that they are in fact both citric acid cycle intermediates, α-ketoglutarate and oxaloacetate. Aspartate, when it is deaminated, thus contributes directly to the insertion of additional molecules of oxaloacetate. Glutamate produces α-ketoglutarate, which, as a component of the citric acid cycle, is a precursor of oxaloacetate.

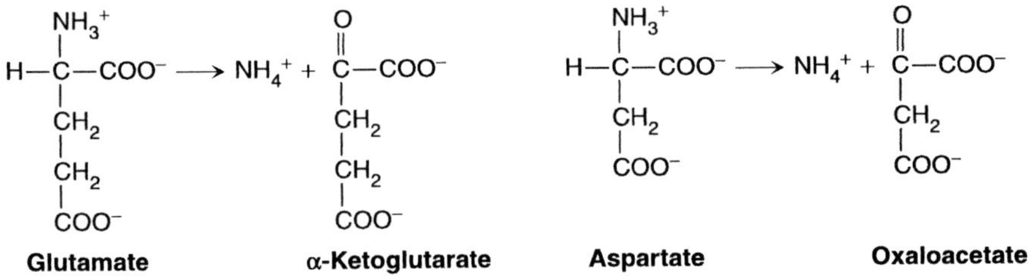

Glutamate   α-Ketoglutarate   Aspartate   Oxaloacetate

10. The entry of acetyl groups from acetyl CoA into the citric acid cycle does not contribute to the net synthesis of oxaloacetate, because two carbons are lost as CO_2 in the pathway from citrate to oxaloacetate. Only the entry of compounds with three or more carbons, like succinate, can increase the relative number of carbon atoms in the pathway. Thus, although odd-numbered fatty acids contribute to the net synthesis of oxaloacetate, compounds with an even number of fatty acids do not.

The Electron-Transport Chain

This is the first of two chapters that describe *respiration* in the *mitochondria*. The word respiration can mean "breathing," and in fact mitochondrial *electron transport* is one of the main reasons why we need to breathe. Mitochondria use up large amounts of oxygen as electron acceptors. This chapter is about the mitochondrial *respiratory chain*, also known as the *electron-transport chain*. A series of reactions take place in the mitochondrial *inner membrane*, removing electrons from cofactors such as NADH and $FADH_2$, and moving the electrons through lower-energy electron carriers until finally they are transferred to oxygen to form water. The process of electron transport is inextricably linked with *pumping of protons* from the inner "matrix" side of the mitochondrial inner membrane over to the outside of the inner membrane, the *intermembrane space*. The pumped protons form a *gradient* which is a source of stored energy. The next chapter will complete the story of respiration by describing how ATP can be made using the energy of the *proton gradient*.

This chapter also shows how to deal with the mathematical connection between *reduction potentials* and the free-energy change of reactions. The structures and actions of electron carriers including *flavin mononucleotide, iron sulfur clusters, heme groups,* and *coenzyme Q* are shown. And whenever molecular oxygen is involved there is some danger of producing *free radicals* via *ROS* or *reactive oxygen species*. This is discussed in some detail.

LEARNING OBJECTIVES

When you have mastered this chapter, you should be able to accomplish the following objectives.

Oxidative Phosphorylation in Eukaryotes Takes Place in Mitochondria
(Text Section 20.1)

1. Compare the amount of ATP required for a typical day's worth of activity to that stored in a sedentary male. Recognize the implications of the disparity and how a human body compensates for it.

2. Describe the *compartments* and *membranes of mitochondria* and locate the *respiratory assemblies* and the *N* and *P sides* of the inner membrane.

3. Provide a hypothesis for the evolutionary origin of mitochondria.

Oxidative Phosphorylation Depends on Electron Transfer (Text Section 20.2)

4. Relate quantitatively *redox potential* ($\Delta E_0'$) and *free-energy change* ($\Delta G^{o'}$).

5. Describe the meaning and the measurement of the redox potential (E_0') for a *redox couple* relative to the *standard reference half-cell*.

6. Explain the meaning of E_0' in electron transfer.

7. Calculate ΔG^o for *oxidation–reduction reactions* from the redox potentials for individual redox couples.

8. Identify the driving force of oxidative phosphorylation and be able to calculate the amount of chemical work that can be coupled to the reduction of O_2 with NADH.

9. Calculate the free energy associated with a proton gradient.

The Respiratory Chain Consists of Proton Pumps and a Physical Link to the Citric Acid Cycle (Text Section 20.3)

10. List the components of the *respiratory chain* and the *electron-carrying molecules*.

11. Describe the entry of electrons from *NADH* into *NADH-Q oxidoreductase (Complex I)* and trace their path through this *proton pump*. State the roles of *flavin mononucleotide (FMN)*, *iron-sulfur clusters*, and *coenzyme Q*.

12. Distinguish among the *quinone, semiquinone,* and *ubiquinol* forms of coenzyme Q. Explain how reduction of a quinone can consume two protons.

13. Discuss the role of coenzyme Q as a mobile electron carrier between *NADH-Q oxidoreductase* and *cytochrome reductase (Complex III)*.

14. Describe the entry of electrons into the respiratory chain at the *succinate-Q reductase complex (Complex II)* from *flavoproteins* such as *succinate dehydrogenase* (a component of Complex II), *glycerol phosphate dehydrogenase*, and *fatty acyl CoA dehydrogenase* by way of $FADH_2$. Appreciate that Complex II is not a proton pump.

15. Describe the prosthetic group and the functions of the *cytochromes* and contrast the features of cytochromes b, c_1, c, a, and a_3.

16. List the components of the *Q-cytochrome c oxidoreductase complex*, and explain how *ubiquinol* transfers its electrons to cytochromes c_1 and b and ultimately to cytochrome c. Describe the roles of *heme* in these processes.

17. Explain the origin of the nomenclature used in cytochrome b (heme b_L and heme b_H). Give a physical explanation for the difference between redox potentials of the two hemes.

18. Explain how a two-electron carrier, ubiquinol, can interact with a one-electron carrier, the *Fe-S cluster*. Describe the steps of the Q cycle and write a balanced reaction for the cycle.

19. Describe the *cytochrome oxidase proton pump (Complex IV)* and its electron-carrying groups. Write a balanced reaction for the process catalyzed by cytochrome c oxidase.

20. Outline the mechanism for the reduction of O_2 to H_2O on cytochrome oxidase. Describe the path of the electrons from the *heme a–CuA* cluster to the *heme a₃–CuB* cluster and state the changes in the oxidation states of Fe and O. Note the formation of a *superoxide anion* intermediate.

21. Describe the salient features of the three-dimensional structure of cytochrome *c* and relate them to its interaction with cytochrome reductase and cytochrome oxidase.

22. List the *reactive oxygen species* that are generated during electron transport. Explain why oxygen is a potentially toxic substance. Summarize the reactions and the biological roles of *superoxide dismutase, catalase,* and the *peroxidases.*

SELF-TEST

Oxidative Phosphorylation in Eukaryotes Takes Place in Mitochondria

1. For a sedentary male weighing 70 kg, how much more ATP is needed each day than than is present in the body?
   (a) 83 kg
   (b) 250 g
   (c) 82.75 kg
   (d) 82.75 g
   (e) None of the above. The body contains the amount needed.

2. Which of the following statements regarding mitochondria and their components are correct?
   (a) Mitochondria are approximately 20 nm in diameter.
   (b) The matrix compartment contains the enzymes of glycolysis.
   (c) Mitochondria are bounded by two membrane systems: an inner membrane and an outer membrane.
   (d) The inner membrane contains pores and is readily permeable to most small metabolites.
   (e) The inner membrane has a large surface area because it is highly folded.

3. Which of the following answers complete the sentence correctly? Mitochondria
   (a) are found in all kingdoms of life.
   (b) are semiautonomous organelles.
   (c) all contain proteins encoded by their own genes and encoded by the nuclear genome.
   (d) likely arose from the engulfment of a virus by a bacterium.

Oxidative Phosphorylation Depends on Electron Transfer

4. Which of the following statements about the redox potential for a reaction are correct?
   (a) It is used to describe phosphate group transfers.
   (b) It is unrelated to the free energy of the reaction.
   (c) It can be used to predict whether a given compound can reduce another.
   (d) It can be used to predict whether a given oxidation will provide sufficient energy for the formation of ATP from ADP and P_i.
   (e) It can be used to predict the rate of O_2 uptake upon the oxidation of a given substrate.

5. The equation for the reduction of cytochrome *a* by cytochrome *c* is

$$Cyt\ a\ (+3) + Cyt\ c\ (+2) \longrightarrow Cyt\ a\ (+2) + Cyt\ c\ (+3)$$

$$where\ Cyt\ a\ (+3) + e^- \longrightarrow Cyt\ a\ (+2): E_0' = 027\ V$$

$$Cyt\ c\ (+3) + e^- \longrightarrow Cyt\ c\ (+2): E_0' = +0.22\ V$$

Which of the following answers completes the sentence correctly? Under standard conditions ([products] = [reactants] = [1M]; pH = 7), the reaction

(a) proceeds spontaneously.
(b) yields sufficient energy for ATP synthesis.
(c) does not alter the absorption spectra of the cytochromes.
(d) involves the transfer of two electrons.

6. What is the $\Delta G^{o'}$ value for the following reaction? Use Table 20.1 in the text for values of $E^{o'}$. Note that 1 kcal = 4.187 kJ.

succinate + FAD $\longrightarrow$ fumarate + FADH$_2$

(a) +5.79 kJ/mol
(b) −2.89 kJ/mol
(c) +0.59 kJ/mol
(d) +2.89 kJ/mol
(e) −5.79 kJ/mol

7. The parameters $\Delta G^{o'}$ and $\Delta E_0'$ can be used to predict the direction of chemical reactions in standard conditions. On the other hand, $\Delta G'$ can be used for any concentration of reactants and products to predict in what direction a chemical reaction will proceed. Using the expressions

$$\Delta G' = \Delta G^{o'} + RT \ln \frac{[products]}{[reactants]}\ and\ \Delta G' = -nF\Delta E_0'$$

derive an expression for $\Delta E'$. Explain the significance of this redox potential.

8. Obtain $\Delta G'$ and $\Delta E'$ for the reaction given in question 6 when the succinate concentration is 2×10^{-3} M, the fumarate concentration is 0.5×10^{-3} M, the FAD concentration is 2×10^{-3} M, the FADH$_2$ concentration is 0.2×10^{-3} M, and the temperature is 37°C. ($R = 8.314$ J/mol K)

9. For each proton transported out of the matrix across the inner membrane and into the inner membrane space of a mitochondrion, how much free-energy potential is generated across the inner membrane?

(a) −220.2 kJ/mol
(b) −30.6 kJ/mol
(c) −2.18 kJ/mol
(d) −21.8 kJ/mol

The Respiratory Chain Consists of Four Complexes: Three Proton Pumps and a Physical Link to the Citric Acid Cycle

10. Place the following respiratory-chain components in their proper sequence. Also, indicate which are mobile carriers of electrons.

(a) cytochrome *c*
(b) NADH-Q oxidoreductase
(c) cytochrome *c* oxidase
(d) ubiquinone
(e) Q-cytochrome *c* oxidoreductase

11. Match the enzyme complexes of the respiratory chain in the left column with the appropriate electron-carrying groups in the right column.

(a) cytochrome c oxidase
(b) Q-cytochrome c oxidoreductase
(c) NADH-Q oxidoreductase
(d) succinate-Q reductase

(1) heme c_1
(2) FAD
(3) heme a_3
(4) heme b_L
(5) iron-sulfur complexes
(6) Cu_A and Cu_B
(7) FMN
(8) heme a
(9) heme b_H

12. Which of the following statements about the enzyme complexes of the electron transport system are correct?

(a) They are located in the mitochondrial matrix.
(b) They cannot be isolated from one another in functional form.
(c) They have very similar visible spectra.
(d) They are integral membrane proteins located in the inner mitochondrial membrane.
(e) They transfer electrons to one another by means of mobile electron carriers.

13. Which of the following statements about ubiquinol are correct?

(a) It is the mobile electron carrier between cytochrome c oxidoreductase and cytochrome c oxidase.
(b) It is an integral membrane protein.
(c) Its oxidation involves the simultaneous transfer of two electrons to the Fe-S center of cytochrome reductase.
(d) It is oxidized to ubiquinone by way of a semiquinone intermediate.
(e) It is a lipid-soluble molecule.

14. Which cytochrome has a protoporphyrin IX heme that is not covalently bound to protein?

(a) cytochrome a
(b) cytochrome a_3
(c) cytochrome b
(d) cytochrome c
(e) cytochrome c_1

15. Explain the roles of cytochrome c_1 and the b cytochromes (b_L and b_H) in the oxidation of ubiquinol to ubiquinone. Are protons pumped across the inner mitochondrial membrane during these reactions?

16. In the reduction of O_2 to H_2O by cytochrome oxidase, four electrons and four protons are used. How can this occur when a single electron at a time is transferred by heme iron and by copper?

17. Which of the following answers correctly complete the sentance? Reactive oxygen species (ROS)

(a) serve as substrates for enzymes that render them less reactive.
(b) arise from intermediates generated in electron transport.
(c) are transported out of the cell on specialized carriers.
(d) include OH·, H_2O_2, O_2^{2-}.

18. How can the $FADH_2$ generated by the succinate-Q-reductase complex participate in electron transport if it is not free to diffuse from the enzyme complex? Does the oxidation of succinate transport protons?

19. Which of the following statements about an aerated, functional mitochondrial preparation in which the reduced substrate is succinate are correct?

    (a) Approximately 1.5 ATP molecules will be formed per succinate oxidized to fumarate.
    (b) Approximately two protons will be pumped across the inner membrane by the succinate-Q reductase complex.
    (c) The addition of CN^- will result in the synthesis of only one ATP per succinate.
    (d) Reduction of NADH-Q oxidoreductase will occur.
    (e) Reduction of Q-cytochrome oxidoreductase will occur.

20. Run-off of artificial fertilizers near the coast of Louisiana causes large blooms of phytoplankton. Phytoplankton are photosynthesizers, so they produce oxygen while they are alive. How can this lead to formation of a "dead zone" where there is not enough oxygen to support shrimp and crab populations?

ANSWERS TO SELF-TEST

1. c. Approximately 83 kg is needed per day but only 250 g (0.250 kg) is present. That means there is a 83 kg − 0.25 kg = 82.75 kg deficit.

2. c, e. Answer (a) is incorrect because mitochrondia are ~500 nm in diameter. They are roughly the size of bacteria.

3. b, c. Answer (d) is incorrect because a bacterium, not a virus, was probably engulfed.

4. c, d

5. a. The $\Delta E_0'$ for the reaction is 0.05 V. Calculating $\Delta G^{o'}$,

$$\Delta G^{o'} = -nF\Delta E_0'$$

where n, the number of electrons transferred, is 1, and F is 96.49 kJ/V·mol.

$$\Delta G^{o'} = -1(96.49 \text{ kJ/V mol})(0.05 \text{ V}) = -4.82 \text{ kJ/mol}$$

Therefore, the reaction will proceed spontaneously. However, when considered by itself, it is insufficiently exergonic to drive ATP synthesis, which requires −30.6 kJ/mol under standard conditions. In the cell, this comparison is relatively meaningless because ATP is not synthesized during oxidative phosphorylation by direct chemical coupling of redox reactions to ATP formation, but rather by being coupled to a proton–motive force. In addition, the concentrations of the reactants can alter the actual free-energy change observed in the reaction. Answer (c) is incorrect because the state of oxidation of a cytochrome alters its absorption spectrum. The heme group contributes significantly to the adsorption spectrum of cytochomes, and the state of oxidation of the heme affects its adsorption spectrum.

6. e. The $\Delta E_0'$ for this reaction is −0.03 V. Calculating $\Delta G^{o'}$,

$$\Delta G^{o'} = -nF\Delta E_0' = -2(96.49 \text{ kJ/V mol})(-0.03 \text{ V}) = -5.79 \text{ kJ/mol}$$

7. The same proportionality constants that relate $\Delta G^{o'}$ and $\Delta E_0'$ can be used to relate $\Delta G'$ and $\Delta E'$. Substituting $\Delta G^{o'} = -nF\Delta E_0'$ and $\Delta G' = -nF\Delta E'$ into the expression for $\Delta G'$,

$$-nF\Delta E' = -nF\Delta E_0' + RT \ln \frac{[\text{products}]}{[\text{reactants}]}$$

$$\Delta E' = \Delta E_0' + \frac{-RT}{nF} \ln \frac{[\text{products}]}{[\text{reactants}]}$$

$\Delta E'$ is a measure of the direction in which an oxidation–reduction reaction will proceed for any given concentration of reactants and products. If $\Delta E'$ is positive the reaction is exergonic in the direction written.

8.
$$\Delta G' = \Delta G^{\circ\prime} + RT \ln \frac{[\text{Fumarate}][\text{FADH}_2]}{[\text{Succinate}][\text{FAD}]}$$

$$\Delta G' = -5.79 \text{ kJ/mol} + (8.314 \text{ J/mol K})(310\text{K}) \ln\left[\frac{(0.5\times10^{-3}\text{M})(0.2\times10^{-3}\text{M})}{(2\times10^{-3}\text{M})(2\times10^{-3}\text{M})}\right]$$

$$\Delta G' = -5.79 \text{ kJ/mol} + -9.51 \text{ kJ/mol} = -15.30 \text{ kJ/mol}$$

9. d. Answers (a) and (b) are incorrect because -220.2 kJ/mol is the free energy released by the oxidation of an NADH by $\frac{1}{2}$ O_2, and -30.6 kJ/mol is the free energy released by the hydrolysis of ATP to ADP + P_i.

10. The proper sequence is b, d, e, a, and c. The mobile carriers are (a) and (d).

11. (a) 3, 6, 8   (b) 1, 4, 5, 9   (c) 5, 7   (d) 2, 5

12. d, e. Answer (c) is incorrect because each enzyme complex has a unique absorption spectrum that reflects the environment of its electron carriers and its oxidation state.

13. d, e

14. c

15. See the Q cycle in Figure 20.12 in the text. Ubiquinol transfers one electron to cytochrome c_1 through a Rieske Fe-S cluster in cytochrome oxidoreductase. The semiquinone derived from the Q in this process donates an electron to cytochrome b_L, giving rise to ubiquinone. In turn, the electron from cytochrome b_L is transferred to cytochrome b_H, which then reduces another semiquinone to ubiquinol. Thus, the b cytochromes act as a recycling device that allows ubiquinol, a two-electron carrier, to transfer its electrons, one at a time, to the Fe-S cluster of cytochrome oxidoreductase. Cytochrome c_1 accepts the electrons (one electron/cytochome c_1) from the Fe-S cluster and transfers them to cytochrome c through the b cytochromes. Protons pumping across the mitochondrial membrane is tightly coupled to the oxidation of ubiquinol. The full oxidation of one QH_2 yields two reduced cytochome c molecules and removes two protons from the matrix.

16. See Figure 20.13 in the text. Molecular O_2 is bound between the Fe^{2+} and Cu^+ ions of the heme a_3-Cu_B center of cytochrome oxidase. The oxygen remains bound while four electrons and four protons are sequentially added to its various intermediates, resulting in the net release of two H_2O. The heme a-Cu_A center supplies the electrons for this process. Although four electrons are used in the reduction of O_2 to 2 H_2O, the individual steps of the reaction cycle involve single electron transfers.

17. a, b, d

18. The $FADH_2$ generated by the succinate-Q-reductase complex upon oxidation of succinate transfers it electrons to iron-sulfur center and finally to ubiquinone. No, this system does not transport protons across the inner mitochondrial membrane.

19. a, e. Answer (b) is incorrect; no protons are pumped by Complex II.

20. As described in the text, it is not the living phytoplankton that cause the problem. The oxygen is all used up by aerobic bacteria that eat the dead phytoplankton that have filtered down to the bottom. Thus the most severely affected animals are the shrimp and crabs, which also live on the bottom of the sea.

PROBLEMS

1. Nitrite (NO_2^-) is toxic to many microorganisms. It is therefore often used as a preservative in processed foods. However, members of the genus *Nitrobacter* oxidize nitrite to nitrate (NO_3^-), using the energy released by the transfer of electrons to oxygen to drive ATP synthesis. Given the following E_0' values, calculate the maximum ATP yield per mole of nitrate oxidized.

$$NO_3^- + 2H^+ + 2\ e^- \longrightarrow NO_2^- + H_2O \qquad E_0' = +0.42\ V$$

$$\tfrac{1}{2}\ O_2 + 2\ H^+ + 2\ e^- \longrightarrow H_2O \qquad E_0' = -0.82\ V$$

2. How are mitochondria thought to have arisen? What evidence suggests a particular bacterium as the origin of the mitochondria in all eukaryotes?

3. A newly discovered compound called *coenzyme U* is isolated from mitochondria.

   (a) Several lines of evidence are presented in advancing the claim that coenzyme U is a previously unrecognized carrier in the electron transport chain.
       (1) When added to a mitochondrial suspension, coenzyme U is readily taken up by mitochondria.
       (2) Removal of coenzyme U from mitochondria results in a decreased rate of oxygen consumption.
       (3) Alternate oxidation and reduction of coenzyme U when it is bound to the mitochondrial membrane can be easily demonstrated.
       (4) The rate of oxidation and reduction of coenzyme U in mitochondria is the same as the overall rate of electron transport.

       Which of the lines of evidence do you find the most convincing? Why?

       Which are the least convincing? Why?

   (b) In addition to the evidence cited in (a), the following observations were recorded when coenzyme U was incubated with a suspension of submitochondrial particles.
       (1) The addition of NADH caused a rapid reduction of coenzyme U.
       (2) Reduced coenzyme U caused a rapid reduction of added cytochrome *c*.
       (3) In the presence of antimycin A, the reduction of coenzyme U by added NADH took place as rapidly as in the absence of antimycin A. However, the reduction of cytochrome *c* by reduced coenzyme U was blocked in the presence of the inhibitor.
       (4) The addition of succinate caused a rapid reduction of coenzyme U.

       Assign a tentative position for coenzyme U in the electron-transport chain.

4. Coenzyme Q can be selectively removed from mitochondria using lipid solvents. If these mitochondria are then incubated in the presence of oxygen with an electron donor that is capable of reducing NAD^+, what will be the redox state of each of the carriers in the electron transport chain?

5. Analysis of the electron-transport pathway in a pathogenic gram-negative bacterium reveals the presence of five electron-transport molecules with the redox potentials listed in Table 20.1.

Table 20.1 Reduction potentials for pathogenic gram-negative bacterium

Oxidant	Reductant	Electrons transferred	E_0' (V)
NAD^+	NADH	2	−0.32
Flavoprotein b (ox)	Flavoprotein b (red)	2	−0.62
Cytochrome c (+3)	Cytochrome c (+2)	1	+0.22
Ferroprotein (ox)	Ferroprotein (red)	2	+0.85
Flavoprotein a (ox)	Flavoprotein a (red)	2	+0.77

(a) Predict the sequence of the carriers in the electron-transport chain.

(b) How many molecules of ATP can be generated under standard conditions when a pair of electrons is transported along the pathway?

(c) Why is it unlikely that oxygen is the terminal electron acceptor?

6. Calculate the minimum value of $\Delta E'_o$ that must be generated by a pair of electron carriers to provide sufficient energy for ATP synthesis. Assume that a pair of electrons is transferred.

7. The value of $\Delta E'_o$ for the reduction of $NADP^+$ is $+0.32$ V.

(a) Calculate the equilibrium constant for the reaction catalyzed by NADPH dehydrogenase:

$$NADP^+ + NADH \rightarrow NADPH + NAD^+$$

(b) What function could NADPH dehydrogenase serve in the cell?

8. Why is it important for the value $\Delta E'_o$ for the NAD^+:NADH redox couple to be less negative than those for the redox couples of oxidizable compounds that are components of the glycolytic pathway and the citric acid cycle?

9. The hemes in cytochrome bc1 have different redox potentials because they are in different polypeptide environments. Speculate on what physical properties of the protein could lead to a higher or lower redox potential in the hemes.

ANSWERS TO PROBLEMS

1. The two reactions that generate nitrate are

$$NO_2^- + H_2O \rightarrow NO_3^- + 2\,H^+ + 2\,e^- \qquad E'_0 = -0.42\ V$$
$$\tfrac{1}{2}\,O_2 + 2\,H^+ + 2\,e^- \rightarrow H_2O \qquad E'_0 = +0.82\ V$$

The net reaction is

$$NO_2^- + \tfrac{1}{2}\,O_2 \rightarrow NO_3^- \qquad E'_0 = +0.40\ V$$

The Nernst equation is used to calculate the free energy liberated by the oxidation of nitrite under standard conditions:

$$\Delta G^{o\prime} = -nF\Delta E'_0 = -2(96.49\ kJ/V \cdot mol)(0.40\ V) = -77.2\ kJ/mol$$

Therefore, each mole of nitrite oxidized yields, in principle, energy sufficient to drive the formation of ~2.5 moles of ATP under standard conditions ($\Delta G^{o\prime} = -30.6$ kJ/mol).

2. Mitochondria probably arose when an ancient free-living organism capable of oxidative phosphorylation invaded another cell and formed a symbiont with enhanced survival capabilities. The sequences of mitochondrial DNAs from a number of eukaryotes indicate an evolutionary relationship. The existence of a common set of encoded proteins in all mitochondrial DNAs, each of which is in the genome of one bacterium, *Rickettsia prowazekii*, is strong evidence for this organism being in the initial symbiont that gave rise to the mitochondria in all eukaryotes.

3. (a) If coenzyme U is a component of the electron-transport chain, it should undergo successive reduction and oxidation in the mitochondrion, and its overall rate of electron transfer should be close to the overall rate. Observations 3 and 4 are therefore the most convincing. In addition to electron carriers, other compounds can be taken up by mitochondria, and some of them, such as pyruvate, can affect the rate of oxygen consumption because they are substrates that donate electrons to carriers. Therefore, observations 1 and 2 are less convincing.

(b) The first two observations show that coenzyme U lies along the electron transport chain between NADH, which can reduce it, and cytochrome c, which is reduced by it. The fact that antimycin A blocks cytochrome c reduction by coenzyme U suggests that the carrier lies before cytochrome reductase. Succinate, which can transfer electrons to Q, can also transfer electrons to coenzyme U, so the position of coenzyme U in the chain is similar to that of Q.

4. The removal of ubiquinone from the electron transport chain means that no electrons can be transferred beyond Q in the pathway. You would therefore expect all carriers preceding Q to be more reduced and those beyond Q to be more oxidized.

5. (a) The carrier with the most negative reduction potential has the weakest affinity for electrons and so transfers them most easily to an acceptor. The carrier with the most positive reduction potential will be the strongest oxidizing substance and will have the greatest affinity for electrons. A carrier should be able to pass electrons to any carrier having a more positive reduction potential. Thus, the probable order of the carriers in the chain is flavoprotein b, NADH, cytochrome c, flavoprotein a, and ferroprotein.

(b) $\Delta E'_0 = +0.85 \text{ V} - (-0.62 \text{ V}) = 1.47 \text{ V}$

The total amount of free energy released by the transfer of two electrons is

$$\Delta G^{\circ\prime} = -nF\Delta E'_0 = -2(96.49 \text{ kJ/V} \cdot \text{mol})(1.47 \text{ V}) = -283.7 \text{ kJ/mol}$$

Because +30.6 kJ/mol is required to drive ATP synthesis under standard conditions, the number of molecules of ATP synthesized per pair of electrons is 283.7/30.6 = 9.3.

(c) It is unlikely that oxygen is the terminal electron acceptor because the reduction potential for the ferroprotein is slightly more positive than that of oxygen, so under standard conditions, the ferroprotein could not transfer electrons to oxygen.

6. The minimum amount of free energy that is needed to drive ATP synthesis under standard conditions is +30.6 kJ/mol. The value of $\Delta E'_0$ needed to generate this amount of free energy can be determined using the equation

$$\Delta G^{\circ\prime} = -nF \, \Delta E'_0$$

$$\Delta E'_0 = \frac{-\Delta G^{\circ\prime}}{nF}$$

If a pair of electrons is transferred, then

$$\Delta E'_0 = -\frac{-30.6 \text{ kJ} / \text{mol}}{2(96.49 \text{ kJ} / \text{Vmol})} = +0.158 \text{ V}$$

7. (a) The transfer of a pair of electrons from NADH to $NADP^+$ occurs with no release of free energy:

$$NAD^+ + H^+ + 2e^- \longrightarrow NADH \qquad E'_0 = -0.32 \text{ V}$$

$$NADP^+ + H^+ + 2e^- \longrightarrow NADPH \qquad E'_0 = -0.32 \text{ V}$$

For the overall reaction, $\Delta E'_0 = 0.00$ V. Because

$$\Delta G^{o\prime} = -nF\,\Delta E'_0,$$

$$\Delta G^{o\prime} = 0 = -RT\ln K'_{eq}$$

$$\ln K'_{eq} = 0$$

$$K'_{eq} = 1$$

$K'_{eq} = 1$ means that this reaction is at equilibrium when the ratio [NADPH] [NAD$^+$]/ [NADP$^+$] [NADH] equals 1. Any combination of concentrations that give a ratio of 1 in this quotient represents an equilibrium condition.

(b) In the cell, NADPH dehydrogenase serves to replenish NADPH when the reduced cofactor is needed for biosynthetic reactions. On the other hand, metabolites such as isocitrate and glucose 6-phosphate are substrates for NADP$^+$-linked dehydrogenases. NAD$^+$ can accept reducing equivalents generated as NADPH through the action of these enzymes.

8. NADH is a primary source of electrons for the respiratory chain. Oxidizable substrates must have a more negative reduction potential to donate electrons to NAD$^+$. A more negative redox potential for the NAD$^+$:NADH couple would make it unsuitable as an electron acceptor.

9. The higher (more positive) the redox potential for a molecule is, the higher its electron affinity. Reduction of cytochrome b converts the iron from the $+3$ state to $+2$, reducing the positive charge and along with the proprionates, giving the heme a net neutral charge. Any physical property that would tend to increase that electron affinity (stabilize the reduced state) would increase the redox potential for the molecule. Placing a heme in an environment with a positive charge nearby would be expected to increase the redox potential of the group by providing a stabilizing force for the additional electron. Conversely, placing the heme in an environment where there is a nearby negative charge should tend to decrease the redox potential. A polar environment would tend to favor the oxidized state (more charged) than the reduced state (more neutral).

The Proton-Motive Force

The reduced coenzymes NADH and $FADH_2$ that are formed during glycolysis (Chapter 16) and as a result of the functioning of the citric acid cycle (Chapter 18, 19) ultimately transfer their electrons via a series of carriers to oxygen and thereby release a large amount of useful energy (Chapter 20). The energy from this electron transfer is coupled to the formation of ATP by means of a transmembrane proton–motive force composed of a pH gradient and an electric potential. This process, known as *oxidative phosphorylation*, produces the bulk of the ATP in aerobic organisms. The chapter begins by discussing the generation of a proton gradient as a consequence of the electron flow and the use of the resulting proton–motive force by ATP synthase to form ATP from ADP and P_i by ATP synthase. The text then introduces the mitochondrial ATP synthase and the chemiosmotic hypothesis, proposed by Peter Mitchell. This model states that electron transport and ATP synthesis are coupled by a proton gradient across the inner mitochondrial membrane. The structure and mechanism of the ATP synthase are described in detail, emphasizing the connection between proton flow and ATP synthesis. Because ATP synthesis occurs inside mitochondria, whereas most of the reactions that utilize ATP take place in the cytosol, the membrane shuttle systems for ATP–ADP and other cofactors and biomolecules are described. The text then discusses the reasons for the variation in the estimation of the number of ATP molecules formed per glucose molecule oxidized. The control of oxidative phosphorylation and the mechanisms that uncouple electron transfer and oxidative phosphorylation as well as disease states resulting from mitochondiral misfunction are disucssed. The chapter ends by stressing the central role of proton gradients in interconverting free energy in cells.

LEARNING OBJECTIVES

When you have mastered this chapter, you should be able to accomplish the following objectives.

1. Write the overall, balanced reactions for the electron transport chain and ATP synthesis, along with their respective values of $\Delta G°'$.

2. Recognize that proton gradients are an interconvertible form of free energy in the cell.

A Proton Gradient Powers the Synthesis of ATP (Text Section 21.1)

3. Describe the *chemiosmotic model* of oxidative phosphorylation and relate experimental evidence that only the proton–motive force links the respiratory chain and ATP synthesis.

4. Describe the mitochondrial location, the subunit structure, and the function of eukaryotic *ATP synthase*.

5. Outline the proposed mechanism of ATP synthesis by ATP synthase during proton flow.

6. Explain the binding-change mechanism for proton-driven ATP synthesis.

7. Describe evidence for *rotational catalysis* in the ATP synthase.

8. Explain how proton flow drives rotation of the γ subunit.

9. Explain the difference between oxidative phosphorylation and the substrate-level phosphorylation occurring in glycolysis and the citric acid cycle.

Shuttles Allow Movement Across the Mitochondrial Membranes (Text Section 21.2)

10. Explain the roles of the *glycerol phosphate* and *malate–aspartate shuttles* in carrying the electrons of cytoplasmic NADH into the mitochondrion. Estimate the ATP yields in each case.

11. Describe the *ATP–ADP translocase* mechanism and state its cost relative to the energy yield from electron transfer by the respiratory chain.

12. List the most important *mitochondrial transport systems* for ions and metabolites.

Cellular Respiration Is Regulated by the Need for ATP (Text Section 21.3)

13. Estimate the net yield of ATP from the complete oxidation of glucose, taking into account the different shuttles for the cytoplasmic reducing equivalents of NADH. Discuss the sources of uncertainty in the estimation.

14. Describe *respiratory control* and relate it to *energy charge*.

15. List compounds that specifically block electron transport and locate their sites of action.

16. Explain the effect of *uncouplers* on oxidative phosphorylation. Note how regulated uncoupling can be used for *thermogenesis*. Give examples of thermogenesis in mammals and describe the physiological consequences for its absence.

17. Relate disorders in energy generation in mitochondria to human disease.

18. List examples of *energy conversions* by proton gradients and appreciate their central roles in free-energy interconversions.

SELF-TEST

1. Which of the following constitute cellular respiration?
   (a) biosynthesis of glycogen in the liver and muscles
   (b) conversion of an electron–motive force into a proton–motive force
   (c) formation of compounds with high electron transfer potential
   (d) conversion of a proton–motive force into a phosphoryl-transfer force

A Proton Gradient Powers the Synthesis of ATP

2. Which of the following experimental observations provide evidence that supports the chemiosmotic model of oxidative phosphorylation?
   (a) A closed membrane or vesicle compartment is required for oxidative phosphorylation.
   (b) A system of bacteriorhodopsin and ATPase can produce ATP in synthetic vesicles when light causes proton pumping.
   (c) A proton gradient is generated across the inner membrane of mitochondria during electron-transport.
   (d) ATP is synthesized when a proton gradient is imposed on mitochondria.

3. Explain why one cannot precisely predict the sites in the electron transport chain where the coupling of oxidation to phosphorylation occurs on the basis of the redox potentials of the electron-transport chain components.

4. Which of the following statements about the mitochondrial ATP-synthesizing complex are correct?
   (a) It contains more than 10 subunits.
   (b) It is located in the intermembrane space of mitochondria.
   (c) It contains a subassembly that constitutes the proton channel.
   (d) It is sensitive to oligomycin inhibition.
   (e) It translocates ATP through the mitochondrial membranes.

5. Match the major units of the ATP-synthesizing system in the left column with the appropriate components and functions in the right column.
   (a) F_0
   (b) F_1
       (1) contains the proton channel
       (2) contains the catalytic sites for ATP synthesis
       (3) contains α, β, γ, δ, and ε subunits
       (4) contains sequences homologous to P-loop NTPase family members
       (5) spans the inner mitochondrial membrane
       (6) is mostly in the matrix

6. Which of the following statements about the proposed mechanism for ATP synthesis by ATP synthase are correct?
   (a) ATP synthase forms ATP only when protons flow through the complex.
   (b) ATP synthase contains sites that change in their affinity for ATP as protons flow through the complex.
   (c) ATP synthase binds ATP more tightly when protons flow through the complex.
   (d) ATP synthase has two active sites per complex.
   (e) ATP synthase has active sites that are not functionally equivalent at a given time.

7. ATP synthase can form ATP in the absence of a proton gradient when it is mixed with ADP and P_i. Explain how this can happen when the formation of ATP from ADP and P_i requires 30.6 kJ/mol of free energy.

8. Identify the similarities in the mechanisms of G proteins and ATP synthase.

Shuttles Allow Movement Across Mitochondrial Membranes

9. The inner mitochondrial membrane contains translocases—that is, specific transport proteins—for which pairs of substances?
   (a) NAD^+ and NADH
   (b) glycerol 3-phosphate and dihydroxyacetone phosphate
   (c) AMP and ADP
   (d) citrate and pyruvate
   (e) glutamate and aspartate

10. Which of the following pairs of molecules are transported in opposition to each other across the mitochondrial membrane in the malate-aspartate shuttle?
    (a) Malate and aspartate
    (b) Aspartate and glutamate
    (c) Malate and α-ketoglutarate
    (d) Malate and glutamate
    (e) Oxaloacetate and glutamate

11. Match each mitochondrial transporter with the molecules it transports.
    (a) Dicarboxylate carrier   (1) Phosphate
    (b) Tricarboxylate carrier   (2) Hydroxide ion
    (c) Pyruvate carrier   (3) Malate
    (d) Phosphate carrier   (4) Citrate
                                    (5) Pyruvate
                                    (6) Protons

12. Explain why the rate of eversion of the binding site from the matrix to the cytosolic side is more rapid for ATP than for ADP when the ATP–ADP translocase functions in the presence of a proton gradient.

Cellular Respiration Is Regulated by the Need for ATP

13. Approximately how many ATP are formed for each extramitochondrial NADH that is oxidized to NAD^+ by O_2 via the electron transport chain. Assume that the glycerol phosphate shuttle is operating.
    (a) 1.0   (c) 2.5
    (b) 1.5   (d) 3.0

14. How many ATP molecules are generated during the complete oxidative degradation of each of the following to CO_2 and H_2O? Assume that the glycerol phosphate shuttle is operating.
    (a) acetyl CoA
    (b) phosphoenolpyruvate
    (c) glyceraldehyde 3-phosphate

15. What is meant by the term *respiratory control*?

16. Which of the following answers completes the sentence more correctly? The rate of flow of electrons through the electron transport chain is most directly regulated by
    (a) the ATP:ADP ratio.
    (b) the concentration of acetyl CoA.
    (c) the rate of oxidative phosphorylation.
    (d) feedback inhibition by H_2O.
    (e) the catalytic rate of cytochrome oxidase.

17. Which of the following answers completes the sentence correctly? Uncouplers, such as dinitrophenol (DNP) or thermogenin, uncouple electron transport and phosphorylation by
    (a) inhibiting cytochrome reductase.
    (b) dissociating the F_0 and F_1 units of ATP synthase.
    (c) blocking electron transport.
    (d) dissipating the proton gradient.
    (e) blocking the ATP-ADP translocase.

18. Which of the following are the products of the reaction of superoxide dismutase?
    (a) O_2^- (d) O_2
    (b) H_2O (e) H_3O^+
    (c) H_2O_2

19. Match each inhibitor in the left column with its *primary effect* in the right column.
    (a) azide   (1) inhibition of electron transport
    (b) atractyloside   (2) uncoupling of electron transport and
    (c) rotenone   (3) oxidative phosphorylation
    (d) 2,4-dinitrophenol (DNP)   (3) inhibition of ADP–ATP translocation
    (e) carbon monoxide   (4) inhibition of ATP synthase
    (f) oligomycin
    (g) antimycin A

20. Proton gradients are used for which of the following?
    (a) generating heat   (d) active transport
    (b) free-energy storage   (e) mechanical movement
    (c) ATP generation

ANSWERS TO SELF-TEST

1. b, c, d. Although glycogen is a molecule that stores energy, answer (a) is incorrect because respiration is defined as the collection of reactions that use the reductive power of $NADH^+$ and $FADH_2$ to form ultimately ATP.

2. a, b, c, d. Answer (d) is true, although not mentioned in the text.

3. The free-energy change ($\Delta G^{o\prime}$) and for each electron transfer step of the respiratory chain can be calculated from the redox-potential change ($\Delta E_0'$) for that step, using the equation $\Delta G^{o\prime} = -nF\Delta E_0'$. Since $\Delta G^{o\prime}$ for the synthesis of ATP from ADP is +30.5 kJ/mol, $\Delta G^{o\prime}$ for an electron transfer reaction in which the coupling of oxidation to phosphorylation could occur must be more negative than +30.6 kJ/mol. However, we cannot conclude that there is a direct, quantitative relationship between a given redox reaction and the phosphorylation of ADP in the cell because the free-energy coupling is by means of a spatially delocalized proton–motive force.

4. a, c, d

5. (a) 1, 5   (b) 2, 3, 4, 6

6. b, e

7. The β subunits of F_1, when in the T form, can bind ATP so tightly that they will condense ADP and P_i to form ATP with the release of water. The binding energy between the protein and the substrates is used to form the chemical bond. The K_{eq} of a reaction can be markedly different when the substrates are bound by an enzyme

compared with when they are free in solution. In such cases, the protein is a stoichiometric part of the reaction and the K_{eq} is for a reaction different from that of the substrates themselves. The proton gradient is used to move, by directional rotation, the β subunits into different environments where their affinities for the substrates and products are different, thereby leading to net synthesis of ATP.

8. Both G proteins and the ATP synthase bind different nucleotides based on interaction with different proteins. The G proteins have a high affinity for GDP until they are activated by interactions with a receptor or an effector protein which can trigger exchange of GDP for GTP. ATP synthase will bind either ADP or ATP depending on which of the three different faces of the γ subunit they interact with.

9. b, e. Answer (a) is incorrect because only the electrons of NADH are transported, not the entire molecule. Answers (c) and (d) are incorrect because these pairs of compounds are not transported by the same translocase.

10. b and c. While all of the molecules listed except oxaloacetate are transported in the shuttle, only certain pairs are transported through the same protein in opposition to each other.

11. (a) 1,3 (b) 3,4,6 (c) 2, 5 (d) 1, 2

12. The proton gradient and the membrane potential make the cytosolic side of the inner mitochondrial membrane more positive than the matrix side; therefore, ATP, which has one more negative charge than ADP, is more attracted to the cytosolic side than is ADP.

13. b. The oxidation of NADH by the electron transport chain leads to the synthesis of approximately 2.5 ATP. However, when the reducing equivalents of an extramitochondrial NADH enter the mitochondrial matrix via the glycerol phosphate shuttle, they give rise to $FADH_2$, which yields 1.5 ATP.

14. (a) About 10 ATP: citric acid cycle (3 NADH → 2.5, 1 $FADH_2$ → 1.5, and 1 GTP)

    (b) About 13.5 ATP: citric acid cycle (10 ATP), pyruvate dehydrogenase reaction (1 NADH, intramitochondrial → 2.5), pyruvate kinase reaction (1 ATP)

    (c) About 16 ATP: citric acid cycle (10 ATP), pyruvate dehydrogenase reaction (1 NADH → 2.5), pyruvate kinase reaction (1 ATP), phosphoglycerate kinase reaction (1 ATP), glyceraldehyde 3-phosphate dehydrogenase reaction (1 NADH, extramitochondrial, which yields 1.5 ATP by the glycerol phosphate shuttle)

15. The regulation of the rate of oxidative phosphorylation by the availability of ADP is referred to as *respiratory control*.

16. a

17. d

18. c, d

19. (a) 1 (b) 3 (c) 1 (d) 2 (e) 1 (f) 4 (g) 1

20. a, b, c, d, e. Answer (b) is correct, but you should realize that free-energy storage by a proton gradient across a membrane is more transient than storage in a molecule such as glucose or NADH.

PROBLEMS

1. The reduction potential for methylene blue is such that it can be reduced by components of the electron transport chain and can itself, when reduced, reduce O_2 to H_2O. Suggest why massive doses of methylene blue might serve to counteract cyanide poisoning.

2. What is the effect on the proton–motive potential across the inner membrane when an ATP is moved from the matrix to the cytosolic side?

3. Predict the relative oxidation–reduction states of NAD^+, NADH-Q reductase, ubiquinone, cytochrome c_1, cytochrome c, and cytochrome a in liver mitochondria that are amply supplied with isocitrate as substrate, P_i, ADP, and oxygen but are inhibited by

   (a) rotenone.
   (b) antimycin A.
   (c) cyanide.

4. Arsenate, AsO_4^{3-}, is an uncoupling reagent for oxidative phosphorylation, but unlike DNP it does not transport protons across the inner mitochondrial membrane. How might arsenate function as an uncoupler?

5. Yeast can grow both aerobically and anaerobically on glucose. Explain why the rate of glucose consumption decreases when yeast cells that have been maintained under anaerobic conditions are exposed to oxygen.

6. The addition of the drug dicyclohexylcarbodiimide (DCCD) to mitochondria markedly decreases both the rate of electron transfer from NADH to O_2 and the rate of ATP formation. The subsequent addition of 2,4-dinitrophenol leads to an increase in the rate of electron transfer without changing the rate of ATP formation. What does DCCD likely inhibit?

7. Mitochondria isolated from the liver of a particular patient will oxidize NADH at a relatively high rate even if ADP is absent. The P:O ratio for oxidative phosphorylation (the ratio of the number of P_i molecules incorporated into organic molecules per atom of oxygen consumed) by these mitochondria is less than normal. Predict the likely symptoms of this disorder.

8. Acidic aromatic compounds like 2,4-dinitrophenol (DNP) act as uncouplers of electron transport and oxidative phosphorylation because they carry protons across the inner mitochondrial membrane, disrupting the proton gradient. The structure of the neutral, protonated form of DNP is shown in Figure 21.1.

FIGURE 21.1

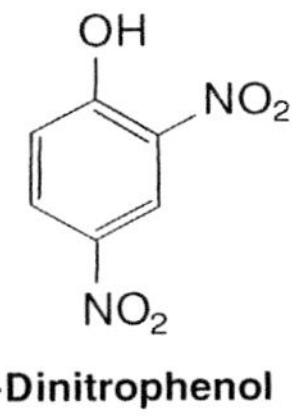

2, 4-Dinitrophenol
(DNP)

   (a) Although you might expect that 2,4-dinitrophenylate anion (pK_a = 4.0) would be unable to cross the inner mitochondrial membrane, the deprotonated form of DNP is membrane-soluble. Explain why, by drawing resonance forms of 2,4-dinitrophenolate anion, showing how negative charge is distributed over the phenyl ring structure.
   (b) Suppose you are studying the effects of DNP on proton transport in an artificial phospholipid membrane system. You observe that the rate of proton transport by DNP increases at temperatures above the transition temperature for the membrane. Explain.

9. Explain why the K_{eq} of the reaction ADP + P_i + H^+ ⇌ ATP is ~1 on the surface of ATP synthase considering that you have been told repeatedly that the $\Delta G^{o'}$ for the formation of ATP is +30.6 kJ/mol.

ANSWERS TO PROBLEMS

1. Cyanide blocks the transfer of electrons from cytochrome oxidase to O_2. Therefore, all the respiratory-chain components become reduced and electron transport ceases; consequently, oxidative phosphorylation stops. An artificial electron acceptor with an appropriate redox potential, such as methylene blue, can reoxidize some components of the respiratory chain, reestablish a proton gradient, and thereby restore ATP synthesis. The methylene blue takes the place of cytochrome oxidase as a means of transferring electrons to O_2, which remains the terminal electron acceptor.

2. The ATP-ADP translocase (ANT) allows the adenosine diphosphate and triphosphates to cross the inner mitochondrial membrane and in so doing brings one ADP in for each exiting ATP. In addition, since ATP bears one more negative charge than does ADP, one negative charge is removed from the matrix by an exchange thereby reducing the membrane potential. Approximately a quarter of the energy yield of electron transport through the respiratory chain is "lost" through the ATP-ADP exchange.

3. Upstream from the inhibitor, reduced respiratory-chain components will accumulate; downstream, oxidized components will be present. The point of inhibition is the crossover point.

   (a) Rotenone inhibits the step at NADH-Q reductase; therefore, NADH and NADH-Q reductase will be more reduced, and ubiquinone, cytochrome c_1, cytochrome c, and cytochrome a will be more oxidized.

   (b) Antimycin A blocks electron flow between cytochromes b and c_1; therefore, NADH, NADH-Q reductase, and ubiquinol will be more reduced, and cytochrome c_1, cytochrome c, and cytochrome a will be more oxidized.

   (c) Cyanide inhibits the transfer of electrons from cytochrome oxidase to O_2, so all the components of the respiratory chain will be more reduced.

4. Arsenate chemically resembles inorganic phosphate; therefore, it can enter into many of the same biochemical reactions as P_i. For example, it substitutes for phosphate in the glyceraldehydes 3-phosphate dehydrogenase reaction forming arsenophosphogylcerate instead of the normally formed bisphosphoglycerate. The arsenate compound is labile to hydrolysis and the free energy resulting from the oxidation forming it is lost, thereby precluding phosphorylation. Arsenate can replace phosphate during oxidative phosphorylation also, presumably forming an arsenate anhydride with ADP. Such compounds are similarly unstable and are rapidly hydrolyzed, effectively causing the uncoupling of electron transport and oxidative phosphorylation.

5. The decrease in glucose consumption when oxygen is introduced is known as the *Pasteur effect*. Under anaerobic conditions, glucose cannot be oxidized completely to CO_2 and H_2O, because NADH and QH_2 generated in the citric acid cycle cannot be reoxidized in the absence of oxygen. In order to regenerate NAD^+, needed for continued operation of the glycolytic pathway, pyruvate is converted to ethanol and CO_2. There is a net production of only two molecules of ATP from each glucose molecule metabolized by the glycolytic pathway. This means that the pace of glycolysis must be relatively high to generate sufficient amounts of ATP for cell maintenance.

   When oxygen is introduced, reduced cofactors in the citric acid cycle can be reoxidized in the electron transport chain and oxidative phosphorylation occurs. Under these conditions the yeast cell can utilize glucose much more efficiently, producing ~30 molecules of ATP for each glucose molecule oxidized completely to CO_2 and H_2O. The rate of glucose consumption is greatly reduced under aerobic conditions because less glucose is needed to provide the amount of ATP needed to maintain the cell.

Other factors that decelerate the pace of glycolysis include increases in concentrations of citrate and ATP under aerobic conditions. Both molecules are key regulators of phosphofructokinase 1, a rate-limiting glycolytic enzyme.

6. The fact that the rate of electron transport increases on addition of DNP without a concomitant increase in ATP synthesis suggests that DCCD inhibits ATP synthase. Experiments show that indeed DCCD blocks proton flow through the C subunit of F_0, inhibiting ATP synthase activity. When DCCD is added to respiring mitochondria, protons cannot move back into the mitochondrial matrix and the rate of ATP synthesis decreases. The flow of electrons through the respiratory chain slows as the need to maintain the proton gradient decreases. The metabolic uncoupler 2,4-dinitrophenol is an effective ion carrier that dissipates the proton–motive force generated by electron transfer by allowing protons to freely cross the inner mitochondrial membrane. Although the rate of electron transport increases in response to the dissipation of the proton gradient, the rate of phosphorylation of ADP through oxidative phosphorylation does not increase because ATP synthase remains inhibited by DCCD.

7. From these observations it appears that electron transfer and ATP synthesis are uncoupled, so there is no way to control electron transport by limiting ADP availability. One would expect the patient to have a very high rate of metabolism, along with a possibly elevated temperature. The fact that much of the energy available from electron transport is not utilized means that the energy is released as heat rather than being utilized for the formation of ATP.

8. (a) See Figure 21.2 for structures. Resonance structures that include the two nitro groups show that the negative charge can be distributed among a number of forms. Therefore the dinitrophenylate anion is soluble in the membrane bilayer. This explains why DNP can rapidly carry protons across the inner mitochondrial membrane.

FIGURE 21.2

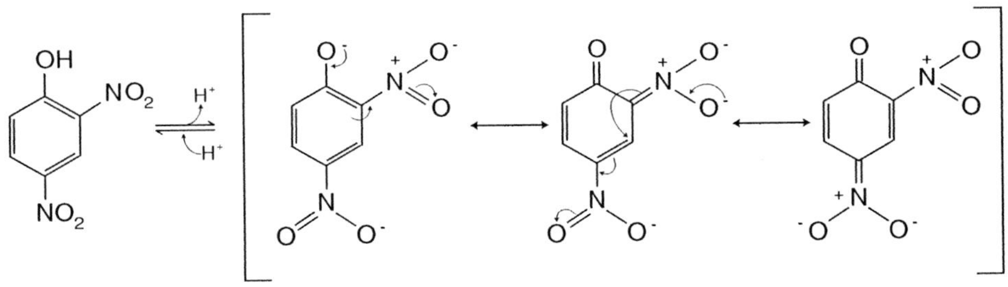

(b) DNP is a mobile proton carrier that is soluble in the membrane bilayer. Below the transition temperature for the phospholipid, the bilayer is in the gel state, where molecules like DNP may not be able to diffuse rapidly from one side of the bilayer to the other. At temperatures above the transition temperature, the bilayer is in the fluid state, in which DNP is more mobile, more rapidly transporting protons across the bilayer.

9. The ATP synthase binds ATP with such high affinity that the reaction is shifted toward synthesis when ADP and P_i are present. The binding is so tight that only rotation of the complex, which is powered by the proton gradient, can release the product ATP. Reactions on the surface of enzymes are not the same as those free in solution. The enzyme is a stoichiometric component of the reaction, and its concentration must be considered when calculating the free-energy change occurring.

Chapter 22

The Light Reactions

To this point, the authors have dealt with the mechanisms by which organisms obtain energy from their environment by oxidizing fuels to generate ATP and reducing power. In this chapter, they describe how light energy is transduced into the same forms of chemical energy, leading to conversion of CO_2 into carbohydrate by photosynthetic organisms. Carbon fixation and sugar synthesis (the dark reactions) will be covered in Chapter 23 of the text.

The authors begin with the basic equation of photosynthesis and an overview of the process. Next come descriptions of the chloroplast, chlorophyll, and the photosynthetic reaction center. The authors then describe the overall structures, components, and reactions of photosystems II and I and the cytochrome *bf* complex, including the absorption of light, charge separation, electron-transport events, and the evolution of O_2. They explain how these light reactions lead to the formation of proton gradients and the synthesis of ATP and NADPH.

A review of the basic concepts of metabolism in Chapter 15 and mitochondrial structure, redox potentials, the proton-motive force, and free-energy changes in Chapters 20 and 21 will help you to understand this chapter.

LEARNING OBJECTIVES

When you have mastered this chapter, you should be able to accomplish the following objectives.

Introduction

1. Describe the purpose of *photosynthesis* and write its overall reaction.
2. Distinguish between the *light* and *dark reactions* of photosynthesis.

Photosynthesis Takes Place in Chloroplasts (Text Section 22.1)

3. Describe the structure of the *chloroplast*. Locate the *outer, inner,* and *thylakoid membranes,* the *intermembrane space,* the *thylakoid space,* the *granum,* and the *stroma.* Associate these structures with the functions they perform.
4. Describe the properties of the thylakoid membrane.
5. Discuss the probable origin of the chloroplast and compare it to theories of the origin of mitochondria.

Photosynthesis Transforms Light Energy Into Chemical Energy (Text Section 22.2)

6. Distinguish between the processes of resonance energy transfer and electron transfer in photosynthesis.
7. List the structural components of chlorophyll *a* and contrast it with the structure of chlorophyll *b*. Explain why chlorophylls are effective *photoreceptors.*
8. Explain the function of the pigments in light-harvesting complexes.

Two Photosystems Generate a Proton Gradient and NADPH (Text Section 22.3)

9. Distinguish the features of photosystems I and II. Indicate the direction of electron flow.
10. Diagram photosystem I. Indicate the components and reactions of photosystem I, including the roles of P700, A_0, A_1, *ferredoxin, FAD, NADPH,* and plastocyanin(Cu^+) in these processes.
11. Diagram photosystem II and identify its major components. Describe the roles of P680, *pheophytin,* and *plastoquinone* in the absorption of light, *separation of charge,* and electron transfer in photosystem II.
12. Explain the function of the *manganese center* in the extraction of electrons from water.
13. Explain the significance of the two plastoquinone binding sites, Q_A and Q_B, in the bacterial reaction center.
14. Describe the composition and function of the *cytochrome bf complex,* and outline the roles of *plastoquinol, plastocyanin (Cu^{2+}),* and *Fe-S clusters* in the formation of a *transmembrane proton gradient.*
15. Compare and contrast the roles of plastocyanin in chloroplasts and cytochrome *c* in mitochondria.
16. List the electron donors utilized by photosynthetic bacteria.

A Proton Gradient Drives ATP Synthesis (Text Section 22.4)

17. Discuss the similarities and differences between the CF_1–CF_0 ATP synthase of chloroplasts and the F_1–F_0 synthase of mitochondria.

18. Explain how photosystem I can synthesize ATP without forming NADPH or O_2.

19. Contrast the formation of ATP by *cyclic photophosphorylation* and by *oxidative phosphorylation*.

20. Write the net reaction carried out by the combined actions of photosystem II, the cytochrome *bf* complex, and photosystem I.

21. Explain how the components of the *light-harvesting complexes* interact to funnel light to the reaction centers.

22. Rationalize the differences in the *photosynthetic assemblies* in the *stacked* and *unstacked* regions of the thylakoid membranes.

23. Explain the mechanisms of common herbicides that work by inhibiting the light reaction.

SELF-TEST

1. Write the basic reaction for photosynthesis in green plants.

Introduction

2. Assign each function or product in the right column to the appropriate structure or pathway in the left column.

   (a) chlorophyll
   (b) light-harvesting complex
   (c) photosystem I
   (d) photosystem II

   (1) O_2 generation
   (2) ATP synthesis
   (3) light collection
   (4) NADPH synthesis
   (5) separation of charge
   (6) light absorption
   (7) transmembrane proton gradient

Photosynthesis Takes Place in Chloroplasts

3. Thylakoid membranes contain which of the following?

   (a) light-harvesting complexes
   (b) reaction centers
   (c) ATP synthase
   (d) electron-transport chains
   (e) galactolipids
   (f) sulfolipids
   (g) phospholipids

4. The similarities between mitochondria and chloroplasts are obvious. In what ways are they opposite?

Photosynthesis Transforms Light Energy Into Chemical Energy

5. Which of the following are constituents of chlorophylls?

   (a) substituted tetrapyrrole
   (b) plastoquinone
   (c) Mg^{2+}
   (d) Fe^{2+}
   (e) phytol
   (f) iron porphyrin

6. Why do chlorophylls absorb and transfer visible light efficiently?

7. After an electron is excited from its ground state to an excited state, several outcomes are possible. Which of the following describes the process of resonance energy transfer?

   (a) The excited electron is transferred to a nearby molecule with a lower excited state.
   (b) The absorbed energy is transferred to a nearby molecule which then moves to a higher energy state.
   (c) The excited electron returns to the ground state and the absorbed energy is transferred to the environment as heat.
   (d) The excited electron returns to the ground state and the absorbed energy is released as light.

8. *Chlorobium thiosulfatophilum* uses hydrogen sulfide as a source of electrons for photosynthesis. The basic equation for this process is given below:

$$CO_2 + 2\,H_2 \rightarrow (CH_2O) + 2S + H_2O$$

   Given the fact that the standard reduction potential for $S + 2\,H^+ \rightarrow H_2S$ is +0.14 V, does it seem likely that two photosystems would be required for this process? Why or why not?

Two Photosystems Generate a Proton Gradient and NADPH

9. Which of the following statements about photosystem II are correct?

   (a) It is a multimolecular transmembrane assembly containing several polypeptides, several chlorophyll molecules, a special chlorophyll (P680), pheophytin, and plastoquinones.
   (b) It transfers electrons to photosystem I via the cytochrome *bf* complex.
   (c) It uses light energy to create a separation of charge whose potential energy can be used to oxidize H_2O and to produce a reductant, plastoquinol.
   (d) It uses an Fe^{2+}-Cu^+ center as a charge accumulator to form O_2 without generating potentially harmful hydroxyl radicals, superoxide anions, or H_2O_2.

10. Which statement about the Mn center of photosystem II is NOT correct?

    (a) The Mn center has four possible oxidation states.
    (b) Electrons are transferred from the Mn center to $P680^+$.
    (c) A tyrosine residue on the D1 protein is an intermediate in electron transfer.
    (d) The O_2 released by the Mn center comes from the oxidation of water.
    (e) Each photon absorbed by the reaction center leads to the removal of an electron from the Mn cluster.

11. Which of the following is not an electron donor in a prokaryotic reaction center?

    (a) Oxygen
    (b) Water
    (c) Hydrogen sulfide
    (d) amino acids

12. Match photosystem I and II in green plants with the appropriate properties listed in the right column.

    (a) photosystem I (PS I)
    (b) photosystem II (PS II)

    (1) Absorbs light with wavelengths less than 700 nm.
    (2) Provides electrons to reduce $NADP^+$ to NADPH.
    (3) Sends electrons through the cytochrome bf proton pump.
    (4) Couples reduction of plastoquinone with transport of two protons across the thylakoid membrane.

(5) Uses an FAD-containing reductase to facilitate electron transfer between the one-electron ferredoxin and the two electron $NADP^+$.

(6) Photolyses water to oxygen.

13. Explain how plastocyanin and plastoquinol are involved in ATP synthesis.

14. Write the net equation of the reaction catalyzed by photosystem I, and describe how NADPH is formed. What is the role of FAD in this process?

A Proton Gradient Drives ATP Synthesis

15. Which of the following statements about cyclic photophosphorylation are correct?
    (a) It doesn't involve NADPH formation.
    (b) It uses electrons supplied by photosystem II.
    (c) It is activated when $NADP^+$ is limiting.
    (d) It does not generate O_2.
    (e) It leads to ATP production via the cytochrome bf complex.
    (f) It involves a substrate-level phosphorylation.

16. What is the overall stoichiometry of photosynthesis in chloroplasts? If eight photons are absorbed, the net yield is _____ O_2, _____ NADPH, and _____ ATP.

17. Which of the following statements about the light-harvesting complex are true?
    (a) It is a single chlorophyll molecule.
    (b) It collects light energy through the absorption of light by chlorophyll molecules.
    (c) It surrounds a reaction center with a specialized chlorophyll pair that contributes to the transduction of light energy into chemical energy.
    (d) It contains chlorophyll molecules that transfer energy from one to another by direct electromagnetic interactions.
    (e) It is the product of Planck's constant h and the frequency of the incident light v.

18. Match the descriptions with the pigments

    A. tetrapyrrole   a. chlorophyll a
    B. polyene   b. β carotene
    C. contains Mg   c. pheophytin

19. Which of the following statements about the thylakoid membrane are correct?
    (a) It contains photosystem I and ATP synthase in the unstacked regions.
    (b) It contains the cytochrome bf complex in the unstacked regions only.
    (c) It contains photosystem II mostly in the stacked regions.
    (d) It facilitates communication between photosystems I and II by the circulation of plastoquinones and plastocyanins in the thylakoid space.
    (e) It allows direct interaction between P680* and P700* reaction centers through its differentiation into stacked and unstacked regions.

ANSWERS TO SELF-TEST

1. The basic reaction for photosynthesis in green plants is

$$H_2O + CO_2 \xrightarrow{\text{Light}} (CH_2O) + O_2$$

where (CH_2O) represents carbohydrate.

2. (a) 3, 5, 6   (b) 3, 6   (c) 2, 3, 4, 5, 6, 7   (d) 1, 2, 3, 5, 6, 7. Chlorophylls are involved in light absorption, light collection in the antennae, and reaction center chemistry. Photosystems I and II cooperate to generate a transmembrane proton-motive force that can synthesize ATP.

3. a, b, c, d, e, f, g

4. Chloroplasts *produce* oxygen from water; mitochondria *use* oxygen and *produce* water. The direction of the proton gradient and ATPase are reversed in the two organelles. Electrons travel only from higher to lower energy in mitochondria, but with the aid of photons, they can travel "uphill" in chloroplasts. Other differences (iron in heme versus. magnesium in chlorophyll; cytochrome *c* versus. plastocyanin) aren't "opposites."

5. a, c, e

6. The polyene structure (alternating single and double bonds) of chlorophylls causes them to have strong absorption bands in the visible region of the spectrum. Their peak molar absorption coefficients are higher than $10^5\ M^{-1}\,cm^{-1}$. Also, although the fact is not emphasized in the text, iron porphyrins (heme groups) return to the ground state much more rapidly than excited magnesium tetrapyrroles. Thus chlorophyll has more time to transfer a high-energy electron before the excitation is dissipated as heat.

7. b. Resource energy transfer occurs without release of a photon or electron so answers (a) and (d) are incorrect.

8. The basic equation for this process is given:

$$CO_2 + 2\ H_2S \longrightarrow (CH_2O) + 2\ S + H_2O$$

Compare the standard reaction potential of $S + 2\ H^+ \longrightarrow H_2S = +0.14$ V with that of water, given in Table 20.1 of the text: $1/2\ O_2 + 2\ H^+ \longrightarrow H_2O = +0.82$ V. Hydrogen sulfide's electrons are much higher in energy than those from water, so it is easier to promote them to the level of NADPH (standard reduction potential $= -0.32$, same as NADH). If we reverse the calculation we see that the free energy change to move two electrons from oxygen to NADH would cost $+220$ kj (or $+52.6$ kcal) of free energy. Starting with hydrogen sulfide cuts this value roughly in half, so a single photosystem suffices.

9. a, b, c. Answer (d) is incorrect because a cluster of four manganese ions serves as a charge accumulator by interactions with the strong oxidant $P680^+$ and H_2O to form O_2.

10. a. Answer (a) is incorrect. The Mn center contains four Mn atoms, and can adopt five oxidation states (S_0–S_4). See Figure 22.15. Each manganese ion can exist in four oxidation states.

11. a. Oxygen is an electron acceptor, not a donor.

12. (a) 1, 2, 5   (b) 3, 4, 6

13. Two electrons from plastoquinol (QH_2) are transferred to two molecules plastocyanin (PC) in a reaction catalyzed by the transmembrane cytochrome *bf* complex; in the process, two protons are pumped across the thylakoid membrane to acidify the thylakoid space with respect to the stroma, and two more protons are contributed by QH_2 (Figure 22.17 in the text). The transmembrane proton gradient is used to synthesize ATP. This process closely resembles the mitochondrial Q cycle except that plastoquinone replaces ubiquinone (CoQ), plastocyanin replaces cytochrome *c*, and "inside" and "outside" are reversed.

14. The net reaction catalyzed by photosystem I is

$$PC(Cu^+) + ferredoxin_{oxidized} \longrightarrow PC(Cu^{2+}) + ferredoxin_{reduced}$$

where PC is plastocyanin. Reduced ferredoxin is a powerful reductant. Two reduced ferredoxins reduce $NADP^+$ to form NADPH and two oxidized ferredoxins in a reaction catalyzed by ferredoxin-$NADP^+$ reductase. FAD is a prosthetic group on the enzyme that serves as an adapter to collect two electrons from two reduced ferredoxin molecules for their subsequent transfer to a single $NADP^+$ molecule.

15. a, c, d, e. Answer (b) is incorrect because photosystem I provides the electrons for photophosphorylation.

16. Eight photons would yield one O_2, two NADPH, and three ATP.

17. b, c, d

18. A: a,c; B: a,b,c; C: a.

19. a, c, d. Answer (b) is incorrect because the cytochrome *bf* complex is uniformly distributed throughout the thylakoid membrane. Answer (e) is incorrect because the differentiation into stacked and unstacked regions probably prevents direct interaction between the excited reaction center chlorophylls P680* and P700*.

PROBLEMS

1. $NADP^+$ and A_0 are two components in the electron-transport chain associated with photosystem I (see Figure 22.11 in the text). A_0^- is a chlorophyll that carries a single electron, whereas NADPH carries two electrons. Write the overall reaction that occurs, and calculate $\Delta E'_0$ and $\Delta G^{o'}$ for the reduction of $NADP^+$ by A_0^- using the fact that the standard reduction potential for A_0 is $\Delta E'_0 = -1.1$ V. See Chapter 20 for similar calculations.

2. Calculate the maximum free-energy change $\Delta G^{o'}$ that occurs as a pair of electrons is transferred from photosystem II to photosystem I, that is from P680* (excited) to P700 (unexcited). Estimate the E'_0 values from Figure 22.11 in the text. Then compare your answer with the free-energy change that occurs in mitochondria as a pair of electrons is transferred from NADH + H^+ to oxygen.

3. Explain the defect or defects in the hypothetical scheme for the light reactions of photosynthesis depicted in Figure 22.1.

FIGURE 22.1 Hypothetical scheme for photosynthesis.

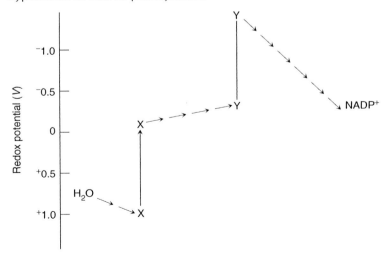

4. Explain why ATP synthesis requires a larger pH gradient across the thylakoid membrane of a chloroplast than across the inner membrane of a mitochondrion.

5. Would you expect oxygen to be evolved when $NADP^+$ is added to an illuminated suspension of isolated chloroplasts? Explain briefly.

6. Would your answer to problem 6 change if the chloroplasts were illuminated with extremely monochromatic light of 700 nm? Explain the basis for your answer.

7. Suppose you were designing spectrophotometric assays for chlorophyll a and chlorophyll b. What wavelengths would you use for the detection of each? (See Figure 22.7 in the text.) Explain your answer very briefly.

8. Green light has a wavelength of approximately 520 nm. Explain why solutions of chlorophyll appear to be green. (See Figure 22.7 in the text.)

9. If you were going to extract chlorophylls a and b from crushed spinach leaves, would you prefer to use acetone or water as a solvent? Explain your answer briefly.

10. The end of Section 22.4 of the text describes inhibitors of the light reaction that are used as herbicides. Inhibiting photosynthesis is a good way to produce compounds that can kill plants while keeping toxicity toward animals to a minimum. Can you think of another way to produce herbicides that would be relatively safe for animals?

11. Why is it considered likely that the photosystems found in chloroplasts evolved from earlier photosynthetic organisms? What is the minimum age for water-based, oxygen-producing photosynthesis?

12. What's so "special" about the special pair? Name three special pairs described in the text chapter, and tell what each one does.

ANSWERS TO PROBLEMS

1. A_0^- is the stronger reductant in the system because it has the more negative standard reducing potential. A_0^- will therefore reduce $NADP^+$ to NADPH under standard conditions. Following the convention for redox problems presented in text Chapter 20, we first write the partial reaction for the reduction involving the weaker reductant (the half-cell with the more positive standard reducing potential):

$$NADP^+ + H^+ + 2\,e^- \longrightarrow NADPH \qquad E'_0 = -0.32 \text{ V} \qquad (1)$$

Next, we write, *again as a reduction*, the partial reaction involving the stronger reductant (the half-cell with the more negative standard reducing potential):

$$A_0 + e^- \longrightarrow A_0^- \qquad E'_0 = -1.1 \text{ V} \qquad (2)$$

To get the overall reaction that occurs, we must equalize the number of electrons by multiplying equation 2 by 2. (We do *not*, however, multiply the half-cell potential by 2.)

$$2\,A_0 + 2\,e^- \longrightarrow 2\,A_0^- \qquad E'_0 = -1.1 \text{ V} \qquad (3)$$

Then we *subtract* equation 3 from equation 1, which yields

$$NADP^+ + H^+ + 2\,A_0^- \longrightarrow NADPH + 2\,A_0 \qquad \Delta E'_0 = +0.78 \text{ V}$$

In calculating $\Delta E'_0$ values, do not make the mistake of multiplying half-cell reduction potentials by factors used to equalize the number of electrons. Remember that $\Delta E'_0$ is a *potential difference* and hence, at least for our purposes, is independent of the *amount* of electron flow. For example, in a house with an adequate electrical power supply, the potential difference measured at the fuse box is approximately 117 V regardless of whether the house is in total darkness or all the lights are turned on.

To get the free-energy change for the overall reaction, we start with the relationship given in Section 20.2 of the text:

$$\Delta G^{o\prime} = -nF\,\Delta E'_0$$

Substitution yields

$$\Delta G^{o\prime} = -2 \times 96.48 \times 0.78 = -151 \text{ kJ/mol}$$

or $\qquad\qquad \Delta G^{o\prime} = -2 \times 23.06 \times 0.78 = -36 \text{ kcal/mol}$

2. In this process, electrons are transferred down an electron-transport chain from P680* to P700. The E'_0 value for P680* is approximately -0.8 V, and that for P700 is approximately 0.4 V; $\Delta E'_0$ is therefore $+1.2$ V. The free-energy change is calculated from the relationship given on in section 20.2 of the text.

$$\Delta G^{o\prime} = -nF\,\Delta E'_0$$

$$= -2 \times 96.48 \times 1.2 = -232 \text{ kJ/mol}$$

or $\qquad\qquad = -2 \times 23.06 \times 1.2 = -55 \text{ kcal/mol}$

In the mitochondrial electron-transport chain, the free-energy change as a pair of electrons is transferred from $NADH + H^+$ to oxygen is -52.6 kcal/mol (see Section 20.2 of the text). In both cases the large "span" of free energy is used to drive the formation of ATP.

3. In the scheme in Figure 22.1, electrons are shown flowing "uphill" from X* to Y as ATP is being formed. This is a thermodynamic impossibility. For electrons to flow spontaneously from X* to Y, the redox potential of X* must be more negative than that of Y. For ATP to be formed as electron transfer occurs, the free-energy change must be of sufficient magnitude to allow for ATP biosynthesis. In order to make electrons flow from X* to Y as depicted in the hypothetical scheme, ATP would be consumed, not generated.

4. The synthesis of ATP in both the chloroplast and the mitochondrion is driven by the proton-motive force across the membrane. In mitochondria, a membrane potential of 0.14 V is established during electron transport. In chloroplasts, the light-induced potential is close to 0. Therefore, there must be a greater pH gradient in the chloroplast to give the same free-energy yield (see Chapter 21 and Section 22.4 of the text).

5. Oxygen would be evolved. $NADP^+$ is the final electron acceptor for photosynthesis; see the summary in Figure 22.21 in the text. Adding $NADP^+$ will drive the process to the right.

6. Yes. Little oxygen would be evolved when 700-nm light is used. Oxygen is evolved by photosystem II, which contains P680 and is therefore not maximally excited by 700-nm light.

7. You would use 430 nm for chlorophyll *a* and 455 nm for chlorophyll *b*. These are the wavelengths of maximum absorbance, so they would provide the most sensitive spectrophotometric assays.

8. Chlorophyll appears to be green because it has no significant absorption in the green region of the spectrum and therefore transmits green light.

9. Acetone is the preferred solvent. Because of the hydrophobic porphyrin ring and the very hydrophobic phytol tail of the chlorophylls, they are soluble in organic solvents like acetone but are insoluble in water.

10. Higher animals tend to have limited biosynthetic abilities because their diet contains plants and sometimes other animals. Thus there are many amino acids that animals can't synthesize. One of the most popular herbicides in use today is glyphosate (Roundup®), which inhibits the synthesis of phenylalanine. See Chapter 31 in the text for more discussion. There are several herbicides that block amino acid biosynthesis. They are not very toxic to animals because they block enzymes we lack.

11. The fact that it requires two separate photosystems to promote electrons from water to NADPH implies that the system evolved from something simpler with a single photosystem, which is why the apparatus from *Rhodopseudomonas viridis* is discussed in the chapter. Also, the 4-manganese center that interacts with water (Figure 22.18 in the text) is quite complex and might relate to a 2-manganese center found in catalase. There is evidence for some O_2 appearing in the atmosphere a little more than 2 billion years ago. Water-based photosynthesis cannot be younger than this, and could be significantly older, assuming the oxygen evolved was scavenged up locally. Stromatolites resembling those found today in Shark Bay, Australia (which use oxygen-producing photosynthesis), can be found in layers dated 3.2 billion years old. One interesting theory about early photosynthesis postulates that a major source of electrons could have been the Ferrous (Fe^{+2}) ions that were abundant in the Earth's oceans before oxygen precipitated most of the iron as banded iron formations (*Trends in Biochem. Sci.* 23[1998]:94).

12 "Special pairs" are so named because they are fundamental to photosynthesis. Photosynthesizing bacteria have one such pair, P960. Green plants have two photosystems, each with a special pair: P680 in photosystem II and P700 in photosystem I. Each pair is named for the wavelength of light it best absorbs; P stands for pigment.

Each special pair consists of two adjacent chlorophyll molecules which absorb light and, when excited, emit an electron. This electron is captured by nearby electron carriers and then sent through a photosynthetic electron transport chain. The departure of an electron leaves the special pair positively charged, producing an initial charge separation without which photosynthesis could not take place. The special pairs are then replenished: P680 gets a replacement electron from a nearby cytochrome, P680 takes its electron from H_2O (generating the oxygen in the Earth's atmosphere), and P700 takes its electron from plastocyanin, which in some cases has been reduced by Photosystem II.

The Calvin Cycle

The Calvin cycle (sometimes referred to as the reductive pentose phosphate pathway) uses NADPH to convert carbon dioxide into hexoses, and the pentose phosphate pathway breaks down glucose into carbon dioxide to produce NADPH. The Calvin cycle constitutes the dark reactions of photosynthesis. The light reactions were discussed in Chapter 22; they transform light energy into ATP and biosynthetic reducing power, nicotinamide adenine dinucleotide phosphate (NADPH). While the dark reactions do not directly require light, they do depend on the ATP and NADPH that are produced by the light reactions. The Calvin cycle synthesizes hexoses from carbon dioxide and water in three stages: (1) fixation of CO_2 by ribulose-5-phosphate to form two molecules of 3-phosphoglycerate, (2) reduction of 3-phosphoglycerate to form hexose sugars, and (3) regeneration of ribulose-5-phosphate so that more CO_2 can be fixed. After a discussion of the reactions of the Calvin cycle, the authors proceed to the regulation of the cycle. Carbon dioxide assimilation by the Calvin cycle operates during the day, and carbohydrate degradation to yield energy occurs at night. The discussion of the Calvin cycle concludes with two environmentally dependent modifications to the pathway used by tropical plants and succulents to respond to high temperatures and drought.

LEARNING OBJECTIVES

When you have mastered this chapter, you should be able to accomplish the following objectives.

Introduction

1. Distinguish between the *dark* and *light reactions* of photosynthesis.
2. Explain the function of the *Calvin cycle*.

The Calvin Cycle Synthesizes Hexoses from Carbon Dioxide and Water
(Text Section 23.1)

3. Outline the three stages of the Calvin cycle.
4. Describe the formation of *3-phosphoglycerate* by *ribulose 1,5-bisphosphate carboxylase* (*rubisco*). Note the two different roles of CO_2 and the role of Mg^{2+} in the reaction.
5. Describe the structure of rubisco. Relate the large amount of rubisco present in plants to its slow catalytic rate.
6. Outline the formation of *phosphoglycolate* by the *oxygenase reaction* of rubisco, and follow its subsequent metabolism. Define *photorespiration*.
7. Give two explanations for why it does not seem possible to remove the *oxygenase* activity from rubisco.
8. Outline the conversion of 3-phosphoglycerate into fructose 6-phosphate and the *regeneration of ribulose 1,5-bisphosphate*.
9. Write a balanced equation for the Calvin cycle, and account for the ATP and NADPH expended to form a hexose molecule.
10. Explain the formation of *starch* and *sucrose*.

The Calvin Cycle Is Regulated by the Environment
(Text Section 23.2)

11. List the four light-dependent changes in the stroma that regulate the Calvin cycle.
12. Outline the role of rubisco and *thioredoxin* in coordinating the light and dark reactions of photosynthesis.
13. Describe the C_4 *pathway* and its adaptive value to tropical plants. Explain how CO_2 transport suppresses the oxygenase reaction of rubisco.
14. Explain the use of *crassulacean acid metabolism* by plants growing in arid climates.

SELF-TEST

The Calvin Cycle Synthesizes Hexoses from Carbon Dioxide and Water

1. Which of the following statements about ribulose 1,5-bisphosphate carboxylase (rubisco) are correct?
    (a) It is present at low concentrations in the chloroplast.
    (b) It is activated by the addition of CO_2 to the ε-amino group of a specific lysine to form a carbamate that then binds a divalent metal cation.

(c) It catalyzes, as one part of its reaction sequence, an extremely exergonic reaction, the cleavage of a six-carbon diol derivative of arabinitol to form two three-carbon compounds.

(d) It catalyzes a reaction between ribulose 1,5-bisphosphate and O_2 that decreases the efficiency of photosynthesis.

(e) It catalyzes the carboxylase reaction more efficiently and the oxygenase reaction less efficiently as the temperature increases.

2. The rubisco-catalyzed reaction of O_2 with ribulose 1,5-bisphosphate forms which of the following substances?

(a) 3-phosphoglycerate
(b) 2-phosphoacetate
(c) phosphoglycolate
(d) glycolate
(e) glyoxylate

3. Which of the following statements about 3-phosphoglycerate (3-PG) produced in the Calvin cycle is NOT true?

(a) It can be used to produce glucose-1-phosphate, glucose-6-phosphate, and fructose-6-phosphate.

(b) It is converted to hexose phosphates in a series of reactions that are identical to those in the gluconeogenic pathway.

(c) It produces glyceraldehyde 3-phosphate, which can be transported to the cytosol for glucose synthesis.

(d) The conversion of 3-PG into hexose phosphates produces energy and reducing equivalents.

(e) Although both glyceraldehyde 3-phosphate (GAP) and dihydroxyacetone phosphate (DHAP) can be produced from 3-PG, only GAP can be used in further sugar-producing reactions.

4. Place the following sugar conversions in the correct order used to regenerate starting material for the Calvin cycle, and name the enzyme that catalyzes each reaction.

(a) C_7-ketose + C_3-aldose $\rightarrow$ C_5-ketose + C_5-aldose
(b) C_6-ketose + C_3-aldose $\rightarrow$ C_4-aldose + C_5-ketose
(c) C_4-aldose + C_3-ketose $\rightarrow$ C_7-ketose

5. Match the two major storage forms of carbohydrates, starch and sucrose, with the appropriate properties listed in the right column.

(a) starch
(b) sucrose

(1) contains glucose
(2) contains fructose
(3) is a polymer
(4) is synthesized in the cytosol
(5) is synthesized in chloroplasts
(6) is synthesized from UDP-glucose

6. Scientists have been unable to create a recombinant rubisco that does not have oxygenase activity. Which of the following are possible explanations as to why?

(a) The enzyme cannot discriminate between oxygen and carbon dioxide.

(b) The oxygenase activity is biochemically important for an unknown reason and cannot be removed.

(c) Because the enzyme is so fast, any diatomic gas will react with it.

(d) Photorespiration is critically important to plants and without the oxygenase activity, it would not be possible.

The Activity of the Calvin Cycle Depends on Environmental Conditions

7. Which of the following statements about the Calvin cycle are true?

   (a) It regenerates the ribulose 1,5-bisphosphate consumed by the rubisco reaction.
   (b) It forms glyceraldehyde 3-phosphate, which can be converted to fructose 6-phosphate.
   (c) It requires ATP and NADPH.
   (d) It is exergonic because light energy absorbed by the chlorophylls is transferred to rubisco.
   (e) It consists of enzymes, several of which can be activated through reduction of disulfide bridges by reduced thioredoxin.
   (f) It is controlled, in part, by the rate of the rubisco reaction.
   (g) Its rate decreases as the level of illumination increases because both the pH and the level of Mg^{2+} of the stroma decrease.

8. Which of these statements about thioredoxin is correct?

   (a) It contains a heme that cycles between two oxidation states.
   (b) Its oxidized form predominates while light absorption is taking place.
   (c) It activates some biosynthetic enzymes by reducing disulfide bridges.
   (d) It activates some degradative enzymes by reducing disulfide bridges.
   (e) Oxidized thioredoxin is reduced by plastoquinol.

9. Answer the following questions about the C_4 pathway in tropical plants.

   (a) What is the three-carbon CO_2 acceptor in mesophyll cells?
   (b) What is the four-carbon CO_2 donor in bundle-sheath cells?
   (c) What is the net reaction for the C_4 pathway?
   (d) Is the C_4 pathway a type of active or passive transport?

10. Plants growing in hot environments have developed adaptations in CO_2 storage and use. Contrast the adaptive differences between plants growing in tropical and arid environments.

ANSWERS TO SELF-TEST

1. b, c, d. Answer (e) is incorrect because the rate of the oxygenase reaction increases relative to that of the carboxylase reaction as the temperature increases; the altered ratio of the two reaction rates decreases the efficiency of photosynthesis as the temperature increases.

2. a, c.

3. The incorrect statements are b, d, and e. Statement (b) is incorrect because the gluconeogenic pathway uses NADH, not NADPH; (d) is incorrect because the conversion requires both ATP and NADPH; e is incorrect because both GAP and DHAP can be used to produce larger sugars.

4. The correct order is b, c, a. Transketolase catalyzes reactions (a) and (b); aldolase catalyzes reaction (c).

5. (a) 1, 3, 5   (b) 1, 2, 4, 6

6. a, b. Answer (c) is incorrect because the enzyme is very slow. Answer (d) is incorrect because photorespiration is harmful to plants, and ideally would be avoided.

7. a, b, c, e, f

8. c. Thioredoxin contains cysteine residues that cycle between two oxidation states. It is reduced by ferredoxin while the light reactions are proceeding. It activates biosynthetic enzymes and inhibits degradative enzymes by reducing their disulfide bridges.

9. (a) Phosphoenolpyruvate is the three-carbon CO_2 acceptor in mesophyll cells.
   (b) Malate is the four-carbon CO_2 donor in bundle-sheath cells.
   (c) CO_2 (in mesophyll cell) + ATP + H_2O → CO_2 (in bundle-sheath cell) + AMP + $2P_i$ + H^+
   (d) It is a type of active transport because it requires ATP to function.

10. Plants in arid environments use crassulacean acid metabolism to store CO_2 absorbed at night in the form of malate until it can be used during the day. Plants in tropical environments use the C4 pathway to increase the concentration of CO_2 in bundle-sheath cells thus accelerating the carboxylase reaction relative to the oxygenase reaction and minimizing photorespiration. In contrast with C4 plants, CAM plants separate CO_2 accumulation from CO_2 utilization temporally rather than spatially.

PROBLEMS

1. Outline the synthesis of fructose 6-phosphate from 3-phosphoglycerate.

2. How many moles of ATP and NADPH are required to convert 6 moles of CO_2 to fructose 6-phosphate?

3. Describe photorespiration, and explain why it decreases the efficiency of photosynthesis.

4. It is said that the C_4 pathway increases the efficiency of photosynthesis. What is the justification for this statement when more than 1.6 times as much ATP is required to convert 6 moles of CO_2 to a hexose when this pathway is used in contrast with the pathway used by plants lacking the C_4 apparatus? Account for the extra ATP molecules used in the C_4 pathway.

5. In addition to the well-understood ferredoxin-thioredoxin couple, NADPH can regulate Calvin cycle enzymes. A recently discovered assembly protein CP12 binds to and inhibits phosphoribulose kinase (PRK) and glyceraldehyde 3-phosphate dehydrogenase (GAPDH) in the dark and releases them in the light (Wedel et al. *Proc. Nat. Acad. Sci.* 94 [1997]:10479–10484). The authors of the paper found that NADPH triggers the release of PRK and GADPH from CP12 and is also necessary for PRK activity after its release. They also noted that PRK is rapidly oxidized in the absence of reduced thioredoxin; it remains reduced when bound to CP12.
   (a) Why would PRK require NADPH for full activity given that is does not catalyze a reduction reaction?
   (b) Given this information, what is a possible role of PRK binding to CP12?

ANSWERS TO PROBLEMS

1. Phosphoglycerate kinase converts 3-phosphoglycerate, the initial product of photosynthesis, to the glycolytic intermediate 1,3-bisphosphoglycerate, which is then converted to glyceraldehyde 3-phosphate (G-3-P) by an NADPH-dependent G-3-P dehydrogenase in the chloroplast. Triosephosphate isomerase converts G-3-P to dihydroxyacetone

phosphate, which aldolase can condense with another G-3-P to form fructose 1,6-bisphosphate. The phosphate ester at C-1 is hydrolyzed to give fructose 6-phosphate. The result of this pathway, which is functionally equivalent to the gluconeogenic pathway, is the conversion of the CO_2 fixed by photosynthesis into a hexose.

2. Eighteen moles of ATP and twelve moles of NADPH are required to fix six moles of CO_2. Two moles of ATP are used by phosphoglycerate kinase to form two moles of 1,3-bisphosphoglycerate, and one mole of ATP is used by ribulose 5-phosphate kinase to form one mole of ribulose 1,5-bisphosphate per mole of CO_2 fixed. Two moles of NADPH are used by G-3-P dehydrogenase to form two moles of G-3-P per mole of CO_2 incorporated. Therefore, three moles of ATP and two moles of NADPH are used for each mole of CO_2 fixed.

3. The oxygenase reaction of rubisco and the salvage reactions that convert two resulting phosphoglycolate molecules into serine are called *photorespiration* because CO_2 is released and O_2 is consumed in the process. Unlike genuine respiration, no ATP or NADPH is produced by photorespiration. Ordinarily, no CO_2 is released during photosynthesis, and all the fixed CO_2 can be used to form hexoses. During photorespiration, no CO_2 is fixed, and the products into which ribulose 1,5-bisphosphate is converted by the oxygenase reaction of rubisco cannot be completely recycled into carbohydrate because of the loss of CO_2 in the phosphoglycolate salvage reactions.

4. Plants lacking the C_4 pathway cannot compensate for the relative increase in the rate of the oxygenase reaction of rubisco with respect to the rate of the carboxylase reaction that occurs as the temperature rises. Plants with the C_4 pathway increase the concentration of CO_2 in the bundle-sheath cell, where the Calvin cycle occurs, thereby increasing the ability of CO_2 to compete with O_2 as a substrate for rubisco. As a result, more CO_2 is fixed and less ribulose 1,5-bisphosphate is degraded into phosphoglycolate, which cannot be efficiently converted into carbohydrate. Thus, the Calvin cycle functions more efficiently in these specialized plants under conditions of high illumination and at higher temperatures than it would otherwise. The concentration of CO_2 is increased by an expenditure of ATP. The collection of one CO_2 molecule and its transport on C_4 compounds from the mesophyll cell into the bundle-sheath cell is brought about by the conversion of one ATP to AMP and PP_i in a reaction in which pyruvate is phosphorylated to PEP. The PP_i is hydrolyzed, and two ATP are required to resynthesize ATP from AMP. Thus, an *extra* ATP/CO_2 × 6 CO_2/hexose = 12 ATP/hexose are used by the C_4 pathway.

5. (a) Since the purpose of PRK is to regenerate ribulose 1,5-bisphosphate for use in the Calvin cycle, it does not make sense to have it active when there is not enough NADPH to run the cycle. The PRK reaction requires ATP and would be wasteful if ribulose 1,5-bisphosphate were not needed.

   (b) In the absence of CP12 complex formation, PRK is rapidly oxidized and becomes inactive. In conditions of low NADPH, if complex formation did not occur, PRK would reoxidze and become inactive before producing ribulose 1,5-bisphosphate. The light energy used to reduce thioredoxin would therefore be wasted. By keeping thioredoxin-reduced PRK bound to CP12 until enough NADPH is present, the light energy is not wasted.

Chapter 24

Glycogen Degradation

The topic of carbohydrate metabolism presented in Chapters 16 and 17 is further developed in Chapters 24 and 25 with a detailed discussion of the metabolism of glycogen, the intracellular storage form of glucose. The breakdown of glycogen, glycogen degradation, is discussed in Chapter 24, while the synthesis of glycogen is covered in Chapter 25. Glycogen is important in the metabolism of higher animals because its glucose residues can be easily mobilized by the liver to maintain blood glucose levels and used by muscle to satisfy its energy needs during bursts of contraction. The text first reviews briefly the structure and the physiologic roles of glycogen and provides an overview of its metabolism. You were introduced briefly to the structure of glycogen, a polymer of glucose, in Chapter 10. Next, the text presents the enzymatic reactions of glycogen degradation. The control of these catabolic reactions by allosteric mechanisms and the phosphorylation and dephosphorylation of the key enzymes in response to hormonal signals is discussed. AMP, ATP, glucose, and glucose 6-phosphate act as allosteric effectors, and the hormones insulin, glucagon, and epinephrine function as signals in transduction pathways that control critical enzyme phosphorylations and dephosphorylations. The text describes relevant structures and control mechanisms for phosphorylase, phosphorylase kinase, glycogen synthase, the branching enzyme, and protein phosphatase 1. The differences in glycogen metabolism in muscle and liver are discussed in the context of the distinct physiologic functions these tissues perform. The text concludes with a discussion of the relevance of glycogen depletion in the onset of fatigue.

LEARNING OBJECTIVES

When you have mastered this chapter, you should be able to accomplish the following objectives.

Introduction

1. Describe the structure of *glycogen* and its roles in the *liver* and *muscle*. Distinguish between *α-1,4 glycosidic linkages* and *α-1,6 glycosidic linkages*.

2. Describe the three steps of *glycogen catabolism* and the three fates of its product, *glucose 6-phosphate*.

3. Explain the role of *allosteric responses* and *hormones* in regulating glycogen breakdown.

Glycogen Breakdown Requires Several Enzymes (Text Section 24.1)

4. Write the phosphorolysis reaction catalyzed by *glycogen phosphorylase*.

5. Explain the advantage of the *phosphorolytic cleavage* of glycogen over *hydrolytic cleavage*.

6 Outline the steps in the degradation of glycogen, and relate them to the action of *phosphorylase, transferase,* and *α-1,6-glucosidase*, which is also known as the *debranching enzyme*. Explain why the glycogen molecule must be remodeled during its degradation.

7. Describe the reaction catalyzed by *phosphoglucomutase* and explain how it helps glycogen breakdown products enter the metabolic mainstream.

8. Explain the importance of *glucose 6-phosphatase* in the release of glucose by the liver. Note the absence of this enzyme in the brain and muscle and rationalize this tissue distribution.

Phosphorylase is Regulated by Allosteric Interactions and Reversible Phosphorylation (Text Section 24.2)

9. Appreciate that the two primary regulatory mechanisms for glycogen phosphorylase are interactions with *allosteric effectors* and *reversible covalent modifications*.

10. Describe the phosphorylation of phosphorylase by *phosphorylase kinase*.

11. Explain the relationships between *phosphorylase a* and *phosphorylase b*, their *T (tense)* and *R (relaxed)* forms, and the allosteric effectors that mediate their interconversions in skeletal muscle. Outline the molecular bases for the relative inactivities of the T states.

12. Contrast the regulation of liver phosphorylase and muscle phosphorylase.

13. Contrast the important structural features of phosphorylase *a* and phosphorylase *b*. Note the variety of binding sites, their functional roles, and the critical location of the phosphorylation and AMP-binding sites near the subunit interface.

14. Describe the major compositional features of phosphorylase kinase and its activation by *protein kinase A (PKA)*. Explain the effects of *calmodulin* and Ca^{2+} on glycogen metabolism in muscle and liver.

15. Explain how a defect in a phosphorylase isozyme can lead to Hers disease.

Epinephrine and Glucagon Signal the Need for Glycogen Breakdown (Text Section 24.3)

16. Compare the effects of *glucagon* and *epinephrine* on glycogen metabolism in liver and in muscle.

17. List the sequence of events from the binding of hormones by their receptors to the

phosphorylation of glycogen phosphorylase. Explain the roles of *G proteins*, *cAMP*, and PKA in these processes.

18. Explain the role of *protein phosphatase 1 (PP1)* in glycogen metabolism.

19. Describe how glycogen depletion is linked to the onset of fatigue.

SELF-TEST

Introduction

1. Answer the questions about the glycogen fragment in Figure 24.1.

   FIGURE 24.1   Fragment of glycogen. (*R* represents the rest of the glycogen molecule.)

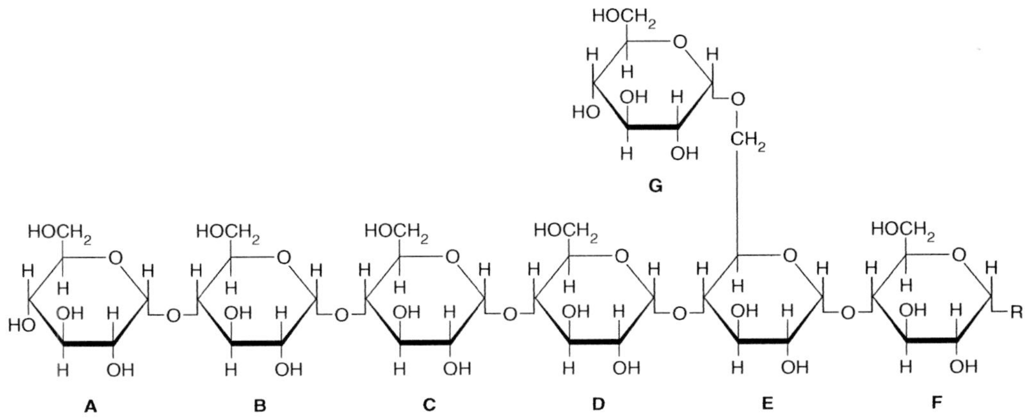

   (a) Which residues are at nonreducing ends?
   (b) An α-1,6 glycosidic linkage occurs between which residues?
   (c) An α-1,4 glycosidic linkage occurs between which residues?
   (d) Is the glycogen fragment a substrate for phosphorylase *a*? Explain.
   (e) Is the glycogen fragment a substrate for the debranching enzyme? Explain.

2. Which of the following statements about glycogen storage are NOT correct?

   (a) Glycogen is stored in muscles and liver.
   (b) Glycogen is a major source of stored energy in brain.
   (c) Glycogen reserves are less rapidly depleted than fat reserves during starvation.
   (d) Glycogen nearly fills the nucleus of cells that specialize in glycogen storage.
   (e) Glycogen storage occurs in the form of dense granules in the cytoplasm of cells.

3. Is the largest total mass of glycogen found in the liver or the muscle?

Glycogen Breakdown Requires Several Enzymes

4. Explain why the phosphorolytic cleavage of glycogen is more energetically advantageous than its hydrolytic cleavage.

5. Match the enzymes that degrade glycogen in the left column with the appropriate properties in the right column.

   (a) Phosphorylase
   (b) α-1,6-Glucosidase
   (c) Transferase

   (1) is part of a single polypeptide chain with two activities.
   (2) cleaves α-1,4 glucosidic bonds.
   (3) releases glucose.
   (4) releases glucose 1-phosphate.
   (5) moves three sugar residues from one chain to another.
   (6) requires ATP.

6. Which of the following are properties of phosphoglucomutase?

   (a) It has a phosphoenzyme intermediate.
   (b) It uses glucose 1,6-bisphosphate intermediate.
   (c) It is an enzyme unique to glycogen metabolism.
   (d) It transfers the phosphate group from one position to another on the same molecule.

7. The activity of which of the following enzymes is NOT required for the release of large amounts of glucose from liver glycogen?

   (a) glucose 6-phosphatase
   (b) fructose 1,6-bisphosphatase
   (c) α-1,6-glucosidase
   (d) phosphoglucomutase
   (e) glycogen phosphorylase

8. Answer the following questions about the enzymatic degradation of amylose, a linear α-1,4 polymer of glucose that is a storage form of glucose in plants.

   (a) Would phosphorylase act on amylose? Explain.
   (b) Would the rates of glucose 1-phosphate release from an amylose molecule by phosphorylase relative to that from a glycogen molecule having an equivalent number of glucose monomers be equal? Explain.
   (c) If the amylose were first treated with an endosaccharidase that cleaved some of its internal glycosidic bonds, how might the rate of production of glucose 1-phosphate be affected?

9. Starting from a glucose residue in glycogen, how many net ATP molecules will be formed in the glycolysis of the residue to pyruvate?

   (a) 1
   (b) 2
   (c) 3
   (d) 4
   (e) 5

Phosphorylase Is Regulated by Allosteric Interactions and Reversible Phosphorylation

10. Consider the diagram of the different conformational states of muscle glycogen phosphorylase in Figure 24.2. Then answer the questions.

    FIGURE 24.2 Conformational states of phosphorylase in muscle.

    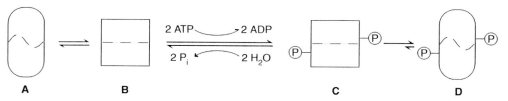

    (a) Which are the active forms of phosphorylase?
    (b) Which form requires high levels of AMP to become activated?
    (c) Which conversion is antagonized by ATP and glucose 6-phosphate?
    (d) What enzyme catalyzes the conversion of C to B?

11. How does the regulation of phosphorylase in the liver differ from the scheme for phosphorylase regulation in muscle shown in Figure 24.2?

12. Indicate which of the following substances have binding sites on phosphorylase. For those that do, give their major roles or effects.
    (a) calmodulin
    (b) glycogen
    (c) Ca^{2+}
    (d) AMP
    (e) P_i
    (f) ATP
    (g) glucose

13. Explain the roles of protein kinase A and calmodulin in the control of phosphorylase kinase in the muscle.

Epinephrine and Glucagon Signal the Need for Glycogen Breakdown

14. Place the following steps of the reaction cascade of glycogen metabolism in the proper sequence.
    (a) phosphorylation of protein kinase A
    (b) formation of cyclic AMP by adenylate cyclase
    (c) phosphorylation of phosphorylase b
    (d) hormone binding to target cell receptors
    (e) phosphorylation of phosphorylase kinase

15. Why are enzymatic cascades, such as those that control glycogen metabolism and the clotting of blood, of particular importance in metabolism?

16. Figure 24.12A in the text shows the decrease in glycogen content of the quadricep muscle in cyclists as a function of time. After 75 minutes if exercise the cyclist becomes fatigued. Answer the following:
    (a) Can we conclude on the basis of this data that the depletion of glycogen was responsible for the onset of fatigue?
    (b) What other changes in metabolic products do you expect at the end of the 75 minutes?
    c) Speculate on the ways in which these metabolic changes might be important in the onset of fatigue.

17. Compare and contrast the action of epinephrine and glucagon in glycogen metabolism.

ANSWERS TO SELF-TEST

1. (a) A and G
   (b) G and E
   (c) All the bonds are α-1,4 glycosidic linkages except for the one between residues G and E.
   (d) No. The two branches are too short for phosphorylase cleavage. Phosphorylase stops cleaving four residues away from a branch point.
   (e) Yes. Residue G can be hydrolyzed by α-1,6-glucosidase (the debranching enzyme).

2. b, c, d

3. Although the concentration of glycogen is higher in liver, the larger mass of muscle stores more glycogen *in toto*.

4. The phosphorolytic cleavage of glycogen produces glucose 1-phosphate, which can enter into the glycolytic pathway after conversion to glucose 6-phosphate. These

reactions do not require ATP. On the other hand, the hydrolysis of glycogen would produce glucose, which would have to be converted to glucose 6-phosphate by hexokinase, requiring the expenditure of an ATP. Therefore, harvesting the free energy stored in glycogen by phosphorolytic cleavage rather than a hydrolytic one is more efficient because it decreases the ATP investment.

5. (a) 2, 4   (b) 1, 3   (c) 1, 2, 5. None of these enzymes requires ATP.

6. a, b

7. b

8. (a) Yes; phosphorylase would act on amylose by removing one glucose residue at a time from the nonreducing end.
   (b) No; the rate of degradation of amylose would be much slower than that of glycogen because amylose would have only a single nonreducing end available for reaction, whereas glycogen has many ends.
   (c) The increased number of ends available to phosphorylase as a result of cleaving the chain into pieces with the endosaccharidase would allow a more rapid production of glucose 1-phosphate by phosphorylase.

9. c. A glucose molecule that is degraded in the glycolytic pathway to two pyruvate molecules yields two ATP; however, the formation of glucose-1-P from glycogen does not consume the ATP that would be required for the formation of glucose-6-P from glucose. Thus, the net yield of ATP for a glucose residue derived from glycogen is three ATP.

10. (a) A and D
    (b) B
    (c) B to A
    (d) protein phosphatase 1

The phosphorylated form of glycogen phosphorylase is phosphorylase *a*, which is mostly present in the active conformation designated D in Figure 24.2. In the presence of high levels of glucose, phosphorylase *a* adopts a strained, inactive conformation, designated C in the figure. The dephosphorylated form of the enzyme is called phosphorylase *b*. Phosphorylase *b* is mostly present in an inactive conformation, labeled B in the figure. When AMP binds to the inactive phosphorylase *b*, the enzyme changes to an active conformation, designated A in the figure. The effects of AMP can be reversed by ATP or glucose 6-phosphate.

11. AMP doesn't activate liver phosphorylase (the B to A conversion shown in Figure 21.2), and glucose shifts the equilibrium between the activated phosphorylase *a* toward the inactivated form (the D to C conversion).

12. (b) Glycogen, as the substrate, binds to the active site; there is also a glycogen particle binding site that keeps the enzyme attached to the glycogen granule.
    (e) AMP binds to an allosteric site and activates phosphorylase *b* in muscle.
    (f) P_i binds to the pyridoxal phosphate at the active site and attacks the α-1,4 glycosidic bond. Another P_i is covalently bound to serine 14 by phosphorylase kinase. This phosphorylation converts phosphorylase *b* into active phosphorylase *a*.
    (g) ATP binds to the same site as AMP and blocks its effects in muscle; therefore, energy charge affects phosphorylase activity.
    (h) Glucose inhibits phosphorylase *a* in the liver by changing the conformation of the enzyme to the inactive T form.

Answers (a) and (d) are incorrect because calmodulin and Ca^{2+} bind to phosphorylase kinase rather than to phosphorylase.

13. Protein kinase A, which is itself activated by cAMP, phosphorylates phosphorylase kinase to activate it. Phosphorylase kinase can also be activated by the binding of Ca^{2+} to its calmodulin subunit. On binding Ca^{2+}, calmodulin undergoes conformational changes that activate the phosphorylase kinase. The activated kinase in turn activates glycogen phosphorylase. These effects lead to glycogen degradation in active muscle.

14. d, b, a, e, c

15. Enzymatic cascades lead from a small signal, caused by a few molecules, to a large subsequent enzymatic response. Thus, small chemical signals can be amplified in a short time to yield large biological effects. In addition, their effects can be regulated at various levels of the cascade.

16. Both epinephrine and glucagon stimulate glycogen breakdown by interacting with 7TM receptors and activating a cAMP signal-transduction cascade that ultimately activates glycogen phosphorylase. Glucagon activates glycogen breakdown in the liver. Epinephrine primarily activates glycogen breakdown in the muscle. Epinephrine can also act on the liver by initiating both the cAMP cascade and a phosphoinositide cascade.

17. (a) No, because although the two events are correlated (they clearly happen at the same time) it does prove that one caused the other.

    (b) The most obvious change is the drop in ATP as it is hydrolyzed during muscle contraction. We'd expect the concentration of ADP, AMP, Pi, and H^+ to increase. Ca^{2+} levels should also increase, activating calmodulin in phosphorylase kinase as well as triggering muscle contraction.

    (c) In addition to the lack of ATP resulting in a slow down of the rate of muscle contraction, it is possible that ADP, Pi, and/or AMP act as inhibitors of muscle contraction. It was long thought that the acidic pH due to lactic acid buildup in anaerobic muscle cells played a role in fatigue, but that has not been conclusively proven.

PROBLEMS

1. A patient can perform nonstrenuous tasks but becomes fatigued with physical exertion. Assays from a muscle biopsy reveal that glycogen levels are slightly elevated relative to normal. Crude extracts from muscle are used to determine the activity of glycogen phosphorylase at various levels of calcium ion for the patient and for a normal person. The results of the assays are shown in Figure 24.3. Briefly explain the clinical and biochemical findings for the patient.

FIGURE 24.3 Response of glycogen phosphorylase to calcium ion in a patient and in a normal person.

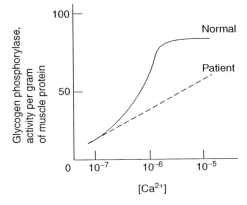

2. A strain of mutant mice is characterized by limited ability to engage in prolonged exercise. After a high-carbohydrate meal, one of these mice can exercise on a treadmill for only about 30% of the time a normal mouse can. At exhaustion, blood glucose levels in the mutant mouse are quite low, and they increase only marginally after rest. When liver glycogen in fed mutant mice is examined before exercise, the polymers have chains that are highly branched, with average branch lengths of about 10 glucose residues in either α-1,4 or α-1,6 linkage. Glycogen from exhausted normal mice has the same type of structure. Glycogen from exhausted mutant mice is still highly branched, but the polymer has an unusually large number of single glucose residues with α-1,6 linkages. Practically all the chains with α-1,4 linkages are still about 10 residues in length. Explain the metabolic and molecular observations for the mutant mice.

3. Your colleague discovers a fungal enzyme that can liberate glucose residues from cellulose. The enzyme is similar to glycogen phosphorylase in that it utilizes inorganic phosphate for the phosphorolytic cleavage of glucose residues from the nonreducing ends of cellulose. Why would you suspect that other types of cellulases may be important in the rapid degradation of cellulose?

4. Consider a patient with the following clinical findings: fasting blood glucose level is 25 mg per 100 ml (normal values are from 80 to 100 mg per 100 ml); feeding the patient glucose results in a rapid elevation of blood glucose level, followed by a normal return to fasting levels; feeding the patient galactose or fructose results in the elevation of blood glucose to normal levels; the administration of glucagon fails to generate hyperglycemia; biochemical examination of liver glycogen reveals a normal glycogen structure.
   (a) What enzyme deficiency could account for these clinical findings?
   (b) What additional experiments would you conduct to provide a specific diagnosis for the patient?

5. Cyclic nucleotide phosphatases are inhibited by caffeine. What effect would drinking a strong cup of coffee have on glycogen metabolism when epinephrine levels are dropping in the blood?

6. During the degradation of branched chains of glycogen, a transferase shifts a chain of three glycosyl residues from one branch to another, exposing a single remaining glycosyl residue to α-1,6-glucosidase activity. Free glucose is released, and the now unbranched chain can be further degraded by glycogen phosphorylase.
   (a) Estimate the free-energy change of the transfer of glycosyl residues from one branch to another.
   (b) About 10 percent of the glycosyl residues of normal glycogen are released as glucose, whereas the remainder are released as glucose 1-phosphate. Give two reasons why it is desirable for cells to convert most of the glycosyl residues in glycogen to glucose 1-phosphate.
   (c) Patients who lack liver glycosyl transferase have been studied. Why would you expect liver extracts from such people to perhaps lack α-1,6-glucosidase activity?

7. You are studying a patient with McArdle's disease, which results from an absence of muscle glycogen phosphorylase. In these patients liver phosphorylase activity is normal. Explain what you would expect to find when you carry out each of the following analyses.
   (a) fasting level of blood glucose
   (b) structure and amount of liver glycogen
   (c) structure and amount of muscle glycogen
   (d) change in blood glucose levels upon feeding the patient galactose
   (e) change in blood lactate levels after vigorous exercise
   (f) change in blood glucose levels after administration of glucagon
   (g) change in blood glucose levels after administration of epinephrine

8. An investigator has a sample of purified muscle phosphorylase *b* that she knows is relatively inactive.

    (a) Suggest two *in vitro* methods that could be used to generate active phosphorylase from the inactive phosphorylase *b*.

    (b) After the phosphorylase is activated, the investigator incubates the enzyme with a sample of unbranched glycogen in a buffered solution. She finds that no glycosyl residues are cleaved. What else is needed for the cleavage of glycosyl residues by active phosphorylase?

9. Arsenate can substitute in many reactions for which phosphate is the normal substrate. However, arsenate esters are far less stable than phosphate esters, and they decompose spontaneously to arsenate and an alcohol:

$$R{-}OAsO_3^{2-} + H_2O \rightarrow R{-}OH + AsO_4^{2-}$$

    (a) In which of the steps of glycogen metabolism might arsenate be used as a substrate?

    (b) What are the energetic consequences of utilizing arsenate as a substrate in glycogen degradation?

10. While muscle cells in tissue culture can be stimulated to break down glycogen only minimally when incubated in a solution containing cyclic AMP, they are more readily stimulated by compounds like dibutyryl cyclic AMP (Figure 24.4). Explain the difference in response of cells to these two substances.

FIGURE 24.4 Dibutyryl-cyclic AMP.

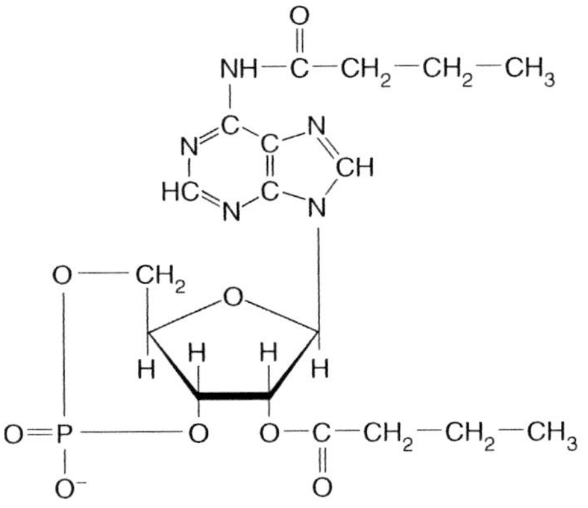

11. Patients with Cori's disease lack debranching enzyme, and therefore the structure of liver and muscle glycogen is unusual, with short outer branches. Design an assay that would enable you to demonstrate the presence of short branches in glycogen from one of these patients. Also explain how you would demonstrate that the debranching enzyme is deficient in these patients.

12. Why is it important for water to be excluded from the active site of glycogen phosphorylase?

13. Amylose is the linear polymer of glucose residues joined by α-1,4 glycosidic linkages found as a form of starch in plants. Why do you think it would serve less well as an energy source in muscle and liver than does glycogen?

ANSWERS TO PROBLEMS

1. Calcium ion normally activates muscle phosphorylase kinase, which in turn phosphorylates muscle phosphorylase. In the patient, glycogen phosphorylase activity is less responsive to Ca^{2+} than it is in the normal subject. It is likely that Ca^{2+} cannot

activate phosphorylase kinase in the patient, perhaps because the δ subunit (calmodulin) of the enzyme is altered in some way. As a result, there are too few molecules of enzymatically active glycogen phosphorylase to provide the rate of glycogen breakdown that is needed to sustain vigorous muscle contraction. Elevated levels of muscle glycogen should be expected when glycogen phosphorylase activity is lower than normal.

2. The longer chains of glucose residues in α-1,4 linkage and the unusually high number of single glucose residues in α-1,6 linkage suggest that although transferase activity is present, α-1,6-glucosidase activity is deficient in the mutant strain. For such chains, far fewer ends with glucose residues are available as substrates for glycogen phosphorylase. (Recall that glycogen phosphorylase cannot cleave α-1,6 linkages.) This limited ability to mobilize glucose residues means that less energy is available for prolonged exercise.

3. Cellulose is an unbranched polymer of glucose residues with β-1,4 linkages. Therefore, each chain has only one nonreducing end that is available for phosphorolysis by the fungal enzyme. Compared with the rate of breakdown of molecules of glycogen, whose branched chains provide more sites for the action of glycogen phosphorylase, the generation of glucose phosphate molecules from cellulose by means of the fungal enzyme alone could be quite slow. Therefore, you would expect to find endocellulases that generate additional nonreducing ends in cellulose chains.

4. (a) A low-fasting blood-glucose level indicates a failure either to mobilize glucose production from glycogen or to release glucose from the liver. However, the elevations in blood-glucose levels after feeding the patient glucose, galactose, or fructose indicate that the liver can release glucose derived from the diet or formed from other monosaccharides. The lack of response to glucagon indicates that the enzymatic cascade for glycogen breakdown is defective. Therefore, you would suspect a deficiency of liver glycogen phosphorylase or phosphorylase kinase.

   (b) The direct assay of the activities of glycogen phosphorylase and phosphorylase kinase would enable you to make a specific diagnosis. For these purposes, a liver biopsy would be necessary.

5. When epinephrine levels in the blood decrease, the synthesis of cyclic AMP decreases. Existing cyclic AMP is degraded by cyclic nucleotide phosphatases. The inhibition of these enzymes by caffeine prolongs the degradation of glycogen because the remaining cyclic AMP continues to activate protein kinase, which in turn activates phosphorylase kinase. Glycogen phosphorylase is, in turn, activated by phosphorylase kinase. Sustained activation of phosphorylase results in continued mobilization of glucose residues from glycogen stores in liver.

6. (a) Because the bonds broken and formed during the transferase action are both α-1,4 glycosidic bonds, the free-energy change is likely to be close to zero.

   (b) The generation of glucose 1-phosphate rather than glucose means that one less ATP equivalent is required for the conversion of a glucose residue to two molecules of pyruvate. The glucose residue released does not have to be phosphorylated for subsequent metabolism when phophorolysis produces it as glucose 1-phosphate directly. In addition, the phosphorylation of glucose ensures that the molecule cannot diffuse across the cell membrane before it is utilized in the glycolytic pathway.

   (c) The glucosidase and the transferase activities are both found on the same 160-kd polypeptide chain. A significant alteration in the structure of the domain for glucosidase in the bifunctional enzyme could also impair the functioning of the transferase domain.

7. (a) In McArdle's disease, muscle phosphorylase is deficient but liver phosphorylase is normal. Therefore, you would expect glucose and glycogen metabolism in the liver to be normal and the control of blood glucose by the liver also to be normal.

 (b) Normal glyogen metabolism in the liver means that both the amount of liver glycogen and its structure would be the same as in unaffected people.

 (c) Defective muscle glycogen phosphorylase means that glycogen breakdown is impaired. Moderately increased concentrations of muscle glycogen could be expected, although the structure of the glycogen should be similar to that in unaffected people.

 (d) Galactose can be converted to glucose 6-phosphate in the liver, which can then export glucose to the blood. Because defective muscle phosphorylase has no effect on galactose metabolism, you would expect similar elevations in blood glucose after the ingestion of galactose in normal and affected people.

 (e) During vigorous exercise, blood lactate levels normally rise as muscle tissue exports the lactate generated through glycogen breakdown. The defect in muscle phosphorylase limits the extent to which glycogen is degraded in the muscle. This in turn reduces the amount of lactate exported during exercise, so the rise in blood lactate levels would not be as great in the affected person.

 (f) Glucagon exerts its effects primarily on liver, not muscle. In patients with McArdle's disease, blood glucose levels increase normally in response to glucagon.

 (g) A slight increase in blood glucose concentration may occur after epinephrine administration, because liver is somewhat responsive to this hormone. Epinephrine does have a greater glycogenolytic effect on muscle, but you would not expect to see any change in blood glucose concentration when it is administered. The reason is that, even if glycogen breakdown is accelerated (which is unlikely to occur in patients with McArdle's disease), the glucose 6-phosphate produced cannot be converted to glucose for export into the circulation, because muscle lacks the enzyme glucose 6-phosphatase.

8. (a) The investigator could activate the phosphorylase by adding AMP to the sample or by using active phosphorylase kinase and ATP to phosphorylate the enzyme.

 (b) Inorganic phosphate is also required for the conversion of glycosyl residues in glycogen to glucose 1-phosphate molecules.

9. (a) Arsenate can substitute for inorganic phosphate in the glycogen phosphorylase reaction, generating glucose arsenate esters.

 (b) When P_i is used as a substrate for glycogen phosphorylase, glucose 1-phosphate is generated. The glucose 1-arsenate esters that are generated when arsenate is used as a substrate spontaneously hydrolyze to yield glucose and arsenate. The conversion of glucose to pyruvate requires one more ATP equivalent than does the conversion of glucose 1-phosphate to pyruvate.

10. Like other nucleotides, cyclic AMP is polar and negatively charged at neutral pH. It therefore crosses plasma membranes at a relatively low rate. The presence of two hydrophobic acyl chains on the molecule make it much more hydrophobic, so that it can more easily dissolve in the bilayer and more readily enter the cytosol.

11. A short outer branch in a glycogen molecule has only a small number of α-1,4-glucosyl residues on the nonreducing side of a branch or an α-1,6 link. Incubating such a glycogen molecule with active phosphorylase and P_i will liberate only limited amounts of glucose 1-phosphate, compared with the number liberated from normal glycogen. Recall that phosphorylase cannot free glucose molecules that are within four residues of a branch point in glycogen. To demonstrate that phosphorylase action is limited by

short outer branches, you can incubate another sample with purified debranching enzyme and phosphorylase, and you would expect to see an increase in production of glucose 1-phosphate. To demonstrate a debranching enzyme deficiency in a patient, you could treat normal glycogen with active muscle phosphorylase and muscle extracts from a patient with Cori's disease. If debranching enzyme activity is low, only limited amounts of glucose 1-phosphate will be produced. Larger numbers of glucose 1-phosphate molecules will be released from a normal glycogen sample treated with active phosphorylase and muscle cell extracts from a normal person.

12. Were water to enter the active site of glycogen phosphorylase, the enzyme would hydrolyze rather than phosphorolyze the glycogen. The result would be the production of a free glucose rather than a glucose 1-phosphate. For the free glucose to be metabolized, even to be catabolized for energy, it would have to be phosphorylated, which would consume an ATP molecule.

13. Because amylose is linear, it has but one nonreducing end per molecule that could be removed by glycogen phosphorylase. Glycogen, which is branched, with α-1,6 linkages every approximately 10 residues, has many more ends on which glycogen phosphorylase can act. Thus, more glucose 1-phosphate molecules can be released quickly per glycogen molecule compared with amylose. In addition, the branches make the glycogen more soluble so that it is more easily accessible to glycogen phosphorylase.

Chapter 25

Glycogen Synthesis

The topic of glycogen degradation was presented in Chapter 24. In this chapter the reverse process, the synthesis of glycogen is discussed, with an emphasis on the reciprocal regulation of both pathways. The text presents first the enzymatic reactions of glycogen synthesis. As with other biosynthetic pathways, an activated biosynthetic precursor is required. In the case of glycogen synthesis, that precursor is UDP-glucose. The control of the anabolic reactions by allosteric mechanisms and the phosphorylation and dephosphorylation of the key enzymes in response to hormonal signals is discussed. The authors also point out the reasons why glycogen is an efficient form of glucose storage. orm. The authors then discuss the reciprocal regulation of glycogen breakdown and synthesis, focussing on the roles that insulin and protein phosphatase 1 play. The text concludes the chapter with a discussion of the biochemical basis of several glycogen storage diseases in humans.

LEARNING OBJECTIVES

When you have mastered this chapter, you should be able to accomplish the following objectives.

Introduction

1. State the benefits in having separate pathways for the forward and reverse directions of a metabolic pathway.
2. Describe the precursors of *glycogen anabolism*.

Glycogen is Synthesized and Degraded by Different Pathways (Text Section 25.1)

3. Explain the roles of *UDP-glucose* and *inorganic pyrophosphatase* in the synthesis of glycogen.
4. Outline the steps in the synthesis of glycogen, name the pertinent enzymes, and note the requirement for a *primer*. Describe the actions of *glycogenin* and *glycogen synthase*.
5. Explain why glycogen lacks *glucose residues* that can be *reduced*.
6. Explain the functional importance of *branching* in the glycogen molecule.
7. Describe the regulation of glycogen synthase by *reversible covalent modification*.
8. Discuss the efficiency of glycogen as a storage form of glucose.

Metabolism in Context: Glycogen Breakdown and Synthesis are Reciprocally Regulated (Text Section 25.2)

9. Contrast the effects of phosphorylation on glycogen synthase and glycogen phosphorylase. Appreciate the *reciprocal regulation strategies* employed and the consequences of *amplification cascades*.
10. Explain the role of *protein phosphatase 1* (PP1) in the control of the activities of glycogen phosphorylase and glycogen synthase.
11. Outline the effects of *insulin* on glycogen metabolism. Rationalize the existence of distinct pathways for the biosynthesis and degradation of glycogen.
12. Describe the events that lead to the inactivation of phosphorylase and the activation of glycogen synthase by glucose in the liver. Note the role of phosphorylase *a* as the glucose sensor in liver cells and the participation of phosphorylase *a* and PP1 in glucose sensing.
13. Provide examples of glycogen storage diseases, and relate the biochemical defects with the clinical observations. Use the disease discovered by von Gierke to show how a deficiency in one of several different enzymes can cause the same disease.

SELF-TEST

Introduction

1. List two reasons why separate pathways are used in glycogen synthesis and degradation.

Glycogen Is Synthesized and Degraded by Different Pathways

2. Which of the following features are common to both glycogen synthesis and glycogen breakdown?
   - (a) Both require UDP-glucose.
   - (b) Both involve glucose 1-phosphate.
   - (c) Both are driven in part by the hydrolysis of pyrophosphate.
   - (d) Both occur on cytoplasmic glycogen granules.
   - (e) Both use the same enzyme for branching and debranching.

3. If glycogen synthase can add a glucose residue to a growing glycogen molecule only if the glucose chain is at least four units long, how does a new glycogen molecule start?

4. Why is the existence of distinct biosynthetic and catabolic pathways for glycogen important for the metabolism of liver and muscle cells?

5. Is it true or false that branching in the structure of glycogen increases the rates of its synthesis and degradation? Explain.

6. Which of the following statements about glycogen synthase are correct?
   - (a) It is activated when it is dephosphorylated.
   - (b) It is activated when it is phosphorylated.
   - (c) It is activated when it is phosphorylated and in the presence of high levels of glucose 6-phosphate.
   - (d) It is activated when it is phosphorylated and in the presence of high levels of AMP.

Metabolism in Context: Glycogen Breakdown and Synthesis Are Reciprocally Regulated

7. Which of the following statements about the hormonal regulation of glycogen synthesis and degradation are correct?
   - (a) Insulin increases the capacity of the liver to synthesize glycogen.
   - (b) Insulin is secreted in response to low levels of blood glucose.
   - (c) Glucagon and epinephrine have opposing effects on glycogen metabolism.
   - (d) Glucagon stimulates the breakdown of glycogen, particularly in the liver.
   - (e) The effects of all three of the regulating hormones are mediated by cyclic AMP.

8. Which of the following are effects of glucose on the metabolism of glycogen in the liver?
   - (a) The binding of glucose to phosphorylase *a* converts this enzyme to the inactive T form.
   - (b) The T form of phosphorylase *a* becomes susceptible to the action of phosphatase.
   - (c) The R form of phosphorylase *b* becomes susceptible to the action of phosphorylase kinase.
   - (d) When phosphorylase *a* is converted to phosphorylase *b*, the bound phosphatase is released.
   - (e) The free phosphatase dephosphorylates and activates glycogen synthase.

9. What would increased epinephrine do to protein phosphatase 1 (PP1) in muscle, and how would muscle glycogen metabolism be affected?

10. Explain the effect of insulin on the activity of protein phosphatase 1 and the subsequent effects on glycogen metabolism.

11. Explain how a defect in phosphofructokinase in muscle can lead to increased amounts of glycogen having a normal structure. Patients with this defect are normal except for having a limited ability to perform strenuous exercise.

12. For the defect in Question 27, explain why there is not a massive accumulation of glycogen.

ANSWERS TO SELF-TEST

1. The two reasons listed in the introduction both relate to flexibility. Two pathways allow the cell to use energetics to its advantage. Both the forward and the reverse direction can occur spontaneously. Secondly, the pathway becomes easier to regulate. By selecting a small number of enzymes to control, reciprocal regulation is possible, where a cellular change that activates one enzyme, inhibits the one catalyzing the reverse reaction.

2. b, d

3. The primer required to start a new glycogen chain is formed by the enzyme glycogenin, which has a glucose residue covalently attached to one of its tyrosine residues. Glycogenin uses UDP-glucose to add approximately eight glucose residues to itself to generate a primer that glycogen synthase can extend.

4. The separate pathways for the synthesis and degradation of glycogen allow the synthesis of glycogen to proceed despite a high ratio of orthophosphate to glucose 1-phosphate, which energetically favors the degradation of glycogen. In addition, the separate pathways allow the coordinated reciprocal control of glycogen synthesis and degradation by hormonal and metabolic signals.

5. True. Since degradation and synthesis occur at the nonreducing ends of glycogen, the branched structure allows simultaneous reactions to occur at many nonreducing ends, thereby increasing the overall rates of degradation or biosynthesis.

6. a, c

7. a, d

8. a, b, d, e

9. Increased epinephrine activates PKA, which phosphorylates a subunit of PP1 and thus reduces the ability of PP1 to act on its protein targets. Furthermore, inhibitor 1 is also phosphorylated by PKA so that it too decreases PP1 activity, albeit by a different mechanism. Inactivated PP1 leads to increased levels of activated (phosphorylated) phosphorylase and inactivated (phosphorylated) glycogen synthase. Glycogen breakdown would be stimulated under these conditions.

10. Insulin results in the activation of PP1. The hormone activates an insulin-sensitive protein kinase that phosphorylates a subunit of PP1, rendering the phosphatase more active. The activated phosphatase dephosphorylates phosphorylase, protein kinase, and glycogen synthase. These changes result in a decrease in glycogen degradation and the stimulation of glycogen synthesis.

11. Since a defect in phosphofructokinase does not impair the ability of muscle to synthesize and degrade glycogen normally, the structure of glycogen will be normal. However, the utilization of glucose 6-phosphate in the glycolytic pathway is impaired, and it equilibrates with glucose 1-phosphate; therefore, some net accumulation of glycogen will occur. The inability to perform strenuous exercise is probably a result of the impaired glycolytic pathway in muscle and the diminished production of ATP.

12. Although the impaired use of glucose 6-phosphate in glycolysis will lead to the storage of extra glycogen, it will not become excessive because the increased concentration of glucose 6-phosphate will inhibit hexokinase and hence the sequestering of glucose in muscle.

PROBLEMS

1. Vigorously contracting muscle often becomes anaerobic when the demand for oxygen exceeds the amount supplied through the circulation. Under such conditions, lactate may accumulate in muscle. Under anaerobic conditions a certain percentage of lactate can be converted to glycogen in muscle. One line of evidence for this synthesis involves the demonstration of activity for malic enzyme, which can use CO_2 to convert pyruvate to malate, using NADPH as an electron donor.

    (a) Why is lactate produced in muscle when the supply of oxygen is insufficient?

    (b) In muscle, pyruvate carboxylase activity is very low. How could malic enzyme activity facilitate the synthesis of glycogen from lactate?

    (c) Why would you expect the conversion of lactate to glycogen to occur only after vigorous muscle contraction ceases?

    (d) Is there an energetic advantage to converting lactate to glycogen in muscle rather than using the Cori cycle for sending the lactate to the liver, where it can be reconverted to glucose and then returned to muscle for glycogen synthesis?

2. The ratio of glycogen phosphorylase to protein phosphatase 1 is approximately 10 to 1. Suppose that in some liver cells the overproduction of the phosphatase results in a ratio of one to one. How will such a ratio affect the cell's response to an infusion of glucose?

3. A young woman cannot exercise vigorously on the treadmill without leg pains and stiffness. During exercise, lactate levels do not increase in her serum, in contrast to results of exercise in normal subjects. As is the case with normal subjects, no significant hypoglycemia is observed when the patient exercises or fasts. Analyses of muscle biopsy samples show that glycogen content is about 10 times greater than normal in the young woman, but the level of muscle phosphorylase activity is normal. Other experiments with biopsy samples show that rapid incorporation of ^{14}C from radioactive glucose into fructose 6-phosphate and glycogen is observed, but very little incorporation of radioisotope into lactate is seen. When ^{14}C-pyruvate is incubated with another sample of the homogenate, the radioisotope is readily incorporated into glycogen.

    What specific deficiency in a metabolic pathway could contribute to these observations? Propose two additional studies that could confirm your conclusion.

4. In 1952, Dr. D. H. Andersen described a seriously ill infant with an enlarged liver as well as cirrhosis. When epinephrine was administered, a relatively low elevation in the patient's blood glucose levels was noted. Several days later when the infant was fed galactose, normal elevation of glucose was observed in the circulation. The infant died at the age of 17 months, and at autopsy Dr. Andersen found that glycogen from the liver, while present in unusually high concentration, was relatively insoluble, making it difficult to extract. She sent a sample of the liver glycogen to Dr. Gerty Cori. In an experiment designed to characterize the glycogen, Dr. Cori incubated a sample with orthophosphate (P_i) and two normal liver enzymes, active glycogen phosphorylase and debranching enzyme. She found that the ratio of glucose 1-phosphate to glucose released from the glycogen sample was 100:1, while the ratio from normal glycogen is 10:1.

(a) What enzyme of glycogen metabolism is most likely to be deficient in the liver tissue of the infant? Write a concise explanation for your answer, and relate it to the relative insolubility of the glycogen in the autopsy sample.

(b) Dr. Andersen, aware that a number of enzyme deficiencies might cause a glycogen-storage disease, sought to rule out a deficiency of a particular enzyme in the infant by studying the elevation of glucose levels after feeding galactose. What is that enzyme, and how does normal elevation of blood glucose after galactose feeding rule out a deficiency of that enzyme in the infant?

5. One method for the analysis of glycogen involves incubating a sample with methyl iodide, which methylates all free hydroxyl groups. Acid hydrolysis of exhaustively methylated glycogen yields a mixture of methyl glucosides, which can be separated and analyzed. Considering the various types of glycogen-storage diseases listed in Table 25.1 of the text, which of them could be diagnosed using exhaustive methylation and acid hydrolysis of glycogen?

6. Table 25.1 in the text lists eight diseases of glycogen metabolism, all of which affect the level of glycogen in muscle and liver or the structure of the polysaccharide in one or both of those tissues. Another rare disease of glycogen metabolism is caused by a deficiency in liver glycogen synthase. After fasting, affected subjects have low blood glucose. Hyperglycemia and high blood lactate are observed after a meal.

(a) Briefly explain how these symptoms could be caused by glycogen synthase deficiency.

(b) Under normal nutritional conditions, glycogen comprises about 4 percent of the wet weight of liver tissue in normal subjects. What proportion of glycogen in liver would you expect in a patient who lacks liver glycogen synthase?

7. Phosphoglucomutase converts the product of glycogen phosphorylase, glucose 1-phosphate, to the glycolytic pathway component glucose 6-phosphate. The reaction catalyzed by phosphoglucomutase proceeds by way of a glucose 1,6-bisphosphate intermediate.

(a) What would happen to phophoglucomutase activity if the glucose 1,6-bisphosphate intermediate were to dissociate from the enzyme before completion of the reaction?

(b) Would glucose 1,6-bisphosphate dissociation be equivalent to the hydrolysis of the serine phosphate on the enzyme? Explain why.

(c) Suppose that a phosphoglucomutase in the dephosphoenzyme form arose. How might the enzyme be reactivated?

8. The reduction of Cu (II) to Cu (I) by the aldehyde group of the open configuration of glucose to form Cu_2O is the defining property of reducing sugars. Predict what would happen if you treated glycogen recently synthesized *de novo* with a Cu(II)-containing solution. Would you expect any reducing sugar reactions?

ANSWERS TO PROBLEMS

1. (a) Muscle cells produce lactate from pyruvate under anaerobic conditions to generate NAD^+, which is required to sustain the activity of glyceraldehyde 3-phosphate dehydrogenase in the glycolytic pathway.

(b) The low activity of muscle pyruvate carboxylase means that other pathways for the synthesis of oxaloacetate must be available. The formation of malate, which is then converted to oxaloacetate, enables the muscle cell to carry out the synthesis of glucose 6-phosphate via gluconeogenesis. Glycogen can then be synthesized through the conversion of glucose 6-phosphate to glucose 1-phosphate, the formation of UDP-glucose, and the transfer of the glucose residue to a glycogen primer chain.

(c) Yes. Energy for vigorous muscle contraction under anaerobic conditions is derived primarily from the conversion of glycogen and glucose to lactate. The simultaneous conversion of lactate to glycogen would simply result in the unnecessary hydrolysis of ATP.

(d) In liver, the conversion of two lactate molecules to a glucose residue in glycogen through gluconeogenesis requires seven high-energy phosphate bonds; six are required for the formation of glucose 6-phosphate from two molecules of lactate, and one is needed for the synthesis of UDP-glucose from glucose 1-phosphate. The conversion of lactate to glycogen in muscle requires two fewer high-energy bonds because the formation of oxaloacetate through the action of malic enzyme does not require ATP. Recall that pyruvate carboxylase requires ATP for the synthesis of oxaloacetate from pyruvate.

2. The normal 10-to-1 ratio means that glycogen synthase molecules are activated only after most of the phosphorylase *a* molecules are converted to the inactive *b* form, which ensures that the simultaneous degradation and synthesis of glycogen does not occur. A phosphorylase to phosphatase ratio of one to one means that, as soon as a few phosphorylase molecules are inactivated, phosphatase molecules that are no longer bound to phosphorylase begin to convert glycogen synthase molecules to the active form. Glycogen degradation and synthesis then occur simultaneously, resulting in the wasteful hydrolysis of ATP.

3. From the clinical observations, it appears that the pathway from pyruvate to glucose 6-phosphate and on to glycogen is functional and that gluconeogenesis is working normally in liver (there is no hypoglycemia during fasting or exercise, when demands for glucose increase). Although muscle glycogen content is higher, normal phosphorylase activity indicates that glycogen could be phosphorylized normally. You should then consider whether there is a deficiency in the glycolytic pathway, because lactate does not accumulate during exercise and it is not labeled when ^{14}C-glucose is administered. Labeled fructose 6-phosphate can be made from radioactive glucose in the biopsy sample, but knowledge about subsequent glycolytic reactions is not available. There could be a significant block at the level of phosphofructokinase or beyond. Such a deficiency would mean that while normal demands for glucose can be taken care of, a high rate of glycolytic activity during vigorous exercise cannot be accommodated. You should consider analyzing for additional radioactive glycolytic intermediates when glucose is administered, then testing for deficiency of one or more glycolytic enzymes using biopsy tissues. The description of the disorder corresponds most closely to a known condition for a deficiency in muscle phosphofructokinase (Type VII glycogen-storage disease). One might also argue that lactate dehydrogenase could be absent, explaining why no lactate is generated during exercise. However, in cases in which muscle lactate dehydrogenase is defective, affected subjects cannot exercise vigorously, but they have no accumulation of glycogen in their muscle tissue.

4. (a) The branching enzyme was deficient in the infant. This enzyme removes blocks of glucosyl residues from a chain of α-1 $\rightarrow$ 4-linked residues and transfers them internally to form a branch with an α-1 $\rightarrow$ 6 link to a polymer chain. The most important clue to the deficiency is found in the ratio of glucose 1-phosphate to glucose, which is 10 times higher in glycogen from the affected infant than from

a normal polymer sample. Recall that glucose 1-phosphate is produced through the action of phosphorylase, which phosphorylizes α-1 ⟶ 4 linkages, while glucose is produced when the glycogen debranching enzyme hydrolyzes a glucose in α-1 ⟶ 6 linkage at a branch point. Normal glycogen has a branch at every 10 or so glycosyl residues, so treatment with a mixture of normal phosphorylase and debranching enzyme will yield a 10:1 ratio of glucose 1-phosphate to glucose. The autopsy sample yielded a ratio of 100:1, suggesting that there are far fewer branches in the sample. This conclusion is consistent with the relative insolubility of the infant's glycogen, which, with fewer branches, is more like amylopectin, a linear glucosyl polymer which has limited solubility in water.

(b) The pathway for galactose metabolism includes its conversion, through steps that include epimerization, to glucose 6-phosphate. Thus feeding galactose should result in an increased concentration of glucose 6-phosphate in the liver cell. If glucose 6-phosphatase were deficient, glucose 6-phosphate would not be converted to glucose, so that the levels of blood glucose would not be elevated after galactose feeding. Dr. Andersen considered a glucose 6-phosphatase deficiency because of the limited increase in blood glucose levels after administration of epinephrine, so she used galactose feeding to increase glucose 6-phosphate levels in liver cells. When glucose levels rose in the blood, she concluded that glucose 6-phosphatase levels were normal. She subsequently considered other deficiencies that would result in storage of abnormal amounts of liver glycogen.

5. Type IV glycogen-storage disease, in which glycogen with a much lower number of α-1,6 glycosidic linkages is produced, could be analyzed using methylation and hydrolysis. Any glucose residue derived from a branch point will have methyl groups at C-2 and C-3, while all other residues (with one exception) will emerge from hydrolysis as 2,3,6-O-trimethyl glucose molecules. The glucose at the reducing end of the glycogen molecule will be converted to a tetramethlyglucoside. In normal subjects, the ratio of trimethylglucose to dimethyl glucose should be about 10 to 1, while glycogen from a person with a deficiency in the branching enzyme will have a much higher ratio.

6. (a) Lack of glycogen synthase implies that the ability of the liver to store glucose as glycogen is impaired. After fasting, when blood glucose concentrations are low, liver glycogen is normally converted to glucose 6-phosphate, which is converted to glucose and exported to the blood. Low glycogen levels in liver tissue would make it impossible for liver to maintain proper glucose levels in the blood. After a meal containing carbohydrates, the liver would be unable to convert glucose to glycogen. Even though glucokinase may convert glucose to glucose 6-phosphate, the high concentration of that substrate may cause accelerated conversion back to glucose through the action of glucose 6-phosphatase. Glucose levels would then increase in the circulation. The elevation of lactate levels in blood suggests that any glucose metabolized in the liver is preferentially converted to lactate rather than to glycogen.

(b) As discussed, liver cells deficient in glycogen synthase would be unable to synthesize large amounts of glycogen. You would therefore expect the percentage of glycogen in affected people to be lower. In the few patients with the disorder, glycogen makes up less than 1 percent of liver tissue.

7. (a) If the glucose 1,6-bisphosphate were to dissociate from the enzyme, the enzyme would not have a phosphate on the serine hydroxyl that is necessary for activity. The dephosphorylated enzyme would lack the phosphate need for transfer to the incoming glucose 1-phosphate to form the bisphosphate intermediate and could not catalyze the mutase reaction.

(b) Yes, both bisphosphate dissociation or phophoenzyme hydrolysis would lead to an inactive, unphosphorylated enzyme.

(c) Since a phophoglucomutase carrying a phosphate group on a specific serine is required for activity, some means of producing the phosphosenzyme is required. A protein kinase could replace the covalently bound enzyme phosphate or a phosphglucokinase enzyme that produced glucose 1,6-bisphospate, which would bind to and phosphorylate phosphglucomutase, could also form the phosphorylated enzyme. The latter is a known mechanism.

8. Glycogen is a treelike molecule in which glucose residues are linked in α-1,4 glycosidic linkages with branches occurring as α-1,6 glycosidic linkages at approximately every tenth residue. Recall also that the free aldehyde at the C-1 position of glucose is the agent that reduces the Cu(II). Since the C-1 of all the sugars in glycogen are in a glycosidic linkage they are unable to react with the divalent copper. Thus, glycogen itself would not act as a reducing sugar. You may ask, What about the first glucose residue that is at the root of the tree—the one to which the first α-1,4 glycosidic-linkage of the chain is formed? Recall that glycogen synthase needs a primer to start a new glycogen chain and that the dimeric protein glycogenin creates that primer by adding the glycosyl moiety of UDP-glucose to itself. The C-1 atom of the first glucose residue of the resultant primer is covalently attached to the protein through a phenolic hydroxyl on a tyrosine residue of the protein. Thus, glycogen that has been synthesized *de novo* has no free aldehyde groups and would itself give no reaction with Cu(II). See Smythe, C., and Cohen, P., *Eur. J. Biochem.* (1991) **200**:625– 631.

The Pentose Phosphate Pathway

In Chapter 23, the Calvin cycle, sometimes referred to as the reductive pentose phosphate pathway, was introduced. The Calvin cycle reactions constitute the dark reactions of photosynthesis and use NADPH to convert carbon dioxide into hexoses. This chapter introduces the pentose phosphate pathway, whose role is to break down glucose into carbon dioxide to produce NADPH. The Calvin cycle and the pentose phosphate pathway, like glycolysis and gluconeogenesis (Chapters 16 and 17), are mirror images of each other.

The role of the pentose phosphate pathway, which is common to all organisms, is to produce NADPH, which is the currency of reducing power utilized for most reductive biosyntheses. In addition, this pathway generates ribose 5-phosphate needed for DNA synthesis and can produce various size sugars for other uses. The pathway can be separated into oxidative steps in which glucose-6-phosphate and $NADP^+$ are converted into ribulose-5-phosphate, CO_2, and NADPH, and nonoxidative steps in which ribulose-5-phosphate is converted into three-, four-, five-, six-, and seven-carbon sugars. The pentose phosphate pathway is linked to glycolysis (Chapter 16) by the common intermediates glucose-6-phosphate, fructose-6-phosphate, and glyceraldehyde 3-phosphate. The authors discuss the mechanisms of the two enzymes that catalyze the conversion of ribose-5-phosphate into glyceraldehyde-3-phosphate and fructose 6-phosphate, transketolase and transaldolase, respectively. The regulation of the pentose phosphate pathway and the ways in which its activity is coordinated with glycolysis are discussed. The chapter concludes with the role of glucose-6-phosphate dehydrogenase in protection against reactive oxygen species and the physiological consequences of deficiencies in the enzyme.

LEARNING OBJECTIVES

When you have mastered this chapter, you should be able to accomplish the following objectives.

Introduction

1. Explain the function of the *pentose phosphate pathway*.

The Pentose Phosphate Pathway Yields NADPH and Five-Carbon Sugars
(Text Section 26.1)

2. List the two phases of the pentose phosphate pathway. List the biochemical pathways that require NADPH from the pentose phosphate pathway.

3. Describe the reactions of the *oxidative branch* of the pentose phosphate pathway.

4. Explain how the pentose phosphate pathway and the glycolytic pathway are linked through reactions catalyzed by *transaldolase* and *transketolase*.

5. Outline the sugar interconversions of the *nonoxidative branch* of the pentose phosphate pathway.

Metabolism in Context: Glycolysis and the Pentose Phosphate Pathway Are Coordinately Controlled (Text Section 26.2)

6. Describe the regulation of *glucose 6-phosphate dehydrogenase* by NADP$^+$ levels.

7. State the different product stoichiometries obtained from the pentose phosphate pathway under conditions in which (1) more ribose 5-phosphate than NADPH is needed, (2) there is a balanced requirement for both, (3) more NADPH than ribose 5-phosphate is needed, and (4) both NADPH and ATP are required.

8. List the tissues with active pentose phosphate pathways and state their functions.

Glucose-6-Phosphate Dehydrogenase Lessens Oxidative Stress (Text Section 26.3)

9. Explain why red blood cells are especially senstive to oxidative stress.

10. Discuss the effects of *glucose 6-phosphate dehydrogenase deficiency* on red cells in drug-induced hemolytic anemia, and relate them to the biological roles of *glutathione*.

11. Discuss the oxidation and reduction of glutathione by *glutathione reductase* and *glutathione peroxidase* respectively.

12. Explain the role of reduced glutathione maintaining the normal structure of red blood cells.

13. Give an example of a benefit in a deficiency of glucose-6-phosphate dehydrogenase.

SELF-TEST

The Pentose Phosphate Pathway Yields NADPH and Five-Carbon Sugars

1. Which of the following compounds is NOT a product of the pentose phosphate pathway?
   (a) NADPH
   (b) glycerate 3-phosphate
   (c) CO_2
   (d) ribulose 5-phosphate
   (e) sedoheptulose 7-phosphate

2. Figure 20.1 shows the first four reactions of the pentose phosphate pathway. Use it to answer the questions.

FIGURE 20.1   Oxidative reactions of the pentose phosphate pathway.

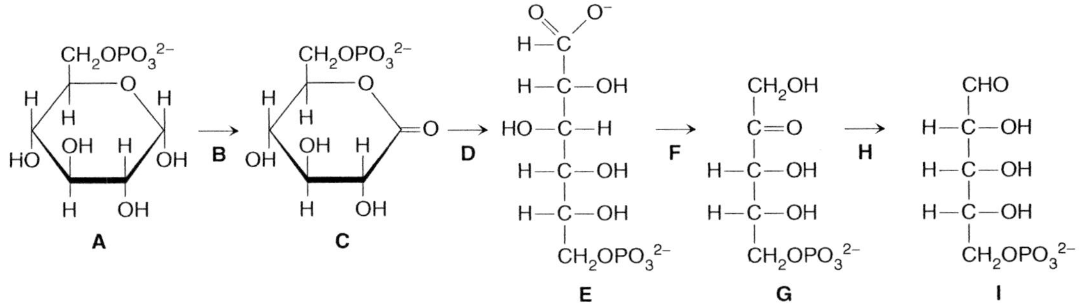

(a) Which reactions produce NADPH?
(b) Which reaction produces CO_2?
(c) Which compound is ribose 5-phosphate?
(d) Which compound is 6-phosphoglucono-δ-lactone?
(e) Which compound is 6-phosphogluconate?
(f) Which reaction is catalyzed by phosphopentose isomerase?
(g) Which enzyme is deficient in drug-induced hemolytic anemia?
(h) Which compound can be a group acceptor in the transketolase reaction?

3. The nonoxidative branch of the pentose phosphate pathway does NOT include which of the following reactions?

(a) Ribulose 5-P $\longrightarrow$ ribose 5-P
(b) Xylulose 5-P + ribose 5-P $\longrightarrow$ sedoheptulose 7-P $\longrightarrow$ glyceraldehyde 3-P
(c) Ribulose 5-P + glyceraldehyde 3-P $\longrightarrow$ sedoheptulose 7-P
(d) Sedoheptulose 7-P + glyceraldehyde 3-P $\longrightarrow$ fructose 6-P + erythrose 4-P
(e) Ribulose 5-P $\longrightarrow$ xylulose 5-P

4. Liver synthesizes fatty acids and lipids for export to other tissues. Would you expect the pentose phosphate pathway to have a low or a high activity in this organ? Explain your answer.

Metabolism in Context: Glycolysis and the Pentose Phosphate Pathway Are Coordinately Controlled

5. Which enzyme catalyzes the rate limiting step in the pentose phosphate pathway?

(a) lactonase
(b) transaldolase
(c) transketolase
(d) glucose 6-phosphate dehydrogenase
(e) 6-phosphogluconate dehydrogenase

6. Which of the following statements about glucose 6-phosphate dehydrogenase are correct?

(a) It catalyzes the committed step in the pentose phosphate pathway.
(b) It is regulated by the availability of NAD^+.
(c) One of its products is 6-phosphogluconate.
(d) It contains thiamine pyrophosphate as a cofactor.
(e) It is important in the metabolism of glutathione in erythrocytes.

7 Which of the following conversions take place in a metabolic situation that requires much more NADPH than ribose 5-phosphate, as well as complete oxidation of glucose 6-phosphate to CO_2? The arrows represent one or more enzymatic steps.

    (a) glucose 6-phosphate $\rightarrow$ ribulose 5-phosphate
    (b) fructose 6-phosphate $\rightarrow$ glyceraldehyde 3-phosphate $\rightarrow$ ribose 5-phosphate
    (c) ribose 5-phosphate $\rightarrow$ fructose 6-phosphate $\rightarrow$ glyceraldehyde 3-phosphate
    (d) glyceraldehyde 3-phosphate $\rightarrow$ pyruvate
    (e) fructose 6-phosphate $\rightarrow$ glucose 6-phosphate

8. List two ways in which the Calvin cycle (Chapter 23) and the pentose phosphate pathway are mirror images of each other.

Glucose-6-Phosphate Dehydrogenase Lessens Oxidative Stress

9. Which of the following statements about reduced glutathione is NOT true?

    (a) It contains one γ-carboxyglutamate, one cysteine, and one glycine residue.
    (b) It keeps the cysteine residues of proteins in their reduced states.
    (c) It is regenerated from oxidized glutathione by glutathione reductase.
    (d) It reacts with hydrogen peroxide and organic peroxides.
    (e) It is decreased relative to oxidized glutathione in glucose 6-phosphate dehydrogenase deficiency.

10. Suggest reasons why glucose 6-phosphate dehydrogenase deficiency may be manifested in red blood cells but not in adipocytes, which also require NADPH for their metabolism.

ANSWERS TO SELF-TEST

1. b

2. (a) B, F (b) F (c) I (d) C (e) E (f) H (g) B (h) I

3. c

4. The activity of the pentose phosphate pathway in the liver is high. The biosynthesis of fatty acids and lipids requires reducing equivalents in the form of NADPH. In all organs that carry out reductive biosyntheses, the pentose phosphate pathway supplies a large proportion of the required NADPH.

5. d

6. a, e

7. a, c, e. Glucose 6-phosphate is converted to ribulose 5-phosphate, producing CO_2 and NADPH in the process. Then ribulose 5-phosphate, via ribose 5-phosphate, is transformed into fructose 6-phosphate and glyceraldehyde 3-phosphate. These two glycolytic intermediates are converted back to glucose 6-phosphate, and the cycle is repeated until the equivalent of six carbon atoms from glucose 6-phosphate are converted to CO_2.

8. (1) Calvin cycle fixes CO_2 and utilizes NADPH to form sugars while the PPP oxidizes a sugar to form CO_2 and generates NADPH. (2) Calvin cycle converts C6 and C3 molecules into a C5 molecule while the PPP converts a C5 molecule into C6 and C3 molecules.

9. a. Answer (a) is incorrect because the glutamate residue in glutathione is not γ-carboxyglutamate; rather, the glutamate in glutathione forms a peptide bond with the adjacent cysteine residue via its γ-carboxyl group.

10. The glucose 6-phosphate dehydrogenase in erythrocytes and that in adipocytes are specified by distinct genes; they have the same function but different structures—that is, they are isozymes. Furthermore, NADPH synthesis by the pentose phosphate pathway may not be as critical in the cells of other tissues as it is in erythrocytes because other tissues have other sources of NADPH.

PROBLEMS

1. The conversion of glucose 6-phosphate to ribose 5-phosphate via the enzymes of the pentose phosphate pathway and glycolysis can be summarized as follows:

$$5 \text{ glucose 6-phosphate} + \text{ATP} \longrightarrow 6 \text{ ribose 5-phosphate} + \text{ADP} + \text{H}^+$$

Which enzyme uses the molecule of ATP shown in the equation?

2. Liver and other organ tissues contain relatively large quantities of nucleic acids. During digestion, nucleases hydrolyze RNA and DNA, and among the products is ribose 5-phosphate.

(a) How can this molecule be used as a metabolic fuel?

(b) Another product formed by the degradation of nucleic acids is 2-deoxyribose 5-phosphate. Can this molecule be converted to glycolytic intermediates through the action of the pentose phosphate pathway? Explain your answer.

3. You have glucose that is radioactively labeled with ^{14}C at C-1, and you have an extract that contains the enzymes that catalyze the reactions of the glycolytic and the pentose phosphate pathways, along with all the intermediates of the pathways.

(a) If the enzymes of the *oxidative* branch of the pentose phosphate pathway are *not* active in your extract, is it possible to obtain labeled sedoheptulose 7-phosphate using glucose labeled with ^{14}C at C-1? Explain.

(b) Suppose that in a second experiment *all* the enzymes of both the oxidative branch and the nonoxidative branch of the pentose phosphate pathway are active. Will the labeling pattern of sedoheptulose 7-phosphate be different? Explain.

(c) Can sedoheptulose 7-phosphate form a heterocyclic ring?

4. Why is the pentose phosphate pathway more active in cells that are dividing than in cells that are not?

5. A bacterium isolated from a soil culture can utilize ribose as a sole source of carbon when grown anaerobically. Experiments show that in the anaerobic pathways leading to ATP production, three molecules of ribose are converted to five molecules of CO_2 and five molecules of ethanol. These organisms also use ribose for the production of NADPH. The assimilation of ribose begins with its conversion to ribose 5-phosphate, with ATP serving as a phosphoryl donor.

(a) Explain how ribose can be converted to CO_2 and ethanol under anaerobic conditions. Write the overall reaction, showing how much ATP can be produced per pentose utilized.

(b) Write an equation for the generation of NADPH using ribose as a sole source of carbon.

6. Mature erythrocytes, which lack mitochondria, metabolize glucose at a high rate. In response to the increased availability of glucose, erythrocytes generate lactate and also evolve carbon dioxide.

   (a) Why is generation of lactate necessary to ensure the continued utilization of glucose?

   (b) In erythrocytes, what pathway is likely to be used for the generation of carbon dioxide from glucose? Can glucose be completely oxidized to CO_2 in erythrocytes? Explain.

7. A biochemist needs to determine whether a particular tissue homogenate has a high level of pentose phosphate pathway activity. She incubates one sample with ^{14}C-1 glucose and another with ^{14}C-6 glucose. Then she measures the specific activity of radioactive CO_2 generated by each sample. Her measurements show that the specific activity of CO_2 from the experiment using glucose labeled at C-1 is much higher than that from the sample in which glucose labeled at C-6 was used. What is her conclusion?

8. Even if glucose 6-phosphate dehydrogenase is deficient, the synthesis of ribose 5-phosphate from glucose 6-phosphate can proceed normally. Explain how this is possible.

ANSWERS TO PROBLEMS

1. Phosphofructokinase uses ATP to convert fructose 6-phosphate to fructose 1,6-bisphosphate, which is then cleaved by aldolase to yield dihydroxyacetone phosphate (DHAP) and glyceraldehyde 3-phosphate. The conversion of DHAP to a second molecule of glyceraldehyde 3-phosphate provides the molecules that are needed for the synthesis of ribose 5-phosphate.

2. (a) The most direct route for the oxidative degradation of ribose 5-phosphate is its conversion to glycolytic intermediates by the nonoxidative enzymes of the pentose phosphate pathway. The overall reaction is

   3 ribose 5-phosphate $\rightarrow$ 2 fructose 6-phosphate $\rightarrow$ glyceraldehyde 3-phosphate

   (b) The formation of glycolytic intermediates from 2-deoxyribose 5-phosphate is not possible, because unlike ribose 5-phosphate, 2-deoxyribose 5-phosphate lacks a hydroxyl group at C-2. It is therefore not a substrate for phosphopentose isomerase, whose action is required to convert ketopentose phosphates to substrates that can be utilized by other enzymes of the pentose phosphate pathway. Most deoxyribose phosphate molecules are used in salvage pathways to form deoxynucleotides.

3. (a) Yes. The most direct route would be the conversion of glucose to fructose 6-phosphate, followed by the condensation of fructose 6-phosphate with erythrose 4-phosphate to form sedoheptulose 7-phosphate and glyceraldehyde 3-phosphate. The labeled carbon of glucose becomes the C-1 of fructose 6-phosphate and C-1 of sedoheptulose 7-phosphate.

   (b) The labeling pattern will be the same, although the amount of labeled carbon incorporated into the heptose will be reduced. In the oxidative branch of the pentose phosphate pathway, the labeled glucose is converted to glucose 6-phosphate with the ^{14}C label on C-1. Glucose 6-phosphate then undergoes successive oxidations and decarboxylation to form ribulose 5-phosphate. The label is lost when the C-1 carbon is removed during decarboxylation.

(c) Sedoheptulose 7-phosphate is a ketose and can form a heterocyclic ring through a hemiketal linkage. The most likely link would be between the keto group at C-2 and the hydroxyl group at C-6.

4. Cells have a high rate of nucleic acid biosynthesis when they grow and divide. Among the precursors needed is ribose 5-phosphate, which is synthesized through the action of the enzymes of the glycolytic and the pentose phosphate pathways. Biosynthetic reactions requiring NADPH occur at a high rate in growing and dividing cells. For these reasons, the enzymes of the pentose phosphate pathway will be extremely active in dividing cells.

5. (a) To generate ATP, ethanol, and CO_2, ribose must first be converted to ribose 5-phosphate, with ATP serving as a phosphate donor. Then, in the nonoxidative branch of the pentose phosphate pathway, three molecules of ribose 5-phosphate are converted to two molecules of fructose 6-phosphate and one molecule of glyceraldehyde 3-phosphate. Two molecules of ATP are required for the production of fructose 1,6-bisphosphate from fructose 6-phosphate. The formation of a total of five molecules of glyceraldehyde 3-phosphate is achieved through the action of aldolase and triose phosphate isomerase. These five molecules are converted to five molecules of pyruvate, yielding ten ATP molecules and five NADH molecules. To keep the anaerobic cell in redox balance, the pyruvate molecules are converted to five molecules of ethanol, with the production of five CO_2 molecules and five NAD^+. The overall reaction is 3 ribose + 5 ADP + P_i → 5 ethanol + 5 CO_2 + 5 ADP.

(b) Ribose 5-phosphate molecules must first be converted to glucose 6-phosphate for the oxidative enzymes of the pentose pathway to generate NADPH. The stoichiometry of the reactions is

6 ribose 5-phosphate → 4 fructose 6-phosphate + 2 glyceraldehyde 3-phosphate

4 fructose 6-phosphate → 4 glucose 6-phosphate

2 glyceraldehyde 3-phosphate → glucose 6-phosphate + P_i

5 glucose 6-phosphate + 10 $NADP^+$ + 5 H_2O → 5 ribose 5-phosphate + 10 NADPH + 10 H^+ + 5 CO_2

The net reaction is

ribose 5-phosphate + 10 $NADP^+$ + 5 H_2O → 10 NADPH + 10 H^+ + 5 CO_2 + P_i

6. (a) Because erythrocytes lack mitochondria, they cannot use the citric acid cycle to regenerate the NAD^+ needed to sustain glycolysis. Instead, they regenerate NAD^+ by reducing pyruvate through the action of lactate dehydrogenase; NAD^+ is then reduced in the reaction catalyzed by glyceraldehyde 3-phosphate dehydrogenase during glycolysis. Failure to oxidize the NADH generated in the glycolytic pathway will cause a reduction in the rate of glucose breakdown.

(b) In erythrocytes, the pentose phosphate pathway is the only route available to yield CO_2 from glucose. Glucose can be completely oxidized by first entering the oxidative branch of the pathway, generating NADPH and ribose 5-phosphate. Transaldolase and transketolase then convert the pentose phosphates to fructose 6-phosphate and glyceraldehyde 3-phosphate. Part of the gluconeogenic pathway is used to convert both the products to glucose 6-phosphate. The net reaction is

glucose 6-P + 12 $NADP^+$ + 7 H_2O → 6 CO_2 + 12 NADPH + 12 H^+ + P_i

7. The experiments show that the activity of the pentose phosphate pathway is high. In the pentose phosphate pathway, glucose labeled at C-1 is decarboxylated, while glucose labeled at C-6 is not. On the other hand, both C-1- and C-6-labeled glucose are decarboxylated to the same extent by the combined action of the glycolytic pathway and the citric acid cycle. Because in these experiments, the specific activity (ratio of labeled CO_2 to total CO_2) is higher for C-1-labeled glucose, much of the glucose in the experiment must be moving through the pentose phosphate pathway.

8. Ribose 5-phosphate can be synthesized from fructose 6-phosphate and glyceraldehyde 3-phosphate, both of which are glycolytic products of glucose 6-phosphate. These reactions are carried out by transketolase and transaldolase in a reversal of the nonoxidative branch of the pentose phosphate pathway and do not involve glucose 6-phosphate dehydrogenase.

Chapter 2

Fatty Acid Degradation

In the discussion of the generation and storage of metabolic energy, the text has thus far focused on the carbohydrates. In Chapters 27 and 28, the authors turn to the fatty acids as metabolic fuels. You should review Chapters 11 and 14 before turning to Chapters 27 and 28. The authors first discuss how stored triacylglycerols are made biochemically accessible through three stages of processing. The first is the degradation of triacylglycerols to fatty acids and glycerol by hormone-stimulated lipases. The second is the activation of fatty acids by attachment to coenzyme A and transport of the fatty acids into the mitochondria of energy-requiring tissues. The third is the breakdown of the fatty acids step-by-step by the β-oxidation pathway into acetyl-CoA which is then processed in the citric acid cycle. The authors then summarize the energy yield derived from oxidation of a fatty acid. Next, the authors discuss how mono- and polyunsaturated and odd-chain fatty acids are oxidized. Each requires additional steps compared to the oxidation of saturated fatty acids. The role of the ketone bodies as acetyl transport molecules in the circulation are discussed. The chapter concludes with discussion of the role of fatty acid metabolism in diabetes and starvation.

LEARNING OBJECTIVES

When you have mastered this chapter, you should be able to accomplish the following objectives.

Introduction

1. State the chemical form in which fatty acids are stored in the human body.

2. Identify the two main locations in the body where adipose tissue is located.

Fatty Acids Are Processed in Three Stages (Text Section 27.1)

3. Summarize the three stages of processing of triacylglycerols by which they are made biochemically accessible.

4. Describe the *lipolysis* of triacylglycerols by *lipases*. Explain the role of *cyclic AMP* in the regulation of lipase in *adipose cells*.

5. Explain the function of *serum albumin* in transport of fatty acids.

6. Outline the conversion of glycerol to *glycerol 3-phosphate* and *dihydroxyacetone phosphate* and appreciate the physiological importance of these reactions.

7. Describe the reaction that links *coenzyme A (CoA)* to a fatty acid. Explain the roles of the *acyl adenylate* and *pyrophosphatase* in the reaction.

8. Explain the involvement of *carnitine* in the transport of fatty acids from the cytoplasm into mitochondria.

9. Explain the effect of carnitine deficiencies on human health and discuss the possible effectiveness of carnitine supplements.

10. List the four reactions of the *β-oxidation pathway* of fatty acid catabolism and identify their substrates and products. Explain the function of NAD^+ and *FAD* in these reactions.

11. Calculate the *energy yield* in ATP molecules for the β oxidation of a given fatty acid.

The Degradation of Unsaturated and Odd-Chain Fatty Acids Requires Additional Steps (Text Section 27.2)

12. Indicate the two reactions, in addition to those of the β-oxidation pathway, used to oxidize naturally occurring unsaturated fatty acids. Explain how they allow the continuation of the β-oxidation pathway.

13. Outline the oxidation reactions of an *odd-numbered fatty acid*.

14. Explain the role of *vitamin B_{12} (cobalamin)* in the pathway by which *propionyl CoA* is converted to succinyl CoA.

Ketone Bodies Are Another Fuel Source Derived from Fats (Text Section 27.3)

15. Name and identify the structures of the *ketone bodies*.

16. Describe the synthesis and normal catabolism of the ketone bodies. Explain why only the liver exports *acetoacetate* and *3-hydroxybutyrate* and appreciate the role of ketone bodies in normal human metabolism.

17. Provide the biochemical basis for the inability of animals to convert fatty acids into glucose.

Metabolism in Context: Fatty Acid Metabolism Is a Source of Insight into Various Physiological States (Text Section 27.4)

18. Describe the effect of high levels of *acetoacetate* on fat metabolism in adipose tissue.

19. Explain the impact that *diabetes* has on fatty acid metabolism.

20. Outline the mechanism by which ketone bodies build up in diabetic patients. Discuss some of the physiological reasons for the symptoms a diabetic can display.

21. Summarize the energy reserves in a typical 70-kg man.

22. Outline the changes in metabolic processes that occur during starvation.

SELF-TEST

Fatty Acids Are Processed in Three Stages

1. Which of the following statements about the triacylglycerols stored in adipose tissue are correct?
   (a) They are hydrolyzed to form fatty acids and dihydroxyacetone.
   (b) They are hydrolyzed by a lipase that is activated by covalent modification.
   (c) They release fatty acids that can be oxidized to CO_2 and H_2O to provide energy to the cell.
   (d) They can yield a precursor of glucose.
   (e) They are mobilized by epinephrine or glucagon.

2. (a) Describe the mechanism for the formation of acyl CoA.
   (b) How is pyrophosphatase involved in the activation of fatty acids for β oxidation?

3. Place the following incomplete list of reactions or locations during the β oxidation of fatty acids in the proper order.
   (a) reaction with carnitine
   (b) fatty acid in cytosol
   (c) activation of fatty acid by joining to CoA
   (d) hydration
   (e) NAD^+-linked oxidation
   (f) thiolysis
   (g) acyl CoA in mitochondrion
   (h) FAD-linked oxidation

4. Explain the involvement of carnitine in the β oxidation of fatty acids.

5. Calculate the approximate yield in ATP molecules of the complete oxidation of hexanoic acid (C6:0).

The Degradation of Unsaturated and Odd-Chain Fatty Acids Requires Additional Steps

6. Place the following steps in the correct order during the degradation of linoleate.
   (a) three rounds of β-oxidation
   (b) Four rounds of β-oxidation
   (c) isomerization of cis-Δ^3 double bond into a trans-Δ^2 double bond
   (d) dehydrogenation of a cis-Δ^4 double bond
   (e) isomerization to form trans-Δ^2-enoyl CoA
   (f) reduction to form trans-Δ^3-enoyl CoA

7. Differentiate between the types enzymes needed to handle the degradation of polyunsaturated fatty acids containing odd- and even-numbered double bonds.

8. Methylmalonyl CoA mutase
   (a) converts D-methylmalonyl CoA to L-methylmalonyl CoA.
   (b) contains biotin.
   (c) involves a homolytic bond cleavage.
   (d) contains a derivative of vitamin B_{12}.
   (e) transforms a *cis*-Δ^3 double bond into a *trans*-Δ^2 double bond.

Ketone Bodies Are Another Fuel Source Derived from Fats

9. Indicate whether the following statement is true or false and explain your answer: After a meal rich in carbohydrates, acetyl CoA levels rise and ketone body synthesis increases.

10. Which of the following statements about acetoacetate and 3-hydroxybutyrate are correct?
    (a) They are normal fuels for heart muscle and the renal cortex.
    (b) They are synthesized in the liver.
    (c) They can give rise to acetone.
    (d) They contain four carbon atoms and require three acetyl CoA molecules for their synthesis.
    (e) They can be regarded as water-soluble, transportable forms of citrate in the blood.

11. Explain how plants are able to synthesize glucose from fatty acids while animals cannot.

Metabolism in Context: Fatty Acid Metabolism Is a Source of Insight into Various Physiological States

12. List the two major roles of insulin in regulating metabolism.

13. Explain the physiological reason for each of the following symptoms in a diabetic patient:
    (a) Smell of alcohol on the breath
    (b) Increased blood pH
    (c) Behavioral changes

14. Describe the two metabolic priorities in starvation and how they are in conflict with each other. Outline the metabolic solution to this conflict.

ANSWERS TO SELF-TEST

1. b, c, d, e. The hydrolysis of triacylglycerols yields glycerol, not dihydroxyacetone, and glycerol can be converted into glyceraldehyde 3-phosphate, which can ultimately give rise to glucose. Several hormones affect the hormone-sensitive lipase of adipose tissue via a cyclic AMP-modulated phosphorylation that activates the enzyme.

2 (a) The carboxyl group of the fatty acid is first activated by reaction with ATP to form an acyl adenylate, which contains a mixed anhydride linkage between the carboxylate and the 5′-phosphate of AMP, with the release of PP_i. In a second step, also catalyzed by acyl CoA synthetase, the acyl group is transferred to the sulfhydryl group of CoA to form the thioester bond and release AMP.

(b) The hydrolysis of PP_i couples the cleavage of a second high-energy bond to the formation of the thioester bond to make its formation exergonic. In effect, two ATPs are used to make one acyl CoA.

3. b, c, a, g, h, d, e, f

4. Acyl CoA is formed in the cytosol, and the enzymes of the β-oxidation pathway are in the matrix of the mitochondrion. The mitochondrial inner membrane is impermeable to CoA and its acyl derivatives. However, a translocase protein can shuttle carnitine and its acyl derivatives across the inner mitochondrial membrane. The acyl group is transferred to carnitine on the cytosol side of the inner membrane and back to CoA on the matrix side. Thus, carnitine acts as a transmembrane carrier of acyl groups.

5. After activation of hexanoic acid to hexanoyl CoA, two rounds of β oxidation are required to produce 3 acetyl CoA molecules. The two cycles also produce 2 $FADH_2$ and 2 NADH molecules. Each acetyl CoA yields 10 ATP molecules on complete oxidation, each $FADH_2$ produces 1.5 ATP, and each NADH makes 2.5 ATP—a total of 38 ATP. Activation uses 2 ATP molecules because AMP is one of the products of the reaction, so the net yield is approximately 36 ATP.

6. a, c, d, f, e, b

7. Polyunsaturated fatty acids containing odd-numbered double bonds require only a cis-Δ^3 isomerase while those containing an even number of double bonds require the isomerase and 2,4-dienoyl CoA reductase. The reason is that the degradation of even-numbered polyunsaturated fatty acids leaves a 2,4-dienoyl intermediate which is not a substrate for the next step in β-oxidation.

8. a, c, d

9. False. When carbohydrates are abundant, oxaloacetate levels are high and condensation of acetyl CoA and oxaloacetate produces citrate. Citrate is used for energy production as well as for fatty acid biosynthesis. Ketone bodies are produced when acetyl CoA is abundant but oxaloacetate is depleted.

10. a, b, c, d. Choice (c) is correct because 3-hydroxybutyrate is in equilibrium with acetoacetate, the actual source of acetone. Choice (e) is incorrect because ketone bodies are the transportable form of acetyl units in blood.

11. Animals cannot synthesize glucose directly from fatty acids because the acetyl CoA generated by fatty acid degradation cannot be converted into pyruvate or oxaloacetate, which are substrates in gluconeogenesis. In contrast, plants have two additional enzymes that allow them to convert acetyl CoA into oxaloacetate, thereby enabling them to synthesize glucose from fatty acids.

12. Insulin stimulates the absorption of glucose in the liver and curtails fatty acid mobilization by adipose tissue.

13. (a) The liver of a diabetic with uncontrolled diabetes releases large amounts of ketone bodies into the blood because fatty acids are being degraded but there is no glucose to replenish the citric acid cycle. One of these ketone bodies, acetoacetate, spontaneously decarboxylates into acetone, which smells somewhat like alcohol.

    (b) The ketone bodies being released into the bloodstream are moderately strong acids, which lowers blood pH.

    (c) Since glucose is not being taken up, the lack of glucose to the brain disrupts function in the central nervous system and will experience behavioral changes.

14. The first priority is to provide sufficient glucose to the brain. The most obvious solution is to move to a new source of energy, primarily protein degradation. The second is to preserve muscle protein, which would normally require glucose. The solution is to have the muscle use fatty acids and ketone bodies as a fuel source which lessens the need to degrade protein. The brain, meanwhile, turns to acetoacetate for fuel in place of glucose.

PROBLEMS

1. (a) Stumpf and his colleagues have described an α-oxidation system in plant leaves and seeds in which fatty acid oxidation occurs at the α carbon. Molecular oxygen is used in the α-oxidative decarboxylation of a free fatty acid, which yields a fatty aldehyde that is one carbon shorter than the original fatty acid. The fatty aldehyde is in turn oxidized to the corresponding fatty acid, with NAD^+ serving as an electron acceptor. These steps are repeated, resulting in the complete oxidation of the fatty acid. Suppose that the NADH generated through the α oxidation of palmitate is reoxidized in the mitochondrial electron transport chain. Compare the yield of ATP generated by the α oxidation of palmitate with that generated by β oxidation of the same fatty acid. Assume that the products of the final round of oxidation are carbon dioxide and acetic acid.

   (b) If fatty acid oxidation occurs via the α-oxidation route, will odd-numbered fatty acids be glucogenic, that is, capable of forming glucose? Why?

2. Although most components of the diet contain fatty acids with unbranched chains, some plant tissues contain fatty acids with methyl groups at odd-numbered carbons in the acyl chain. These fatty acids cannot be broken down through β oxidation.

   (a) Which step in β oxidation is likely to be blocked when branched-chain fatty acids are substrates?

   (b) Some tissues, including brain tissue, can carry out the limited α oxidation of a fatty acid with one or more methyl groups at odd-numbered carbons. Using the pathway discussed in problem 2, show how one round of α oxidation enables a cell to bypass the block to β oxidation. Use as your substrate a molecule of palmitate with a methyl branch at C-3.

3. The oxidation by microbes of long-chain alkanes, which are found in crude oil, is a subject of study because of concern about oil spills. In many bacteria, alkane oxidation occurs within the outer membrane. A monooxygenase enzyme uses molecular oxygen and an oxidizable substrate, such as NADH, to convert an alkane to a primary alcohol. Studies show that three additional reactions are required for the primary alcohol to undergo β oxidation. Propose a pathway for the conversion of a long-chain primary alcohol to a substrate that can undergo β oxidation. Include cofactors and electron acceptors that might be required.

4. A deficiency of carnitine acyltransferase I in human muscle causes cellular damage and recurrent muscle weakness, especially during fasting or exercise. A deficiency of the enzyme in the liver causes an enlarged and fatty liver, hypoglycemia, and a reduction in the levels of ketone bodies in blood. Explain the likely causes of these symptoms.

5. Plant seeds contain triacylglycerols in organelles called *spherosomes*. During germination, lipases located in the spherosome membrane convert triacylglycerol to monoacylglycerols, free fatty acids, and glycerol. Both free fatty acids and monoacylglycerols enter the glyoxysome, whereas most of the glycerol is metabolized in the plant cell cytosol. A membrane-bound lipase in the glyoxysome converts monoacylglycerols to free fatty acids and glycerol.

   (a) Describe two possible metabolic fates of glycerol in the cytosol.

   (b) What is the fate of fatty acids in the glyoxysome?

   (c) When a germinating plant begins to carry out photosynthesis, the number of glyoxysomes in the germinating plant decreases rapidly. Why?

(d) Plant tissues with high numbers of mitochondria also have high concentrations of carnitine, but there is little correlation between numbers of glyoxysomes and carnitine concentrations in germinating tissue. What does this observation suggest about the role of carnitine in fatty acid metabolism in these two organelles?

(e) Another difference between plant glyoxysomes and plant mitochondria is that glyoxysomes cannot oxidize acetyl CoA, whereas mitochondria can. How is this observation related to the metabolism of fatty acids in these two organelles?

6. Many of the enzymes of the β-oxidation pathway have relatively broad specificities for fatty acyl chain lengths. Why is this important for the economy of the cell?

7. Liver tissue carries out the synthesis of ketone bodies from fatty acids. Suppose a liver cell converts palmitic acid to acetoacetate and then exports it to the circulation. How many molecules of ATP per molecule of palmitate converted to acetoacetate are available to the liver cell?

8. Hydrogenating oils to saturate the double bonds in their fatty acids (see problem 13) in order to increase their melting temperatures causes some of the cis double bonds to convert into the trans conformation. Predict what would happen if a monoenoic fatty acid with a trans-Δ^{10} bond were produced, ingested, and degraded by the β-oxidation pathway. If another of the ingested fatty acids contained a cis-Δ^{11} double bond, what would be the outcome of these processes? What effect would the presence of the double bond have on the yield of ATP obtained by the β oxidation of these fatty acids?

9. Certain desert mammals can survive long periods of drought by consuming plants and seeds and then generating water by metabolizing the fuels they provide.

(a) Briefly describe how water is generated through intermediary metabolism. Include the sources of oxygen and hydrogen and describe reactions that lead to the formation of water.

(b) While parts of mature plants are a reliable source of carbohydrates and proteins, plant seeds contain high quantities of triacylglycerols and free fatty acids. Would plants or seeds be better for generating metabolic water? Why?

(c) Suppose that a desert rat metabolizes 30 g of palmitoyl CoA from seeds. How many milliliters of water can be generated from the process?

10. Explain why the metabolism of a C_{15} fatty acid can lead to the net synthesis of glucose, but the metabolism of a C_{16} fatty acid cannot.

11. You are examining mitochondria from muscle cells of an infant who has a deficiency in one of the enzymes in the fatty acid oxidative pathway. The mitochondria consume oxygen normally when incubated with pyruvate and malate, with succinate, or with palmitoyl CoA (in the presence of carnitine), but the rate of oxygen utilization is decreased when the mitochondria are incubated with linoleoyl CoA in the presence of carnitine. Blood levels of carnitine in the patient are low, while the levels of an unusual acylcarnitine derivative are present in blood and urine. Analysis of this acylcarnitine species using mass spectroscopy reveals that it is trans-Δ^2, cis-Δ^4 decadienoyl (C10:2)-acylcarnitine. The infant suffers from hypotonia (lack of muscle tone) and slow weight gain.

What enzyme is deficient in the cells of the infant? Explain the observed symptoms on the basis of such a deficiency and how you might treat such a disorder.

12. In mammals, acetyl CoA from fatty acid oxidation cannot be used for the net synthesis of pyruvate or oxaloacetate, which in turn means that net glucose synthesis from acetyl CoA is impossible. However, glucose can be radioactively labeled when ^{14}C-labeled acetate is introduced into human tissue culture cells and converted to acetyl CoA by

acetyl CoA synthetase. Radioactive fatty acids can also be used to label glucose. Why? If the methyl carbon of acetate is labeled, where will glucose be labeled?

13. To improve the shelf life (resistance to oxidation) and "crunchiness" of baked products, partially hydrogenated fatty acids are used in recipes. Vegetable oils containing unsaturated fatty acids are treated at high temperature (typically 260°C) and high pressure with hydrogen to reduce the double bonds to single bonds. If the hydrogenation process went to completion, no double bonds would remain and the fatty acids would be fully saturated. However, incomplete reduction leads to isomerization of some of the remaining double bonds from their normal, natural cis configuration to the trans configuration, which confers the desired properties on the oil. Assuming that the original oil had palmitoleate (cis-Δ^9- hexadecanoate) as its only unsaturated fatty acid and that after partial hydrogenation some of the remaining cis-Δ^9 double bonds were now trans-Δ^9 double bonds, what would you predict concerning the β oxidation of the mixture of fully saturated palmitate (16:0) and the remaining 16:1 fatty acid isomers? What do you think trans fatty acids might do to the physical properties of the oil?

ANSWERS TO PROBLEMS

1. (a) The net yield from the β oxidation of palmitate is 106 molecules of ATP, as discussed on pages 470 and 471 of the text. If 1 molecule of NADH is generated for 15 of the 16 carbons of palmitate, then the yield of ATP is 2.5 × 15, or 37.5. For α oxidation, activation of the acetate molecule requires 2 ATP. Subsequent oxidation of acetyl CoA generates 10 ATP molecules. Thus 45.5 molecules of ATP are generated by the α oxidation of a molecule of palmitate.

   (b) In β oxidation of odd-numbered fatty acids, the products include propionyl CoA, which can be converted to succinyl CoA, a glucogenic substrate. However, α oxidation of an odd-numbered fatty acid would yield carbon dioxide as well as a single molecule of acetate or acetyl CoA, neither of which is glucogenic.

2. (a) As shown in Figure 27.1, the oxidation of a fatty acid with a methyl group at C-3 proceeds to the formation of the L-hydroxymethylacyl CoA derivative. Subsequent oxidation of the β carbon to the ketoacyl derivative is blocked by the methyl group. Compare this pathway with the one shown in Figure 27.5 of the text (page 469).

FIGURE 27.1 Formation of L-hydroxymethylacyl CoA through β oxidation of branched-chain acyl CoA.

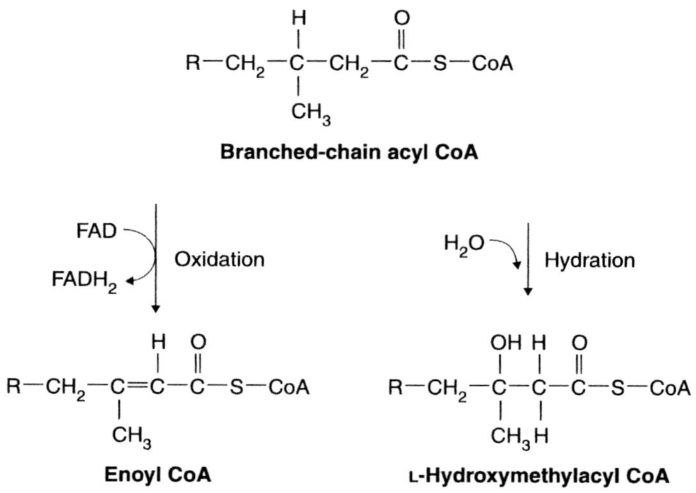

(b) As shown in Figure 27.2, the oxidation of the α carbon in the palmitate derivative followed by decarboxylation of the molecule yields a fatty acid that has a methyl group at an even-numbered carbon. Activation of the fatty acid to form an acyl CoA derivative followed by oxidation at the β carbon results in the generation of propionyl CoA and a shortened acyl derivative, lauroyl CoA (C:12).

FIGURE 27.2 The α oxidation and oxidative decarboxylation of a branched-chain fatty acid allow generation of intermediates that can enter normal oxidative pathways.

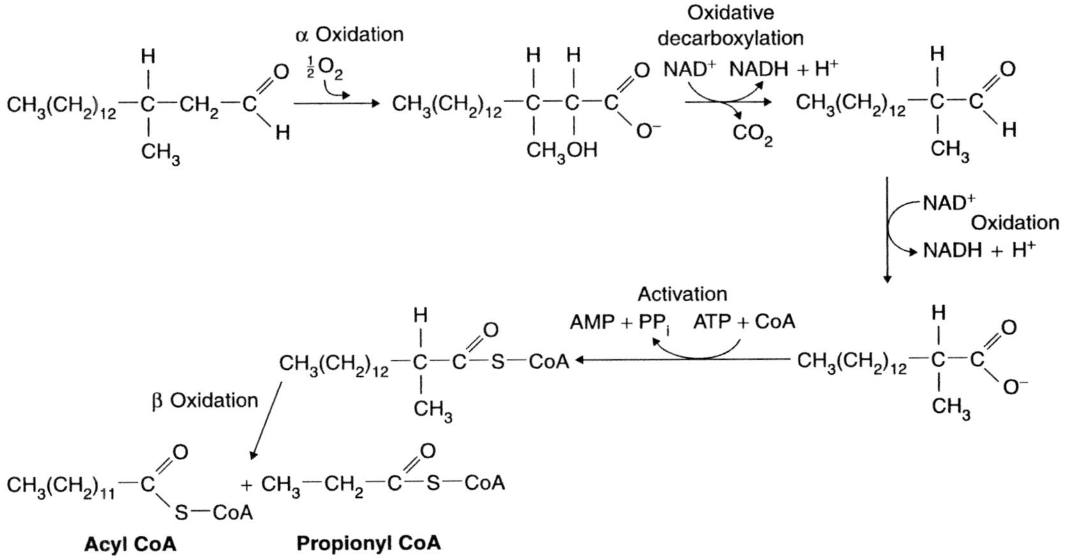

3. The normal route for β oxidation in bacteria utilizes acyl CoA derivatives, which are formed from free fatty acids. To convert a primary alcohol to a free fatty acid, two oxidative steps are needed, each requiring an electron acceptor. In *Corynebacterium*, NAD^+-dependent dehydrogenases catalyze the sequential conversion of a primary alcohol to a fatty acid, with the corresponding aldehyde as an intermediate. Conversion of the free fatty acid to an acyl CoA derivative requires two equivalents of ATP (because ATP is converted to AMP and PP_i), as well as coenzyme A. The reaction is catalyzed by acyl CoA synthase.

4. Carnitine acyltransferase I facilitates the transfer of long-chain fatty acids into the mitochondrion by catalyzing the formation of fatty acyl carnitine molecules. The failure to form such molecules means that long-chain fatty acids are not available for cellular oxidation. In muscle, exercise or fasting increases dependence on fatty acids as a source of energy, so the inability to metabolize them interferes with cellular functions, causing cramps, weakness, and muscle damage. Liver cells also require formation of fatty acyl carnitine molecules to oxidize fats in mitochondria. If fatty acids cannot be utilized, they will remain in the cytosol, where high concentrations of them cause cell enlargement and interfere with other functions. Liver cells must then use glucose as a source of energy instead of exporting it to other cells. Because liver cells use acetyl CoA, which is derived primarily from fatty acid oxidation, as a precursor of ketone bodies, the failure to oxidize fatty acids will result in a reduction in the rate of ketone body synthesis. This in turn will exacerbate the symptoms of hypoglycemia because tissues that normally use ketone bodies as a source of energy, such as cardiac muscle and renal cortex, will have to rely more heavily on glucose as a source of energy.

5. (a) Glycerol is converted to dihydroxyacetone phosphate, which in turn can serve as a source of glucose or can be converted to acetyl CoA.

   (b) Fatty acids serve as a source of acetyl CoA, which is used in the glyoxylate cycle and gluconeogenesis.

(c) The primary function of glyoxysomes is to utilize fatty acids from triacylglycerols for the synthesis of glucose, which is used as a source of other molecules by the developing plant. Once leaf development enables the plant to generate glucose by photosynthesis, glyoxysomes are no longer needed.

(d) Carnitine functions in the transport of long-chain fatty acids from the cytosol to the interior of the mitochondrion. The observation suggests that, although carnitine may be important in mitochondrial transport of fatty acyl chains, the compound is not involved in the movement of fatty acyl chains into the glyoxysome. It is also possible that glyoxysomes metabolize fatty acids with shorter acyl chains, for which transport facilitated by carnitine is not necessary.

(e) The fate of fatty acids is different in glyoxysomes and in mitochondria. Both organelles carry out β oxidation of fatty acids to acetyl CoA; however, in glyoxysomes, acetyl CoA is a precursor of glucose, whereas mitochondria oxidize acetyl CoA to CO_2 and H_2O to generate ATP.

6. If each enzyme could operate only on fatty acyl CoA derivatives of a particular chain length, then as many as eight sets of enzymes would be required to carry out the β oxidation of palmitate. The fact that most enzymes of the β-oxidation pathway can use acyl CoA molecules of different chain lengths as substrates means that the cell needs to synthesize fewer different enzymes to carry out fatty acid oxidation.

7. To synthesize acetoacetate from palmitate, liver cells must carry out β oxidation of the 16-carbon acyl chain, generating 8 molecules of acetyl CoA, which will in turn generate 4 molecules of acetoacetate. A total of 7 NADH and 7 FADH$_2$ molecules are generated per molecule of palmitate converted to acetyl CoA. The 14 reduced cofactors are equivalent to 28 ATP molecules. Because 2 molecules of ATP are needed to activate palmitate, the net yield of ATP per palmitate is 26.

8. Four rounds of β oxidation of a fatty acid with a trans-Δ^{10} double bond would yield a *trans*-Δ^2-enoyl CoA derivative. This compound is the natural intermediate formed by an acyl CoA dehydrogenase. It would be hydrated by enoyl CoA hydratase to form the L-3-hydroxyacyl CoA derivative. For the fatty acid with a cis-Δ^{11} double bond, four rounds of β oxidation would produce a cis-Δ^3 double bond, which would not serve as a substrate for enoyl CoA hydratase. An isomerase would convert this bond into the trans-$\Delta 2$ configuration to allow subsequent metabolism. Since the double bond already exists in the fatty acids and does not arise from β oxidations, one less FADH$_2$ would be formed. Consequently, approximately 1.5 fewer ATP molecules would be produced for each preexisting double bond.

9. (a) The source of oxygen for formation of water during respiration is atmospheric oxygen, whereas the sources of hydrogen include oxidizable foodstuffs such as carbohydrates and fats. These substances are oxidized to generate "energy-rich" electrons, which are in turn used to reduce oxygen to generate water. The principal terminal reaction in the process occurs in the mitochondrion, where electrons are transferred from cytochrome *c* to oxygen to generate oxidized cytochrome *c* and water. Also important in water generation is the formation of ATP from ADP and inorganic phosphate, where a molecule of water is generated during the formation of each ATP molecule.

(b) The more reduced the carbons of a substrate, the larger the number of electrons available during metabolism and the more water generated. Most carbon atoms of fatty acids are saturated and therefore highly reduced, so that they are a better source of available electrons. Carbohydrate molecules like glucose, whose carbons are at the alcohol level of oxidation or, in the case of the C-1 atom, at the aldehyde level, provide fewer electrons during terminal oxidation. Seeds, which contain a high percentage of fats, are therefore a better source than mature plants for the generation of water.

(c) First determine the number of moles of palmitate that are converted to CO_2 and water. The molecular weight of the molecule ($C_{16}H_{31}O_2$) is 255 g mol^{-1}.

$$30 \text{ g}/255 \text{ g mol}^{-1} = 0.12 \text{ mole palmitate oxidized}$$

Then, calculate the number of moles of water produced by the complete oxidation of palmitate.

For palmitoyl CoA, the text shows on page 471 that oxidation of the molecule gives 7 $FADH_2$, 7 NADH, and 8 acetyl CoA molecules, utilizing 7 molecules of water.

On page 335, the text shows that oxidation of acetyl CoA in the citric acid cycle yields 3 NADH, 1 $FADH_2$, and 1 GTP, equivalent to 1 ATP, utilizing 2 water molecules. Thus, the 8 acetyl CoA molecules produced from palmitoyl CoA give 24 NADH, 8 $FADH_2$, and 8 ATP equivalents, utilizing 16 water molecules.

The total number of reduced electron carriers from the oxidative process is 31 NADH and 15 $FADH_2$. Recall that 2.5 ATP molecules are produced when NADH is oxidized in the electron transport chain, and 1.5 ATP are generated from $FADH_2$ oxidation.

One water molecule is gained per ATP molecule formed plus 1 water molecule per pair of e^- molecules oxidized.

The overall equation for the production of NAD$^+$, ATP, and water from palmitoyl CoA is

$$31 \text{ NADH} + 15.5 \text{ O}_2 + 77.5 \text{ ADP} + 77.5 \text{ P}_i + 108.5 \text{ H}^+ \longrightarrow$$
$$31 \text{ NAD}^+ + 77.5 \text{ ATP} + 108.5 \text{ H}_2\text{O}$$

and for $FADH_2$ it is

$$15 \text{ FADH}_2 + 7.5 \text{ O}_2 + 22.5 \text{ ADP} + 22.5 \text{ Pi} + 37.5 \text{ H}^+ \longrightarrow$$
$$15 \text{ FAD} + 22.5 \text{ ATP} + 37.5 \text{ H}_2\text{O}$$

The total number of water molecules produced is 146, and the net water produced is $(146 - 23) = 123$ molecules of water per palmitate oxidized or 123 moles of water per mole of palmitate. The molecular weight of water is 18.0 g mol^{-1}.

Thirty grams of palmitoyl CoA is equivalent to 0.12 mole of palmitate, which generates $0.12 \times 123 = 14.8$ moles of water when oxidized. At 18 g mol^{-1}, 14.8 moles of water equals 266 g, or 266 ml, of water.

10. The oxidation of a C_{16} fatty acid (palmitate) leads to the formation of eight molecules of acetyl CoA. Acetyl CoA, which contains two carbon atoms, is oxidized to two CO_2 in the citric acid cycle, so the net number of carbons entering and leaving the cycle is zero. Thus, no net carbons are available to enter the gluconeogenic pathway. On the other hand, oxidation of a C_{15} fatty acid generates seven acetyl CoA molecules plus one molecule of propionyl CoA. This compound is converted by carboxylation, epimerization, and conversion to succinyl CoA, a *four*-carbon compound that is an intermediate in the citric acid cycle. Succinyl CoA contributes two extra carbons to the gluconeogenic pathway, leading to the net synthesis of glucose.

11. The most likely deficiency is a lack of 2,4-dienoyl CoA reductase, an enzyme that is essential for the degradation of unsaturated fatty acids with double bonds at even-numbered carbons. Such fatty acids include linoleate (9-*cis*,12-*cis* 18:2). Four rounds of oxidation of linoleoyl CoA generate a 10-carbon acyl CoA that contains a *trans*-Δ^2 and a *cis*-Δ^4 double bond. This intermediate is a substrate for the reductase, which converts the 2,4-dienoyl CoA to *cis*-Δ^3-enoyl CoA. A deficiency of 2,4-dienoyl reductase leads to an accumulation of *trans*-Δ^2,*cis*-Δ^4-decadienoyl CoA molecules in the mitochondrion. The observation that carnitine derivatives of the 2,4-dienoyl CoA are found in blood and urine provides evidence that these molecules accumulate in the mitochondrion and are then attached to carnitine. Formation of carnitine decadienoate allows the acyl molecules to be transported across the inner mitochondrial membrane into the cytosol and then into the circulation.

Mitochondria from the patient function normally, taking up oxygen as they carry out oxidation of various substrates including palmitate, a saturated fatty acid. However, incubation of those mitochondria with linoleate results in reduced oxygen uptake, because the absence of the reductase molecule allows only a limited number of rounds of β oxidation to occur before the 2,4-dienoyl molecule is formed. Lack of muscle tone could mean that there are difficulties in oxidizing fuel molecules needed to provide energy for muscle contraction. If carnitine levels in cells are lower because many of them are esterified to decadienoate molecules, the result is a virtual deficiency of carnitine. The ability of the cell to transport other long-chain fatty acids across the inner mitochondrial membrane is limited under these conditions. Impairment of fatty acid oxidation means that fewer ATP molecules are available for muscular activity.

One immediate strategy for dealing with this disorder is to limit linoleate in the diet. However, linoleate is a starting point for other unsaturated fatty acids including arachidonate, a precursor of eicosanoid hormones. Limiting linoleate in the diet of a person with the reductase deficiency would have to be carried out carefully, to avoid a deficiency of an essential fatty acid.

12. Radioactive acetyl CoA can be generated by direct synthesis from ^{14}C-acetate or from β oxidation of radioactive fatty acids, such as uniformly labeled palmitate. Examination of the reactions of the citric acid cycle reveals that neither of the two carbons that enter citrate from acetate is removed as carbon dioxide during the first pass through the cycle. Labeled carbon from ^{14}C-methyl-labeled acetate appears in C-2 and C-3 of oxaloacetate because succinate is symmetrical, with either methylene carbon in that molecule labeling C-2 or C-3 of oxaloacetate. The conversion of oxaloacetate to phosphoenolpyruvate yields PEP labeled at C-2 or C-3 as well. Formation of glyceraldehyde 3-phosphate and its isomer dihydroxyacetone phosphate gives molecules both labeled at carbons 2 and 3. Condensation by aldolase gives fructose 1,6-bisphosphate radioactively labeled at carbons 1, 2, 5, and 6. The corresponding four carbons will then be labeled in glucose 6-phosphate or glucose. No net synthesis of glucose will have occurred, but the label will have been incorporated.

13. The β-oxidation pathway would convert the palmitate to eight acetyl CoA molecules. The natural palmitoleate (*cis*-Δ^9- hexadecanoate) would have three two-carbon units removed until it became *cis*-Δ^3- enoyl CoA)—a 10-carbon compound. A *cis*-Δ^3 double bond cannot be further metabolized as such, so the enzyme *cis*-Δ^3- CoA isomerase converts it into *trans*-Δ^2-enoyl CoA, which is a normal constituent in the β oxidation pathway. The *trans*-Δ^2-enoyl CoA can be further oxidized to completion to yield five more CoA molecules. The situation is different for the *trans*-Δ^9-hexadecanoate. It would be

oxidized by β oxidation to yield *trans*-Δ^3-enoyl CoA. The *cis*-Δ^3- CoA isomerase converts the *trans*-Δ^3-enoyl CoA to *trans*-Δ^2-enoyl CoA that would then be subject to further, normal catabolism. Thus with the partial hydrogenation of this particular oil, the presence of a trans double bond causes no problem for complete catabolism because enzymes exist to isomerize them to metabolizable forms. Some trans fatty acids arising from partial hydrogenation of other oils are not recognized as normal physiological components and are deposited in blood vessels.

Trans fatty acids are more extended than those with *cis* double bonds giving them properties more like fully saturated fatty acids. They would increase the melting temperature of the oil (hardening it) and, if incorporated into the phospholipids of membranes, would decrease the fluidity of the lipid membrane.

Fatty Acid Synthesis

In this chapter the authors build on Chapter 27 by discussing the synthesis of lipids. The chapter begins with the three stages of fatty acid synthesis, analogous to the three stages of fatty acid degradation. In the first step acetyl CoA is transferred from the mitochondrial to the cytoplasm, the site of fatty acid synthesis. The second step begins with the activation of acetyl CoA to form malonyl CoA. In the last step the reaction intermediates are attached to an acyl carrier protein, and the fatty acid is synthesized in a five-step elongation cycle. The authors then discuss the elongation and desaturation of palmitate to form other fatty acids. The regulation of fatty acid synthesis and degradation through allostery and covalent modification are then discussed, centering around acetyl CoA carboxylase. The chapter ends by discussing the ways in which ethanol alters energy metabolism in the liver.

LEARNING OBJECTIVES

When you have mastered this chapter, you should be able to accomplish the following objectives.

Introduction

1. List some circumstances in which a human would need to synthesize fatty acids de novo.
2. Identify acetyl CoA and palmitate as the precursors for virtually all fatty acids.

Fatty Acid Synthesis Takes Place in Three Stages (Text Section 28.1)

3. Outline the three stages of fatty acid synthesis.

4. Describe the transport of acetyl groups across the inner mitochondrial membrane in the form of *citrate* and explain its purpose. Account for the synthesis of *NADPH* during the conversion of oxaloacetate into pyruvate in the cytosol.

5. List the sources of the NADPH used in fatty acid synthesis.

6. List the substrates and products of the committed step in fatty acid synthesis and describe its catalytic mechanism. Appreciate the role of *biotin* in the *acetyl CoA carboxylase* reaction.

7. Name the common component of *acyl carrier protein* (*ACP*) and CoA, give its functions, and describe the overall functions of ACP and CoA in fatty acid metabolism.

8. Describe the four reactions of the elongation cycle of fatty acid synthesis. Explain how *malonyl CoA* provides the driving force for the condensation of acetyl units with the growing acyl chain.

9. Calculate the energy cost of the synthesis of a given fatty acid.

10. Contrast the enzymatic machinery for fatty acid biosynthesis in bacteria with that in eukaryotes. Outline the movements of the elongating acyl chain on the mammalian *fatty acid synthetase* dimer during fatty acid biosynthesis.

11. Describe how fatty acid synthase inhibitors may be used as drugs.

12. Contrast the structure and physiological function of β-hydroxybutyric and γ-hydroxybutyric acids.

Additional Enzymes Elongate and Desaturate Fatty Acids (Text Section 28.2)

13. Describe the elongation and desaturation reactions that can occur on preformed fatty acids. Explain why linoleate and linolenate are essential in the diet.

14. List the different kinds of *eicosanoid hormones*. Outline their metabolic relationships and biological functions.

15. Describe the effects of *acetylsalicylate* (*aspirin*) on the synthesis of eicosanoids.

Acetyl CoA Carboxylase Is a Key Regulator ofFatty Acid Metabolism
(Text Section 28.3)

16. Discuss the different modes of regulation of *acetyl CoA carboxylase*. Explain the reciprocal control of fatty acid synthesis and degradation through local (intracellular), hormonal, and adaptive regulation.

Metabolism in Context: Ethanol Alters Energy Metabolism in the Liver
(Text Section 28.4)

17. Explain the process of metabolism of ethanol in humans. Include the biochemical basis for the adverse effects of ethanol consumption.

SELF-TEST

Fatty Acid Synthesis Takes Place in Three Stages

1. Which of the following statements about citrate are correct?

    (a) It transports reducing power from the mitochondria into the cytosol.
    (b) It inhibits gluconeogenesis.
    (c) It activates the first enzyme of fatty acid biosynthesis.
    (d) It transports acetyl groups from the mitochondria into the cytosol.
    (e) It supplies the CO_2 required for formation of malonyl CoA.

2. For each of the following metabolic pathways indicate whether it contributes NADPH or ATP for fatty acid synthesis.

    (a) Citric acid cycle
    (b) Citrate transport system
    (c) Glycolysis
    (d) Oxidative phosphorylation
    (e) Pentose phosphate pathway

3. Explain the requirement for bicarbonate (HCO_3^-) in fatty acid biosynthesis.

4. (a) Do condensation, reduction, dehydration, and reduction occur during fatty acid degradation or synthesis?

    (b) How many carbon atoms are added to or removed from a fatty acid during its synthesis or degradation, respectively?

5. Match the reactant or characteristic in the right column with the appropriate pathway in the left column.

    (a) fatty acid oxidation
    (b) fatty acid synthesis

    (1) acyl CoA
    (2) occurs in the cytosol
    (3) uses NAD^+
    (4) D-3-hydroxyacyl derivative involved
    (5) pantetheine involved
    (6) malonyl CoA
    (7) single polypeptide with multiple activities involved
    (8) uses FAD

6. Calculate the ATP and NADPH requirements for the synthesis of lauric acid (C12:0) from acetyl CoA.

7. The fatty acid synthase of mammals is a dimer consisting of identical subunits, each of which contains all the activities necessary to synthesize fatty acids from malonyl CoA and acetyl CoA. Why is a single subunit unable to carry out the reactions?

8. Possible advantages of multifunctional polypeptide chains, that is, polypeptide chains having more than one active site, include which of the following?

   (a) enhanced stability beyond that expected for a noncovalent complex of the same activities on separate polypeptide chains

   (b) fixed stoichiometric relationships among the different enzymatic activities because of their coordinate synthesis

   (c) enhanced specificity and decreased side reactions because the product of each active site is in the immediate vicinity of the active site carrying out the next reaction in the sequence

   (d) enhanced versatility because the product of any one active site could be used by any other active site in its immediate vicinity to generate a variety of products

   (e) accelerated overall reaction rate because of the proximity of the active sites

Additional Enzymes Elongate and Desaturate Fatty Acids

9. Which of the following answers completes the sentence correctly? The major product of the fatty acid synthase complex in mammals is

   (a) oleate.
   (b) stearate.
   (c) stearoyl CoA.
   (d) linoleate.
   (e) palmitate.
   (f) palmitoyl CoA.

10. Which of the following statements about desaturases in humans are correct?

    (a) They cannot introduce double bonds into a fatty acid that already contains a double bond.

    (b) They cannot introduce double bonds between the Δ^9 position and the ω end of the chain.

    (c) They convert the essential fatty acid linoleate into arachidonate.

    (d) They use an isozyme of the FAD-linked dehydrogenase of the β-oxidation cycle to form double bonds.

11. Which of the following statements about the eicosanoid hormones are NOT correct?

    (a) The major classes of eicosanoid hormones include prostaglandins, leukotrienes, thromboxanes, and prostacyclins.

    (b) The eicosanoid hormones are derived from arachidonic acid.

    (c) The eicosanoid hormones are very potent and exert global effects because they are widely distributed by the circulatory system.

    (d) The prostaglandins have a variety of physiologic effects.

    (e) Prostaglandins are derived directly from phospholipids.

12. Explain why aspirin is a potent anti-inflammatory agent.

Acetyl CoA Carboxylase Is a Key Regulator of Fatty Acid Metabolism

13. Which of the following statements about acetyl CoA carboxylase are correct?

    (a) It is active in the phosphorylated form.
    (b) It is partially active in the phosphorylated form in the presence of citrate.
    (c) It is phosphorylated by a cAMP-dependent protein kinase.

(d) It is stimulated by a high-energy charge.

(e) It is converted from an inactive form to an active form by protein phosphatase 2A.

14. For each situation place the physiological responses in the correct order.

    (a) low glycogen stores, high energy needs.

    (b) low energy needs, lots of fuel available.

    (1) Activation of Acetyl CoA Carboxylase

    (2) Dephosphorylation of Acetyl CoA Carboxylase

    (3) Glucagon and epinephrine released

    (4) Inactivation of Acetyl CoA Carboxylase

    (5) Inhibition of fatty acid synthesis

    (6) Phosphorylation of Acetyl CoA Carboxylase

    (7) Release of insulin

    (8) Stimulation of fatty acid synthesis

Metabolism in Context: Ethanol Alters Energy Metabolism in the Liver

15. Match each metabolite of ethanol with its physiological effect.

    (a) NADH

    (b) Acetadehyde

    (c) Acetate

    (1) covalent modification of proteins

    (2) fatty liver

    (3) formation and release of ketone bodies

    (4) gluconeogenesis inhibition

    (5) hypoglycemia

    (6) lactic acidosis

    (7) liver cell death

ANSWERS TO SELF-TEST

1. c, d

2. NADPH: a,b, and e; ATP: c and d

3. The irreversible and committed step of fatty acid biosynthesis is the formation of malonyl CoA from acetyl CoA and HCO_3^- by acetyl CoA carboxylase. HCO_3^- is fixed to form a dicarboxylic acid at the expense of an ATP cleavage. This facilitates the subsequent condensation reactions with activated acyl groups to form an acetoacyl-ACP by releasing CO_2 to help drive the reaction.

4. (a) Synthesis. These four steps result in the addition of a 2-carbon alkane unit to a growing fatty acid.

    (b) Two.

5. (a) 1, 3, 5, 8   (b) 1, 2, 4, 5, 6, 7. Acyl CoA is involved in both the synthesis and the oxidation of fatty acids.

6. For a C12:0 fatty acid, 6 acetyl CoA molecules are required. One serves as a primer forming the ω end of the chain and five undergo condensation reactions as their malonyl CoA derivatives. Formation of each malonyl CoA requires 1 ATP molecule, and each cycle of elongation uses 2 NADPH molecules. Thus, 5 ATP and 10 NADPH are required.

7. The reactions of elongation require the interactions of domains from different sub-units of the dimer to form active sites at the interfaces of the subunits. One monomer holds the growing acyl chain while the other is linked to the incoming activated acetyl unit.

8. a, b, c, e. For a discussion relevant to the correct answers, see pages 486–487 in the text.

9. e

10. b, c. For (c) additional elongations as well as desaturations are required.

11. c. Answer (c) is incorrect because the eicosanoid hormones have very short half-lives and therefore exert local rather than global effects. Answer (e) is correct because phospholipids supply the arachidonate for prostaglandin synthesis.

12. Aspirin acetylates a specific Ser residue in the cyclooxygenase component of prostaglandin synthase. Thus aspirin inhibits the synthesis of prostaglandins, thromboxanes, and prostacyclins, which mediate the inflammatory response.

13. b, d, e. Acetyl CoA carboxylase is inactivated by phosphorylation. This effect is partially abolished by citrate, which acts as an allosteric activator. Phosphorylation–dephosphorylation of this enzyme is under the control of hormones, whose action is mediated by a protein kinase that is dependent on AMP, not cAMP. High-energy charge stimulates acetyl CoA carboxylase, while low-energy charge, that is, high AMP levels, inhibits it.

14. (a) 3, 6, 4, 5 (b) 7, 2, 1, 8

15. (a) 2, 4, 5, 6 (b) 1, 7 (c) 3

PROBLEMS

1. Many plants have enzyme systems that catalyze the formation of a cis double bond in oleic acid at one or more positions between C-9 and the terminal methyl group. The fact that these enzyme systems exist in plants is of great significance to animals. Why?

2. Malonyl CoA, labeled with ^{14}C in the methylene carbon, is used in excess as a substrate in a system in vivo for the synthesis of palmitoyl CoA, which is catalyzed by a yeast fatty acid synthase complex. Acetyl CoA and other substrates are also present in the system, but acetyl CoA carboxylase is not. Which carbons in palmitoyl CoA will be labeled?

3. One intermediate in the conversion of propionyl CoA to succinyl CoA is methylmalonyl CoA, the structure of which follows. This compound is an analog of malonyl CoA. In people who are unable to convert propionyl CoA to succinyl CoA, high levels of methylmalonyl CoA are observed. What effect could such levels of methylmalonyl CoA have on fatty acid metabolism?

$$H_3C-\underset{\underset{\underset{O}{\overset{|}{C}}-S-CoA}{\overset{|}{\underset{|}{C}}-H}}{\overset{\overset{COO^-}{|}}{}}$$

L-Methylmalonyl CoA

4. Animals cannot synthesize glucose from even-numbered fatty acids, which make up the bulk of the fatty acids in their diet.

   (a) How can odd-numbered fatty acids be used for the net synthesis of glucose in animals?

(b) Triacylglycerols can be used as precursors of glucose. Give two reasons why this is possible.

(c) Why are most of the fatty acids found in animal tissues composed of an even number of carbon atoms?

(d) Some bacteria synthesize odd-numbered fatty acids. What CoA derivative is required, in addition to acetyl CoA and malonyl CoA, for the synthesis of an odd-numbered fatty acid?

5. (a) Describe how malonyl CoA affects the balance between the rates of synthesis and β oxidation of fatty acids in a liver cell.

(b) Show that failure to regulate these two processes reciprocally could result in the wasteful hydrolysis of ATP.

6. People concerned about their weight must pay attention not only to triacylglyceride intake but also to the consumption of starch, glucose, and other carbohydrates. Although carbohydrates can be converted to glycogen in liver, muscle, and other tissues, only about 5 percent of the energy stored in the body is present as glycogen. What happens to most carbohydrates that are consumed in excess of caloric need?

7. Wakil's pioneering studies on fatty acid synthesis included the crucial observation that bicarbonate is required for the synthesis of palmitoyl CoA. He was surprised to find that very low levels of bicarbonate could sustain palmitate synthesis; that is, there was no correlation between the amount of bicarbonate required and the amount of palmitate produced. Later he also found that ^{14}C-labeled bicarbonate is not incorporated into palmitate. Explain these observations.

8. In tissue culture, cells that are deficient in $NADP^+$-linked malate enzyme can be isolated. They exhibit a slightly lower rate of fatty acid synthesis when compared with normal cells. However, cells lacking citrate lyase are very difficult to isolate. Why?

9. An unusual sphingolipid contains a 22-carbon, polyunsaturated fatty acid called *clupanodonic acid,* or *7,10,13,16,19-docosapentaenoic acid.* In mammals, both the mitochondrial and endoplasmic reticular acyl chain elongation and desaturation systems can synthesize clupanodonate from linolenate.

(a) What steps are required to synthesize clupanodonate from linolenate?

(b) Why are mammals unable to synthesize clupanodonate from linoleate?

10. Compare the effects of high levels of intracellular citrate on pathways of fatty acid and carbohydrate metabolism. Explain how its transport from the mitochondrion to the cytosol is essential for the action of citrate on both sets of pathways.

ANSWERS TO PROBLEMS

1. Because animals lack an enzyme that can introduce double bonds beyond the C-9 position in a fatty acid, they cannot synthesize linoleate and linolenate *de novo.* These unsaturated fatty acids are precursors for a number of other necessary fatty acids, as well as the eicosanoid hormones. Animals therefore rely on their diet as the source of linoleate and linolenate, which are synthesized only in plants.

2. As shown in Figure 28.4 of the text, acetyl-ACP and malonyl-ACP condense to form acetoacetyl-ACP. Carbons 4 and 3 of acetoacetyl-ACP are not labeled because they are derived from acetyl CoA. These two carbons will become carbons 15 and 16 of palmitate. Only C-2 of acetoacetyl-ACP will be labeled because it is derived from the methylene carbon of malonyl-ACP. When the second round of synthesis begins, butyryl-ACP condenses with a second molecule of methylene-labeled malonyl-ACP, which contributes

C-1 and C-2 of the newly formed six-carbon ACP derivative. In this compound, C-2 and C-4 will be labeled. Chain elongation continues until palmitoyl-ACP is formed. Each even-numbered carbon atom, except for carbon 16 (at the ω end), will be labeled.

3. Because malonyl CoA is a substrate for fatty acid synthase, competition from methyl-malonyl CoA could cause a decrease in the rate of palmitoyl CoA synthesis in the cytosol, which could in turn lead to an increase in the concentration of acetyl CoA because palmitoyl CoA inhibits acetyl CoA carboxylase. In addition, high levels of methyl-malonyl CoA could interfere with transport of long-chain fatty acyl chains into mitochondria by inhibiting carnitine acyltransferase, as does malonyl CoA. Thus, both the synthesis and the oxidation of fatty acids could be inhibited by methylmalonyl CoA.

4. (a) The oxidation of an odd-numbered fatty acid yields acetyl CoA molecules as well as one molecule of propionyl CoA, which can be converted to succinyl CoA, a component of the citric acid cycle. Although two-carbon compounds like acetyl CoA cannot be used for the net synthesis of glucose, succinyl CoA can contribute net carbons to the citric acid cycle, enabling oxaloacetate and ultimately glucose to be formed through gluconeogenesis.

    (b) Triacylglycerols are converted to glycerol and three free fatty acids through the action of lipases. Glycerol can be converted to glucose by way of dihydroxyacetone phosphate. Odd-numbered fatty acids found in triacylglycerols can also be used for net synthesis of glucose, whereas even-numbered fatty acids cannot.

    (c) During fatty acid synthesis, most organisms use acetyl CoA as a source of the ω carbon and its adjacent carbon in the acyl chain. Two of the three carbons of malonyl CoA are incorporated during each cycle of acyl chain elongation. Thus the resulting fatty acid will contain an even number of carbon atoms.

    (d) To produce an odd-numbered fatty acid, at least one odd-numbered CoA intermediate must be incorporated in its entirety during fatty acid synthesis. Propionyl CoA can be used by certain bacteria for the initial condensation step with malonyl CoA in fatty acid synthesis. The resulting five-carbon acyl intermediate is then extended in two-carbon units to yield an odd-numbered fatty acid.

5. (a) Malonyl CoA is a key substrate for the synthesis of fatty acids; when it is abundant, synthesis is stimulated. In addition, high levels of this intermediate inhibit carnitine acyltransferase I, thereby limiting the entry of fatty acyl chains into the mitochondrion, where they are oxidized. A decrease in the concentration of malonyl CoA leads to a decrease in the rate of fatty acid synthesis and an increase in the rate of fatty acid oxidation in the mitochondrion.

    (b) The overall equation for the synthesis of palmitoyl CoA is

    $$8 \text{ acetyl CoA} + 7 \text{ ATP} + 14 \text{ NADPH} \rightarrow$$
    $$\text{palmitoyl CoA} + 14 \text{ NADP}^+ + 7 \text{ CoA} + 7 \text{ H}_2\text{O} + 7 \text{ ADP} + 7 \text{ P}_i$$

    The overall equation for the oxidation of palmitoyl CoA is

    $$\text{palmitoyl CoA} + 7 \text{ FAD} + 7 \text{ NAD}^+ + 7 \text{ CoA} + 7 \text{ H}_2\text{O} \rightarrow$$
    $$8 \text{ acetyl CoA} + 7 \text{ FADH}_2 + 7 \text{ NADH} + 7 \text{ H}^+$$

    Assuming that NADPH is equivalent in reducing power to NADH, that a molecule of FADH$_2$ yields 1.5 ATP during electron transport and oxidative phosphorylation, and that a molecule of NADH yields 2.5 ATP, then 42 ATP molecules are required to synthesize a molecule of palmitoyl CoA, whereas 28 ATP are generated by the conversion of palmitoyl CoA to 8 molecules of acetyl CoA. There is a net loss of 14 ATP molecules if the two processes occur simultaneously.

6. Carbohydrates consumed in excess of caloric need are converted to acetyl CoA, which in turn serves as a source of fatty acids. The concurrent synthesis of glycerol from carbohydrates such as glucose and fructose provides the second precursor needed for the synthesis of triacylglycerols, which are the primary storage form of energy in humans. Excess carbohydrate is converted to fat.

7. Bicarbonate is a source of carbon dioxide for the reaction catalyzed by acetyl CoA carboxylase, in which malonyl CoA is formed. Malonyl CoA is then used as a source of two-carbon units for fatty acyl chain elongation, and the carbon atom derived originally from bicarbonate is released as CO_2. Carbon dioxide is then rapidly converted to bicarbonate, which is used again for the synthesis of another molecule of malonyl CoA. Thus, the carbon atom derived from bicarbonate can be used many times for the production of malonyl CoA, but it is never incorporated into the growing acyl chain, so it does not appear in palmitate.

8. Both malate enzyme and citrate lyase are part of the shuttle system that transports two-carbon units from the mitochondrion to the cytosol. Malate enzyme also generates reducing power in the form of NADPH, which is used for fatty acid synthesis; however, the pentose phosphate pathway also serves as a source of NADPH, so fatty acid synthesis can continue even if malate enzyme is deficient. Citrate lyase is more critical to fatty acid synthesis because it is required to generate acetyl CoA from citrate in the cytosol. Without cytosolic acetyl CoA, fatty acid synthesis cannot take place, and the cells cannot grow and divide.

9. (a) To synthesize clupanodonate from linolenate, the acyl chain must be elongated from 18 to 22 carbons, and two new double bonds must be introduced into the chain. Although the details of the various mammalian desaturation systems are not completely understood, it appears that a double bond at C-6 can be introduced when a double bond at C-9 is available, and a double bond at C-5 can be introduced when one at C-8 is available. Thus, the probable sequence of reactions includes the introduction of a double bond at C-6 of linolenate (yielding a 18:4 cis-Δ^6, Δ^9, Δ^{12}, Δ^{15}-acyl chain) followed by chain elongation to a 20-carbon derivative. The introduction of a double bond at C-5 then gives an acyl chain denoted as 20:5 cis-Δ^5, Δ^8, Δ^{11}, Δ^{14}, Δ^{17}. The final reaction required to yield clupanodonate is chain elongation to the 22-carbon fatty acyl chain.

    (b) Linoleate has cis double bonds at C-9 and C-12. Elongation to a 22-carbon chain would yield an acyl chain with double bonds at C-13 and C-16. To form clupanodonate, a double bond at C-19 is needed, but mammals lack the enzymes required to introduce double bonds beyond C-9. Thus, linoleate cannot be used for the synthesis of clupanodonate.

10. High levels of citrate signal that glucose utilization is no longer necessary and that adequate carbon atoms are available for synthesis of palmitoyl CoA. Citrate inhibits phosphofructokinase 1 activity, decelerating the rate of glycolysis. On the other hand, citrate stimulates the activity of acetyl CoA carboxylase, so increased production of malonyl CoA leads to stimulation of fatty acid synthesis. The transport of citrate from the mitochondrial matrix to the cytosol is important because both phosphofructokinase 1 and acetyl CoA carboxylase are located in the cytosol.

Lipid Synthesis

This chapter describes the biosynthesis of membrane lipids, steroids, and other important lipid molecules, such as bile salts, and vitamin D. As background material for this chapter, you should review the earlier chapters on cell membranes (Chapter 12) and fatty acid metabolism (Chapter 12), paying particular attention to the structure and properties of lipids and the central role of acetyl CoA in the metabolism of lipids. Chapter 29 begins with a discussion of the formation of triacylglycerols, phosphoglycerides, and sphingolipids from the simple precursors glycerol 3-phosphate, fatty acyl CoAs, and polar alcohols, for example, choline, inositol, and sugars. The text also emphasizes the importance of phosphatidic acid phosphatase and diacylglycerol kinase in the regulation of lipid synthesis. The text then describes the synthesis of cholesterol from acetyl CoA via the important intermediate isopentenyl pyrophosphate. The regulation of a key enzyme in the biosynthetic pathway as well as other modes of regulation of cholesterol metabolism are also outlined. The cholesterol and triacylglycerols synthesized in the liver and intestines are transported by lipoproteins to peripheral tissues. Cholesterol from dietary sources is also moved from the intestine to the liver by lipoproteins. Therefore, the classification, the properties, and the mechanisms by which the lipoproteins deliver lipids to cells are discussed next. A biochemically based strategy for controlling one form of abnormal cholesterol metabolism is also described. Finally, the authors describe the synthesis of bile salts, steroid hormones, and vitamin D from cholesterol.

LEARNING OBJECTIVES

When you have mastered this chapter, you should be able to accomplish the following objectives:

Introduction

1. Name the three major lipid-based components of biological membranes.
2. Explain the biological significance of *cholesterol*.
3. List the primary biological functions of *triacylglycerols* and *phospholipids*.

Phosphatidate Is a Precursor of Storage Lipids and Many Membrane Lipids
(Text Section 29.1)

4. Describe the roles of *phosphatidate, glycerol 3-phosphate, lysophosphatidate,* and *diacylglycerol (DAG)* in the synthesis of triacylglycerols and phospholipids and identify their sources.
5. Note the significance of *CDP-diacylglycerol* and *CDP-ethanolamine*, the activated precursors in the biosyntheses triacylglycerols and phospholipids.
6. Describe the biosyntheses of *phosphatidyl serine, phosphatidyl ethanolamine, phosphatidyl choline,* and *phosphatidyl inositol*.
7. Restate the physiologic roles of phosphatidyl inositol and its degradation products, *inositol 1,4,5-trisphosphate* and *diacylglycerol* (Chapter 13).
8. Summarize the steps in the biosynthesis of *sphingosine* from *palmitoyl CoA* and *serine*.
9. Outline the synthesis of *sphingomyelin, cerebrosides,* and *gangliosides* from sphingosine. Note the use of activated sugars and acidic sugars.
10. Provide examples of how sphingolipids confer diversity on lipid structure and function.
11. Discuss the general degradation pathway of gangliosides and the biochemical basis of *Tay-Sachs disease* and *respiratory distress syndrome*.
12. Discuss the proposed role of *phosphatidic acid phosphatase (PAP)* and *diacylglycerol kinase* in regulation of lipid synthesis, including the consequences of an abundance or lack of PAP function in mammals.

Cholesterol Is Synthesized from Acetyl Coenzyme A in Three Stages
(Text Section 29.2)

13. Describe the physiologic roles of *cholesterol*.
14. List the major stages in cholesterol biosynthesis and give the key intermediates. Recognize the structure of cholesterol.
15. Compare the synthetic paths leading from acetyl CoA to *mevalonate* and to the *ketone bodies* (Chapter 27). Note the role of *3-hydroxy-3-methylglutaryl CoA reductase (HMG CoA reductase)* as the major regulatory enzyme in cholesterol biosynthesis.
16. Describe the conversion of mevalonate into *isopentenyl pyrophosphate*.
17. Outline the condensation reactions leading from isopentenyl pyrophosphate to *squalene*. Describe the mechanisms of these condensation reactions.

18. Discuss the *cyclization* of squalene and the formation of cholesterol from *lanosterol*. Note the role of O2 in the formation of cholesterol.

The Regulation of Cholesterol Synthesis Takes Place at Several Levels
(Text Section 29.3)

19. List the sources of cholesterol and the locations of its synthesis in mammals.

20. List the four mechanisms of regulation of cholesterol biosynthesis through HMG CoA reductase.

21. Discuss how the rate of synthesis of HMG CoA reductase mRNA is controlled by SREBP, including the role of SCAP as a cholesterol sensor.

22. Describe the structural changes that occur in SCAP upon binding cholesterol that control its sub-cellular localization.

23. Give an explanation as to how HMG CoA reductase proteolysis is facilitated by the presence of sterols.

24. Compare the regulation of HMG CoA reductase through covalent modification with that of Acetyl CoA carboxylase (Chapter 28).

Lipoproteins Transport Cholesterol and Triacylglycerols Throughout the Organism (Text Section 29.4)

25. List the various classes of *lipoproteins* together with their lipid and protein components. Describe their lipid transport functions.

26. Discuss the diagnostic value of measuring serum levels of LDL and HDL. Explain the mechanism by which HDL protects against *arteriosclerosis*.

27. Summarize the steps in the delivery of cholesterol to cells *via the low-density-lipoprotein (LDL) receptor*. Discuss the regulation of cellular functions by the *LDL pathway*.

28. Describe the proposed domain structure of the LDL receptor derived from the primary sequence of this protein.

29. Discuss the biochemical defects of the LDL receptor that result in *familial hypercholesterolemia*.

30. Summarize approaches used to reduce *serum cholesterol*.

Cholesterol Is the Precursor of Steroid Hormones (Text Section 29.5)

31. Describe the physiologic roles and the general structures of the *bile salts*.

32. List the five major classes of *steroid hormones*, their physiologic functions, and their sites of synthesis. Outline their biosynthetic relationships.

33. Discuss the synthesis and the physiologic role of *vitamin D*. Explain the consequences of a deficiency in vitamin D.

34. Explain the side effects resulting from the use of *anabolic steroids*. Compare the structures of *androstendione* and *dianabol*.

35. Describe the *hydroxylation reactions* involving *cytochrome P450*. Indicate the role of these *monooxygenase reactions* in steroid biosynthesis and the metabolism of foreign substances, including ethanol.

SELF-TEST

Introduction

1. Which of the following are components of biological membranes?
   (a) free fatty acids
   (b) sphingolipids
   (c) triacylglycerols
   (d) phospholipids
   (e) cholesterol
   (f) proteins

Phosphatidate Is a Precursor of Storage Lipids and Many Membrane Lipids

2. Which of the following reactions are significant sources of glycerol 3-phosphate that is used in lipid synthesis?
   (a) reduction of dihydroxyacetone phosphate
   (b) oxidation of glyceraldehyde 3-phosphate
   (c) phosphorylation of glycerol
   (d) dephosphorylation of 1,3-bisphosphoglycerate
   (e) reductive phosphorylation of pyruvate

3. Match the lipids in the left column with the major synthetic precursors or intermediates in the right column.

   (a) triacylglycerol
   (b) phosphatidyl ethanolamine (mammals)

   (1) phosphatidate
   (2) diacylglycerol
   (3) acyl CoA
   (4) glycerol 3-phosphate
   (5) CDP-diacylglycerol
   (6) CDP-ethanolamine

4. Explain the role of the CDP derivatives in the synthesis of phosphoglycerides.

5. Calculate the number of "high-energy" phosphate bonds that are expended in the formation of phosphatidyl choline from diacylglycerol and choline in mammals.

6. Which of the following is a common reaction used for the formation of phosphatidyl ethanolamine?
   (a) decarboxylation of phosphatidyl serine
   (b) reaction of CDP-ethanolamine with a diacylglycerol
   (c) demethylation of phosphatidyl choline
   (d) reaction of ethanolamine with CDP-diacylglycerol
   (e) reaction of CDP-ethanolamine with CDP-diacylglycerol

7. Which of the following is a lipid with a signal-transducing activity?
   (a) phosphatidyl choline
   (b) phosphatidyl serine
   (c) plasminogen activator
   (d) phosphatidyl inositol 4,5-bisphosphate
   (e) phospholipase A_2

8. Which of the following structural components is found in glyceryl ester phospholipids?
   (a) two long hydrocarbon chains
   (b) acetyl group
   (c) phosphate group

(d) ether linkage
(e) α, β-double bond
(f) glycerol group
(g) long fatty acyl chain

9. Which of the following phospholipases would you expect to cleave the R_1-containing chain from the phospholipid shown in Figure 29.1?

(a) phospholipase A_1
(b) phospholipase A_2
(c) phospholipase C
(d) phospholipase D
(e) none of the above

FIGURE 29.1 A phospholipid.

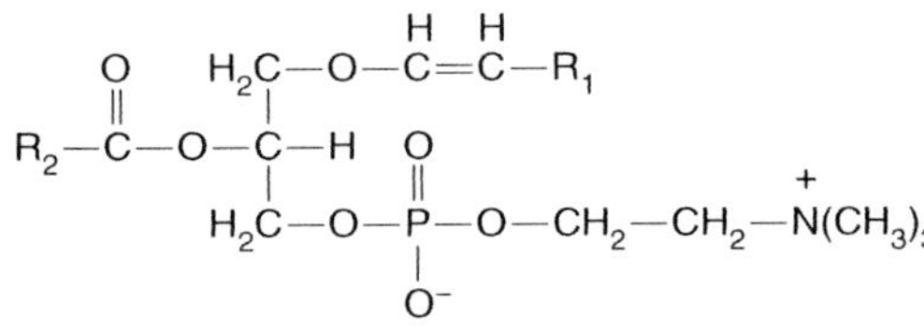

10. Which of the following is NOT a precursor or intermediate in the synthesis of sphingomyelin?

(a) palmitoyl CoA
(b) lysophosphatidate
(c) CDP-choline
(d) acyl CoA
(e) serine

11. Match the lipids in the left column with the appropriate activated precursors in the right column.

(a) sphingomyelin
(b) ganglioside
(c) phosphatidyl serine

(1) acyl CoA
(2) CDP-choline
(3) CDP-diacylglycerol
(4) CMP-N-acetylneuraminate
(5) UDP-sugar

12. In which compartment of the cell does ganglioside G_{M2} accumulate in Tay-Sachs patients? What is the biochemical defect?

13. When phosphatidic acid phosphatase (PAP) activity is high,

(a) phosphatidate is dephosphorylated.
(b) phosphatidylethanolamine, phosphatidylserine, and phosphatidylcholine are produced.
(c) phosphatidylinositol and cardiolin are produced.
(d) expression of genes in phospholipid synthesis is increased.
(e) obesity can result.

Cholesterol Is Synthesized from Acetyl Coenzyme A in Three Stages

14. From the following compounds, identify the intermediates in the synthesis of cholesterol and list them in their proper sequence.

(a) geranyl pyrophosphate
(b) squalene
(c) isopentenyl pyrophosphate
(d) mevalonate
(e) farnesyl pyrophosphate
(f) lanosterol

15. Which of the following are common features of the syntheses of mevalonate and ketone bodies?

    (a) Both involve 3-hydroxy-3-methylglutaryl CoA (HMG CoA).
    (b) Both require NADPH.
    (c) Both require the HMG CoA cleavage enzyme.
    (d) Both occur in the mitochondria.
    (e) Both occur in liver cells.

16. Select the appropriate characteristics in the right column for the three stages in the synthesis of cholesterol in the left column.

    (a) mevalonate to isopentenyl pyrophosphate   (1) releases PP_i
    (b) isopentenyl pyrophosphate to squalene   (2) requires NADPH
    (c) squalene to cholesterol   (3) requires O_2
       (4) releases CO_2
       (5) requires ATP

17. Yeast cells growing aerobically synthesize sterols and incorporate them into membranes. However, under anaerobic conditions, yeast cells do not survive unless they are provided with an exogenous source of sterols. Explain the metabolic basis for this nutritional requirement.

The Regulation of Cholesterol Synthesis Takes Place at Several Levels

18. The key step in cholesterol biosynthesis is the conversion of 3-hydroxy-3-methylglutaryl CoA to mevalonate. Which of the following are ways in which this reaction can be modulated?

    (a) covalent modification of HMG CoA reductase through phosphorylation
    (b) controlling the rate of translation of the mRNA encoding HMG CoA reductase
    (c) controlling the rate of transcription of the gene encoding HMG CoA reductase
    (d) proteolytic degradation of HMG CoA reductase
    (e) deletion and duplication of the gene encoding HMG CoA reductase

19. Which of the following is correct about SCAP and SREBP regulation of cholesterol biosynthesis?

    (a) SCAP and SREBP form a complex when cholesterol levels are high.
    (b) Binding of cholesterol to SREBP leads to nuclear translocation, where SREBP binds to an SRE on the 5' side of the HMG CoA reductase gene.
    (c) Proteases are used to release SREBP to the nucleus.
    (d) The cytoplasmic domain of SREBP is a nuclear transcription factor for HMG CoA reductase.

Lipoproteins Transport Cholesterol and Triacylglycerols Throughout the Organism

20. Match the appropriate components or properties in the right column with the lipoproteins in the left column.

    (a) chylomicron   (1) contains apoprotein B-100
    (b) VLDL   (2) contains apoprotein B-48
    (c) LDL   (3) contains apoprotein A
    (d) HDL   (4) transports endogenous cholesterol esters
       (5) transports dietary triacylglycerols

(6) transports endogenous triacylglycerols
(7) is degraded by lipoprotein lipase
(8) is taken up by cells via receptor-mediated mechanisms
(9) is a precursor of LDL
(10) may remove cholesterol from cells

21. Which of the following events occur in the LDL pathway in fibroblasts? Place them in their proper sequential order.

(a) breakdown of LDL in lysosomes
(b) endocytosis of LDL along with LDL receptors
(c) degradation of LDL receptors in lysosomes
(d) binding of LDL to LDL receptors
(e) return of LDL receptors to the plasma membrane

22. Exons in the gene for the LDL receptor give rise to structurally diverse domains. What is the likely function of the cysteine-rich amino-terminal domain?

(a) carbohydrate binding
(b) LDL Binding
(c) Ca^+ binding
(d) growth-factor binding
(e) clathrin binding
(f) structure stabilization

23. Explain how LDL regulates the cholesterol content in fibroblasts.

24. Assume that LDL is produced normally in a patient but that the apoprotein B-100 domain that recognizes the receptor is functionally defective, which prevents the binding of LDL to its receptor. What outcome would this defect have on cholesterol metabolism in peripheral cells?

Cholesterol Is the Precursor of Steroid Hormones

25. The physiologic roles of bile salts include which of the following?

(a) They aid in the digestion of lipids.
(b) They aid in the digestion of proteins.
(c) They facilitate the absorption of sugars.
(d) They facilitate the absorption of lipids.
(e) They provide a means for excreting cholesterol.

26. Which of the following are common features in the structures of cholesterol and glycocholate?

(a) Both have three hydroxyl groups.
(b) Both contain four fused rings.
(c) Both have a hydrocarbon side chain.
(d) Both contain a carboxylate group.
(e) Both contain double bonds.
(f) Both contain a sulfur atom.

27. Explain the structural characteristics of bile salts that make them effective biological detergents.

28. For the sterol structure in Figure 29.2, answer the questions that follow the figure.

FIGURE 29.2 A sterol.

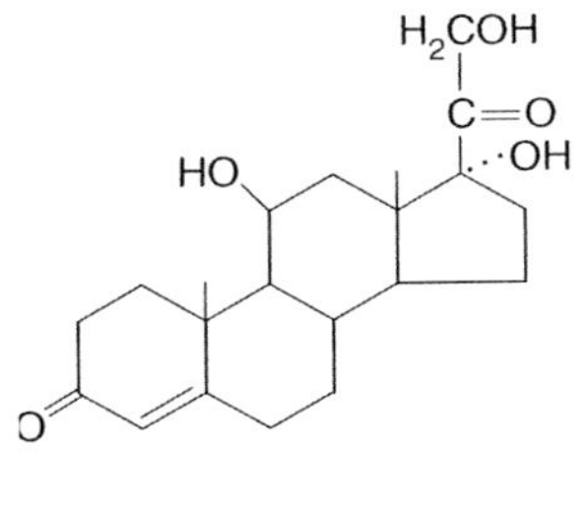

(a) Name the sterol.

(b) It is synthesized from what *via* three hydroxylation reactions?

(c) It has how many fewer carbon atoms than cholesterol?

(d) Its concentration will be diminished if there is a deficiency of 21-hydroxylase-true or false? Explain why.

29. Hydroxylation reactions involving cytochrome P450 have which of the following characteristics?

(a) They require a proton gradient.

(b) They involve electron transport from NADPH to O_2.

(c) They activate O_2 by binding it to adrenodoxin.

(d) They transfer one oxygen atom from O_2 to the substrate and form water from the other oxygen atom.

(e) They occur in adrenal mitochondria and liver microsomes.

30. Match the steroid hormones in the left column with the characteristics in the right column that distinguish them from one another.

(a) aldosterone	(1) has 18 carbon atoms
(b) estrogen	(2) has 19 carbon atoms
(c) testosterone	(3) has 21 carbon atoms
	(4) contains an aromatic ring
	(5) contains an aldehyde group at C-18

31. Which of the following statements about active vitamin D are NOT correct?

(a) It has the same fused ring system as cholesterol.

(b) It requires hydroxylation reactions for its synthesis from cholecalciferol.

(c) It is important in the control of calcium and phosphorus metabolism.

(d) It can be synthesized from cholesterol in the presence of UV light.

(e) It can be derived from the diet.

32. List the physiological consequences of a deficiency in Vitamin D.

ANSWERS TO SELF-TEST

1. b, d, e, f. Answers (a) and (c) are incorrect because neither neutral fats nor free fatty acids appear in membranes.

2. a, c. Reduction of dihydroxyacetone phosphate is the primary route.

3. (a) 1, 2, 3, 4 (b) 1, 2, 3, 4, 6. Phosphatidyl ethanolamine can also be formed through an exchange reaction of ethanolamine with phosphatidyl serine.

4. CDP-diacylglycerol and the CDP-alcohols are activated intermediates that allow the formation of phosphate ester bonds in phosphoglycerides, a process that is otherwise highly exergonic. ATP supplies the energy to form these compounds. Recall that UDP-sugars are used in a similar manner in the synthesis of carbohydrates (see pages 628–629 of the text).

5. Summing the individual reactions:

Choline + ATP $\rightarrow$ phosphorylcholine + ADP

Phosphorylcholine + CTP $\rightarrow$ CDP–choline + PP_i

CDP–choline + diacylglycerol $\rightarrow$ CMP + phosphatidyl choline

_____

Choline + ATP + CTP + diacylglycerol $\rightarrow$ ADP + PP_i + CMP + phosphatidyl choline

Two high-energy bonds (from ATP and CTP) are directly consumed in these reactions. In addition, pyrophosphate is hydrolyzed by pyrophosphatase, driving the net reaction farther to the right. A total of three high-energy bonds would be consumed to regenerate ATP and CTP from ADP and CMP.

6. b

7. d

8. a, c, f, g

9. e. Phospholipases are specific for *ester* bonds; therefore, none will cleave the *ether* bond on the C-1 carbon of this plasmalogen phospholipid. Phospholipases A_2, C, and D cleave specific ester linkages: A_2 cleaves the R_2-containing chain to release the fatty acid, C cleaves the phophodiester bond to produce the choline (R_3) -phosphate, and D cleaves the phosphodiester bond to produce the R_3-alcohol. If the phospholipid had been a glycerol ester phospholipid, *e.g.*, phosphatidyl ethanolamine, phospholipase A_1 would have cleaved the ester bond to yield the R_1-contining fatty acid. Phospholipase C hydrolyzes phosphatidyl inositol 4, 5-bisphosphate to produce inositol 1, 4, 5,-trisphosphate and diacylglycerol, which are intracellular second messengers (Chapter 14).

10. b

11. (a) 1, 2   (b) 1, 4, 5   (c) 1, 3

12. The degradative enzymes for gangliosides are located in lysosomes; therefore, ganglioside G_{M2} will accumulate in the lysosomes of Tay-Sachs patients. The enzyme, a specific β-N-acetylhexosaminidase that removes the terminal sugar GalNAc from the ganglioside is deficient in these people.

13. a, b, and e.

14. The proper sequence is d, c, a, f, b, g.

15. a, e

16. (a) 4, 5   (b) 1, 2   (c) 2, 3

17. A key intermediate in the biosynthesis of cholesterol and related sterols is squalene, an open-chain isoprenoid hydrocarbon. It is converted to squalene 2,3-epoxide, which in turn is converted to lanosterol. The conversion of squalene to the 2,3-epoxide is catalyzed by a monooxygenase, and molecular oxygen is a required component for this reaction. Under anaerobic conditions, yeast cells cannot synthesize sterols because they lack oxygen, a substrate for the monooxygenase reaction.

18. a, b, c, d

19. c, d

20. (a) 2, 5, 7   (b) 1, 6, 7, 9   (c) 1, 4, 8   (d) 3, 4, 10

21. All the events except (c) occur in the LDL pathway. The proper sequence is d, b, a, e.

22. c

23. The main source of cholesterol for cells outside the liver and intestine is from circulating LDL. Cholesterol released during the degradation of LDL suppresses the formation of new LDL receptors, thereby decreasing the uptake of exogenous cholesterol by the cell.

24. A defect in apoprotein B-100 that prevents the binding of LDL to the cell-surface receptor would result in the stimulation of the synthesis of endogenous cholesterol and LDL receptors and a decrease in the synthesis of cholesterol esters via the ACAT reaction. Indeed, the cellular and physiologic consequences of such a mutation may be similar to those seen in familial hypercholesterolemia.

25. a, d, e

26. b, e

27. Bile salts are effective detergents because they contain both polar and nonpolar regions. They have several hydroxyl groups, all on one side of the ring system, and a polar side chain that allow interactions with water. The ring system itself is nonpolar and can interact with lipids or other nonpolar substances. Bile salts are planar, amphipathic molecules, in contrast with such detergents as sodium dodecyl sulfate (see page 72 of the text), which are linear.

28. (a) cortisol
    (b) progesterone
    (c) six
    (d) true. A deficiency of 21-hydroxylase will impair hydroxylation at C-21 of progesterone, which will prevent the normal synthesis of cortisol and mineralocorticoids from progesterone.

29. b, d, e

30. (a) 3, 5   (b) 1, 4   (c) 2

31. a

32. The most well-known consequence of a lack of vitamin D in childhood is the disease rickets, which results in inadequate calcification of cartilage and bone. In adults a deficiency can lead to bone softening and weaking called osteomalacia. New research suggests that a lack of vitamin D can impead muscle performance, play a role in cardiovascular disease, and increase risk of developing cancer and some autoimmune diseases.

PROBLEMS

1. An infant has an enlarged liver and spleen, cataracts, and anemia and exhibits general retardation of development. Mevalonate is found in the urine. Investigation reveals a deficiency of mevalonate kinase, which catalyzes the formation of 5-phosphomevalonate from mevalonate.
   (a) Why is urinary excretion of mevalonate consistent with a deficiency of mevalonate kinase?
   (b) How would a deficiency of mevalonate kinase affect cholesterol synthesis in this infant?
   (c) What level of HMG CoA reductase activity, relative to normal, would you expect to find in cells isolated from the infant? Briefly explain your answer.

2. Normally, most of the bile acids that are secreted into the intestine undergo reabsorption and are returned to the liver. Cholestyramine is a positively charged resin that binds bile acids in the intestinal lumen and prevents their reabsorption.
   (a) To examine the effects of cholestyramine on LDL metabolism, two fractions of LDL were prepared: one was covalently labeled on tyrosine residues with ^{125}I; the other was labeled with ^{131}I and treated with cyclohexanedione, which interferes with LDL binding to the LDL receptor. When rabbits were given cholestyramine, hepatic uptake of ^{125}I-labeled LDL was enhanced relative to normal, whereas the uptake of ^{131}I-labeled LDL was unchanged relative to that in rabbits that had not been given cholestyramine. Briefly explain the relationship between the action of cholestyramine and LDL uptake in the liver.

(b) The administration of cholestyramine usually results in a 15 to 20% reduction in levels of circulating LDL, whereas the administration of a combination of cholestyramine and mevacor (lovastatin) can often yield a 30 to 40% reduction. Why?

3. The presence of apoprotein E in lipoproteins enables them to be taken up by hepatic cells. Provide a brief explanation for each of the following observations made of a person with a deficiency in apoprotein E synthesis.

(a) elevated levels of plasma triacylglycerols and cholesterol, coupled with the presence of chylomicron remnants and IDL. The latter particles persist in the bloodstream much longer than in normal people
(b) abnormally low levels of LDL in the blood
(c) abnormally high levels of LDL receptors in liver cells
(d) a marked reduction in levels of circulating chylomicron remnants and IDL when the diet is low in cholesterol and fat

4. Pregnant women often have increased rates of triacylglycerol breakdown and, as a result, have elevated levels of ketone bodies in their blood. Why do they also often exhibit an increase in plasma lipoprotein levels?

5. Hopanoids are pentacyclic molecules that are found in bacteria and in some plants. As an example, a typical bacterial hopinoid is shown below. Organisms that make hopanoids use a pathway similar to that for cholesterol synthesis. The biosynthetic pathway for hopane includes the formation of squalene, followed by more steps to form the final product itself, a C30 compound. Hopane is similar to lanosterol (page 506 of the text), but it lacks the hydroxyl group.

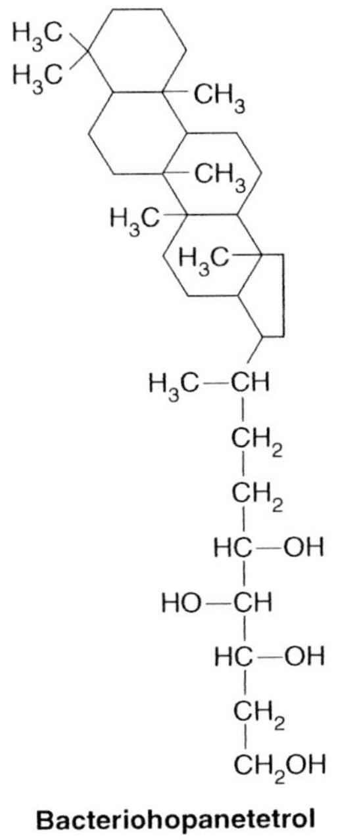

Bacteriohopanetetrol

(a) How many molecules of mevalonic acid are required for the synthesis of hopane?
(b) Squalene can undergo concerted cyclization to form hopane in a reaction that is catalyzed by a unique type of squalene cyclase. The reaction is initiated by a proton and does not require oxygen. Compare this step with the formation of lanosterol from squalene. Why could it be argued that the synthesis of hopanoids preceded the synthesis of sterols in evolution?

6. Your colleague has discovered a compound that is a very powerful inhibitor of HMG CoA reductase, and she has evidence that the drug will completely block the synthesis of mevalonate in liver. Why is this compound unlikely to be useful as a drug?

7. The liver is the site of the synthesis of plasma phospholipids and lipoproteins. Rats maintained on a diet deficient in choline often develop fat deposits in liver tissue. How could choline deficiency be related to this aberration in lipid metabolism?

8. Among the sugar residues found in a blood group ganglioside is fucose. Experiments utilizing isolated Golgi membranes and ribonucleoside triphosphates show that fucose can be incorporated into the ganglioside only when GTP is available. What is the role of GTP in fucose incorporation?

9. Suppose a cell is deficient in phosphatidate phosphatase, which catalyzes the formation of diacylglycerol from phosphatidate. What effects on lipid metabolism would you expect?

10. In the adult form of Gaucher's disease, glucosylcerebrosides accumulate in liver, spleen, and bone-marrow cells. Although the common galactosylceramides and their derivatives are found in the tissues of affected patients, accumulations of galactosylcerebrosides or their metabolites are not found, nor do ceramides accumulate. What enzyme activity is probably deficient in patients with Gaucher's disease?

11. Cells of the adrenal cortex have very high concentrations of LDL receptors. Why?

12. At low concentrations of phospholipid substrates in water, the reaction catalyzed by a phospholipase occurs at a rather low rate. The reaction rate accelerates when the concentrations of the phospholipid substrates increase to the point that micelles are formed. How is this property of phospholipases related to their activity in the cell?

13. Glucagon has been shown to reduce the activity of HMG CoA reductase. Why is this observation consistent with the overall effect of glucagon on cellular metabolism?

14. People who have elevated levels of low-density lipoproteins (LDL) in their serum can be treated in a number of ways. These include restriction of dietary intake of cholesterol, ingestion of positively charged resin polymers that inhibit intestinal reabsorption of bile salts, and administration of lovastatin, a competitive inhibitor of 3-hydroxy-3-methylglutaryl CoA reductase.

    (a) Briefly explain how each of these treatments reduces serum LDL levels.
    (b) Why should none of these treatments be used for patients who are homozygous for a defect in LDL receptors?

15. Currently there are two established methods for dealing with hypercholesterolemia in patients homozygous for LDL receptor deficiency.

    (a) The first is plasma apheresis, whereby the plasma and blood cells of a patient are separated in a continuous flow device, and the plasma is passed over a column that removes lipoproteins containing apoprotein B-100. Which lipoproteins are removed by this procedure, and how could their removal lower plasma cholesterol levels?
    (b) A more extreme method of dealing with extreme hypercholesterolemia in FH homozygotes is liver transplantation. The rationale for this procedure is based on the observation that over 70% of total body LDL receptors are in the liver. In the small group of patients who have undergone liver transplants, LDL cholesterol levels are substantially reduced. In one particular case, the rate of LDL turnover increased about threefold, and one patient became responsive to lovastatin after the transplant. Why did increased LDL turnover and lovastatin response indicate that the transplantation procedure was successful?

16. Provide a physiologic rationale for each of the following responses to an increase in the rate of transport of unesterified cholesterol into a mammalian cell:
    (a) stimulation of the synthesis of cholesteryl oleate esters
    (b) suppression of the activity of HMG CoA reductase
    (c) suppression of the synthesis of LDL receptors

17. Glycerol phosphate acyltransferase can convert 3,4-dihydroxybutyl-1-phosphonate, an analog of glycerol 3-phosphate, to diacylbutyl-1-phosphonate, which is an analog of phosphatidate. Would this analog be more likely to inhibit triglyceride synthesis or CDP-diacylglycerol synthesis? Briefly explain your answer.

$$H_2C-OH$$
$$HO-C-H$$
$$CH_2-CH_2-\overset{O}{\underset{O^-}{\overset{\|}{P}}}-O^-$$

3, 4-Dihydroxybutyl-1-phosphonate

18. During the uptake of low-density lipoprotein (LDL) by a liver cell, LDL-receptor protein complexes are internalized by endocytosis. The endosomes then fuse with lysosomes, where protein components of LDL are hydrolyzed to free amino acids, while cholesterol esters are hydrolyzed by a lysosomal acid lipase. The LDL receptor itself is not affected by lysosomal enzymes.
    (a) Briefly describe what would happen to cholesterol metabolism in a cell deficient in lysosomal acid lipase.
    (b) Why is it important that LDL receptors are not degraded by lysosomal enzymes?

19. Glycerol kinase catalyzes the conversion of free glycerol into glycerol 3-phosphate, using ATP as a phosphoryl donor. Although liver tissue has high levels of the enzyme, the activity of glycerol kinase in adipose tissue is low. How do these differences contribute to the balance between carbohydrate and triglyceride metabolism in mammals?

20. Niemann-Pick disease is an inherited disorder of sphingomyelin breakdown due to a deficiency of sphingomyelinase. This enzyme, found in all tissues and easily assayed in white blood cells collected from a patient, converts sphingomyelin to ceramide and phosphocholine. Phosphocholine is highly soluble in water, while sphingomyelin is more soluble in chloroform. Assuming that you can obtain sphingomyelin labeled with 14C in any desired carbon atoms, design an assay that would allow you to confirm a diagnosis of Niemann-Pick disease.

21. Chronic alcoholics derive a significant fraction of their calories from the metabolism of ethanol in the liver, the first step of which is its reaction with NAD^+ to form acetaldehyde and $NADH + H^+$—a reaction catalyzed by liver alcohol dehydrogenase. The acetaldehyde is itself oxidized to acetate in a reaction by an NAD^+-dependent acetaldehyde dehydrogenase that produces more NADH. Thus, excessive metabolism of ethanol leads to a marked increase in the $NADH/ NAD^+$ ratio. Relate this fact to the development of "fatty" liver (droplets of triacylglycerol are deposited in the liver) in alcoholics.

ANSWERS TO PROBLEMS

1. (a) A deficiency of mevalonate kinase activity means that mevalonate cannot be used as a precursor of 5-phosphomevalonate. If no other pathways can use mevalonate, its concentration in the liver will increase until it spills into the blood and

then, in turn, into the urine. Furthermore, because the activity of HMG CoA reductase is increased in this infant (see answer c), the rate of mevalonate synthesis will be stimulated.

(b) You would expect the rate of cholesterol synthesis to be depressed because the pathway is blocked at the step in which 5-phosphomevalonate is formed.

(c) You would expect to find a higher-than-normal level of HMG CoA reductase activity. A depressed rate of cholesterol synthesis lowers the amount of cholesterol in the cell. HMG CoA reductase activity increases because cholesterol reduces both its synthesis and its activity.

2. (a) The experiments show that rabbits given cholestyramine have higher rates of removal of LDL from the blood and that hepatic uptake of LDL depends on the ability of the lipoprotein to bind to the LDL receptor. One explanation for this is that cholestyramine interferes with the return of bile acids to the liver, stimulating the synthesis of more bile acids from cholesterol. An increased demand for cholesterol stimulates the synthesis of LDL receptors, which take up more cholesterol-containing LDL particles from the blood.

(b) Cholestyramine stimulates the hepatic uptake of cholesterol-containing LDL, but it has no direct effect on cholesterol synthesis de novo in the liver. Mevacor inhibits HMG CoA reductase, thereby depressing the rate of cholesterol biosynthesis. The subsequent requirement for cholesterol leads to a further increase in the number of LDL receptors, which in turn can take up more LDL from the circulation.

3. (a) Chylomicrons, chylomicron remnants, and IDL normally contain apoprotein E. A deficiency of the apoprotein means that hepatic uptake of chylomicron remnants and IDL is impaired, so these particles persist in the circulation. Because both these types of particles contain triacylglycerols and cholesterol, circulating levels of these compounds are also elevated.

(b) Both chylomicron remnants and IDL particles serve as precursors of VLDL in the liver. When the uptake of the VLDL precursors by hepatic tissue is impaired by an apoprotein E deficiency, the rate of synthesis and export of VLDL particles is reduced. Since VLDL are LDL precursors in circulation, LDL are reduced.

(c) As discussed in answer (b), VLDL synthesis in the liver is impaired. Additional LDL receptors are synthesized because their synthesis is no longer repressed by VLDL-derived cholesterol.

(d) A diet low in cholesterol and fat will reduce the rate of formation of chylomicrons, which are precursors of chylomicron remnants.

4. Increased levels of ketone bodies, such as acetoacetate, imply that the levels of acetyl CoA and HMG CoA, both precursors of cholesterol, are also elevated. Cholesterol synthesis is stimulated by an increase in the availability of these substrates. The subsequent decreased demand for dietary cholesterol results in an elevation in cholesterol-containing lipoproteins.

5. (a) Mevalonic acid, a six-carbon compound, is a precursor of isopentenyl pyrophosphate (IPP), which contains five carbon atoms. IPP serves as the basic unit for the formation of squalene, a 30-carbon compound. Six molecules of IPP are needed for the synthesis of a molecule of squalene, which is in turn the precursor of hopane. Thus, six molecules of mevalonic acid are required.

(b) Aerobic processes, such as the synthesis of sterols, probably evolved later than anaerobic processes and only after free oxygen became available. Thus, the synthesis of hopane from squalene, an anaerobic process, probably preceded the synthesis of sterols, such as lanosterol, from squalene.

6. The synthesis of mevalonate is required not only for the synthesis of cholesterol but also for the synthesis of a number of other important compounds derived from isopentenyl pyrophosphate, including ubiquinone (CoQ), an important component of the electron transport chain. Therefore, the complete blockage of mevalonate synthesis, even if adequate cholesterol is available in the diet, would be ill-advised.

7. Choline, which is ordinarily supplied by the diet and is synthesized only to a limited extent in mammals, is a constituent of phosphatidyl choline, an important component of membranes and lipoproteins. A deficiency in dietary choline, which could not be completely replaced by the endogenous methylation of phospatidyl ethanolamine, could interfere with the synthesis and export of lipoproteins like VLDL, which is a carrier of triacylglycerols to peripheral tissues. Failure to export fats such as triacylglycerols leads to their accumulation in the liver.

8. Nucleotide sugars, such as UDP-glucose, serve as donors during the incorporation of sugar residues into gangliosides. In this case, it appears that the donor of fucose residues is GDP-fucose, which is synthesized from fucose and GTP.

9. You would expect to see reduced rates of synthesis of triacylglycerols, which use diacylglycerols as acceptors of activated acyl groups. In addition, phosphatidyl choline synthesis is dependent on the availability of diacylglycerols as acceptors of choline phosphate from CDP-choline.

10. Because glucosylcerebrosides accumulate but galactosylcerebrosides do not, you would suspect that the defect involves ganglioside breakdown rather than ganglioside synthesis. The defect involves the step that removes glucose from the cerebroside to yield free ceramide, or N-acyl sphingosine. The enzyme that carries out this step is a glycosyl hydrolase; it is also called *β-glucosidase*.

11. Cells of the adrenal cortex utilize cholesterol for the synthesis of a number of steroid hormones, including cortisol. Although these cells can themselves synthesize cholesterol, it is often also necessary for additional cholesterol to be obtained from plasma lipoproteins. A high concentration of LDL receptors enables cortical cells to take up LDL, which contains cholesterol, rapidly.

12. In the cell, a phospholipase would most often encounter substrates that are part of an aggregate, such as those phospholipids found in membranes. Thus, the enzyme should be expected to function at a higher rate with aggregates or assemblies of lipid molecules because their local concentrations would be higher than if they were individually free in solution.

13. The presence of glucagon is a signal that carbohydrate and triacylglycerol catabolism is needed to generate energy in the organism. Under such conditions, one would expect biosynthetic reactions to be suppressed because energy charge is low. Low energy charge means high AMP levels that would activate an AMP-dependent protein kinase leading to the phosphorylation of HMG CoA reductase.

14. (a) Restricting the level of dietary cholesterol lowers the input of exogenous cholesterol into lipoproteins, so fewer LDL molecules are present in serum. Compounds that inhibit bile salt reabsorption from the gut stimulate additional synthesis of bile acids from cholesterol in the liver, decreasing concentrations of the sterol in liver cells and, by causing an increase in the number of receptors on the cell surface, stimulating LDL uptake from the circulation. Finally, mevacor reduces the rate of cholesterol biosynthesis de novo, which can also stimulate uptake of LDL

from the bloodstream. Any of these treatments could help in reducing circulating levels of cholesterol as LDL.

(b) Homozygotes have virtually no functional LDL receptors. Such people are unable to internalize significant amounts of LDL, which means that circulating levels of that lipoprotein are elevated in the blood. In addition, an absence of LDL receptors means that endogenous cholesterol fails to enter the liver cell to suppress de novo synthesis. Dietary restriction could reduce exogenous LDL levels somewhat but would not prevent formation of LDL and other lipoproteins arising from cell turnover of cholesterol. Sequestrants of bile salts could cause some depletion of liver cell cholesterol but again would not stimulate LDL uptake from the circulation. Mevacor will suppress cholesterol synthesis de novo, but this suppression would again not be compensated for by uptake from the circulation. Homozygotes with two nonfunctional receptor genes are therefore resistant to compounds that inhibit LDL synthesis and stimulate uptake. Thus, none of these measures has a great effect on reducing circulating LDL levels in these patients.

15. (a) Protein B-100 is found in VLDL, IDL, and LDL, and all three lipoproteins are removed from the plasma. Each contains cholesterol, and, in addition, VLDL and IDL are regarded as precursors of LDL, so that total cholesterol concentration in the blood would be lowered by apheresis. This method can reduce LDL cholesterol levels by 70%. Treatment must be repeated about every two weeks, and the effects of long-term apheresis are problematic.

(b) Increased LDL turnover indicates that the transplanted liver is producing normal LDL receptors that can take up LDL from the circulation and can facilitate its conversion to other lipoproteins. A response to lovastatin also indicates that functional LDL receptors are available to accelerate uptake in response to diminished de novo cholesterol synthesis, which is inhibited by lovastatin. It should be noted that liver transplant operations are hazardous, especially in FH homozygotes who usually have advanced atherosclerosis. The capability of normal liver cells to contribute functional LDL receptors has stimulated interest in gene therapy designed to target a normal LDL gene to liver cells of FH homozygotes.

16. (a) Formation of cholesteryl esters provides the cell with a means of storing cholesterol until it is needed for membrane biosynthesis or other purposes.

(b) Suppression of the activity of HMG CoA reductase leads to a decrease in cholesterol synthesis de novo, which occurs when the cell has sufficient endogenous cholesterol to not need to synthesize the steroid on its own.

(c) Suppression of LDL receptor synthesis leads to a gradual reduction in the number of LDL receptors in the cell because the receptors undergo a relatively constant rate of degradation. Reduction in LDL receptor levels means that fewer LDL particles will be able to enter the cell, resulting in a decrease in the entry of endogenous cholesterol.

17. The conversion of phosphatidate to a triacylglycerol is initiated by hydrolysis of the phosphate group and the formation of diacylglycerol. The C—P bond in the phosphonate cannot be cleaved by the phosphatase (also known as *phosphatidate phosphohydrolase*), so it is likely that triglyceride synthesis could be impaired by the analog. On the other hand, formation of CDP-diacylglycerol involves the formation of an anhydride bond between the phosphates of phosphatidic acid and cytidylic acid (see page 761 of the text). Since the phosphonate is not cleaved in this reaction, formation of the phosphonyl analog of CDP-diacylglycerol seems possible even if at a much slower rate, or at least the synthesis of normal substrates would not be impaired. Phosphonolipids are

known in trace amounts in mammals but are found more extensively in some invertebrates, including the protozoan *Tetrahymena*, where they may represent up to 25% of total phospholipid (see D. E. Vance and J. Vance [eds.], *Biochemistry of Lipids, Lipoproteins and Membranes.* Elsevier, 1991, p. 205).

18. (a) Both the LDL receptor gene and the gene for HMG CoA reductase contain sterol regulatory elements that are responsive to free cholesterol. A reduction in free cholesterol release from the lysosome leads to an increase in LDL receptor production and to increased HMG CoA reductase activity. Both these consequences lead to an increase in cholesterol concentrations in the cell through an increased rate of LDL entry and accelerated cholesterol synthesis. Lysosomal accumulation of cholesteryl esters and triglycerides can eventually destroy the cell. One form of this disorder, termed *Wolman disease*, is characterized by liver enlargement, digestive difficulties, and enlargement and deterioration of the adrenal glands. The disease is usually fatal within a year after birth.

    (b) LDL receptors, after their release from lysosomes, return to the cell surface, where they take up other LDL particles and bring them back to lysosomes. A round trip takes about 10 minutes. Destruction of LDL receptors by lysosomal enzymes would make it necessary to synthesize the 115-kd glycoprotein at a much faster and energetically wasteful rate.

19. Free glycerol in mammals is produced in adipocytes when triglycerides are converted to free fatty acids and glycerol by hormone-sensitive lipases. Hormone-responsive lipolysis occurs when glucose levels are low and fatty acids are needed as fuels. Under these conditions, the low activity of glycerol kinase in adipocytes prevents unnecessary resynthesis of triacylglycerols from free fatty acids and glycerol 3-phosphate via phosphatidic acid. Triacylglycerol synthesis is more likely to occur when glucose levels are high. Adipocytes can then synthesize glycerol 3-phosphate from dihydroxyacetone phosphate produced from glucose during glycolysis. Thus, adipocytes are unable to synthesize triglycerides unless glucose or another suitable carbon source is available.

20. Extracts of white cells from the blood of a person suspected of having a sphingomyelinase deficiency are incubated in a buffered solution with radioactive sphingomyelin labeled with ^{14}C in the methyl groups of the phosphocholine moiety. Then the incubation mixture is extracted with chloroform. Any radioactive phosphocholine liberated by the enzyme will remain in the upper aqueous layer while intact radioactive sphingomyelin will be extracted into the lower chloroform layer. Using white cells from patients with Neimann-Pick disease, incubation with cell extracts followed by chloroform extraction results in little or no radioactivity in the aqueous phase, confirming the deficiency of sphingomyelinase activity.

21. As stated, the metabolism of ethanol leads to a more reduced state in the hepatocyte; that is, the ratio of NADH to NAD^+ is increased. Increased NADH levels lead to inhibition of fatty acid oxidation (NADH is a product of fatty acid oxidation) and signal the capacity for biosynthesis requiring reducing equivalents. Decreased fatty acid oxidation leads to the accumulation of triacylglycerols. In addition, the increased levels of acetate and NADH promote the synthesis of fatty acids and subsequently triacylglycerol to exacerbate the problem. The excess triacylglycerols coalesce into droplets in the fatty liver.

Amino Acid Degradation and the Urea Cycle

Organisms derive energy from both stored and exogenous fuels. The catabolism of carbohydrates (Chapter 16 and 17) and fats (Chapter 27 and 28) have been discussed in previous chapters. In Chapter 30, the authors explain the role of proteins in energy metabolism. Although proteins are not stored as fuels per se as carbohydrates and fats are, supplies of proteins in excess of those needed to provide biosynthetic precursors are degraded for energy or are converted into fats or carbohydrates. Most of the amino groups of excess amino acids are converted into urea through the urea cycle, whereas their carbon skeletons are transformed into acetyl CoA, pyruvate, or one of the citric acid cycle intermediates.

The authors first discuss how dietary proteins are degraded. Once a protein is cleaved into individual amino acids, the amino acids are either incorporated into newly synthesized proteins or degraded to specific compounds for entry into an energy transduction pathway. If entry into an energy transduction pathway is its fate, the nitrogen(s) must first be removed. The α-amino groups of most amino acids are transferred to α-ketoglutarate to form glutamate by transamination (catalyzed by aminotransferases), and the α-amino group of glutamate is then converted to ammonia by an oxidative deamination. The authors then describe the glucose-alanine cycle in which nitrogen is transported from peripheral tissues to the liver. The urea cycle is introduced next, which carries out the condensation of ammonia, the α-amino group of aspartate, and CO_2 to form urea—a nontoxic excretory product of nitrogen in higher animals. The urea cycle is linked to the citric acid cycle (Chapter 18 and 19) due to its production of the citric acid cycle intermediate fumarate. The physiological effects of defects in the urea cycle are also explored.

Because there are 20 amino acids, the catabolic pathways of their carbon skeletons are numerous and of varied types. The authors describe how the carbon atoms of each amino acid are funneled into one or more of seven primary products. Two of these, acetyl CoA and acetoacetyl CoA, can be converted to ketone bodies (Chapter 27), and the remaining five can be converted into glucose (Chapter 17), all of which can be oxidized in energy-generating pathways. The two groups of products lead to the glycogenic-ketogenic classification of the amino acids. The chapter ends emphasizing the importance of carrying out amino acid catabolism by examining the pathological consequences of defects or deficiencies in some of the enzymes involved in catabolism of amino acids and the synthesis of urea.

LEARNING OBJECTIVES

When you have mastered this chapter, you should be able to accomplish the following objectives.

INTRODUCTION

1. State the fate of exogenously supplied amino acids that are not used for biosynthesis.

Nitrogen Removal Is the First Step In the Degradation of Amino Acids
(Text Section 30.1)

2. Name the major organ responsible for *amino acid degradation* in mammals.

3. Describe the reactions catalyzed by the *aminotransferases (transaminases)* and state the major function of these reactions.

4. Write the equations for the transamination reactions catalyzed by *aspartate aminotransferase* and *alanine aminotransferase*.

5. Describe the reaction catalyzed by *glutamate dehydrogenase*, outline its regulation, and state its major function. Note that the participation of NAD^+ in the reaction links nitrogen metabolism and energy generation.

6. Explain how the α-amino groups of serine and threonine can be directly converted into NH_4^+.

7. Describe the transport of nitrogen from muscle to liver.

Ammonium Ion Is Converted into Urea in Most Terrestrial Vertebrates
(Text Section 30.2)

8. Define the terms *ureotelic*, *uricotelic*, and *ammonotelic*.

9. Name the molecule that brings nitrogen and carbon into the *urea cycle*.

10 Describe the caramoyl phosphate synthetase reaction. Account for the ATP requirement of the urea cycle.

11. Name the enzymes of the urea cycle, note their intracellular locations, and indicate the molecular connection between this cycle and the citric acid cycle. Recognize the reaction catalyzed by each enzyme.

12. Explain how deficiencies in several different enzymes of the urea cycle give rise to *hyperammonemia* and outline strategies for coping with deficiencies in urea synthesis.

13. Discuss the disposal of nitrogen in hibernating bears.

Carbon Atoms of Degraded Amino Acids Emerge as Major Metabolic Intermediates (Text Section 30.3)

14. State the strategy used by humans for catabolizing the carbon atom skeletons of amino acids and name the seven major metabolic products formed.

15. Describe the basis for the *glycogenic-ketogenic* designation of the amino acids and classify each amino acid accordingly. Appreciate the limitations of this classification.

16. List the amino acids that give rise to *pyruvate, oxaloacetate, fumarate, succinyl CoA, acetyl CoA,* and *acetoacetyl CoA* respectively.

17. List the amino acids that give rise to α-*ketoglutarate.*

18. Describe the role of *tetrahydrobioprotein* and *S-adenosylmethionine* in amino acid degredation.

19. Explain the biochemical bases of *phenylketonuria* and *maple syrup urine disease.* Describe some of the consequences of these diseases and other diseases of amino acid metabolism.

SELF-TEST

Introduction

1. Which of the following answers complete the sentence correctly? Surplus dietary amino acids may be converted into

   (a) proteins.
   (b) fats.
   (c) ketone bodies.
   (d) glucose.
   (e) a variety of biomolecules for which they are precursors.

Nitrogen Removal Is the First Step In the Degradation of Amino Acids

2. Which of the following compounds serves as an acceptor for the amino groups of many amino acids during catabolism?

   (a) glutamine   (c) α-ketoglutarate
   (b) asparagine   (d) oxalate

3. Which of the following answers completes the sentence correctly? The removal of α-amino groups from amino acids for conversion to urea in animals may occur by

   (a) transamination.   (c) oxidative deamination.
   (b) reductive deamination.   (d) transamidation.

4. From which of the following amino acids are α-amino groups removed by dehydratases?

   (a) histidine   (d) glutamine
   (b) tryptophan   (e) threonine
   (c) serine

5. Which of the following answers completes the sentence correctly? The products of an aminotransferase-catalyzed reaction between pyruvate and glutamate would be

   (a) aspartate and oxaloacetate.
   (b) aspartate and α-ketoglutarate.
   (c) alanine and oxaloacetate.
   (d) alanine and α-ketoglutarate.

6. Choose from the list below molecules that transport nitrogen from the muscle to the liver. Place them in the correct order of their occurrence in the transport chain.

   Alanine, Glucose, Glutamate, Glutamine, Isoleucine, Leucine, Pyruvate, Urea, Valine

Ammonium Ion Is Converted into Urea in Most Terrestrial Vertebrates

7. Considering all forms of life, which of the following are major excretory forms of the α-amino groups of amino acids?

   (a) urea   (c) ammonia
   (b) uracil   (d) uric acid

8. How many moles of ATP are required to condense two moles of nitrogen and one mole of CO_2 into one mole of urea via the urea cycle? How many high-energy bonds are used in this process? Do both atoms of nitrogen enter the cycle as NH_4^+?

9. What would be the net effect of linking the following two transamination reactions, and why would such coupling be useful when excess proteins were being catabolized for energy generation?

   Alanine + α-ketoglutarate → pyruvate + glutamate
   Oxaloacetate + glutamate → aspartate + α-ketoglutarate

10. Describe the role of ornithine in the urea cycle.

11. Explain how hyperammonemia, the increased concentration of NH_4^+ in the serum, can arise from defects in more than one enzyme of the pathway that forms urea.

12. How do hibernating bears dispose of urea?

Carbon Atoms of Degraded Amino Acids Emerge as Major Metabolic Intermediates

13. Match the catabolic products in the right column with the amino acids in the left column from which they can be derived.

    (a) alanine   (1) succinyl CoA
    (b) aspartate   (2) acetoacetate
    (c) glutamine   (3) α-ketoglutarate
    (d) phenylalanine   (4) oxaloacetate
    (e) leucine   (5) pyruvate
    (f) valine   (6) acetyl CoA
                             (7) fumarate

14. Classify the following amino acids as glycogenic (G), ketogenic (K), or both (GK).

    (a) leucine   (e) histidine
    (b) alanine   (f) isoleucine
    (c) tyrosine   (g) aspartate
    (d) serine   (h) phenylalanine

15. What common feature is shared by the catabolism of fatty acids having an odd number of carbon atoms and the catabolism of the amino acids isoleucine, methionine, and valine?

16. Catabolism of which of the following amino acids requires the direct involvement of O_2?

   (a) histidine
   (b) phenylalanine
   (c) tyrosine
   (d) isoleucine
   (e) glutamine

17. For each of the following types of chemical reactions, list one enzyme in an amino acid degragative pathway that catalyzes that type of reaction.

   (a) dehydration
   (b) oxidative deamination
   (c) transamination
   (d) hydroxylation
   (e) hydrolysis
   (f) oxidative decarboxylation

18. Which of the following statements is true of the metabolic disease phenylketonuria?

   (a) The disease is caused by an inability to synthesize phenylalanine.
   (b) The disease can be caused by a deficiency in phenylalanine hydroxylase.
   (c) The disease can be caused by a deficiency in tetrahydrobiopterin.
   (d) The disease is treated with a high phenylalanine diet.
   (e) The disease leads to a buildup of phenylalanine in the body.

ANSWERS TO SELF-TEST

1. All are correct. The amino acids that are needed for protein synthesis and as precursors for other biomolecules are used directly for those purposes. The carbon skeletons of any in excess can be converted into acetyl CoA or glucose, depending on the particular amino acid, and thus into products that are derivable from these two basic molecules.

2. c. The transamination of several different amino acids with α-ketoglutarate forms glutamate and α-keto acids that can subsequently be catabolized.

3. a, c

4. c, e. Serine and threonine are deaminated by dehydratases that take advantage of the β-hydroxyl of these amino acids to carry out a dehydration followed by a rehydration to release NH_4^+.

5. d. A five-carbon amino acid will yield a five-carbon ε-keto acid as a result of a transamination; in this case, glutamate yields ε-ketoglutarate. The other partner in the reaction, pyruvate, will yield alanine as a product.

6. The molecules involved are alanine, glutamate, urea and the branched amino acids (valine, isoleucine and leucine). The correct order is:

   1) (Isoleucine, Leucine, Valine)
   2) Alanine
   3) Glutamate
   4) Urea

   Glucose, pyruvate, and glutamine are either not involved at all (glutamine) or don't contain nitrogen (glucose, pyruvate).

7. a, c, d. Uracil is a pyrimidine component of RNA and is not a nitrogen excretory product. Uric acid is a purine derivative excreted by uricotelic organisms.

8. Three moles of ATP are directly involved in the synthesis of urea. Two are converted to ADP and P_i by carbamoyl phosphate synthetase, and one is converted to AMP and PP_i by argininosuccinate synthetase. Two ATP would be required to convert AMP back into ATP, so a total of four high-energy bonds are used. Only one molecule of nitrogen enters as NH_4^+; the other enters in the α-amino group of aspartate, which can be formed by a transamination between oxaloacetate and glutamate.

9. The sum of the two reactions would be alanine + oxaloacetate $\rightarrow$ aspartate + pyruvate, and the net effect would be that the α-amino group of alanine would appear as the α-amino group of aspartate, one of the two direct donors of nitrogen into the urea cycle—the other is carbamoyl phosphate. The α-amino groups of many other amino acids can be similarly collected on aspartate and fed into the cycle.

10. Ornithine serves as the carrier on which the urea molecule is constructed. The α-amino group of ornithine has a carbamoyl group added to it by ornithine transcarbamoylase to form citrulline. Subsequent steps of the cycle add aspartate to bring in the second nitrogen atom and also regenerate ornithine when arginase cleaves arginine to form urea.

11. A defect in carbamoyl phosphate synthesis would cause increased NH_4^+ concentrations, as would a defect in any of the four reactions that condense carbamoyl phosphate with ornithine and regenerate the ornithine. Essentially, blocking a biochemical pathway at any of its steps may lead to increased concentrations of any of the precursors or members of the pathway.

12. Hibernating bears do not excrete urea through their urine and must utilize other means to dispose of nitrogen. Bacteria in the intestine hydrolyze urea, generating ammonia which is used to synthesize amino acids and proteins.

13. (a) 5 (b) 4, 7. Aspartate can be converted to fumarate via the urea cycle. (c) 3 (d) 2, 7 (e) 2, 6 (f) 1

14. (a) K   (b) G   (c) GK   (d) G   (e) G   (f) GK (g) G   (h) GK

15. Both give rise to methylmalonyl CoA, which can, in turn, be converted into succinyl CoA and ultimately into glucose.

16. b, c. Monoxygenases and dioxygenases are involved in the conversion of phenylalanine to tyrosine and the subsequent opening of the aromatic ring during tyrosine catabolism.

17. (a) serine and threonine dehydratase
    (b) glutamate dehydrogenase
    (c) aspartate and alanine aminotransferases
    (d) phenylalanine hydroxylase
    (e) asparaginase
    (f) branched-chain α-ketoacid dehydrogenase complex

18. Answers (b), (c), and (e) are correct. Phenylketonuria is a metabolic disorder arising from an absence or deficiency in the enzyme phenylalanine hydroxylase or (more rarely) its cofactor tetrahydrobiopterin. It results in the buildup of phenylalanine in the body and is treated with a diet low in phenylalanine.

PROBLEMS

1. Birds require arginine in their diet. Would you expect to find the production of urea in these animals? Explain.

2. Which would you expect to have a greater effect on the rate of urea biosynthesis, a defect in fumarase activity or a defect in alanine aminotransferase?

3. Pyridoxal phosphate or related metabolites are required growth factors for *Lactobacillus* species (Morishita et al., *J. Bacteriol.* 148[1981]:64–71). For example, when amino acids such as alanine or glutamate are used as the sole source of nutrition, these bacilli do not grow nor do they generate metabolic energy unless pyridoxal phosphate or its metabolites are supplied. Explain these observations.

4. Why is glutamate dehydrogenase a logical point for the control of ammonia production in cells?

5. During the process of glomerular filtration in the kidney, amino acids, as well as other metabolites, enter the lumen of the kidney tubule. Normally, a large portion of these amino acids are reabsorbed into the blood through the action of membrane-bound carrier systems that are specific for different classes of amino acids. Cystinuria is a disorder whose symptoms include urinary excretion with unusually high concentrations of cystine as well as excess amounts of ornithine, lysine, and arginine. Cystine is a dibasic amino acid composed of two cysteine molecules joined by a disulfide linkage. Patients with this disorder often have urinary tract stones, which are caused by the limited solubility of cystine. A related disorder found in other people is characterized by the appearance of ornithine, lysine, and arginine in the urine, although the levels of urinary cystine are normal.

    (a) What is the most likely source of cystine in cells?
    (b) What common structural feature of the four amino acids—cystine, ornithine, lysine, and arginine—is recognized by the carrier in the kidney tubule membrane?
    (c) How many carrier systems may exist for these molecules?
    (d) Other amino acidurias are due to a deficiency in one or more of the enzymes in the catabolic pathway for an amino acid. This deficiency leads to higher concentrations of the amino acid in the blood and a corresponding increase in the concentrations in the glomerular filtrate. In this case, the capacity of the reabsorption system is surpassed, causing some amino acid to be lost in the urine. How could you distinguish between a defect in amino acid metabolism and a defect in a renal transport system?

6. Why is the catabolism of isoleucine said to be both glucogenic and ketogenic?

7. Brain cells take up tryptophan, which is then converted to 5-hydroxytryptophan by tryptophan hydroxylase, an enzyme whose activity is similar to that of phenylalanine hydroxylase. Aromatic amino acid decarboxylase then catalyzes the formation of the potent neurotransmitter 5-hydroxytryptamine, also called *serotonin*. In the blood, tryptophan is bound to serum albumin, with an affinity such that about 10% of the tryptophan is freely diffusable. The rate of tryptophan uptake by brain cells depends on the concentration of free tryptophan. In these cells, tryptophan concentration is normally well below that of the K_M for tryptophan hydroxylase. Aspirin and other drugs displace tryptophan from albumin, thereby increasing the concentration of free tryptophan.

    (a) What cofactor is required for the activity of tryptophan hydroxylase?
    (b) What effect does aspirin have on tryptophan metabolism in brain cells?

8. In many microorganisms, glutamate dehydrogenase (GDH) participates in the catabolism of glutamate by generating ammonia and α-ketoglutarate, which undergoes oxidation in the citric acid cycle. However, when *E. coli* is grown with glutamate as the sole source of carbon, the synthesis of GDH protein is strongly repressed. Under these conditions, aspartase, an enzyme that catalyzes the removal of ammonia from aspartate to form fumarate, is required for the cell to grow in glutamate. Propose a cyclic pathway for the catabolism of glutamate that includes aspartate.

9. When *E. coli* is grown in glucose and ammonia, GDH synthesis is accelerated and the enzyme is active. Under these conditions, what role does GDH play in bacterial metabolism?

10. After an overnight fast, muscle tissue proteolysis generates free amino acids, many of which pass into the blood. Among the amino acids that are found in the blood are alanine, glutamate, and glutamine, all of which are rapidly taken up by the liver. What happens to these amino acids when they enter hepatic cells?

11. Propionyl CoA and methylmalonyl CoA both inhibit N-acetylglutamate synthase activity in slices of liver tissue. What clinical symptom would you expect to see in patients suffering from methylmalonic aciduria as a result of this inhibition?

12. Early work by Esmond Snell on the enzymes that employ pyridoxal phosphate included experiments in which free pyridoxal was heated with amino acids like glutamate. Snell found that the α-amino group of glutamate was transferred to pyridoxal, generating pyridoxamine. Why was this an important clue to the function of pyridoxal as a cofactor?

13. A small number of infants who have phenylketonuria have normal levels of phenylalanine hydroxylase activity, but on normal diets they continue to accumulate phenylalanine as well as other metabolites, including phenylpyruvate, phenyllactate, and phenylacetate. They also have high levels of quinonoid dihydrobiopterin.
    (a) What is the probable enzyme deficiency in these infants? Rationalize the deficiency with the observed clinical symptoms.
    (b) Write brief pathways for the formation of the phenylalanine metabolites found in these infants.

Phenylpyruvate   **Phenyllactate**   **Phenylacetate**

14. The mechanism of proteolysis by the β subunits of the proteosome is through a threonine-dependent nucleophilic attack. In addition to the catalytic threonine, conformational changes in a loop outside the active site are critical to catalysis. Using chymotrypsin and HIV protease as a model, speculate on ways in which an inhibitor could be designed that would inactivate the proteosome. How could the *Mycobacterium tuberculosis* proteoseome be targeted without also inhibiting the human proteosome?

ANSWERS TO PROBLEMS

1. In the urea cycle, arginine is cleaved to yield urea and ornithine. The fact that birds require arginine in their diet indicates that they are unable to synthesize it for utilization in protein synthesis. As a result, they are also unable to synthesize urea to dispose of ammonia; instead, they synthesize uric acid. Birds do have carbamoyl phosphate synthetase activity; however, it is located in the cytosol, and it catalyzes the formation of carbamoyl phosphate, which is then utilized for pyrimidine synthesis.

2. Fumarase activity has an effect on the urea cycle because it is needed, along with malate dehydrogenase, for the regeneration of oxaloacetate, which in turn undergoes transamination to form aspartate. The amino group of aspartate contains one of the two nitrogen atoms that are used to synthesize urea. Alanine aminotransferase is one of a number of aminotransferases that can transfer amino groups from amino acids to α-ketoglutarate to generate glutamate. Subsequent deamination of glutamate provides ammonia for the urea cycle. If all the other aminotransferases in the cell are active, then alanine aminotransferase would not be particularly essential. Thus, a defect in fumarase activity would have the greater effect on the rate of urea biosynthesis.

3. To utilize amino acids as sources of oxidative energy or to generate glucose through gluconeogenesis, the bacilli must carry out transamination reactions to dispose of ammonia (or to use it for the biosynthesis of other nitrogen-containing compounds) as well as to generate α-keto acids that can be used in the citric acid cycle or other pathways. Pyridoxal phosphate is a required cofactor for the aminotransferase enzymes, and in bacteria in which it cannot be synthesized, it must be derived from the growth medium. Otherwise, amino acids cannot be metabolized. In this case, where an amino acid is the only source of carbon and of nitrogen, the bacilli will not be able to introduce the amino acid into any catabolic pathway. Pyridoxal phosphate also functions as a cofactor for a large number of other enzymes, including decarboxylases, racemases, aldolases, and deaminases. Therefore, deficiencies in pyridoxal phosphate would also adversely affect a large number of other pathways.

4. The deamination of amino acids occurs through the action of transaminases as well as through the action of glutamate dehydrogenase (GDH). GDH is the only enzyme that catalyzes the oxidative deamination of an L amino acid. It deaminates glutamate, whose precursor, α-ketoglutarate, is the ultimate acceptor of amino groups from almost all the amino acids. In addition, while the reactions catalyzed by the transaminases are freely reversible, the GDH reaction is far from equilibrium; it is therefore a logical activity to control because large changes in its velocity can be achieved with small changes in the concentrations of allosteric effectors like ATP or NADH. Thus, GDH is the enzyme of choice for the control of ammonia synthesis.

5. (a) Disulfide linkages exist in many proteins, and when they are hydrolyzed by proteases to yield free amino acids, cystine is often one of the products.
   (b) Like cystine, the other three amino acids—arginine, ornithine, and lysine—have two basic groups. The carrier systems probably recognize and bind these groups for transport.
   (c) From the disorders described, it is likely that there are two transport systems. One carries all four dibasic acids; when it is defective, reabsorption of all four species fails, allowing all four to spill over into the urine. Another system transports ornithine, arginine, and lysine but not cystine; its failure to function accounts for the appearance of these three amino acids but not cystine in the urine.
   (d) A defect in the catabolic pathway for a particular amino acid causes elevation in the concentration of that single amino acid in blood and in urine as well, unless other amino acids carried by the same kidney transport system are lost to the urine. A defect in renal reabsorption means that all those amino acids that share the affected carrier system will be lost to the urine. Their concentration in blood will be lower than normal, while their concentration in urine will be higher.

6. The catabolic pathway for isoleucine leads to the formation of acetyl CoA and propionyl CoA. Acetyl CoA can be utilized for the net synthesis of fatty acids or ketone bodies, but it cannot be used for the net synthesis of glucose; thus, it is said to be ketogenic. In contrast to acetyl CoA, propionyl CoA is converted to succinyl CoA, which

can be utilized through part of the citric acid cycle and the gluconeogenic pathway to give the net formation of glucose. The distinction between the two types of substrates is somewhat arbitrary, however. For example, succinyl CoA can also be converted via pyruvate and acetyl CoA to citrate, which, when transported to the cytosol, serves as the source of carbons for the synthesis of fatty acids. Thus, glucogenic substrates can, under certain conditions, be ketogenic; however, ketogenic substrates cannot be glucogenic, unless a cell has a functional glyoxylate pathway.

7. (a) Tetrahydrobiopterin is utilized as a reductant by many hydroxylase enzymes, including phenylalanine hydroxylase and tryptophan hydroxylase.

   (b) The higher the concentration of free tryptophan, the greater the rate of uptake of the amino acid by the brain cells. Because the normal concentration of tryptophan in these cells is below that of the K_M for tryptophan hydroxylase, an influx of more tryptophan into the cells provides more substrate for the enzyme. You would therefore expect an increase in the level of 5-hydroxytryptophan production.

8. A possible catabolic pathway for glutamate that includes aspartate follows:

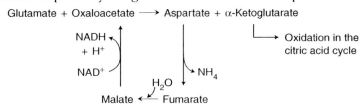

Glutamate undergoes transamination with oxaloacetate to generate α-ketoglutarate and aspartate. Oxidation of α-ketoglutarate is carried out in the citric acid cycle, whereas aspartate is cleaved to yield ammonia and fumarate. Fumarate is converted to malate, which is then oxidized to oxaloacetate in the citric acid cycle so that it can be regenerated to serve as an acceptor of the amino group from glutamate. It should be noted that glutamate will also be used as a source of amino groups by the aminotransferases and other enzymes involved in biosynthesis.

9. In cells grown in glucose and ammonia, GDH catalyzes the assimilation of ammonia by incorporating it into α-ketoglutarate to yield glutamate, which serves as a source of amino groups for other biosynthetic reactions.

10. In the liver, alanine, glutamate, and glutamine are utilized as sources of carbon for gluconeogenesis. Glutamine is deaminated to yield glutamate and ammonia. Glutamate undergoes oxidative deamination to form ammonia and α-ketoglutarate, a substrate for gluconeogenesis. Pyruvate is generated from the transamination of alanine, and carboxylation of the α-keto acid yields oxaloacetate, another source of carbon for gluconeogenesis. The ammonia generated by the conversion of the amino acids to their corresponding α-keto acids is used for the synthesis of urea. Glucose synthesized by liver can be returned through the blood to the muscle, where it serves as a source of energy. Thus, muscle uses the amino acids as a means of contributing to the generation of glucose in liver as well as a means of transporting ammonia to the liver, where the synthesis of urea can be carried out.

11. The activity of mitochondrial carbamoyl phosphate synthetase (CPS) depends on the availability of N-acetylglutamate, which is generated from glutamate and acetyl CoA. A reduction in the availability of the activating molecule will lead to a decrease in the activity of CPS, which utilizes ammonia and bicarbonate for the synthesis of carbamoyl phosphate. This, in turn, leads to an increase in the level of ammonia in blood and urine. Over two-thirds of patients with methylmalonic aciduria are hyperammonemic.

12. Snell's observations of the formation of pyridoxamine by heating with α-amino acids suggested that pyridoxal is involved in transamination reactions. As an enzyme co-factor, it could transfer an α-amino group from an amino acid to the α-keto group of an α-keto acid. It is now established that the action of pyridoxal phosphate in aminotransferase enzymes includes formation of pyridoxamine phosphate during the catalytic cycle (see page 682 of the text).

13. (a) The enzyme that is deficient in these infants is dihydropteridine reductase, which converts quinonoid dihydrobiopterin to tetrahydrobiopterin, using NADH as a substrate. In the phenylalanine hydroxylase reaction, tetrahydrobiopterin, the reductant in the conversion of phenylalanine to tyrosine, is oxidized to quinonoid dihydrobiopterin. The reductase enzyme regenerates tetrahydrobiopterin so that it can be used for further use in tyrosine formation. Cells that are deficient in the reductase cannot carry out efficient conversion of phenylalanine to tyrosine because they cannot regenerate tetrahydrobiopterin.

    (b) Phenylpyruvate can be generated from phenylalanine by transamination, and reduction of phenylpyruvate by NADH or NADPH generates phenyllactate, in a reaction similar to that catalyzed by lactate dehydrogenase. Phenylacetate can be generated by oxidative decarboxylation of phenylpyruvate, in a reaction reminiscent of the conversion of pyruvate to acetyl CoA, catalyzed by pyruvate dehydrogenase.

14. An irreversible, mechanism-based inhibitor such as diisopropylfluorophosphate (DIPF) or a sulfonyl fluoride could be used to covalently label a reactive threonine in much the same way as they modify the serine in serine proteases. The rest of the molecule would have to be designed to bind specifically to the proteosome active site. Since both eukaryotic and archaeal proteosomes contain the reactive threonine, some other feature might need to be used to target it specifically. Some inhibitors of the HIV protease use interactions with flexible regions of the protein to add specificity. This method could be used to differentiate the eukaryotic and archaeal proteosomes by way of the conformational changes in the loop. This approach has indeed been followed in research such as that published by Lin et al. in *Nature* 461, 621–626 (1 October 2009).

Chapter 31

Amino Acid Synthesis

In this chapter, the biosynthetic origins of the amino acids are explained, beginning with the need for a source of nitrogen for the amino acids. This need is met by nitrogen fixation, which is the process of converting atmospheric nitrogen in the form of N_2 to NH_4^+. The enzyme that carries out this difficult task, nitrogenase, is discussed in detail, including the role of an unusual molybdenum-iron cofactor. The authors then explain how NH_4^+ is incorporated into the amino acids glutamate and glutamine via the enzymes glutamate dehydrogenase and glutamine synthetase. These two amino acids are major nitrogen donors in a range of biosynthetic pathways, including those of the remaining amino acids whose synthesis is discussed next. While the pathways for the synthesis of the amino acids are diverse, they have in common the fact that their carbon skeletons come from intermediates in glycolysis, the pentose phosphate pathway or the citric acid cycle. This leads to a grouping of the amino acids into one of six biosynthetic families based on their starting material: oxaloacetate, pyruvate, ribose-5-phosphate, α-ketoglutarate, 3-phosphoglycerate, and phosphoenolpyruvate/erythrose 4-phosphate. The role of three important cofactors involved in some of the syntheses: pyridoxal phosphate, tetrahydrofolate, and S-adenosylmethionine is discussed. The latter two are carriers of single carbon atoms in metabolism. The authors also explain that the lack of some biosynthetic pathways in humans has led to the dietary requirement for nine amino acids. The examination of amino acid synthesis concludes with a general discussion of how metabolic pathways are controlled via feedback inhibition, using examples from amino acid metabolism to illustrate the relevant principles.

LEARNING OBJECTIVES

When you have mastered this chapter, you should be able to accomplish the following objectives.

Introduction

1. Recognize that nitrogen in the form of *ammonia* is the source of nitrogen for all amino acids, and amino acids, in turn, are the nitrogen source for many other biomolecules.

2. Appreciate the need for amino acids to be synthesized in the correct enantiomeric form, and that the stereochemistry at the α-carbon is established by a *transamination* reaction that includes *pyridoxal phosphate (PLP)*.

3. Define *nitrogen fixation* and name the groups of organisms that can carry out this conversion. Compare the reduction of N_2 in industrial reactions with that carried out in biology.

The Nitrogenase Complex Fixes Nitrogen (Text Section 31.1)

4. Describe the *nitrogenase complex* and explain the roles of its *reductase* and *nitrogenase* components. Note the function of the *FeMo-cofactor*.

5. Explain the energy requirement for nitrogen fixation and write the equation giving the *stoichiometry* of the overall reaction.

6. Outline the key roles of *glutamate* and *glutamine* in the assimilation of NH_4^+ into amino acids and describe the reactions of *glutamate dehydrogenase, glutamine synthetase,* and *glutamate synthase.* Recognize the functions of *ATP* and *NADPH* in these processes.

Amino Acids Are Made from Intermediates of Major Pathways (Text Section 31.2)

7. Classify the amino acids into six *biosynthetic families* and identify their *seven precursors.* Name the metabolic pathways from which these precursors originate.

8. Identify the *essential* amino acids for humans and explain why they are essential.

9. Describe the single-step biosyntheses of alanine, aspartate, and glutamate.

10. Compare the formation of asparagine from aspartate to that of glutamine from glutamate.

11. Outline the syntheses of glutamine, proline, and arginine from *α-ketoglutarate.*

12. Outline the syntheses of serine, glycine, and cysteine from *3-phosphoglycerate.*

13. Explain the roles of pyridoxal phosphate, *tetrahydrofolate,* and S-adenosylmethionine in amino acid biosyntheses.

14. Identify the structure of tetrahydrofolate and indicate the reactive part of the molecule. Draw the structures of the single-carbon groups that can be carried on tetrahydrofolate and provide examples of reactions that generate and use them. Describe the sources of this cofactor in humans.

15. Draw the structure of S-adenosylmethionine and describe its synthesis. Indicate the reactive part of the molecule and describe the basis of its *high methyl group–transfer potential.*

16. Outline the *activated methyl cycle* and describe the roles of *methylcobalamin* and *ATP* in the cycle. Give examples of important derivatives from S-adenosylmethionine.

17. Describe the synthesis of cysteine from *homocysteine* and serine. Explain the most common cause and consequences of elevated levels of homocysteine in humans.

18. Outline the biosyntheses of phenylalanine, tyrosine, and tryptophan in *E. coli*. Describe the roles of *phosphoenolpyruvate*, *erythrose 4-phosphate*, and *phosphoribosylpyrophosphate* in these reactions.

19. Point out the locations of shikimate and chorismate in the shikimate pathway.

20. Describe the structure of *tryptophan synthetase* and the role of *substrate channeling* in its catalytic reaction.

Feedback Inhibition Regulates Amino Acid Biosynthesis (Text Section 31.3)

21. Define the *committed step* of a metabolic pathway and recognize that it is often the target of *feedback regulation*.

22. Note the main features of control of branched pathways by *feedback inhibition and activation, enzyme multiplicity,* and *cumulative feedback.*

23. Describe the cumulative feedback control of *glutamine synthetase* from *E. coli*. Explain the mechanisms and functions of the *reversible covalent modifications* and describe the advantage of employing an *enzymatic cascade* in regulating this reaction.

SELF-TEST

The Nitrogenase Complex Fixes Nitrogen

1. Define *nitrogen fixation* and explain why it is crucial to the maintenance of life on earth.

2. Place the following components, reactants, and products of the nitrogenase complex reaction in their correct sequence during the electron transfers of nitrogen fixation:

   (a) oxidized ferredoxin
   (b) reductase component
   (c) nitrogenase component
   (d) NH_3

   (e) N_2
   (f) reduced ferredoxin
   (g) electron source

3. Write the net equation for nitrogen fixation and describe the sources of the electrons and ATP.

4. Match the structural components or features in the right column with the appropriate component of the nitrogenase reaction.

   (a) reductase component
   (b) nitrogenase component

   (1) MoFe-cofactor
   (2) [4Fe-4S] cluster
   (3) ATP-ADP binding site
   (4) N_2-binding site
   (5) $\alpha_2\beta_2$ tetramer
   (6) dimer of identical subunits

5. Match the enzyme with the reaction it catalyzes.

   (a) glutamine synthetase
   (b) glutamate dehydrogenase
   (c) glutamate synthase

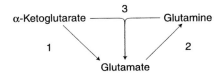

6. Which of the reactions shown in question 5 require the following?
   (a) NH_4^+
   (b) ATP
   (c) NADH
   (d) NADPH

7. All organisms can incorporate NH_4^+ into glutamate and glutamine using glutamate dehydrogenase and glutamine synthetase. Why do prokaryotes have an additional enzyme, glutamate synthase, to perform this function?

Amino Acids Are Made from Intermediates of Major Pathways

8. Which of the following amino acids are essential dietary components for an adult human?
   (a) alanine
   (b) aspartate
   (c) histidine
   (d) tryptophan
   (e) leucine
   (f) phenylalanine
   (g) glutamine
   (h) asparagine
   (i) glutamate
   (j) threonine
   (k) methionine

9. Which of the following amino acids are derived from pyruvate?
   (a) phenylalanine
   (b) alanine
   (c) tyrosine
   (d) histidine
   (e) valine
   (f) leucine
   (g) cysteine
   (h) glycine

10. Which of the following amino acids are derived from α-ketoglutarate?
    (a) glutamate
    (b) proline
    (c) cysteine
    (d) aspartate
    (e) glutamine
    (f) arginine
    (g) ornithine
    (h) serine

11. Which of the following compounds provide the carbon skeletons of the six biosynthetic families of amino acids? Name the metabolic pathways from which each of the precursor compounds originates.
    (a) pyruvate
    (b) oxaloacetate
    (c) α-ketoglutarate
    (d) succinate
    (e) 2-deoxyribose
    (f) 3-phosphoglycerate
    (g) ribose 5-phosphate

(h) glucose 6-phosphate
(i) phosphoenolpyruvate
(j) erythrose 4-phosphate
(k) α-ketobutyrate

12. Explain the role of the conserved lysine and arginine residues in the active site of transaminases. Be sure to include how they aid in the stereochemical specificity of the reaction.

13. Three coenzymes are involved in carrying activated one-carbon units. Match the activated group in the right column with the appropriate coenzyme in the left column.

    (a) tetrahydrofolate   (1) $-CH_3$
    (b) S-adenosylmethionine   (2) $-CH_2-$
    (c) biotin   (3) $-CHO$
                                    (4) $-CHNH$
                                    (5) $-CH=$
                                    (6) $-CO_2^-$

14. Which of the following answers completes the sentence correctly? The major source of one-carbon units for the formation of the tetrahydrofolate derivative N^5,N^{10}-methylenetetrahydrofolate is the conversion of

    (a) methionine to homocysteine.
    (b) deoxyuridine 5′-phosphate to deoxythymidine 5′-phosphate.
    (c) 3-phosphoglycerate to serine.
    (d) serine to glycine.

15. Why does S-adenosylmethionine have a higher methyl group–transfer potential than N^5-methyltetrahydrofolate?

16. S-adenosylmethionine is involved directly in which of the following reactions?

    (a) methyl transfer to phosphatidyl ethanolamine
    (b) synthesis of glycine from serine
    (c) DNA methylation
    (d) conversion of homocysteine into methionine
    (e) synthesis of ethylene in plants

17. How many high-energy bonds are expended during the synthesis of S-adenosylmethionine from ATP and methionine?

18. The conversion of homocysteine into methionine involves which of the following cofactors?

    (a) N^5-methyltetrahydrofolate
    (b) N^5,N^{10}-methylenetetrahydrofolate
    (c) methylcobalamin
    (d) pyridoxal phosphate

19. Which of the following statements about vitamin treatment for patients suffering from high homocysteine levels is correct?

    (a) They help reduce oxidative damage caused by an excess of homocysteine.
    (b) Folic acid helps activate cystathionine β-synthase, decreasing the concentration of homocysteine.
    (c) They decrease the activity of two major metabolic pathways involving homocysteine.
    (d) Vitamins B6 and B12 support conversion of homocysteine into other metabolites.

Feedback Inhibition Regulates Amino Acid Biosynthesis

20. In the following biosynthetic pathway A → B → C → D → E → F → G, which is likely to be the committed step? Which compound is likely to inhibit the committed step?

21. Since glutamine is an important source of nitrogen in biosynthetic reactions, the enzyme that synthesizes it is carefully regulated. Which of the following compounds act as inhibitors of glutamine synthetase in *E. coli*?

    (a) tryptophan
    (b) histidine
    (c) carbamoyl phosphate
    (d) glucosamine 6-phosphate
    (e) AMP
    (f) CTP
    (g) alanine
    (h) glycine

ANSWERS TO SELF-TEST

1. Nitrogen fixation is the process by which nitrogen present in the atmosphere as N_2 is enzymatically converted to NH_3 by some bacteria and blue-green algae. This process is crucial to all other organisms because they can use only NH_4^+, and not N_2, as the source of nitrogen for biosynthesis.

2. g, f, a, b, c, e, d

3. The net equation for nitrogen fixation is

$$N_2 + 8\ e^- + 16\ ATP + 16\ H_2O \rightarrow 2\ NH_3 + 16\ ADP + 16\ P_i + 8\ H^+ + H_2$$

   The eight electrons needed to reduce N_2 are supplied by oxidative processes in non-photosynthetic nitrogen-fixing organisms and by light energy from the sun in photosynthetic nitrogen-fixing organisms. The ATP requirement is met by the usual oxidative or photosynthetic mechanisms of the cells.

4. (a) 2, 3, 6 (b) 1, 2, 4, 5

5. (a) 2 (b) 1 (c) 3

6. (a) 1, 2 (b) 2 (c) None (d) 1, 3. Glutamate dehydrogenase uses NADPH when catalyzing reductive aminations and NAD^+ when carrying out oxidative deaminations.

7. Glutamate synthase catalyzes the reductive amination of α-ketoglutarate in a reaction with glutamine to form two glutamates. Glutamate can also be made from NH_4^+ and α-ketoglutarate using glutamate dehydrogenase. However, this route requires high concentrations of NH_4^+ because of the high K_M of the enzyme for NH_4^+. Prokaryotes can use glutamine synthetase, which has a low K_M for NH_4^+, to form glutamine when NH_4^+ concentrations are low. Thus, by using an additional enzyme, they can form glutamate from glutamine and α-ketoglutarate when NH_4^+ is scarce.

8. c, d, e, f, j, k

9. b, e, f

10. a, b, e, f, g. Recall that ornithine is a precursor of arginine in the urea cycle and is derived from α-ketoglutarate.

11. The biosynthetic precursors are a, b, c, f, g, i, and j. The pathways they originate from are as follows:

Glycolysis: pyruvate (a)
3-phosphoglycerate (f)
phosphoenolpyruvate (i)

Citric acid cycle: oxaloacetate (b)
α-ketoglutarate (c)

Pentose phosphate pathway: ribose 5-phosphate (g)
erythrose 4-phosphate (j)

12. The lysine forms a Schiff base with the PLP cofactor and the arginine interacts with the α-carboxylate group of the ketoacid. The interaction between the arginine and the α-carboxylate helps orient the substrate so that the lysine residue transfers a proton to the bottom face of the quinonoid intermediate, generating an aldimine with an L configuration at the Ca center.

13. (a) 1, 2, 3, 4, 5   (b) 1   (c) 6

14. d. Furthermore, since 3-phosphoglycerate can give rise to serine, you can see how carbohydrates can provide activated one-carbon units via a glucose $\rightarrow$ 3-phosphoglycerate $\rightarrow$ serine $\rightarrow$ glycine pathway.

15. The positive charge on the sulfur atom of S-adenosylmethionine activates the methyl sulfonium bond and makes methyl group transfer from S-adenosylmethionine energetically more favorable than from N^5-methyltetrahydrofolate.

16. a, c, e. The cofactor for reactions (b) and (d) is tetrahydrofolate.

17. Three high-energy bonds are expended. The adenosyl group of ATP is condensed with methionine to form a carbon-to-sulfur bond with the release of P_i and PP_i, which is hydrolyzed to 2 P_i.

18. a, c. Homocysteine transmethylase uses a vitamin B_{12}–derived cofactor.

19. d

20. A $\rightarrow$ B. Control of the first step conserves the first compound, A, in the sequence and also saves metabolic energy by preventing subsequent reactions in the pathway. Compound G would likely inhibit the committed step. The end product of a biosynthetic pathway often controls the committed step.

21. All the choices are correct. When all eight compounds are bound to the enzyme, it is almost completely inactive. The control of this enzyme is an excellent example of cumulative feedback inhibition.

PROBLEMS

1. The essential amino acids are those that cannot be synthesized de novo in humans. Given an abundance of other amino acids in the diet, the α-keto acid

analogs that correspond to the essential amino acids can substitute for these compounds in the diet.

(a) What do these observations tell you about the steps in the synthesis of essential amino acids that may be missing in humans?

(b) If ^{15}N-labeled alanine is supplied in the diet, many other amino acids in the body will contain at least a small amount of the label within 48 hours. What enzymes are primarily responsible for this observation?

2. In muscle, glutamine synthetase is very active, catalyzing the formation of glutamine from glutamate and ammonia at the expense of a molecule of ATP. In the liver, the rate of formation of glutamine is very low, but a high level of glutaminase activity, which generates ammonia and glutamate, is observed. How would you explain the difference in the levels of enzyme activity in these two organs?

3. Glutamine synthetase in mammals is not subject to the same type of complex regulation that is seen in bacteria. Why?

4. Most of the proteins synthesized in mammals contain all 20 common amino acids. More protein is degraded than is synthesized when even one essential amino acid is missing from the diet.

(a) Under such conditions, how could an increase in the rate of protein degradation provide the missing amino acid?

(b) How does an increase in the rate of protein degradation contribute to increased levels of nitrogen excretion?

5. The diagram below outlines the biosynthesis of a compound that is required for the oxidation of fatty acids in the mitochondrion.

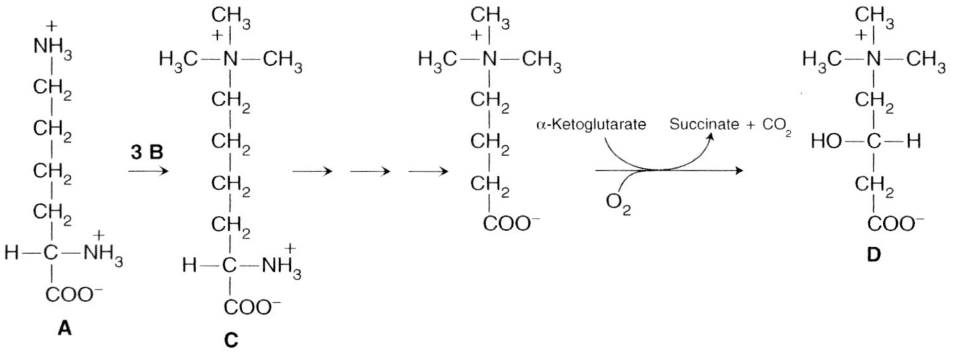

(a) Name compound D and briefly explain its role in fatty acid metabolism.

(b) Name compound A. Why is it considered essential in human diets?

(c) Three molecules of compound B are required for the formation of compound C. Its synthesis depends on the availability of an essential amino acid. Name that amino acid and then name compound B and compound C.

6. A pathway for the synthesis of ornithine from glutamate is shown in Figure 31.1.

FIGURE 31.1 Biosynthesis of ornithine from glutamate.

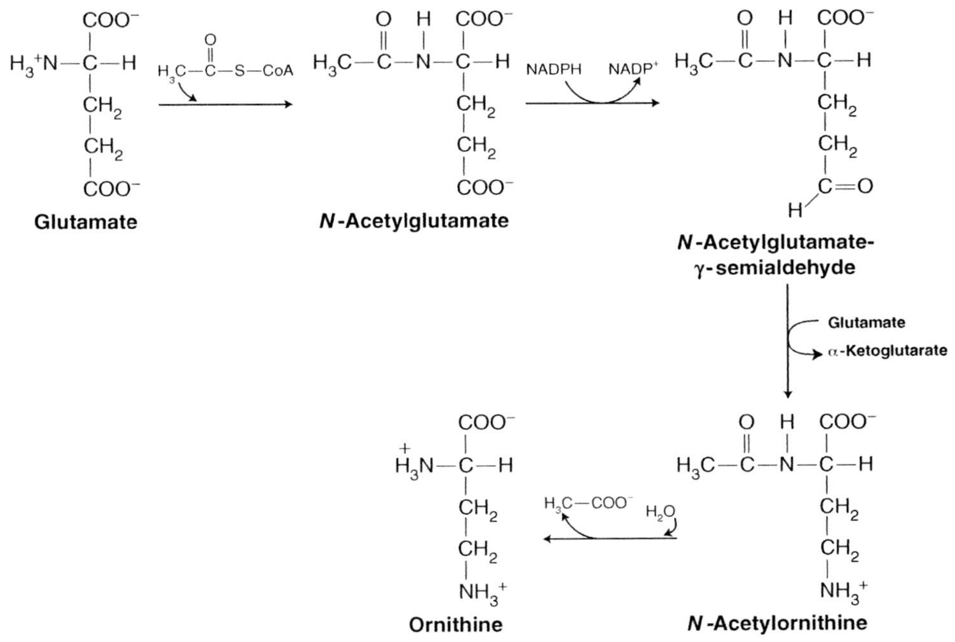

(a) Why can this pathway also be considered to be part of the de novo pathway for the synthesis of arginine?

(b) Given that glutamate-γ-semialdehyde cyclizes in the proline biosynthetic pathway, speculate on the role of acetylation in the ornithine pathway.

7. Elevated levels of ammonia in blood can result from deficiencies in one or another of the enzymes of the urea cycle. Measures taken to relieve hyperammonemia have included limiting intake of dietary proteins, administering α-keto analogs of several of the naturally occurring L-amino acids, or administering other compounds designed to exploit pathways of nitrogen metabolism and excretion.

(a) In trying to determine why a patient has hyperammonemia, which organ should you check first for normal function? Why?

(b) Why would limiting protein intake assist in relieving chronic hyperammonemia? Why would eliminating dietary proteins *altogether* (without any other supplement) probably increase the level of hyperammonemia?

(c) Write a brief rationale for using α-keto acid analogs in treating hyperammonemia, mentioning a particular group of enzymes essential to your explanation. Would it be better to use α-keto analogs of essential or nonessential amino acids? Why?

8. Plants synthesize all 20 common amino acids de novo. Glyphosate, a weed killer sold under the trade name Roundup, is an analog of phosphoenolpyruvate that specifically inhibits 3-enolpyruvylshikimate 5-phosphate synthase, a key enzyme of the pathway for chorismate biosynthesis, a precursor of the aromatic amino acids. This compound is a very effective plant herbicide, but has virtually no effect on mammals. Why?

ANSWERS TO PROBLEMS

1. (a) The fact that α-keto acid analogs can substitute for essential amino acids means that the carbon skeletons of the essential amino acids are not synthesized in humans. Many studies have shown that one or more of the enzymes needed for the synthesis of these structures are missing.

   (b) The enzymes that are primarily responsible for the distribution of the ^{15}N label among the other amino acids are the aminotransaminases, which catalyze the interconversions of amino acids and their corresponding α-keto acids. The redistribution of the label begins with the transamination of alanine, with α-ketoglutarate serving as the amino acceptor to yield pyruvate and glutamate. Glutamate then serves as an amino donor for other α-keto acids. In order for an essential amino acid to be labeled, you must postulate the transamination of that amino acid to yield the corresponding α-keto acid analog, followed by the donation of a labeled amino group from glutamate or another donor of amino groups.

2. Ammonia, which is generated as part of the process of amino acid catabolism in muscle, is toxic and must be removed from the cells. This could be done through the synthesis of urea, but that process occurs only in the liver. In muscle cells, therefore, glutamine synthetase catalyzes the formation of glutamine, which is an efficient and nontoxic carrier of ammonia. This accounts for the high activity of that enzyme in muscle. The glutamine is transported by the blood to the liver, where glutaminase and aspartate aminotransferase work together to generate aspartate and two molecules of ammonia from glutamine, hence the high activity of glutaminase in the liver. Aspartate and ammonia are both used by the liver for the synthesis of urea, a nontoxic and disposable form of ammonia.

3. Mammals acquire many nitrogen-containing compounds, such as tryptophan and histidine, in their diet rather than through de novo biosynthesis, so glutamine synthetase does not play so prominent a role in the nitrogen metabolism of mammals as it does in that of bacteria. Complex regulation of the enzyme is therefore not needed in mammals.

4. (a) Many experiments have shown that under normal conditions cells continuously synthesize and degrade proteins. Although both essential and nonessential amino acids are continuously recycled during these processes, reutilization is not completely efficient; thus, additional amino acids are needed. In mammals, there are no reservoirs of free amino acids; the only sources of essential amino acids are dietary proteins or the proteins of the body tissues. If an essential amino acid is not available from the diet, cells appear to accelerate the hydrolysis of their own proteins in order to generate the missing essential amino acid. How the rate of cellular proteolysis is accelerated in response to a deficiency of an essential amino acid is not understood.

   (b) An increased rate of protein degradation generates a higher concentration of free amino acids. During the oxidation of those amino acids not used for synthesis of other proteins, ammonia will be produced. An elevation in ammonia concentration in the body stimulates the formation of urea, causing the level of nitrogen excretion to increase.

5. (a) Compound D is carnitine, which, when esterified to the acyl group of a long-chain fatty acid, shuttles it from the cytosol to the matrix of the mitochondrion, where fatty acid oxidation takes place.

   (b) Compound A is the essential amino acid lysine; it is termed *essential* because it cannot be synthesized de novo in humans. Lysine and other essential amino acids must be obtained from the diet.

(c) Compound C is trimethyllysine, and the methyl groups that are attached to lysine are likely to be derived from compound B, *S*-adenosylmethionine, the major donor of methyl groups in biosynthetic reactions. The methyl group of *S*-adenosylmethionine is derived from methionine, an essential amino acid.

6. (a) Ornithine is a precursor of arginine, as part of the pathway for the synthesis of urea. Thus the pathway for the synthesis of ornithine from glutamine, along with part of the urea cycle pathway, can together be considered as a de novo pathway for the synthesis of arginine. Arginine can in turn be used for the synthesis of urea, or it can serve instead as one of the amino acids used for polypeptide synthesis.

(b) The N-acetyl group blocks the condensation of the amino group with the aldehyde group, thereby preventing the formation of the pyrroline ring. This allows the pathway to proceed toward the synthesis of ornithine.

7. (a) You should assess liver function, because enzymes of the urea cycle are found primarily in this organ. In addition, liver takes up amino acids such as alanine, glutamate, and glutamine, which are in effect nontoxic forms of ammonia generated by muscle and other tissues. Amino groups of these compounds, along with carbon dioxide from carbamoyl phosphate, are precursors of urea in the liver.

(b) During digestion, dietary proteins are hydrolyzed to their component amino acids. Those amino acids that are not needed immediately for protein synthesis or for the biosynthesis of other nitrogen-containing compounds are degraded. One of the products of amino acid degradation is ammonia. Usually ammonia is metabolized through conversion to nitrogen carriers such as alanine, glutamate, and glutamine, and it is ultimately utilized for the synthesis of urea when the urea cycle is operating. Thus limiting protein intake in a patient with a deficiency in urea synthesis would be expected to reduce ammonia production in liver and other tissues.

Protein turnover and amino acid degradation constantly take place in the tissues, and essential amino acids (those that cannot be synthesized de novo in human tissues) must be generated either from dietary sources or from additional breakdown of body proteins. A complete restriction of dietary protein would accelerate body protein breakdown and would exacerbate the condition of hyperammonemia.

(c) The α-keto acid analogs can serve as acceptors for amino groups from glutamate and other amino acids in reactions catalyzed by transaminases or aminotransferases. Nonessential amino acids formed as the result of this process may be themselves eliminated, degraded (often generating more ammonia), or else used for biosynthesis of other nitrogen-containing compounds. Employing analogs of essential amino acids might be preferable, because tissues are more likely to require them for protein synthesis or other biosyntheses.

8. Chorismate is an intermediate in the biosynthesis of the aromatic amino acids tryptophan, phenylalanine, and tyrosine. Mammals do not synthesize these amino acids from chorismate. Instead, they obtain the essential aromatic amino acids tryptophan and phenylalanine from the diet, and they can synthesize tyrosine from phenylalanine. Glyphosate is an effective herbicide because it prevents synthesis of aromatic amino acids in plants. But the compound has no effect on mammals because they have no active pathway for de novo aromatic amino acid synthesis.

Nucleotide Metabolism

In this chapter, the authors complete their treatment of the biosyntheses of the major classes of macromolecular precursors by describing the synthesis of the purine and pyrimidine nucleotides. Besides being the precursors of RNA and DNA, these compounds serve a number of other important roles that are reviewed in the opening paragraph of the chapter. Nucleotide nomenclature is reviewed in the introduction to the chapter, as is an outline for the synthesis of nucleotides through de novo and salvage pathways.

The chapter begins with the synthesis of the pyrimidine nucleotides. The pyrimidine ring is synthesized de novo from bicarbonate, aspartate, and ammonia (usually from glutamine) prior to attachment to a ribose sugar. The authors go through the synthesis step by step, paying particular attention to the enzyme carbamoyl phosphate synthetase (CPS), which synthesizes carbamoyl phosphate from bicarbonate and ammonia and catalyzes the committed step in eukaryotic pyrimidine synthesis. The next step in the synthesis is catalyzed by aspartate transcarbamoylase (ATCase). This reaction, the formation of carbamoylasparate from carbamoyl phosphate and aspartate, is the committed step in prokaryotic pyrimidine synthesis. A condensation and an oxidation reaction complete the formation of orotate, which is then coupled to a phosphoribose by reaction with 5-ribosyl-1-pyrophosphate (PRPP) to form the pyrimidine nucleotide orotidylate. Decarboxylation of orotidylate gives uridine monophosphate (UMP), which can be phosphorylated by nucleoside mono- and diphosphate kinases to form UDP and UTP, respectively. Amination of UTP forms cytidine triphosphate (CTP) and completes the synthesis of the pyrimidine ribonucleotides.

Next the authors turn to synthesis of the purine nucleotides. Unlike synthesis of pyrimidines, synthesis of purine nucleotides builds upon the ribose ring. As in the pyrimidine ring system, the ribose sugar is donated by the activated form of ribose 5-phosphate, 5-phosphoribosyl-1-pyrophosphate (PRPP). The two purine nucleotides AMP and GMP have a common precursor, inosine 5′-monophosphate (IMP). The authors discuss the synthesis of this initial purine product and then formation of AMP and GMP. The reactions that allow cells to salvage free purines and the control of purine biosynthesis are presented. The regulation of nucleotide biosynthesis through feedback inhibition is discussed later in the chapter.

Two reactions that are required to form the precursors of DNA are described in detail: ribonucleotide reductase converts ribonucleotides to deoxyribonucleotides, and thymidylate synthase methylates dUMP to form dTMP. The authors present the mechanisms and cofactors of these enzymes and explain how some anticancer drugs and antibiotics function by inhibition of dTMP synthesis and thus the growth of cells. Nucleotides also serve important roles as constituents of NAD^+, $NADP^+$, FAD, and coenzyme A (CoA), so the syntheses of these cofactors are described briefly. The chapter concludes with an explanation of how the purines are catabolized and some of the pathological conditions that arise from defects in the catabolic pathway of the purines.

LEARNING OBJECTIVES

When you have mastered this chapter, you should be able to accomplish the following objectives.

Introduction

1. List the major biochemical roles of the *nucleotides*.

An Overview of Nucleotide Biosynthesis and Nomenclature (Text Section 32.1)

2. Distinguish among the *purine* and *pyrimidine nucleosides* and *nucleotides*.

3. Define *de novo* and *salvage pathways* for biosynthesis of nucleotides.

The Pyrimidine Ring Is Assembled and Then Attached to a Ribose Sugar
(Text Section 32.2)

3. Draw the structure of a pyrimidine ring and identify the precursors that provide each carbon and nitrogen atom of the ring. Note the numbering of the ring atoms.

4. Discuss the reaction catalyzed by *carbamoyl phosphate synthetase (CPS)*. Explain the role of *carbamoyl phosphate* in pyrimidine biosynthesis.

5. Write the *aspartate transcarbamoylase* reaction and outline the remaining reactions that form *orotate*. Outline the conversion of orotate to *uridylate (UMP)*.

6. Explain how nucleoside *mono-* and *diphosphate kinases* interconvert the nucleoside mono-, di-, and triphosphates.

7. Describe the reaction that converts *UTP* to *CTP*.

8. Use the example of *thymine* to discuss the use of salvage pathways to recover pyrimidine bases from breakdown products of DNA and RNA. Discuss why *thymidine kinase* is a good therapeutic target for viral therapy.

The Purine Ring Is Assembled on Ribose Phosphate (Text Section 32.3)

9. Draw the structure of a purine ring and identify the precursors that provide each carbon and nitrogen atom of the ring. Note the numbering of the ring atoms.

10. Describe the committed step in de novo purine biosynthesis and the enzyme that catalyzes it.

11. Outline the synthesis of *inosine 5'-monophosphate (IMP)*, noting the sources of the atoms and the cofactors involved. List the steps that require ATP.

12. Describe the synthesis of *adenylate (AMP)* and *guanylate (GMP)* from IMP. List the cofactors and intermediates of the reactions.

13. Discuss the evidence that enzymes involved in many metabolic pathways are physically associated with each other. Explain how assembly of enzymes in purine biosynthesis is thought to be controlled.

14. Outline the synthesis of purine nucleotides by the *salvage reactions* and explain why these reactions are energetically advantageous.

Ribonucleotides Are Reduced to Deoxyribonucleotides (Text Section 32.4)

15. Outline the *ribonucleotide reductase* reaction.

16. Explain the roles of *NADH, thioredoxin,* and *thioredoxin reductase* in the ribonucleotide reductase mechanism. Include the role of disulfide bonds in the reaction.

17. Describe the *thymidylate synthase* reaction. Account for the source of the methyl group and describe the change in the oxidation state of the transferred carbon atom that occurs during the reaction.

18. Explain the role of *dihydrofolate reductase* in the synthesis of deoxythymidylate.

19. Account for the ability of *fluorouracil* to act as a *suicide inhibitor*. Describe the inhibitory mechanism of *methotrexate* and *aminopterin*. Explain how these three compounds interfere with the growth of cancer cells. List the mechanisms by which a cell could become resistant to methotrexate. Explain the antibiotic activity of *trimethoprim*.

Nucleotide Biosynthesis Is Regulated by Feedback Inhibition (Text Section 32.5)

20. Outline the regulation of the biosynthesis of the purine and pyrimidine nucleotides and name the committed steps in the pathways.

21. Describe the subunit structure of ribonucleotide reductase.

22. Describe the control of deoxyribonucleotide synthesis by ribonuclease reductase regulation.

Disruptions in Nucleotide Metabolism Can Cause Pathological Conditions (Text Section 32.6)

23. Describe the reactions of the *nucleotidases* and *nucleoside phosphorylases*.

24. Describe the link between *adenosine deaminase* and *severe combined immunodeficiency (SCID)*.

25. Outline the conversions of AMP and *guanine* to *uric acid*. Describe the role of *xanthine oxidase* in these processes.

26. Describe the major clinical findings in patients with *gout* and explain the rationale for the use of *allopurinol* to alleviate the symptoms of the disease.

27. Describe the *antioxidant* role of *urate*.

28. Name the biochemical lesion that leads to the *Lesch-Nyhan syndrome* and describe the symptoms of the disease.

29. Explain the role of folate in the prevention of *spina bifida*.

SELF-TEST

Introduction

1. Describe the physiological roles of the nucleotides.

An Overview of Nucleotide Biosynthesis and Nomenclature

2. Which of the following answers completes the sentence correctly? Cytosine is a
   (a) purine base.
   (b) pyrimidine base.
   (c) purine nucleoside.
   (d) pyrimidine nucleoside.

3. Which of the following are nucleotides?
   (a) deoxyadenosine
   (b) cytidine
   (c) deoxyguanylate
   (d) uridylate

The Pyrimidine Ring Is Assembled and Then Attached to a Ribose Sugar

4. Which of the following statements about the carbamoyl phosphate synthetase of mammals, which is used for pyrimidine biosynthesis, are true?
   (a) It requires one mole of ATP per mole of carbamoyl phosphate synthesized.
   (b) CPS II catalyzes a three-step reaction.
   (c) It uses NH_4^+ as a nitrogen source.
   (d) It uses glutamine as a nitrogen source.
   (e) It requires N-acetylglutamate as a positive effector.

5. Which of the following statements about 5-phosphoribosyl-1-pyrophosphate (PRPP) are true?
   (a) It is an activated form of ribose 5-phosphate.
   (b) It is formed from ribose 1-phosphate and ATP.
   (c) It has a pyrophosphate group attached to the C-1 atom of ribose in the α configuration.
   (d) It is formed in a reaction in which PP_i is released.

6. How is orotate, a free pyrimidine, converted into a nucleotide? Is this reaction considered to be a salvage reaction or a biosynthetic one?

7. Which of the following enzymes are involved in converting the nucleoside 5′-monophosphate (NMP) products of the purine or pyrimidine biosynthetic pathways into their 5′-triphosphate (NTP) derivatives?

(a) purine nucleotidase
(b) nucleoside diphosphate kinase
(c) nucleoside monophosphate kinases
(d) nucleoside phosphorylase

8. How is the exocyclic amino group on the N-4 position of cytosine formed?

9. Which of the following is not true about the thymine salvage pathway?
   (a) Thymine is converted into the nucleoside thymidine by thymidine phosphorylase in the first step of the pathway.
   (b) The activity of thymidine phosphorylase fluctuates with the cell cycle.
   (c) Thymidine kinase phosphorylates thymidine to form thymine monophosphate.
   (d) The mammalian and viral versions of thymidine kinase are highly homologous.

The Purine Ring Is Assembled on Ribose Phosphate

10. Which of the following compounds directly provide atoms to form the purine ring?
    (a) aspartate
    (b) carbamoyl phosphate
    (c) glutamine
    (d) glycine
    (e) CO_2
    (f) N^5,N^{10}-methylenetetrahydrofolate
    (g) N^{10}-formyltetrahydrofolate
    (h) NH_4^+

11. Which of the following answers completes the sentence correctly? The first product of purine nucleotide biosynthesis that contains a complete purine ring (hypoxanthine) is
    (a) AMP.
    (b) GMP.
    (c) IMP.
    (d) xanthylate (XMP).

12. The conversion of IMP to AMP requires which of the following?
    (a) ATP
    (b) GTP
    (c) aspartate
    (d) glutamine
    (e) NAD^+

13. The conversion of IMP to GMP requires which of the following?
    (a) ATP
    (b) GTP
    (c) aspartate
    (d) glutamine
    (e) NAD^+

14. Which of the following reactants and products are involved in the salvage reactions of purine biosynthesis?
    (a) IMP $\longrightarrow$ AMP
    (b) IMP $\longrightarrow$ GMP
    (c) adenine $\longrightarrow$ AMP
    (d) guanine $\longrightarrow$ GMP

15. During a purine salvage reaction, what is the source of the energy required to form the C–N glycosidic bond between the base and ribose?

16. Show which of the nucleotides in the right column regulate each of the conversions in the left column.
    (a) ribose 5-phosphate $\longrightarrow$ PRPP
    (b) PRPP $\longrightarrow$ 5-phosphoribosylamine
    (c) phosphoribosylamine $\longrightarrow$ IMP
    (d) IMP $\longrightarrow$ adenylosuccinate
    (e) IMP $\longrightarrow$ xanthylate (XMP)
    (1) AMP
    (2) GMP
    (3) IMP

17. Explain how GFP has been used to study enzyme association in purine biosynthesis.

Ribonucleotides Are Reduced to Deoxyribonucleotides

18. Which of the following statements about ribonucleotide reductase are true?

    (a) It converts ribonucleoside diphosphates into 2′-deoxyribonucleoside diphosphates in humans.
    (b) It catalyzes the homolytic cleavage of a bond.
    (c) It accepts electrons directly from $FADH_2$.
    (d) It receives electrons directly from thioredoxin.
    (e) It contains two kinds of allosteric regulatory sites—one for control of overall activity and another for control of substrate specificity.

19. Select from the following those compounds that are precursors of 2′-deoxythymidine-5-triphosphate (dTTP) in mammals and place them in their correct biosynthetic order.

    (a) OMP
    (b) UMP
    (c) UDP
    (d) UTP
    (e) dUMP

    (f) dUDP
    (g) dUTP
    (h) dTMP
    (i) dTDP
    (j) dTTP

20. Define *suicide inhibitor* and give an example from pyrimidine biosynthesis.
21. Methotrexate and trimethoprim are both inhibitors of dihyrofolate reductase. Why is trimethoprim the drug of choice in treating a human microbial infection?

Nucleotide Biosynthesis Is Regulated by Feedback Inhibition

22. What is the committed step in purine biosynthesis and which of the following compounds are involved in the control of the purine biosynthetic pathway?

    (a) IMP
    (b) AMP
    (c) OMP

    (d) GMP
    (e) PRPP

23. For each of the following, indicate the effect it would have on ribonucleotide reductase activity

    (a) dATP
    (b) ATP

    (c) TTP
    (d) dGTP

Disruptions in Nucleotide Metabolism Can Cause Pathological Conditions

24. What is the biochemical deficiency that leads to severe combined immunodeficiency disease?

    (a) nucleoside phosphorylase
    (b) xanthine oxidase
    (c) adenosine deaminase
    (d) all of the above.

25. Which of the following compounds would give rise to urate if they were catabolized completely in humans?

    (a) ADP-glucose
    (b) GDP-mannose
    (c) CDP-choline
    (d) UDP-galactose

    (e) CoA
    (f) FAD
    (g) UMP

26. What is the benefit of high serum levels of urate in humans, given that too much urate leads to gout?

ANSWERS TO SELF-TEST

1. The nucleotides (1) are the activated precursors of DNA and RNA; (2) are the source of derivatives that are activated intermediates in many biosyntheses; (3) include ATP, the universal currency of energy in biological systems, and GTP, which powers many movements of macromolecules; (4) include the adenine nucleotides, which are components of the major coenzymes NAD^+, FAD, and CoA; and (5) serve as metabolic regulators.

2. b

3. c, d. Nucleotides are nucleosides that contain one or more phosphate substituents on their ribose or deoxyribose moieties.

4. b, d. The mitochondrial carbamoyl phosphate synthetase used for urea synthesis is activated by N-acetylglutamate and uses NH_4^+ as the nitrogen source. CPS II uses 2 moles of ATP in the synthesis of CP.

5. a, c

6. Orotate condenses with PRPP in a reaction catalyzed by orotate phosphoribosyl transferase to form the nucleotide orotidylate (OMP). Orotidylate decarboxylase converts OMP to the more abundant nucleotide UMP. The reaction occurs during de novo pyrimidine biosynthesis and is therefore not a salvage reaction.

7. b, c. Several different specific nucleoside monophosphate kinases phosphorylate dNMPs and NMPs, using ATP as the phosphoryl donor. A single enzyme, nucleoside diphosphate kinase, uses the phosphorylation potential of ATP to convert the dNDPs and NDPs to dNTPs and NTPs. The ubiquitous adenylate nucleotides are interconverted by adenylate kinase (myokinase).

8. CTP is formed by amination of UTP. The carbonyl oxygen at C-4 of UTP is replaced with an amino group via the formation of an enol phosphate ester intermediate. In *E. coli*, NH_4^+ serves as the source of the nitrogen atom that displaces the phosphate group, whereas the amide group of glutamine serves this purpose in mammals.

9. d. Answer d is incorrent because the mammalian and viral versions of TK are quite different, a fact that has been utilized in the development of anti-viral drugs.

10. a, c, d, e, g

11. c

12. b, c

13. a, d, e

14. c, d

15. The activated form of ribose 5-phosphate (R-5-P), PRPP, reacts with the purine base to form the nucleotide and release PP$_i$. The displacement and subsequent hydrolysis of PP$_i$ drives the formation of the N-glycosyl bond. ATP ultimately provides the energy through its reaction with R-5-P to form PRPP.

16. (a) 1, 2, 3   (b) 1, 2, 3   (c) none   (d) 1   (e) 2

17. Researchers have fused different enzymes of the purine biosynthetic pathway with the fluorescent protein GFP. They then observed the GFP in cells that had been switched to growth media lacking in purines to see how the cellular localization would change upon initiation of purine synthesis. They observed that the enzymes were spread diffusely throughout the cell in the absence of purine synthesis, but were localized to cytoplasmic granules called purinosomes upon intiation of purine synthesis. Additional evidence suggests a role for phosphorylation in the assembly.

18. a, b, d, e. NADPH provides electrons via thioredoxin.

19. a, b, c, f, g, e, h, i, j. In mammals, NDPs are converted to dNDPs by ribonucleotide reductase. Thus, UDP is converted to dUDP, which is converted to dUTP by nucleoside diphosphate kinase. A specific pyrophosphatase hydrolyzes dUTP to dUMP, which is then converted to dTMP by thymidylate synthase. The dTMP is converted to dTTP. A priori, you might have expected the dUDP product of the ribonucleotide reductase reaction to be converted directly to dUMP. However, in fact, cells contain a dUTP pyrophosphatase to prevent dUTP from serving as a DNA precursor, and it is this enzyme that functions in the dTTP biosynthetic pathway.

20. A suicide inhibitor is a substrate that is converted by an enzyme into a substance that is capable of reacting with and inactivating the enzyme. In pyrimidine biosynthesis, thymidylate synthase converts fluorouracil into a derivative that becomes covalently attached to the enzyme and thereby inactivates it.

21. Since trimethoprim binds to the mammalian dihydrofolate reductase much less tightly than to the enzyme of susceptible microorganisms, it causes fewer deleterious effects to humans than does methotrexate.

22. The conversion of PRPP into phosphoribosylamine by *glutamine phosphoryl amidotransferase* is the committed step in purine biosynthesis. Compounds a, b, and d are involved in the regulation.

23. All of the molecules bind to the specificity site, but only ATP and dATP bind to the activity site.
    (a) Lowers activity when bound to activity site; enhances reduction of UDP and CDP when bound to specificity site.
    (b) Reverses effect of dATP on activity site; same effect as dATP on specificity site.
    (c) Enhances reduction of GDP; inhibits pyrimidine reduction.
    (d) Enhances reduction of ATP.

24. a, b, e, f. Each of these compounds contains a heterocyclic purine base.

25. Urate levels in humans are often close to the solubility limit, which leads to gout when salts of urate crystallize (resulting in damage to joints and kidneys). There is a significant benefit to high concentrations of urate, however, as urate is a highly effective scavenger of reactive oxygen species (ROS). ROS can cause damage in cells contributing to cancer and the effects of aging. Urate is about as effective as ascorbate (vitamin C) as an antioxidant.

26. (c)

PROBLEMS

1. Why might covalently linked (multifunctional) enzymes, such as those of the pyrimidine biosynthetic pathway of mammals, be advantageous to an organism?

2. Mammalian lymphocytes that lack adenosine deaminase neither grow nor divide. The level of dATP in these cells is 100 times higher than that in normal lymphocytes, and the synthesis of DNA in the cells is impaired.
   (a) How is adenosine converted to dATP? Assume that the first step is catalyzed by a specific nucleoside kinase.
   (b) How does the elevation in dATP concentration in the abnormal lymphocytes affect the synthesis of DNA?

3. Clinicians who use F-dUMP and methotrexate *together* in cancer treatment find that the combined effects on cancer cells are not synergistic. Suggest how the administration of methotrexate could interfere with the action of F-dUMP.

4. Elevated levels of ammonia in the blood can be caused by a deficiency of mitochondrial carbamoyl phosphate synthetase or a deficiency of any of the urea cycle enzymes. These two types of disorders can be distinguished by the presence of orotic acid or related metabolites in the urine.

   (a) Why is it possible to determine the basis of hyperammonemia in this way?
   (b) Why would a deficiency of cytoplasmic carbamoyl phosphate synthetase not cause hyperammonemia? What problems would such an enzyme deficiency cause? How would you treat a patient who has a deficiency in cytoplasmic carbamoyl phosphate synthetase?

5. The degradation of thymine yields β-aminoisobutyrate, as shown in the figure below, which can be converted to succinyl CoA and then degraded in the citric acid cycle. What cofactors are needed to convert β-aminoisobutyrate to succinyl CoA?

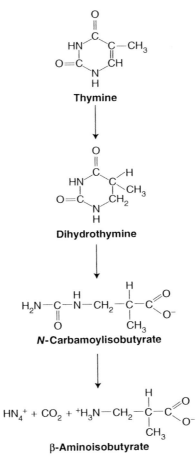

6. You wish to prepare 14C-labeled purines by growing bacteria in a medium containing a suitably labeled precursor. The only precursors available are amino acids that are all uniformly labeled to the same specific activity per carbon atom. Which of the amino acids would you use to obtain purine rings that are labeled to the highest specific activity?

7. 6-Mercaptopurine (6-MP) can be converted to the corresponding nucleotide 6-thioinosine-5′-monophosphate (tIMP) through the purine salvage pathway. tIMP can

then be converted to 6-thioguanine nucleotides (6-TNG) or methylated to form Me-tIMP. Methotrexate (MTX) increases incorporation of 6-TNGs through the salvage pathway (Bokkerink et al., *Hematol. Blood Transf.* 33(1990):110–117). Both 6-MP and MTX are clinically useful anticancer agents and have been used together for many years in the treatment of childhood leukemia in part because of the synergistic effect they have on each other.

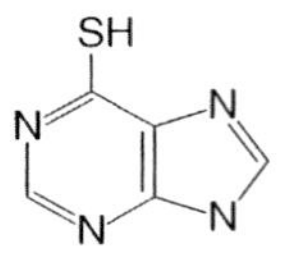

6-Mercaptopurine

(a) Briefly describe the salvage reactions required to convert 6-MP to the corresponding nucleotide.

(b) What step in the de novo biosynthesis of purines is likely to be inhibited by tIMP?

(c) How could the presence of MTX increase the incorporation of 6-TNG into DNA and RNA?

8. Methotrexate, a folate antagonist, interferes with nucleic acid biosynthesis. Would you expect it to inhibit purine or pyrimidine biosynthesis or both processes? Explain.

9. Nucleoside phosphorylases catalyze the interconversion of bases and nucleosides through the following reactions:

$$\text{Ribose 1-phosphate} + \text{base} \longrightarrow \text{ribonucleoside} + P_i$$

or

$$\text{Deoxyribose 1-phosphate} + \text{base} \longrightarrow \text{deoxyribonucleoside} + P_i$$

The equilibrium constant for each of these reactions is close to 1.

(a) The pathway for the incorporation of radioactive thymine into bacterial DNA includes a step catalyzed by nucleoside phosphorylase. It has often been observed that the incorporation of thymine into DNA is enhanced when deoxyadenosine or deoxyguanosine is added to the medium. Can you explain this observation? Why might deoxyguanosine be preferable to deoxyadenosine?

(b) In cells that cannot carry out de novo synthesis of IMP, inosine can be utilized to produce IMP but only through an indirect salvage route because of the absence of inosine kinase. Suggest an alternative pathway for the formation of IMP from inosine. Among the enzymes you will need are nucleoside phosphorylase and phosphoribomutase, which isomerizes ribose 1-phosphate to ribose 5-phosphate.

10. Hypoxanthine-guanine phosphoribosyl transferase (HGPRT), a salvage enzyme of nucleotide metabolism, uses 5′-phosphoribosylpyrophosphate (PRPP) to convert hypoxanthine to IMP and guanine to GMP. A deficiency of this enzyme can lead to an increased level of purine synthesis, excess formation of uric acid, and hyperuricemia, or gout.

(a) How might a deficiency in HGPRT stimulate purine synthesis?

(b) Under what conditions might one expect a deficiency of hypoxanthine-guanine phosphoribosyl transferase to affect the rate of *pyrimidine* nucleotide synthesis? How could you estimate the rate of pyrimidine nucleotide synthesis in humans?

11. In mammals, the committed step for pyrimidine synthesis is catalyzed by carbamoyl phosphate synthetase, while in bacteria, the committed step is the formation of N-carbamoyl-aspartate, catalyzed by aspartate transcarbamoylase.

    (a) Account for these differences in mammals and bacteria.
    (b) Bacterial carbamoyl phosphate synthetase is only partially inhibited by UMP. Why?

12. The synthesis of deoxythymidylate can proceed not only from dUMP but also from dCMP. The route from dCMP begins with the formation of dCDP from CDP, catalyzed by ribonucleotide reductase, followed by dephosphorylation to dCMP, and the deamination of dCMP to form dUMP, catalyzed by dCMP deaminase.

$$dCMP \; + \; H_2O \; + \; H^+ \longrightarrow dUMP \; + \; NH_3^+$$

dCMP deaminase is an allosteric enzyme that is stimulated by dCTP and inhibited by dTTP. Account for these effects and relate them to the regulation of ribonucleotide reductase by deoxynucleoside triphosphates.

ANSWERS TO PROBLEMS

1. The clustering of two or more enzymes (active sites) in a single polypeptide chain ensures that their synthesis is coordinated and helps assure that they will assemble into a coherent complex. Also, the proximity of the active sites means that side reactions are minimized as substrates are channeled from one active site to another. Finally, a multifunctional complex with covalently linked active sites is likely to be more stable than a complex formed by noncovalent interactions.

2. (a) Adenosine is phosphorylated to AMP, with ATP serving as the phosphoryl donor, in a reaction carried out by a specific nucleoside kinase. The conversion of AMP to ADP through the action of a specific nucleoside monophosphate kinase is accomplished, with ATP again utilized as a phosphate donor. Ribonucleotide reductase catalyzes the reduction of ADP to dADP, which is then converted to dATP by nucleotide diphosphokinase.

   (b) High concentrations of dATP displace ATP from the overall activity site on ribonucleotide reductase, which lowers the rate of synthesis of all four deoxyribonucleoside diphosphates. This, in turn, leads to a depletion of deoxyribonucleoside triphosphates, which are the substrates for DNA synthesis.

3. Methotrexate blocks the regeneration of tetrahydrofolate from dihydrofolate, which is produced during the synthesis of thymidylate. The failure to regenerate tetrahydrofolate means that those biochemical reactions in the cell that depend on one-carbon metabolism cannot be carried out. One of the products of tetrahydrofolate is methylenetetrahydrofolate, which is used as a substrate by thymidylate synthetase and is required for inhibition of the enzyme by F-dUMP. A deficiency of methylenetetrahydrofolate means that F-dUMP cannot irreversibly inactivate thymidylate synthetase. Conversely, F-dUMP prevents the formation of dihydrofolate, thereby abolishing the adverse effects caused by the depletion of tetrahydrofolate in the cell.

4. (a) The presence of orotic acid, a precursor of pyrimidines, in the urine suggests that carbamoyl phosphate synthesized in mitochondria is not utilized there. Instead, carbamoyl phosphate enters the cytosol, where it stimulates an increase in the rate of synthesis of precursors of pyrimidines, including orotic acid. An excess

of carbamoyl phosphate arises in mitochondria whenever any of the urea cycle enzymes are deficient. Such a condition will lead to hyperammonemia, as well as to the accumulation of carbamoyl phosphate. Although a deficiency in mitochondrial carbamoyl phosphate synthetase leads to hyperammonemia, it cannot lead to an accumulation of mitochondrial carbamoyl phosphate and therefore does not stimulate pyrimidine synthesis in the cytosol.

(b) Cytoplasmic carbamoyl phosphate synthetase is involved primarily in the pathway for pyrimidine synthesis, not for the assimilation of ammonia. Recall that, in the cytosol, the substrate for the formation of carbamoyl phosphate is glutamine, not ammonia. A deficiency of carbamoyl phosphate synthesis in the cytosol would cause a depletion of pyrimidines. Such a deficiency is treated by administration of uracil or uridine, which are precursors of UMP and CMP.

5. The transamination of β-aminoisobutyrate to form methylmalonate semialdehyde requires pyridoxal phosphate as a cofactor. This reaction is similar to the conversion of ornithine to glutamate γ-semialdehyde. Then NAD+ serves as an electron acceptor for the oxidation of methylmalonate semialdehyde to methylmalonate. The conversion of methylmalonate to methylmalonyl CoA requires coenzyme A. The final reaction, in which methylmalonyl CoA is converted to succinyl CoA, is catalyzed by methylmalonyl CoA mutase, an enzyme that contains a derivative of vitamin B_{12} as its coenzyme.

6. Examination of the pathway for purine synthesis shows that only glycine is incorporated intact into the purine ring at the C-4 and C-5 positions. Therefore, glycine is a good choice as the radiolabeled precursor. Serine can also be considered because it is a precursor of glycine and the ultimate donor of C-1 groups to tetrahydrofolate, and activated tetrahydrofolate derivatives participate in two reactions in the formation of purines. Whether serine is a better choice than glycine depends on the relative amounts of the two unlabeled amino acids in the cell.

7. (a) 6-Mercaptopurine is converted to the mononucleotide through the action of hypoxanthine-guanine phosphoribosyl transferase (HGPRT), which uses PRPP to add 5′-phosphoribose to the purine ring. The resulting compound is 6-thioinosine-5′-monophosphate, an analog of IMP.

(b) IMP (and presumably its analog 6-MP) inhibits Gln-PRPP aminotransferase, which catalyzes the committed step of purine biosynthesis. The 6-MP metabolite Me-tIMP may be involved in the inhibition of Gln-PRPP aminotransferase as well (Stet et al., *Biochem. Journal* 304(1994):163–168).

(c) MTX inhibits folate-dependent enzymes in the de novo purine biosynthetic pathway leading to an accumulation of PRPP. This increase in substrate availability for the salvage pathway leads to a greater conversion of 6-MP into 6-TNG and therefore a higher level of incorporation of 6-TNGs into DNA. Also, since 6-MP is a substrate for HGPRT—see part (a)—it can compete with endogenous purine bases for HGPRT, leading to a decrease in the synthesis of AMP and GMP.

8. Methotrexate and aminopterin, a similar compound, are analogs of dihydrofolate (DHF) and inhibitors of dihydrofolate reductase, an enzyme that converts DHF to tetrahydrofolate (THF). The thymidylate synthase reaction converts N^5,N^{10}-methylenetetrahydrofolate to DHF in the process of methylating dUMP to form dTMP. In the presence of one of the inhibitors, this reaction functions as a sink that reduces the THF level of the cell by converting THF to DHF. Since THF derivatives are substrates in two reactions of purine metabolism and one of pyrimidine metabolism, both pathways are affected by the inhibitor.

9. (a) Deoxyribonucleosides such as deoxyadenosine can be converted to the free base and deoxyribose 1-phosphate by nucleoside phosphorylase. Increased levels of deoxyribose 1-phosphate are then available for the formation of deoxythymidine from thymine in the reverse reaction catalyzed by nucleoside phosphorylase. Deoxyguanosine might be preferable to deoxyadenosine because the conversion of elevated levels of deoxyadenosine to dAMP and then to dATP could lead to the inactivation of ribonucleotide reductase, which is sensitive to the concentration of dATP.

   (b) Inosine is cleaved to produce hypoxanthine and ribose 1-phosphate through the action of nucleoside phosphorylase; note that inorganic phosphate is required for this reaction. Hypoxanthine-guanine phosphoribosyl transferase converts free hypoxanthine to IMP by condensation with PRPP. PRPP can be derived from ribose 1-phosphate in two steps: (1) the conversion of ribose 1-phosphate to ribose 5-phosphate, which is catalyzed by phosphoribomutase; and (2) the formation of PRPP from ribose 5-phosphate and ATP, which is catalyzed by PRPP synthetase.

10. (a) When active, HGPRT consumes PRPP as it catalyzes the synthesis of GMP and IMP. Decreased flux through this reaction raises the steady-state level of PRPP, thereby increasing the activity of PRPP amidotransferase, which catalyzes the initial step in purine synthesis. Increased activity may make the amidotransferase resistant to feedback inhibition by AMP and GMP, the end products of the purine biosynthetic pathway.

    (b) As noted above, decreased activity of HGPRT increases the concentration of PRPP. This increases the rate of pyrimidine synthesis at the orotate phosphoribosyl transferase reaction, if PRPP levels are normally subsaturating for that enzyme. Orotate incorporation into nucleotide pools or into nucleic acids would give a reasonable estimate of de novo pyrimidine nucleotide synthesis.

11. (a) Bacteria use a single form of carbamoyl phosphate synthetase not only for the synthesis of pyrimidines but also for the synthesis of arginine. Arginine biosynthesis begins with glutamate and includes formation of citrulline from ornithine and carbamoyl phosphate, a pathway that resembles urea formation in mammals. Two forms of carbamoyl phosphate synthetase, a cytoplasmic form for pyrimidine synthesis and a mitochondrial form for arginine and urea synthesis, are employed in mammals. Because the two pathways are compartmentalized, the formation of carbamoyl phosphate in the cytosol is regarded as the committed step for pyrimidine synthesis.

    (b) UMP does not completely inhibit bacterial carbamoyl phosphate synthetase because that inhibition would interfere with arginine production.

12. An increase in dCTP levels signals that the cell has ample deoxynucleotides for DNA synthesis and that there is a need for thymidylate synthesis. An increase in dTTP levels signals that the activity of thymidylate synthase can be decreased, and the inhibition of dCMP deaminase by dTTP reduces the input of dUMP into the pathway. While ribonucleotide reductase is subject to regulation by other deoxynucleotides, it is not subject to allosteric regulation by dCTP. Instead it appears that regulation of dCMP deaminase provides a second control point for the generation of deoxynucleotides in the cell.

The Structure of Informational Macromolecules

In this chapter the authors begin to look at nucleic acids, which serve as the storage forms of genetic information and are critical participants in the elaboration of this information into functional forms. First, they describe the structures of the nucleoside building blocks of DNA and the phosphodiester bond that links them together. Following this, the Watson-Crick DNA double helix is presented, an overview of how the strands of DNA separate for replication is given, and some of the various conformations and structures that nucleic acids can assume are described. Next the authors discuss the binding of proteins to eukaryotic DNA, particularly the basic proteins known as histones. The formation of nucleosomes from DNA and histones and the formation of chromatin from nucleosomes is detailed.

The chapter finishes with a discussion of the structures that RNA can adopt, emphasizing the role of non-Watson-Crick basepairing.

LEARNING OBJECTIVES

When you have mastered this chapter, you should be able to accomplish the following objectives.

Introduction

1. State the names of the four bases posing DNA and their relative ratios.

A Nucleic Acid Consists of Bases Linked to a Sugar Phosphate Backbone

(Text Section 33.1)

2. Locate the structural components of DNA, namely, the *nitrogenous bases*, the *sugar,* and the *phosphate* group. Know the various conventions used to represent these components and the structure of DNA. Know how the carbon atoms are numbered.

3. Differentiate *purines, pyrimidines, ribonucleosides, deoxyribonucleosides, ribonucleotides,* and *deoxyribonucleotides.*

4. Recognize the *deoxyadenosine, deoxycytidine, deoxyguanosine,* and *deoxythymidine* constituents of DNA, and describe the *phosphodiester* bond that joins them together to form DNA.

5. Compare the *phosphodiester backbones* of RNA and DNA. Contrast the composition and structures of RNA and DNA. Distinguish *thymine* from *uracil* and *2′-deoxyribose* from *ribose.* Understand the effect that a 2′-OH has on structure and base lability.

6. Relate the *polarity of the DNA* chain (5′→3′) to the convention for writing a single-letter DNA sequence abbreviation.

7. Compare the lengths of the DNA molecules in polyoma virus, the bacterium *E. coli,* and the average human chromosome.

Nucleic Acid Strands Can Form a Double-Helical Structure (Text Section 33.2)

8. List the important features of the *Watson-Crick DNA double helix* including its dimensions. Relate the *base pairing* of *adenine* with *thymine* and of *cytosine* with *guanine* to the duplex structure of DNA and to the replication of the helix. Explain the molecular determinants of the specific base pairs in DNA.

9. Explain the forces that stabilize the double helix.

10. Outline the *Meselson-Stahl experiment* and relate it to *semiconservative replication.*

11. Define *the melting temperature* (T_m) for DNA and relate it to the separation of the strands of duplex DNA. Describe *annealing.*

DNA Double Helices Can Adopt Multiple Forms (Text Section 33.3)

12. Describe the variety of structures that double stranded and *single-stranded nucleic acids* can assume.

13. Explain the structural origin of the major and minor grooves of B-DNA. Describe the hydrogen bond donors and acceptors in each group and explain why the major groove binds more DNA-binding proteins than the minor groove.

14. Describe *supercoiling* and state its biological consequences.

15. Define *topoisomers* and explain why negative supercoiling is the most common in naturally occurring DNA.

Eukaryotic DNA Is Associated With Specific Proteins (Text Section 33.4)

16. Describe the composition of chromatin. List the types of *histones* and describe their general characteristics. Note the evolutionary stability of the sequences of the H2A, H2B, H3, and H4 histones and assign the types of histones to their locations within the *nucleosome.*

17. Describe the composition and structure of the nucleosome and relate the nucleosome to the proposed structure of the chromatin fiber.

18. Distinguish between the DNA associated with the nucleosome core and that in the internucleosome linker.

19. Explain how cisplatin disrupts the structure of DNA and leads to its use as a chemotherapy drug.

RNA Can Adopt Elaborate Structures (Text Section 33.5)

20. Describe the stem-loop structure and explain the role of nonstandard Watson-Crick base pairing in the stabilization of the structure.

SELF-TEST

A Nucleic Acid Consists of Bases Linked to a Sugar Phosphate Backbone

FIGURE 33.1

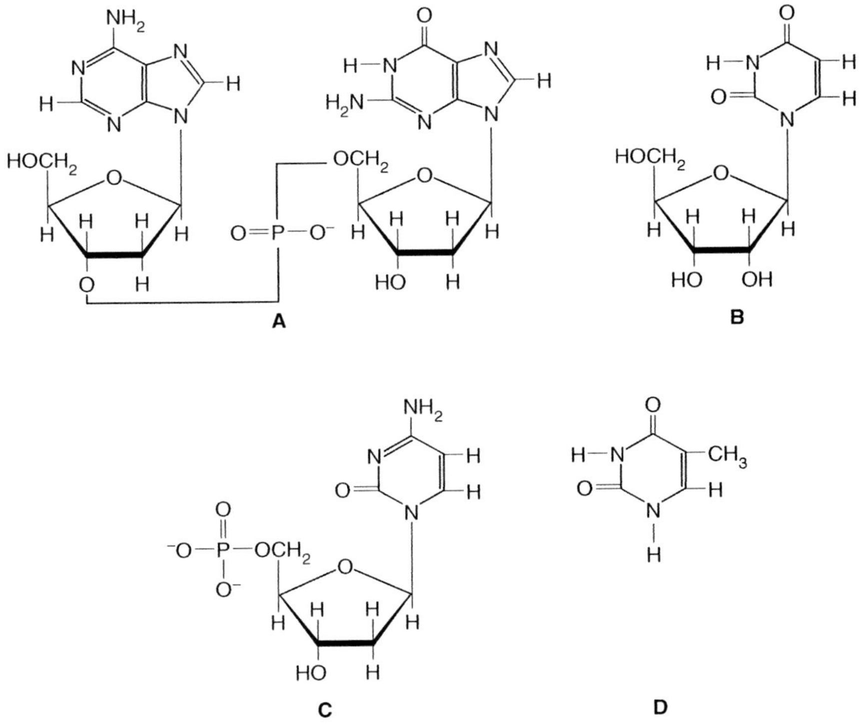

1. Which of the preceding structures in Figure 33.1
   (a) contains ribose?
   (b) contains deoxyribose?
   (c) contains a purine?
   (d) contains a pyrimidine?
   (e) contains guanine?
   (f) contains a phosphate monoester?
   (g) contains a phosphodiester?
   (h) is a nucleoside?
   (i) is a nucleotide?
   (j) would be found in RNA?
   (k) would be found in DNA?

Nucleic Acid Strands Can Form a Double-Helical Structure

2. Which of the following are characteristics of the Watson-Crick DNA double helix?

   (a) The two polynucleotide chains are coiled about one another and about a common axis.
   (b) Hydrogen bonds between A and C and between G and T help hold the two chains together.
   (c) The helix makes one complete turn every 34Å because each base pair is rotated by 36° with respect to adjacent base pairs and is separated by 3.4Å from them along the helix axis.
   (d) The purines and pyrimidines are on the inside of the helix and the phosphodiester-linked backbones are on the outside.
   (e) Base composition analyses of DNA duplexes isolated from many organisms show that the amounts of A and T are equal as are the amounts of G and C.
   (f) The sequence in one strand of the helix varies independently of that in the other strand.

3. If a region of one strand of a Watson-Crick DNA double helix has the sequence ACGTAACC, what is the sequence of the complementary region of the other strand?

4. Explain why A · T and G · C are the only base pairs possible in normal double-strand DNA.

5. Match the appropriate characteristics in the right column with the structures of double-strand or single-strand DNA.

   (a) double-strand DNA
   (b) single-strand DNA

   (1) is a rigid rod
   (2) shows a greater hyperchromic effect upon heating
   (3) contains equal amounts of A and T bases
   (4) may contain different amounts of C and G bases
   (5) contains U rather than T bases
   (6) may contain stem-loop structures

6. Haploid human DNA has 3×10^6 kilobase pairs (a kilobase pair, abbreviated kb, is 1000 base pairs). What is the total length of human haploid DNA in centimeters?

7. Outline the basic process by which a Watson-Crick duplex replicates to give two identical daughter duplexes. Explain the molecular reasons for the accuracy of the process.

8. The DNA in a bacterium is uniformly labeled with ^{15}N, and the organism shifted to a growth medium containing ^{14}N-labeled DNA precursors. After two generations of

growth, the DNA is isolated and is subjected to density-gradient equilibrium sedimentation. What proportion of light-density DNA to intermediate-density DNA would you expect to find?

9. Purified duplex DNA molecules can be
   (a) linear.
   (b) circular and supercoiled.
   (c) linear and supercoiled.
   (d) circular and relaxed, that is, not supercoiled.

10. You are given two solutions containing different purified DNAs. One is from the bacterium *P. aeruginosa* and has a G + C composition of 68%, whereas the other is from a mammal and has a G + C composition of 42.5%.
    (a) You measure the absorbance of ultraviolet light of each solution as a function of increasing temperature. Which solution will yield the higher T_m value and why?
    (b) After melting the two solutions, mixing them together, and allowing them to cool, what would you expect to happen?
    (c) Would appreciable amounts of bacterial DNA be found associated in a helix with mammalian DNA? Explain.

Eukaryotic DNA Is Associated with Specific Proteins

11. What is a primary consequence of the folding of chromatin on gene regulation?

12. Which of the following statements about histones are correct?
    (a) They are highly basic because they contain many positively charged amino acid side chains.
    (b) They are extensively modified after their translation.
    (c) In combination with DNA, they are the primary constituents of chromatin.
    (d) They account for approximately one-fifth of the mass of a chromosome.

13. Which of the following statements about nucleosomes are correct?
    (a) They constitute the repeating units of a chromatin fiber.
    (b) Each contains a core of eight histones.
    (c) They contain DNA that is surrounded by a coating of histones.
    (d) They occur in chromatin in association with approximately 200 base pairs of DNA, on average.

14. Describe the structure of the nucleosome.

15. Does the formation of nucleosomes account for the observed packing ratio of human metaphase chromosomes? Explain.

RNA Can Adopt Elaborate Structures

16. Answer the following questions about RNA.
    (a) What is the name of the bond joining the ribonucleoside components of RNA to one another?
    (b) Is this bond between the 2'- or the 3'-hydroxyl group of one ribose and the 5'-hydroxyl of the next?
    (c) Intramolecular base pairs form what kinds of structures in RNA molecules?
    (d) What bases pair with one another in RNA?

17. If you have samples of pure RNA and duplex DNA, how can you tell whether they have any complementary nucleotide sequences?

18. If all the RNA referred to in Question 17 turns out to have sequences that were complementary to the DNA, will its percentage of G and C be identical to that of the DNA? Explain.

ANSWERS TO SELF-TEST

1. (a) B (b) A, C (c) A (d) B, C, D (e) A (f) C (g) A (h) B (i) C; strictly speaking, A is called a dinucleotide, not a nucleotide (j) B (k) A, C, D

2. a, c, d, and e. Answer (b) is not correct because A pairs with T and G pairs with C. Answer (f) is not correct because the sequence of one strand determines the sequence of the other by base pairing.

3. GGTTACGT. The convention for indicating polarity is that the 5′-end of the sequence is written to the left. The two chains of the Watson-Crick double helix are antiparallel, so the correct complementary sequence is not TGCATTGG.

4. The space between the two deoxyribose-phosphodiester strands is precisely defined. This distance is not large enough for two purines to hydrogen-bond. Conversely, two pyrimidine bases would not be close enough to form stable hydrogen bonds. Furthermore, in the double-strand structure the hydrogen-bond donor and acceptor groups are not properly aligned to form stable G · T or A · C base pairs.

5. (a) 1, 2, 3 (b) 4, 6. Answer (5) does not apply because DNA does not contain uracil.

6. 102 cm. The math is as follows:

$$(3 \times 10^6 \text{ kb} \times 10^3 \text{ bases/kb} \times 3.4 \text{ Å/base} \times 10^{-8} \text{ cm/Å}) = 102 \text{ cm}$$

7. When replication occurs, the two strands of the Watson-Crick double helix must separate so that each can serve as a template for the synthesis of its complement. Since the two strands are complementary to one another, each bears a definite sequence relationship to the other. When one strand acts as a template, it directs the synthesis of its complement. The product of the synthesis directed by each template strand is therefore a duplex molecule that is identical to the starting duplex. The process is accurate because of the specificity of base pairing and because the protein apparatus that catalyzes the replication can remove mismatched bases.

8. After two generations, you should expect to find equal amounts of light-density DNA, in which both strands of each duplex were synthesized from ^{14}N precursors, and intermediate-density DNA, in which each duplex consists of a heavy ^{15}N strand paired with a light ^{14}N strand.

9. a, b, and d. Answer (d) is correct because, if at least one discontinuity exists in the phosphodiester backbone of either chain of a circular duplex molecule, the chains are free to rotate about one another to assume the relaxed circular form. Answer (c) is incorrect because supercoiling requires closed circular molecules. In a linear molecule, the ends of each strand are not constrained with respect to rotation about the helical axis; therefore, the molecule cannot be supercoiled.

10. (a) The bacterial DNA solution has the higher T_m value because it has the higher G + C content and is therefore more stable to the thermal-induced separation of its strands because G · C base pairs are more stable than A · T base pairs.

    (b) The complementary DNA strands from each species will anneal to form Watson-Crick double helices as the solution cools.

    (c) No; each strand will find its partner because the perfect match between the linear arrays of the bases of complementary strands is far more stable than the mostly imperfect matches in duplexes composed of one strand of bacterial and one strand of mammalian DNA would be.

11. The tight folding of chromatin renders many of the sites on DNA inaccessible to the proteins that must be assembled to form an active transcription complex. Chromatin structure decreases the amount of DNA available to nonchromatin proteins. Remodeling of chromatin makes some of these sites accessible.

12. a, b, c. Answer (d) is incorrect because histones make up nearly half the mass of a chromosome.

13. a, b, d. A nucleosome core consists of ~145 base pairs of DNA wrapped around a histone octamer. The nucleosome cores are connected by linker DNA, which contains from fewer than 20 to more than 100 base pairs (bp), the exact length depending on the organism and the tissue. The average length is ~200 bp.

14. The nucleosome core has a disk shape and is composed of eight histone molecules. The octameric core of histones has ~145 base pairs of DNA wound about it in approximately 1 3/4 turns of a left-handed torroidal supercoil. Two copies each of histones H2A, H2B, H3, and H4 are on the inside of the toroidal coil, whereas histone H1 is associated with the DNA where it emerges from the core. Each core histone has a basic tail that protrudes from the core structure. In total, ~200 bp of DNA is present per nucleosome.

15. No. As mentioned, each nucleosome is associated with approximately 200 base pairs of DNA. If this DNA were coiled into a sphere with a diameter of approximately 100 Å, it would be condensed from 200 base pairs × 3.4 Å per base pair = 680 Å of linear DNA to 100 Å, which is a packing ratio of about 7. The chromatin fiber, which is composed of a helical array of nucleosomes, must be formed, and the resulting 360 Å coils must themselves be looped and folded. Scaffolding proteins, topoisomerases, and small basic molecules, such as the polyamines, also contribute to the ultimate compaction of 104 that is observed in metaphase chromosomes.

16. (a) The bond is called the phosphodiester bond.

    (b) The bond joins the 3'-hydroxyl to the 5'-hydroxyl to form a 3' $\longrightarrow$ 5' phosphodiester bond.

    (c) Hairpin loops are formed when the RNA chain folds back upon itself and some of the bases become hydrogen bonded to form an antiparallel duplex stem with unpaired bases forming a loop at one end.

    (d) A pairs with U, and G pairs with C; G can also pair with U, but the association is weaker than that of the G · C base pair.

17. You could sequence the RNA and DNA and compare the sequences of each to see if the two are complementary; this method provides definitive evidence of identity. An easier but less precise way would be to use hybridization. You would mix the samples, heat the mixture to melt the double-strand DNA and RNA hairpins, slowly cool the solution, and then examine it to see if it contains double-strand DNA-RNA hybrids. Such hybrids would indicate that the RNA and DNA sequences are complementary.

18. Not necessarily; RNA synthesis is asymmetric, and generally only one strand of any region of the DNA serves as a template. This can lead to RNA with a G + C composition different from that of the duplex DNA.

PROBLEMS

1. A number of factors influence the behavior of a linear, double-strand DNA molecule in a 0.25M sodium chloride solution. Considering this, explain each of the following observations.

   (a) The T_m increases in proportion to length of the molecule.
   (b) As the concentration of sodium chloride decreases, the T_m decreases.
   (c) Renaturation of single strands to form double strands occurs more rapidly when the DNA concentration is increased.
   (d) The T_m value is reduced when urea is added to the solution.

2. (a) Many proteins that interact with double-strand DNA bind to specific sequences in the molecule. Why is it unlikely that these enzymes operate by sensing differences in the diameter of the helix?
   (b) What other features of the double-strand helix might be recognized by the protein?

3. Certain deoxyribonucleases cleave any sequence of single-strand DNA to yield nucleoside monophosphates; these enzymes do not hydrolyze base-paired DNA sequences. What products would you expect when you incubate a solution containing a single-strand specific deoxyribonuclease and the following oligodeoxyribonucleotide?

   5'-ApGpTpCpGpTpApTpCpCpTpCpTpApCpGpApCpTp-3'

4. Formaldehyde reacts with amino groups to form hydroxymethyl derivatives. Would you expect formaldehyde to react with bases in DNA? Suppose you have a solution that contains separated complementary strands of DNA. How would the addition of formaldehyde to the solution affect reassociation of the strands?

5. When double-strand DNA is placed in a solution containing tritiated water (^3H_2O), hydrogens associated with the bases readily exchange with protons in the solution. The greater the percentage of AT base pairs in the DNA, the greater the rate of exchange. Why?

6. The value of the T_m for DNA in degrees Celsius can be calculated using the formula, $T_m = 69.3 + 0.41(G + C)$, where G + C is the mole percentage of guanine plus cytosine.

   (a) A sample of DNA from E. coli contains 50 mole percent G + C. At what temperature would you expect this DNA molecule to melt?
   (b) The melting curves for most naturally occurring DNA molecules reveal that their T_m values are normally greater than 65°C. Why is this important for most organisms?
   (c) What problem concerning replication does a T_m value > 65°C imply?

7. During early studies of the denaturation of double-strand DNA, it was not known whether the two strands unwind and completely separate from each other. Suppose that you have double-strand DNA in which one strand is labeled with ^{14}N and the other is labeled with ^{15}N. If density-gradient equilibrium sedimentation can be used to distinguish between both double- and single-strand molecules of different densities, how can you determine whether DNA strands separate completely after denaturation?

8. Under strongly acidic conditions, several atoms of DNA bases are protonated; these include the N-1 of adenine, the N-3 of cytosine, and the O-4 of thymine. Predict the effects of such protonations occurring at low pH on the stability of double-strand DNA.

9. The microbiologist Sol Spiegelman found that some types of single-strand RNA can associate with single-strand DNA to form double-strand molecules. What is the most

important condition that must be satisfied in order to allow the formation of these hybrid molecules?

10. Many cells can synthesize deoxyuridine 5′-triphosphate (dUTP). Can dUTP be used as a substrate for DNA polymerase? If so, with which base will uracil pair in newly replicated DNA?

11. The DNA of bacteriophage λ is a linear double-strand molecule that has complementary single-strand ends. These molecules can form closed-circular molecules when two "cohesive" ends on the same molecule join, and they can form linear dimers, trimers, or longer molecules when sites on different molecules are joined.

    (a) What conditions should be chosen *in vitro* to ensure that λ phage DNA molecules form closed-circular monomers?

    (b) Under certain conditions, λ phage DNA molecules are infective. When a very low concentration of λ phage DNA is incubated with DNA polymerase I and the four deoxyribonucleoside triphosphates, the infectious activity of λ phage DNA is destroyed. Brief treatment of λ phage DNA with bacterial exonuclease III, an enzyme that removes 5′-mononucleotides from the 3′-ends of double-strand DNA molecules also destroys infectivity, but subsequent treatment of the DNA with DNA polymerase I and dNTP substrates can restore infectivity. Describe more completely the structure of λ phage DNA, and provide an interpretation of the action of the two enzymes on the molecule.

12. The isolation of viral DNA from animal cells that have been infected with adenovirus yields linear double-strand molecules that, when denatured and allowed to reassociate under conditions favoring intramolecular annealing, form single-strand circles. Although circular molecules can be detected using the electron microscope, resolution is not sufficient to visualize the ends of the molecule. Other analyses of the single-strand molecule show that each end has a sequence that allows the structure shown in Figure 33.2 to form.

FIGURE 33.2   A single-strand circle formed by intra-molecular annealing of adenovirus DNA.

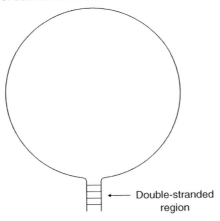

Double-stranded region

    (a) Suppose that the base sequence at one end of the single-strand molecule is 5′-ACTACGTA.... What is the corresponding sequence at the other end? Show how these sequences would allow full-length, double-strand linear molecules to be formed.

(b) An alternate suggestion for the formation of the single-strand molecules was also proposed; it is shown in Figure 33.3. Why is this proposed pairing scheme unlikely?

FIGURE 33.3 Another proposal for formation of single-stranded molecules of adenovirus DNA.

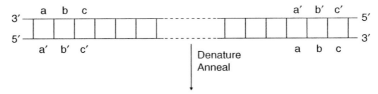

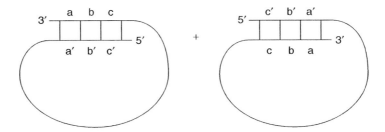

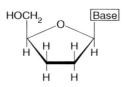

13. The 2′,3′-dideoxynucleosides can be used as reagents to inhibit DNA replication. These analogs must be converted to dideoxynucleoside triphosphates in order to have a measurable effect on DNA synthesis. When incorporated into a growing DNA chain, a single dideoxyribonucleoside residue can effectively block subsequent chain extension.

(a) Why must a 2′,3′-dideoxyribonucleoside be converted to a dideoxyribonucleoside triphosphate to be incorporated into DNA?

(b) What feature of a 2′,3′-dideoxynucleoside is most likely to account for inhibition of DNA chain extension?

FIGURE 33.4

$$HOCH_2 \quad \boxed{Base}$$

2′, 3′-Dideoxyribonucleoside

14. In his studies of DNA in the late 1940s, Erwin Chargaff established that DNA from all organisms has equal numbers of adenine and thymine bases and equal numbers of guanine and cytosine bases. Considering that thymine and uracil are equivalent in their abilities to form hydrogen bonds with adenine, state whether you would expect similar constraints on base composition to be found in the following:

(a) single-strand RNA from tobacco mosaic virus.

(b) the DNA-RNA hybrid molecule synthesized by reverse transcriptase.

(c) RNA from a virus in the reovirus family, which have large genomes composed of double-strand RNA molecules.

15. Certain DNA endonucleases degrade double-strand DNA to yield mononucleotides and dinucleotides, but these enzymes do not degrade those duplex sequences to which other proteins are tightly bound.

(a) How can you use such a DNA endonuclease and RNA polymerase to locate a promoter site?

(b) Why should this process be performed in the absence of ribonucleoside triphosphates?

16. During their formation or processing, microRNA (miRNA) and small interfering RNA (siRNA) molecules, which have sequences determined by the DNA sequence of the organism, involve short duplex, self-complementary RNA structures. Propose two ways in which a self-complementary RNA duplex might be formed in the cell.

17. To gain an appreciation for the length of duplex DNA that is in an organism, calculate the distance the DNA of a human adult would cover were the DNA molecules (chromosomes) in each cell connected end-to-end. Use data in Chapter 4 of the text as well as the following possibly useful facts or approximations: 1) the distance from San Francisco, USA, to Chicago, USA, is 2000 miles; 2) the haploid human genome is 3×10^9 base pairs; 3) the distance from London, UK, to Sydney, Australia, is 10,500 miles; 4) 1 mile = 1.6 km; 5) each human cell is diploid; 6) the distance from the earth to the sun is 1.5×10^{11} m; 7) the Sears Tower building in Chicago is 1400 ft. high; 8) the distance from the Earth to the Moon is 384,000 km; 9) the human adult has 10^{14} cells (assume all have nuclei with chromosomes); 10) a typical plastic drinking water bottle is 8 inches tall; 11), the average man is about 6 ft tall; 12) each human cell has 23 pairs of chromosomes (neglect sex differences); and 13) one Ångstrom equals 10^{-8} cm.

18. Many biochemical techniques that replicate or detect DNA sequences rely on the binding of pieces of DNA or RNA called oligonucleotides. (Oligonucleotides are just short DNA or RNA single strands). These methods are known as hybridization-based techniques. When the oligonucleotide is mixed (hybridized) with the longer strand, the mixture is incubated at a temperature well below the T_m for that sequence. A "rule of thumb" is to incubate at 5°C below the T_m. Why incubate at this temperature?

19. A DNA-RNA hybrid double strand is placed in a solution of NaOH. What products result?

20. Extremophiles are organisms that live in environments that would normally not be conducive to life—hot springs and geysers, submarine vents in the ocean floor, the low-pH, high-sulfur run-off of metal mines, etc. When the DNA from extremophiles that live in high-temperature environments was analyzed, it was found to be GC-rich and more extensively positively supercoiled (overwound) than DNA from other organisms. What advantage do these particular adaptations bring the extremophiles?

ANSWERS TO PROBLEMS

1. (a) The longer the DNA molecule, the larger the number of base pairs it contains. As a result, more thermal energy is required to disrupt entirely the helical structure of the longer DNA molecule. Experiments show that such a relationship is true for molecules up to ~4000 base pairs in length.

   (b) Sodium ions neutralize the negative charges of the phosphate groups in both strands. As the concentration of NaCl decreases, repulsion between the negatively charged phosphate groups increases, making it easier to separate the two strands. The tendency for the strands to separate more easily means that dissociation occurs at a lower temperature, which is reflected in a lower T_m value of the molecule.

   (c) The reassociation of single strands begins when a short sequence of bases in one strand forms hydrogen bonds with a complementary sequence in another-a process called nucleation. Once a nucleation occurs, reassociation to form the longer double-strand molecule occurs rapidly. The higher the concentration of DNA, the greater the number of complementary sequences in the solution, and thus the quicker the complementary sequences will find and pair with each other.

(d) Urea, which contains hydrogen bond donors ($-NH_2$) and hydrogen bond acceptors ($\supset C = O$), disrupts the hydrogen bonds between bases. Because hydrogen bonds are partly responsible for the stability of the double helix, the disruption of these bonds makes the structure more sensitive to denaturation by thermal energy and thereby reduces the T_m value. In addition to hydrogen bonding, the tendency of bases to stack also contributes significantly to the stability of the helix. Base stacking minimizes the contact of the relatively insoluble bases with water, and it also allows the sugar-phosphate chain to be located on the outside of the helix, where it can be highly solvated. Urea may also cause destabilization of the helix by allowing bases to associate more readily with water by disrupting its structure.

2. (a) The four base pairs found in the DNA double helix are almost identical in size and shape, so the diameter of the double helix is essentially uniform all along its length. It is therefore unlikely that a protein can identify a specific sequence by sensing differences in the diameter of the helix.

   (b) Proteins that interact with specific sequences might do so by forming hydrogen bonds with the bases; in some cases, it might be necessary for the double strand to undergo local unwinding or melting in order for the bases to form hydrogen bonds with a protein. However, hydrogen-bond donors and acceptors are also found in the grooves of the intact helix. A protein could also bind to a specific location on DNA by forming hydrogen bonds with a particular group of atoms in one of the grooves of the helix. Hydrophobic interactions between amino acid side chains and the methyl group of thymine or the edges of the bases can also contribute to the specificity of the interaction.

3. In solution, the oligodeoxyribonucleotide forms an interchain double-strand molecule with flush ends and a small single-strand loop containing the sequence 5′-pTpCpCpTpCp-3′. The deoxyribonuclease hydrolyzes the phophodiester bonds in this single-strand region to form nucleoside monophosphates, leaving a small double-strand linear molecule remnant containing seven base pairs.

4. Formaldehyde could react with the exocyclic amino groups on the C-6 carbon of adenine, the C-2 of guanine, and the C-4 of cytosine to form hydroxymethyl derivatives. Because these derivatives cannot form hydrogen bonds with complementary bases, formaldehyde-treated single strands would reassociate to a lesser extent than would untreated single strands. All the actual sites of the reaction of formaldehyde with DNA are not precisely known; these sites may also include the ring nitrogen atoms in pyrimidines.

5. The hydrogen bonds of base-paired regions of double-strand DNA may undergo reversible dissociation to form single-strand regions, often known as bubbles. The transient disruption of these hydrogen bonds allows the exchange of protons with the tritiated water. A · T pairs open more easily than G · C pairs. Thus, the greater the percentage of A · T pairs, the greater the rate of proton exchange.

6. (a) The expected melting temperature for *E. coli* DNA containing 50% GC base pairs is

$$T_m = 69.3 + 0.41(G + C)$$
$$= 69.3 + 0.41(50)$$
$$= 69.3 + 20.5$$
$$= 89.8°C$$

(b) Most organisms live at temperatures that are considerably lower than 65°C. Because both the transmission and expression of genetic information depends on the integrity of the double-strand DNA molecule, it is important that the molecule not be disrupted by thermal energy.

(c) Some mechanism other than thermal denaturation must be involved in order to separate the strands for replication. Proteins that unwind and separate the strands will be described later.

7. First, you must determine the temperature at which the hydrogen bonds are disrupted and single strands are formed. You can do this by heating the double-strand DNA to various temperatures and measuring the extent of hyperchromicity. Once the DNA has been melted, centrifuge the sample using the density-gradient equilibrium sedimentation technique to attempt to separate the ^{14}N-labeled DNA strands from the ^{15}N-labeled DNA strands, which will be the denser of the two. If you are successful, this would suggest that the strands separate completely during thermal denaturation.

8. The protonation of the N-1 of adenine, the N-3 of cytosine, and the O-4 of thymine makes normal hydrogen bonding at these locations impossible because the atoms can no longer serve as hydrogen-bond acceptors. Therefore, at low pH, where proton concentrations are high and protonation of these atoms occurs, double-strand DNA is less stable than at neutral pH values. At high pH values (> 11) DNA is also denatured by deprotonation of other ring atoms.

9. The association of a molecule of RNA with a molecule of DNA to form a hybrid molecule depends primarily on the two molecules having complementary sequences of bases. The formation of hydrogen bonds between complementary bases will allow the formation of a double helix composed of RNA and DNA. Thus, an mRNA will anneal with the denatured DNA template from which it was made to form a DNA-RNA hybrid duplex.

10. The deoxyribonucleoside triphosphate dUTP can be used as a substrate for DNA polymerase during DNA replication because the structure and hydrogen-bonding properties of uracil are very similar to those of thymine. When incorporated into a double-strand DNA polymer, uracil pairs with adenine, as does thymine.

11. (a) To ensure that λ phage DNA molecules form closed-circular monomers, the concentration of λ phage DNA should be relatively low so that the intrachain formation of hydrogen bonds is favored. At higher concentrations, the probability of interchain joining to form multimers is enhanced.

(b) The most reasonable model for the structure of the λ phage DNA molecule is a double-strand molecule having single-strand protrusions at the 5'-ends, as illustrated below. The 3'-ends have hydroxyl groups, which allow them to serve as primers for DNA synthesis catalyzed by DNA polymerase I. This enzyme fills in the single-strand regions of the molecule, producing a molecule with flush ends. Such a molecule no longer has cohesive ends that can form the required circular molecule needed for infectivity.

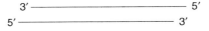

Molecules treated with exonuclease III have a longer single-strand sequence at both ends; they may not be infective because the newly exposed bases may not be fully complementary to each other, which would mean that the ends could no longer be joined. When the exonuclease-treated DNA is treated with DNA polymerase I, the single-strand regions are sufficiently filled in to reform a molecule that has protruding single strands that are approximately the same length as those in the native molecule. Hence, the molecule once again becomes infective. Further treatment of the molecule with DNA polymerase I will once again produce a molecule that has flush ends and is no longer infective.

12. (a) The sequence at the other end of the single-strand molecule must be composed of complementary bases. It must therefore be

...TACGTAGT-3′

The structure of the full-length, double-strand, linear molecule would be

5′-ACTACGTA————TACGTAGT-3′

3′-TGATGCAT————ATGCATCA-5′

Each single strand has a pair of inverted repeats.

(b) The formation of double-strand helical segments depends upon hydrogen bond formation between bases in nucleotide chains that are antiparallel, as follows:

5′...PuPyPuPyPu...3′

3′...PyPuPyPuPy...5′

where Py = pyrimidine and Pu = purine. When the suggested structure is labeled using this scheme, as in Figure 33.5, it can be seen that it would require the formation of base pairs between parallel chains, and such pairing cannot readily take place.

FIGURE 33.5 Base pairing between parallel nucleotide chains, required to form the circular structures shown in Figure 4.3, is unlikely in DNA.

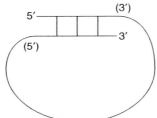

13. (a) DNA polymerase requires deoxyribonucleoside triphosphates as substrates for DNA chain extension. Nucleosides like the 2′,3′-dideoxy analogs must be converted to nucleoside triphosphates in order to serve as substrates for DNA polymerase. Studies on inhibition of DNA synthesis in living cells involve incubating those cells with the nucleoside forms of the analogs instead of their nucleoside triphosphate forms, because negatively charged phosphate anions cannot pass across the plasma membrane, while relatively neutral nucleosides can. Once inside the cell, nucleoside analogs are phosphorylated by cellular enzymes that normally function to "salvage" nucleosides generated by turnover of nucleotides from RNA and DNA.

(b) Dideoxynucleosides lack a free 3′-hydroxyl group, which would normally serve as an acceptor for incorporation of the next nucleotide into the growing polynucleotide chain. The lack of a 3′-OH group also interferes with excision by the error-correcting exonuclease activity of some DNA polymerases, so that chain extension is blocked.

14. (a) The ratios observed by Chargaff can be attributed to the requirement that in a double-strand polynucleotide, only certain bases can form hydrogen bonds with one another. Although a single-strand polynucleotide might form some hydrogen bonds between bases as it folds, the overall base ratios will not conform to Chargaff's established rules. This is also true for single-strand DNA in a virus like ΦX174.

(b) Because hydrogen bonding between A and T (or U, in the case of RNA) and between G and C can occur in a duplex molecule formed by one strand of DNA and a complementary strand of RNA, you would expect to see base ratios like those observed by Chargaff.

(c) Double-strand RNA molecules form hydrogen bonds between bases in a manner similar to those in DNA helices. Therefore, bearing in mind that U, not T, would normally be found in RNA, the number of uracil residues would equal the number of adenines, and the number of guanine bases would be expected to be the same as those of cytosine.

15. (a) To locate a promoter site, you would first incubate the double-strand DNA with RNA polymerase; the RNA polymerase will bind tightly to the promoter site. Next, you would add the DNA endonuclease, which will degrade the DNA that is not protected by the bound RNA polymerase. Electrophoresis can then be used to determine the size of the protected fragments of DNA, and the base sequence can be determined using methods discussed in Chapter 5 of the text.

(b) Ribonucleoside triphosphates are substrates for RNA polymerase transcription. If present when this process is performed, they would allow the polymerase molecule to move from the promoter site to the site on the template where transcription begins, as well as beyond, as transcription progresses. As a result, the promoter site would no longer be protected from endonuclease degradation.

16. RNA duplexes might be formed as a result of an RNA polymerase transcribing both strands of a segment of DNA, and the resulting two product RNA chains annealing with each other to form a duplex. This would be contrary to the usual transcription to form mRNA, tRNA, or rRNA because RNA polymerase transcribes only one of the two strands at a given locus on the DNA. Alternatively, an RNA polymerase might produce a single RNA molecule by transcribing the DNA and this RNA might have self-complementary regions that anneal to one another to form a base-paired hairpin (Figure 4.31 in the text). For either duplex segment of RNA, hydrolytic enzymes could cut initial product to form a duplex of the needed size.

17. There are 3×10^9 base pairs of DNA/haploid set of human chromosomes/cell $\times$ 3.4 Ångstrom/base pair $\times 10^{-8}$ cm/Ångstrom $\times$ 2 haploid sets of chromosomes/diploid cell $\times 10^{-2}$ meter/cm = 2 meters of total DNA/cell; 2 meters DNA/cell $\times 10^{14}$ cells/adult = 2×10^{14} meters/1.5×10^{11} meters to sun = 1.3×10^3 distances to the sun or ~ 650 round trips to the Sun!

18. The T_m is the temperature at which the DNA is 50% denatured. To have complete annealing, it is crucial to be *below* this temperature. The quantity of five degrees is enough to ensure that the majority of the DNA is hybridized.

19. The products are single-stranded DNA and individual ribonucleotides. First, the high pH changes the ionization state of the bases, causing the helix to denature. Second,

remember that RNA is base-labile. The NaOH causes the 2'-OH of the RNA to be deprotonated. The resulting 2'-alkoxide attacks the 3'-phosphate, resulting in hydrolysis of the phosphodiester bond and creating individual RNA nucleotides.

20. The increased G-C content means that there are more base pairs with three hydrogen bonds rather than two. Thus, it takes more thermal energy to denature this DNA. Secondly, positive supercoiling (overwinding) stores energy in DNA, so the DNA has a higher T_m when in the more highly positively supercoiled state. Thus, both of these adaptations increase the thermal stability of DNA and make the organism able to withstand higher temperatures.

DNA Replication

The text returns to the topic of the flow of genetic information and considers the detailed biochemical mechanisms underlying this complex process. Chapter 33 introduced DNA and RNA and outlined the structure of genetic information and describes how DNA is replicated. The chapter opens by pointing out the need for faithful copying and the obstacles to fidelity that a cell must overcome to duplicate its duplex DNA. The biochemistry of DNA polymerases is discussed, explaining the roles the template, primer, and metal ions play in their activities. The chemical basis for the fidelity of DNA chain extension by the polymerases is also presented, and the helicases that unwind DNA are described. The text also explains the role that topoisomerases play in relieving the stress that is introduced during strand separation. The authors then discuss the replication fork; replication initiation; and RNA-primed, semidiscontinuous DNA elongation. The structure and important roles of DNA polymerases I and III in replication are described in detail. The special problems of replication arising from the sheer amount of DNA and number of linear DNA molecules in a eukaryotic cell are introduced, and the nature and functions of telomeres and telomerase are described. The precise organization and timing of the origination of DNA replication in eukaryotes and in prokaryotes are explained and contrasted. The chapter ends with a discussion of the enzyme telomerase and the role it plays in healthy and cancerous cells.

LEARNING OBJECTIVES

When you have mastered this chapter, you should be able to accomplish the following objectives:

Introduction

1. Reprise the Watson-Crick hypothesis for DNA replication and outline some problems facing a cell in creating an exact duplicate copy of its double-strand DNA genome. Appreciate that enzymes and DNA-binding proteins play essential roles in solving the challenges of DNA replication.

DNA Is Replicated by Polymerases (Text Section 34.1)

2. Summarize the functions and enzyme activities of the five *E. coli* DNA *polymerases*.

3. Outline the key features of the reactions catalyzed by *DNA polymerases*. Define *template* and *primer* as they relate to DNA polymerases.

4. Relate the $3' \rightarrow 5'$ *nuclease* activity of DNA polymerases to the fidelity of DNA replication.

5. Appreciate the common structures and the evolutionary relationships among DNA polymerases.

6. Account for the fidelity with which a DNA polymerase selects the correct incoming *deoxyribonucleotide triphosphate (dNTP)* substrate in terms of *shape complementarity* and *hydrogen-bond donors* and *acceptors*.

7. Describe how *helicases* separate the strands of duplex DNA.

8. Describe the function of *topoisomerases*; distinguish between *type I* and *type II* topoisomerases; and describe the substrates, products, and mechanisms of *topoisomerase I* and *II*.

9. List antibiotics that act through inhibition of bacterial *Topoisomerase II* and recognize that the enzyme is also known as *DNA gyrase*.

10. Describe the *exonuclease* activity of *DNA polymerase I*, including how the enzyme senses whether a newly added base is correct.

11. State the accuracy enhancement of replication through *proofreading*.

DNA Replication Is Highly Coordinated (Text Section 34.2)

12. Describe the function and features of the nucleotide sequence of *oriC* and note that it is the unique site of *bidirectional replication initiation* in *E. coli*. List the proteins that interact with the DNA in this region of the chromosome, and give the reactions they catalyze and functions they serve.

13. Explain the roles of *RNA* in DNA replication and describe the enzymes that form and remove *RNA primers* from the genome.

14. Define *continuous replication* and *discontinuous replication* and relate these processes to the *leading* and *lagging strands* of replicating DNA. Describe an *Okazaki fragment*.

15. Draw a *replication fork* and describe the reactions and the movements of the DNA strands that occur during replication.

16. Define *processivity* as it relates to DNA polymerases and describe the role of the *sliding-clamp β₂* subunit of DNA polymerase III in retarding dissociation of the enzyme from the template.

17. List the distinctive features of the *DNA polymerase III holoenzyme,* and describe how an asymmetric dimer of the enzyme, along with other proteins, coordinates the synthesis of the leading and lagging strands of the daughter duplexes. Appreciate the structural complexity of the replication machinery and explain the essential role of *DNA polymerase I* and DNA ligase in this process.

18. Summarize the reactions and identify the proteins at the replication fork that carry out DNA replication using the trombone model.

19. Describe the function of *DNA ligases*

20. Describe the special problems arising from DNA length and the *cell cycle* in eukaryotes. Define *replication* and explain the roles of *multiple replication origins* and the *telomeres* in eukaryotic DNA replication.

21. Describe how *telomerase* makes DNA of defined sequence in the absence of a DNA template.

22. Explain why telomerase is a potential target for anti-cancer therapy.

SELF-TEST

DNA Is Replicated by Polymerases

1. Which of the following statements about DNA polymerases are correct?
   (a) They add deoxyribonucleotide units to the 3′-hydroxyl of a primer.
   (b) They use the template strand to help determine which deoxyribonucleotide unit to add to the growing DNA chain.
   (c) They contain a 3′ → 5′ nuclease that cleaves phosphodiester bonds of misincorporated deoxyribonucleotides.
   (d) They check the size of an incoming deoxyribonucleotide triphosphate (dNTP) to help ensure that the correct, complementary choice is made.
   (e) They bind one complementary dNTP and add a second complementary dNTP to initiate a new DNA chain.

2. DNA polymerase activity requires
   (a) a template
   (b) a primer with a free 5′ hydroxyl group
   (c) dATP, dCTP, dGTP and dTTP (which is the same as TTP).
   (d) ATP
   (e) Mg^{2+}

3. Why are helicases required during DNA replicaton? Is ATP required for their action?

4. The topological features of circular DNA may affect which of the following?
   (a) the electrophoretic mobility of the DNA
   (b) the sedimentation properties of the DNA
   (c) its affinities toward proteins that bind to the DNA
   (d) the susceptibility of the strands of the DNA to unwinding
   (e) the susceptibility of the DNA to the action of DNA ligase

5. Which of the following statements about DNA molecules that are topoisomers are correct?
   - (a) They are bound to topoisomerases.
   - (b) They differ from one another topologically only in that they have different linking numbers.
   - (c) They may be separated from one another by electrophoresis.
   - (d) They have identical molecular weights.
   - (e) They are topological or spatial isomers.

6. Which of the following statements about topoisomerases are correct?
   - (a) They alter the linking numbers of topoisomers.
   - (b) They break and reseal phosphodiester bonds.
   - (c) They require NAD^+ as a cofactor to supply the energy to drive the conversion of a supercoiled molecule to its relaxed form.
   - (d) They form covalent intermediates with their DNA substrates.
   - (e) They can, in the case of a particular type of topoisomerase, use ATP to form negatively supercoiled DNA from relaxed DNA in E. coli.

7. Why are the antibiotics novobiocin, ciprofloxin, and nalidixic acid, which inhibit DNA gyrase, useful in treating bacterial infections in humans?

DNA Replication Is Highly Coordinated

8. Match the properties or functions in the right column with a DNA polymerase in the left column.

   - (a) DNA polymerase I
   - (b) DNA polymerase III

   - (1) involved in replication
   - (2) requires a primer and a template
   - (3) involved in DNA repair
   - (4) makes most of the DNA phosphodiester bonds during replication
   - (5) removes the primer and fills in gaps during replication

9. Which of the following statements about DNA replication in E. coli are correct?
   - (a) It occurs at a replication fork.
   - (b) It starts at a unique locus on the chromosome.
   - (c) It proceeds with one replication fork per replicating molecule.
   - (d) It is bidirectional.
   - (e) It involves discontinuous synthesis on the leading strand.
   - (f) It uses RNA transiently as a template.

10. Which of the following statements about DNA polymerase III holoenzyme from E. coli are correct?
    - (a) It elongates a growing DNA chain hundreds of times faster than does DNA polymerase I.
    - (b) It associates with the parental template, adds a few nucleotides to the growing chain, and then dissociates before initiating another synthesis cycle.
    - (c) It maintains a high fidelity of replication, in part, by acting in conjunction with a subunit containing a $3' \rightarrow 5'$ exonuclease activity.
    - (d) When replicating DNA, it is a molecular assembly composed of at least 10 different kinds of subunits.

11. Explain how the β_2 subunit of DNA polymerase III holoenzyme contributes to the processivity of the DNA synthesis machinery.

12. Which of the following statements about DNA ligase are correct?

    (a) It forms a phosphodiester bond between a 5′-hydroxyl and a 3′-phosphate in duplex DNA.
    (b) It requires a cofactor, either NAD^+ or ATP, depending on the source of the enzyme, to provide the energy to form the phosphodiester bond.
    (c) It catalyzes its reaction by a mechanism that involves the formation of a covalently linked enzyme adenylate.
    (d) It catalyzes its reaction by a mechanism that involves the activation of a DNA phosphate through the formation of a phosphoanhydride bond with AMP.
    (e) It is involved in DNA replication, repair, and recombination.

13. Why is RNA synthesis essential to DNA synthesis in *E. coli*?

14. Match the functions or features related to DNA replication in *E. coli* listed in the right column with the molecules or structures in the left column.

    (a) replication fork
    (b) *oriC*
    (c) lagging strand
    (d) leading strand
    (e) Okazaki fragment
    (f) DnaB helicase
    (g) single-strand binding protein (ssb)
    (h) DNA gyrase
    (i) primase
    (j) DNA polymerase III holoenzyme
    (k) ε subunit of DNA polymerase III
    (l) DNA polymerase I
    (m) DNA ligase

    (1) synthesis direction is opposite that of replication fork movement
    (2) unwinds strands at the origin of replication in association with dnaA and dnaC proteins
    (3) is synthesized continuously
    (4) synthesizes most of DNA
    (5) is synthesized discontinuously
    (6) relieves positive supercoiling
    (7) is the locus of DNA unwinding
    (8) hydrolyzes ATP to reduce the linking number of DNA
    (9) binds dnaA, dnaB, and dnaC proteins
    (10) fills in gaps where RNA existed
    (11) is the point of initiation of synthesis
    (12) joins lagging strand pieces to each other
    (13) contains a $5' \rightarrow 3'$ exonuclease that removes RNA primers
    (14) is an RNA polymerase
    (15) performs "proofreading" on most of the DNA synthesized
    (16) stabilizes unwound DNA
    (17) uses NAD^+ to form phosphodiester bonds

15. The duplication of the ends of linear, duplex DNA in humans presents a problem to the replicative machinery of a cell. Describe this problem, its cause, and the way the cell overcomes it.

16. Give two reasons why eukaryotes must use multiple origins of replication (in contrast to prokaryotes, which usually use one).

ANSWERS TO SELF-TEST

1. a, b, c, d

2. a, c, and e. Answer (b) is incorrect because, although the enzyme requires a primer, the nature of its 5′-end is irrelevant since dNMP residues are added to its 3′-end. A

primer with a 3'-OH is required. Answer (d) is not correct because the enzyme uses dNTP and not NTP molecules, where N means A, C, G, T, or U. Note that dTTP is used interchangeably with TTP.

3. Duplex B-DNA is a stable molecule at physiological temperature and helicases are required to unwind the two strands of the helix so that each can serve as a template for DNA polymerases. Because DNA is so stable, energy is required in the form of ATP hydrolysis to drive helicase action.

4. a, b, c, d. In regard to answer (e), supercoiling is ordinarily a property of covalently closed circular DNA—that is, of DNA in which there are no discontinuities in either strand of the helix. Hence, these molecules are not substrates for DNA ligase, because they lack ends.

5. b, c, d, e. Answer (a) is not correct because the DNA topoisomer need not necessarily be bound by a topoisomerase.

6. a, b, d, e. Although all topoisomerases break and reseal phosphodiester bonds, an external energy source is not always required. Relieving the torsional stress in a negatively supercoiled DNA molecule by relaxing it with topoisomerase I is exergonic and requires no energy input, whereas introducing negative supercoils with DNA gyrase is endergonic and must be coupled to ATP hydrolysis. The particular catalytic mechanisms of given topoisomerases determine whether they are coupled to ATP hydrolysis.

7. These compounds interfere with the essential helix-destabilizing function of DNA gyrase in bacterial DNA replication. By inhibiting its action, they prevent the gyrase from relieving the positive supercoils that build up ahead of the moving replication fork. Human cells lack an enzyme similar to gyrase, and thus they are relatively unharmed by these antibiotics.

8. (a) 1, 2, 3, 5   (b) 1, 2, 4

9. a, b, d. Answer (c) is incorrect because, although not explicitly stated in the text, the replicating E. coli chromosome has two replication forks that synthesize the DNA bidirectionally from the unique oriC origin. Answer (e) is incorrect because only the lagging strand is synthesized discontinuously. Answer (f) is incorrect because RNA serves as a primer and not as a template.

10. a, c, d. Answer (b) is incorrect because DNA polymerase III holoenzyme is a highly processive enzyme that synthesizes extensively before dissociating from its template.

11. The β_2 subunit forms a torus, with the duplex DNA in its aperture. The β_2 ring acts as a sliding clamp that holds the replication machinery on the DNA.

12. b, c, d, e. Answer (a) is incorrect because the enzyme joins a 3'-hydroxyl to a 5'-phosphate. Answer (d) is correct because, although not completely described in the text, DNA ligase activity is required to seal the discontinuities in DNA arising during DNA replication, repair, and recombination.

13. Because DNA polymerases are unable to initiate DNA chains de novo and because they require a primer with a 3'-hydroxyl group, short RNA chains are used as primers to start DNA replication on the leading strand at the origin of replication and to initiate the Okazaki fragments of the lagging strand. RNA polymerases can start RNA chains by adding a nucleotide to an initiating NTP, but they do so with relatively low accuracy. RNA-initiated DNA chains facilitate high-fidelity replication at the beginning sequences of new chains because they allow DNA polymerase I to replace the RNA with DNA, using the information in the complementary strand and both of its exonucleases in a nick translation reaction (page 823 of the text).

14. (a) 7 (b) 7, 9, 11 (c) 1, 5 (d) 3 (e) 1, 3 (f) 2 (g) 16 (h) 6, 8 (i) 14 (j) 4 (k) 15 (l) 1, 10, 13 (m) 12, 17. Answer (5) is not a correct match with (e) because each Okazaki fragment is synthesized continuously.

15. Because DNA polymerases extend their growing polynucleotide chains only in the 5′ → 3′ direction and because the two strands of the parental DNA duplex are antiparallel, removal of the RNA primer that is paired with the 3′ end of the parental template DNA would leave an overhanging 3′ DNA strand with no means of having its complement synthesized. Ordinary DNA polymerases are unable to initiate DNA chains de novo. Each round of replication would consequently shorten the DNA because a portion could not be copied. To circumvent this problem, human DNA chromosomes have a segment of repeating G-rich DNA (telomeres) at their ends. In addition, a special enzyme, telomerase, which is an RNA-dependent DNA polymerase (reverse transcriptase) that carries its own RNA template, can extend the uncompleted end at each round of replication. The RNA template renews the repeating telomere sequence so that the DNA is not shortened.

16. The great amount of genomic DNA in eukaryotes (6×10^9 bp in a human) requires that polymerases start at multiple sites in order to complete the DNA synthesis in a biologically relevant period of time. In addition, the genome of eukaryotes comprises multiple separate DNA molecules—23 pairs of chromosomes in a human, so sites must be provided on each molecule. The first requirement accounts for the vast majority of the ~30,000 origins in a human cell.

PROBLEMS

1. The helicase described in the text (Figure 34.7) has the same "P-loop NTPase" structure as the proteins described in Chapter 8. What purpose does this structure serve in the action of a helicase?

2. Suppose that two polynucleotide chains are joined by DNA ligase in a reaction mixture to which ATP labeled with ^{32}P in the α-phosphoryl (the innermost) group has been added as an energy source. What products of the reaction would be expected to carry the radioactive label? Explain.

3. What property of DNA polymerase I leads to the observation that *polA1* mutants of *E. coli* are more sensitive to ultraviolet light than are the wild-type cells? [Hint: The 5′ → 3′ exonuclease activity of DNA polymerase I can remove damaged nucleotides from DNA as well as destroying the RNA primers on Okazaki fragments.]

4. Suppose that a single-strand circular DNA with the base composition 30% A, 20% T, 15% C, and 35% G serves as the template for the synthesis of a complementary strand by DNA polymerase.
   (a) Give the base composition of the complementary strand.
   (b) Give the overall base composition of the resulting double-helical DNA.

5. Suppose that a plasmid with a single origin of replication on its circular chromosome and containing only genes A, B, C, and D begins to replicate rapidly at time $t = 0$. At $t = 1$, there are twice as many copies of genes B and C as there are copies of genes D and A. Is it possible to establish the order of the four genes on the plasmid? Explain.

6. Suppose that a bacterial mutant is found to replicate its DNA at a very low rate. Upon analysis, it is found to have normal levels of activity of DNA polymerases I and III, DNA gyrase, and DNA ligase. It also makes normal amounts of the wild-types of

dnaA, dnaB, dnaC, and SSB proteins. The sequence of the *oriC* region of its chromosome is found to be wild type. What defect might account for the abnormally low rate of DNA replication in this mutant? Explain.

7. Physical studies on the interaction of the β_2 subunit of DNA polymerase III holoenzyme show that the β_2 subunit binds much more tightly to circular than to linear DNA molecules.

   (a) Propose an explanation for this observation.
   (b) What do you think would happen if the circular DNA were treated with a double-strand hydrolyzing endonuclease?

8. Thermoacidophilic bacteria can grow in volcanic sulfur springs at pH 2 and at temperatures as high as 85°C. DNA polymerase purified from the thermophile *Sufolobus acidocaldarius* has an optimal activity at 70°C and is stable at 80°C. When incubated with a circular DNA template at 100°C, the isolated polymerase can extend a 20-nucleotide primer by more than 100 nucleotides. These experiments require that enzyme-to-primer concentration be at least 1:1. The T_m value for the double-strand DNA used in the experiment is about 60°C. Unlike DNA polymerase I from *E. coli*, DNA polymerase from *S. acidocaldarius* has no demonstrable exonuclease activity to correct mistakes in DNA by removing mismatched nucleotides (such an enzyme activity is often referred to as *proofreading*).

   (a) Why should the ratio of enzyme to primer be 1 in order for primer extension to take place at 100°C?
   (b) Would you expect to find an auxiliary proofreading enzyme in *S. acidocaldarius*? Why?
   (c) Would you expect DNA from the genome of *S. acidocaldarius* to have a G + C content higher or lower than that from a bacterium that grows at a more normal temperature? Why?

9. Terminal deoxynucleotidyl transferase (TdT), an enzyme found in bone marrow and thymus tissue, can extend a DNA primer by 5′ to 3′ polymerization using deoxyribonucleoside triphosphates as substrates. The primer must be at least three nucleotides in length and must have a free 3′-OH end. The enzyme does not require a template nor does it copy one.

   (a) Compare TdT with DNA polymerase I.
   (b) Would TdT be useful for synthesizing DNA molecules that carry genetic information? Why?

10. In each chain-elongation reaction catalyzed by DNA polymerase, a phosphodiester bond is formed and pyrophosphate is concomitantly released. Hydrolysis of pyrophosphate to two molecules of inorganic phosphate occurs rapidly because most cells have a potent pyrophosphorylase. By removing one of the products of the chain-elongation reaction, pyrophosphate cleavage in the cell is partially responsible for the forward progress of polymerization. However, isolated DNA polymerases can efficiently carry out chain extension in the absence of pyrophosphate cleavage, as long as the double-strand helix is allowed to form during elongation. What forces resulting from DNA helix formation might contribute to driving polymerization forward?

11. Acyclovir is an antiviral agent used to reduce the pain and promote the healing of skin lesions resulting from adult chicken pox. Its structure is shown in Figure 34.1.

FIGURE 34.1   Structure of acyclovir.

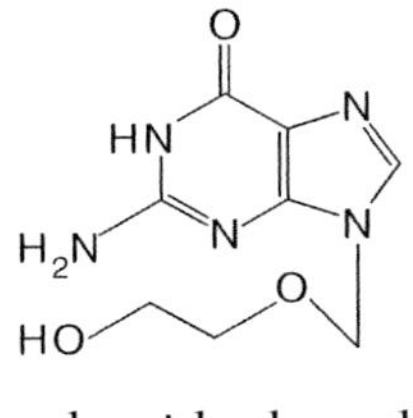

(a)   What nucleoside does this drug resemble?

(b)   Why must the drug be administered in dephosphorylated form?

(c)   Acyclovir has very few side effects because it inhibits DNA replication only in herpes-infected cells. This is because all herpes viruses encode a thymidine kinase gene that is able to activate the drug. What is this activating reaction?

(d)   Once acyclovir is activated, how does it inhibit DNA replication?

(e)   Why are cells uninfected by virus relatively unaffected by acyclovir?

(f)   The herpes virus can become insensitive to acyclovir therapy by mutations in either of two genes. What might they be?

12. You have a double-strand linear DNA molecule, the appropriate primers, all the enzymes required for DNA replication, four ^{32}-P-labeled deoxyribonucleoside triphosphates, Mg^{2+} ion, and the means to detect newly synthesized radioactive DNA. Why is this system not sufficient to distinguish between conservative and semi-conservative replication of the DNA molecule?

13. While many experiments were suggesting DNA in chromosomes is very long and continuous, it was established that DNA polymerase adds deoxyribonucleotides to the 3'-hydroxyl terminus of a primer chain and that a DNA template is essential. Why did investigators interested in DNA replications initially focus a great deal of attention on determining whether chromosomal DNA contained breaks in the sugar-phosphate backbone?

14. In cells, the DNA replication process begins with RNA polymerase generating a short piece of RNA that is complementary to the 3'-end of the template DNA strand. DNA polymerase then extends this primer to begin replication. Why is RNA polymerase used to make the DNA primer?

ANSWERS TO PROBLEMS

1. At the end of Chapter 9 there is a discussion of the "P-loop NTPase" superfamily, which describes a wide variety of proteins and enzymes that use this structure to propel "springs, motors, and clocks." Suffice it to say that the P-loop binds to the phosphates in ATP or other nucleoside triphosphates, and that the binding can lead to large conformational changes. So the task of a helicase, which is like unraveling two twisted threads, is accomplished by binding single strands and pulling them apart. And this is accomplished by binding and hydrolyzing molecules of ATP at the P-loops. The wide variety of other proteins and enzymes in this family all make use of NTP binding and concomitant conformational changes.

2. In the overall reaction, ATP is hydrolyzed to AMP and pyrophosphate. Only AMP would be labeled. The phosphate involved in the formation of the phosphodiester bond is furnished by the polynucleotide chain and does not arise from ATP.

3. The *polA1* mutants are extraordinarily sensitive to ultraviolet irradiation because they are deficient in the $5' \rightarrow 3'$ exonuclease activity of DNA polymerase I and are therefore impaired in DNA repair. They have only 1% of the activity of their wild-type counterpart and cannot efficiently remove thymine dimers formed by UV light. They can, however, replicate their DNA at normal rates because DNA polymerase III is the enzyme that is primarily responsible for DNA replication. An enzyme, RNaseH, which hydrolyzes RNA only when it is base paired to DNA, likely replaces the $5' \rightarrow 3'$ exonuclease in processing the Okazaki fragments.

4. (a) 30% T, 20% A, 15% G, 35% C
   (b) 25% A, 25% T, 25% C, 25% G. The base composition of the double strand is the average of that of the two single strands.

5. The order cannot be unambiguously established from the information given. Two possibilities are shown in Figure 34.2.

FIGURE 34.2   Two possible gene arrangements for problem 11.

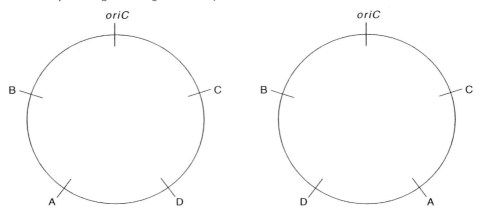

6. A decrease in the activity of primase would account for the low rate of DNA replication. Synthesis of DNA itself requires the prior synthesis of RNA primers. Also, decreased rates of dNTP synthesis could slow replication.

7. (a) A possible explanation is that the β_2 subunit falls off the end of a linear molecule whereas it is trapped on the circular molecule because it forms a torus around the DNA.
   (b) Treatment of circular DNA with an endonuclease cleaving both strands would convert it to a linear DNA, and the β_2 protein could dissociate from the free end, thereby decreasing its apparent affinity.

8. (a) Each enzyme molecule probably tightly clamps the primer as well as the extended, newly synthesized chain to the template, thereby protecting the helix from denaturation at high temperature. One primer would be required for each template strand. The association between primer and enzyme may protect the enzyme from thermal denaturation as well. There are many examples in biochemistry where substrate binding stabilizes protein structure.
   (b) During polymerization of a new DNA chain, the chance that base incorporation errors can occur will increase at high temperatures. Even though a proofreading or error-correcting activity is not found in the *S. acidocaldarius* polymerase polypeptide, you would expect an auxiliary enzyme to be present in the cells in

order for the bacterial genome to be accurately replicated so that the genetic integrity of the organism is maintained.

(c) The higher the G + C content of double-strand DNA, the higher the melting point at which the helix is denatured. Therefore, you might expect DNA from a thermophile to have a higher G + C composition. Surprisingly, DNA base ratios are sometimes not very different from those in bacteria living at lower temperatures, so that DNA isolated from these thermophilic bacteria melts at temperatures lower than those encountered in the hot springs where they grow. There must be proteins or other molecules in the bacterial cells that protect the genomic DNA of these thermophiles from thermal denaturation.

9. (a) Like DNA polymerase I, TdT can extend a DNA primer by using deoxynucleoside triphosphates as substrates. However, TdT does not use a template and cannot copy from one, so that the base composition of the newly synthesized single strand of DNA will depend solely on the relative concentrations of the deoxynucleoside triphosphate substrates. For chains synthesized by DNA polymerase I, the base composition will be complementary to that of the template strand. Although DNA polymerase has an exonuclease activity that removes mismatched bases from newly synthesized strands, TdT has no such activity and does not need one.

(b) DNA molecules that carry genetic information must be synthesized as faithful copies of template strands; TdT cannot copy a template and would not be useful in genomic DNA synthesis. However, in cases where variability is desired, TdT is used to introduce sequence variation into DNA during antibody formation.

10. Noncovalent forces also contribute to driving the reaction forward. Hydrogen bonds form between opposing A and T bases and between G and C molecules in the antiparallel chains. There are also significant hydrophobic interactions between adjacent bases on the same strand, and these stacking interactions may in fact contribute significantly to helix formation and stability. In vivo, it is likely that these noncovalent forces, along with the cleavage of the product, account for the forward progress of chain elongation.

11. (a) guanosine

(b) The phosphorylated form could not cross cell membranes.

(c) The activation involves adding phosphates onto the distal $-OH$ group at the expense of ATP hydrolysis by kinases to produce a compound resembling 5′-GTP. (Although one of the enzymes responsible for the activation is called *thymidine kinase*, it can activate other nucleosides and some of their analogs as well.)

(d) The triphosphate of acyclovir will serve as a substrate for DNA polymerase, and acyclovir nucleotide residues will be incorporated into growing polynucleotide chains in the place of guanosine resiues. Acyclovir will, however, cause premature termination of nascent polynucleotide chains because it lacks a free $-OH$ group onto which further nucleotides can be linked by phosphodiester bonds.

(e) Thymidine kinase is encoded by a viral, not a host, gene. Therefore, uninfected cells will lack the susceptible enzyme.

(f) Mutations that impair the ability of either the viral thymidine kinase or DNA polymerase to use the analog would render infected cells insensitive to the agent.

12. Although the system described could yield ^{32}P-labeled daughter DNA molecules, chemical methods cannot distinguish DNA in which both strands are radioactively labeled from DNA in which one strand is labeled and one strand is unlabeled. In their experiments, Meselson and Stahl used a physical technique, density gradient

equilibrium sedimentation, to separate the labeled molecules according to their content of ^{14}N and ^{15}N, which differ in their specific densities.

13. A continuous, linear double-strand DNA molecule has only two 3'-OH groups available for the initiation of DNA synthesis by DNA polymerase; because each is located at opposite ends of the molecule, no template sequence is available. In order to construct a relatively simple mechanism for chromosomal replication, one could postulate that the enzyme initiates DNA replication at a number of breaks along the chromosome, with each of the breaks offering the 3'-OH group required for the initiation of the new DNA strand. The template required for replication would then be located on the strand opposite the break, thus ensuring that DNA synthesis could continue. It is now well established that DNA in chromosomes is very long and continuous. The fact that there are initially no breaks in the molecule makes the mechanism of replication complex. It involves a number of enzyme activities, as well as the use of RNA to prime the synthesis of DNA. Thus, the initial conjecture that the long molecules might have single-strand breaks where replication could initiate was not confirmed.

14. DNA polymerase requires a primer to initiate replication; RNA polymerase does not. So the RNA polymerase generates the primer for DNA polymerase.

Chapter 35

DNA Repair and Recombination

In Chapter 34, the authors discussed the replication of DNA, including some of the mechanisms that a cell uses to avoid errors. In this chapter, the errors that can occur during DNA replication as well as errors that can arise from DNA damage are discussed. The authors then turn to mechanisms by which the errors can be corrected, reiterating the role that exonuclease activity in DNA polymerases plays in DNA repair.

Examples of pathological deficiencies of DNA repair in humans, the relationship of mutations and DNA repair impairments to carcinogenesis, and a test system for detecting potential carcinogens through their mutagenic action on bacteria is outlined.

To provide the new sequences of nucleotides in DNA upon which evolution can act, not only mutation, but also recombination between different DNA molecules occurs. The breakage and joining of fragments of DNA with similar sequences also rearrange gene orders within the chromosome and are mechanisms for repairing damaged DNA and regulating gene expression. The activity of the RecA protein and a description of a key intermediate in recombination, the Holliday junction, and the recombinases that form and resolve it are presented.

LEARNING OBJECTIVES

When you have mastered this chapter, you should be able to accomplish the following objectives:

Introduction

1. Summarize some of the consequences of DNA damage in a cell.

Errors Can Arise in DNA Replication (Text Section 35.1)

2. Outline the ways in which the DNA of an organism can be damaged or the DNA of its progeny be an unfaithful copy.

3. Explain why the formation of *mismatched base pairs* during replication can cause a mutation. List other types of errors that occur during replication of DNA. Describe the involvement of *error-prone* DNA polymerases in repairing replication errors and appreciate their limitations.

4. Describe *trinucleotide-repeat expansions* during DNA replication and relate them to *Huntington disease*.

5. List some agents that damage DNA and describe the nature of the damage.

6. Explain the role of cytochrome P450 enzymes in activating carcinogens and mutagens.

7. Describe the structure of the *pyrimidine dimer* formed by *ultraviolet light*. Distinguish among *substitution*, *insertion*, and *deletion mutations*.

DNA Damage Can Be Detected and Repaired (Text Section 35.2)

8. Outline the general strategies for repairing damaged DNA and relate them to the *repair* of particular damage, for instance, *mismatches*, *pyrimidine dimers*, alkylated bases. Distinguish between *base-excision* repair and *nucleotide-excision* repair.

9. Explain why *thymine* rather than *uracil* is used in DNA.

10. Relate defective DNA repair to *cancer* and relate *tumor-suppressor genes* to DNA repair. List two defining features of cancer cells and relate them to DNA damage.

11. Describe *xeroderma pigmentosum* and *hereditary nonpolyposis colorectal cancer*, their causes, pathological consequences, and relationships to DNA repair.

12. Relate *mutagens* and *carcinogens* and outline the *Ames Salmonella mutagen assay*.

DNA Recombination Plays Important Roles in Replication and Repair
(Text Section 35.3)

13. Explain when *recombination* plays a role in DNA repair, normal cellular processes, and DNA technology.

14. Describe the *Holliday model* for *homologous recombination*. Explain how resolution of the *Holliday junction intermediate* can form different recombinant DNA products.

15. Describe the role that recombination plays in generating genetic diversity.

16. Define "gene knockout" and "knock in" mice. Give an example of the use of gene-knockouts in studying gene transcription in muscle cells.

SELF-TEST

Errors Can Arise in DNA Replication

1. How could the tautomerization of a keto group on a guanine residue in DNA to the enol form lead to a mutation?

2. Explain why most nucleotides that have been misincorporated during DNA synthesis in *E. coli* do not lead to mutant progeny.

3. Match the usual type of mutation or physiologic consequence in the right column with the appropriate mutagen or mutagenic process in the left column.

   (a) alkylating agents (activated aflatoxin B_1)
   (b) deaminating agents
   (c) ultraviolet light
   (d) psoralens
   (e) x-rays
   (f) oxidizing agents (hydroxyl radicals)

   (1) interstrand cross-links
   (2) intrastrand cross-links
   (3) single-strand and double-strand breaks
   (4) mispaired base pairs
   (5) replication and transcription blockage

4. What general property of DNA allows the repair of some residues damaged through the action of mutagens?

5. Which of the following enzymes or processes can be involved in repairing DNA in *E. coli* damaged by UV light–induced formation of a thymine dimer?

   (a) DNA ligase seals the newly synthesized strand to undamaged DNA to form the intact molecule.
   (b) The UvrABC enzyme (excinuclease) hydrolyzes phosphodiester bonds on both sides of the thymine dimer.
   (c) DNA polymerase I fills in the gap created by the removal of the oligonucleotide bearing the thymine dimer.
   (d) The UvrABC enzyme recognizes a distortion in the DNA helix caused by the thymine dimer.
   (e) A photoreactivating enzyme absorbs light and cleaves the thymine dimer to re-form two adjacent thymine residues.

6. Which of the following is true about cytochrome P450 enzymes?

   (a) They catalyze the formation of reactive epoxides, which modify DNA.
   (b) They alkylate DNA, which leads to mutations.
   (c) They catalyze the conversion of guanine to adenine.
   (d) Their substrates include polyaromatic hydrocarbons found in automobile exhaust and cigarette smoke.

DNA Damage Can Be Detected and Repaired

7. What role does N^5, N^{10}-methenyltetrahydrofolate play in the action of direct repair of DNA by DNA photolyase?

   (a) It methylates uracil to produce thymine
   (b) It adds a methylene bridge to the thymine dimmer
   (c) It absorbs a photon to provide the energy for the reaction
   (d) It has no actual role in the reaction.

8. Given that the base T requires more energy to synthesize than U, and A pairs equally well with U or T, what is the probable reason that DNA contains A·T base pairs instead of A·U base pairs?

9. Explain how mutations in genes encoding proteins likely to be involved in DNA repair, such as those defective in xeroderma pigmentosum and hereditary nonpolyposis colorectal cancer, may contribute to the onset of cancer.

10. How might a trinucleotide expansion in a gene affect the primary structure of the protein normally encoded by that gene?

11. Explain how some strains of *Salmonella* are used to detect carcinogens. How is an extract from human liver involved in this test?

DNA Recombination Plays Important Roles in Replication and Repair

12. Which of the following statements about genetic recombination are correct?
    (a) It generates new combinations of genes.
    (b) It can move a segment of DNA from one chromosome to another (for example, from a virus to a host cell).
    (c) It is mediated by the breakage of DNA and the rejoining of the resulting fragments.
    (d) It generates genome sequence variability upon which natural selection can act.

13. How many strands of DNA are present at the junction of a Holliday junction?

14. Explain how a gene knock out of myogenin demonstrated the importance of the level of its expression in muscle.

ANSWERS TO SELF-TEST

1. The rare enol tautomer of G could base-pair with a T in the template to allow its incorporation into a growing DNA strand during replication. If the proofreading process missed this erroneous incorporation, the resulting daughter DNA duplex would contain a G·T base pair. During the next round of replication, the T would direct the incorporation of an A into its complementary daughter strand. The final result would be the substitution of an A·T base pair for the original G·C base pair.

2. The proofreading $3' \rightarrow 5'$ nuclease of the ε subunit of DNA polymerase III holoenzyme removes most of the misincorporated nucleotides that do not form a base pair with the template. The polymerase activity of the enzyme then has a second chance to incorporate the correct nucleotide. Additionally, DNA repair systems exist that can detect and repair a mismatched base pair resulting from a misincorporation during synthesis.

3. (a) 4 (b) 4 (c) 2, 5 (d) 1, 5 (e) 3, 5 (x-rays also generate hydroxyl radicals, and thus can lead to mispairing of oxidized bases; in addition, double-stranded breaks can prevent replication and transcription) (f) 4

4. Since DNA is double-strand, damage to one strand of the DNA can often be repaired by using the undamaged complementary strand as a template to direct new incorportion of correct deoxynucleotides in place of the removed incorrect ones.

5. a, b, c, d, e. Although not mentioned in the text, the uvrD protein is a helicase that removes the 12-nucleotide-long oligonucleotide bearing the thymine dimer.

6. a and d. Answer b is not true because the reaction described is an epoxidation, which then leads to alkylation of the DNA. Answer c is not true because although a guanine to adenine mutation may result, it is not directly catalyzed by the cytochrome.

7. C. Tetrahydrofolate is generally a cofactor for one-carbon transfers, and in fact one derivative (methylene or CH_2) is used in the synthesis of thymine. But DNA photolyase uses this cofactor in an unusual way, as a collector of photons, as described in the text.

8. C spontaneously deaminates to form U in DNA. This change would lead to a mutation during the next round of replication of the DNA, since U would pair with A, changing what was a C·G base pair into an A·U base pair. The repair machinery of a cell that used U normally in its DNA would be unable to distinguish the U in an A·U base pair arising from a C deamination from one formed during "normal" replication. The methyl group on T, which is almost universally used in DNA, distinguishes it from the uracils formed by deamination so that the uracils can be repaired.

9. The inability to effectively repair mutagenic lesions in DNA may lead to their accumulation. As a consequence, genes regulating cellular proliferation may malfunction and thereby cause cancer.

10. The increased number of triplet sequences would give rise to a protein with a corresponding repeat of the amino acid encoded by the trinucleotide. In the case of Huntington disease, the sequence CAG is increased in number within the coding region of the gene. This leads to the gene product protein huntingtin, which has an inserted stretch of glutamine residues that were encoded by the increased number of CAG codons. These extra amino acids alter the function of the protein.

11. Special strains of *Salmonella* have been developed to detect substitution, insertion, and deletion mutations in their DNA as a result of exposure to exogenously supplied chemicals. Mutagens can alter the DNA in these strains and thus convert them from auxotrophs, which are unable to grow in the absence of histidine, to prototrophs. The revertants can grow on media lacking histidine and are detected with high sensitivity. Since there is a correlation between mutagenicity and carcinogenicity, these strains are used as an inexpensive initial test of the carcinogenic potential of a compound. Because animals sometimes metabolize innocuous compounds and convert them to carcinogens, incubation of a suspect chemical with a human liver extract before using the bacterial test can sometimes mimic what would happen to the chemical in vivo. This adjunct to the test expands its capacity to detect potential human carcinogens.

12. a, b, c, d

13. Four. The Holliday junction is formed from the four strands of two interacting duplex DNA molecules that, as a result of the initial reactions of recombination, become joined to form one molecule. The Holliday junction is resolved when recombination is completed and two separate duplexes are reformed. Although not mentioned in the text, the products can sometimes have regions of duplex where one strand of DNA is from one parent and the other strand from the other parent, that is, a heteroduplex is formed.

14. When both genes coding for myogenin was knocked out in mice, the animals die at birth because muscle cells that have failed to differentiate fully. When only one gene is disrupted, the animal appears normal. This implies that the level of gene expression is unimportant, just that some amount is present.

PROBLEMS

1. Mismatch repair is a DNA repair system in which non-Watson Crick base pairs are detected, and one of the nucleotides is replaced to fix the mismatch. But with this process happening independently of replication, how can the enzymes determine which base is likely to be correct and which is an error?

2. An early and initially attractive mechanism proposed for genetic recombination was the copy-choice model. It suggested that recombination between two parental DNA duplexes occurs during DNA replication when DNA polymerase switches or jumps from one parental duplex to the other, producing a recombinant daughter DNA duplex that contains sequences derived from the templates of two different DNA duplexes. The copy-choice model is now known to act infrequently. One experimental finding inconsistent with the copy-choice model is the observation that when *E. coli* bacteria are infected by T4 bacteriophage of two different genotypes whose DNAs are distinctly marked, one by ^{32}P and the other by bromouracil, recombinant DNAs containing both markers are found under conditions in which DNA synthesis is blocked. How are these findings inconsistent with the copy-choice model but consistent with the breakage–reunion model for genetic recombination?

3. Relate genetic recombination to exon shuffling, that is, the rearrangement of exons to form new proteins.

4. The drug fluorouracil is used as an anticancer agent. It irreversibly inactivates the enzyme thymidylate synthase. Explain how this treatment retards the growth of tumor tissue. Will the growth of normal cells be affected as well?

5. Mammalian cells of two differing genotypes can be fused, usually in the presence of Sendai virus, to form multinucleate cells (heterokaryons) containing nuclei of both genotypes. When fibroblasts from two patients suffering from xeroderma pigmentosum were fused, the resulting heterokaryons showed no deficiency in DNA repair. What conclusions can be drawn from this observation? Explain.

6. Eukaryotic DNA can be highly methylated at the C-5 position of cytosine. The degree of methylation is inversely correlated with gene expression. Although the exact role of C-5 methylation in gene expression has not been determined, it is known that these C-5–methylated cytosines can cause mutations. How?

ANSWERS TO PROBLEMS

1. In the text there is a description of the system in which MutS and MutL detect a mismatch and then recruit MutH to cut the strand with the incorrect nucleotide. While it is not spelled out in the textbook, many forms of both DNA and RNA are extensively methylated. At least in gram negative bacteria, "hemimethylated" DNA provides a clue. The older strand has been around long enough to accumulate methyl groups, whereas the newly made strand has not. Therefore the mismatch repair system (in E. coli and other bacteria) "believes" the older strand and the MutH nicks and initiates repair in the newer, unmethylated strand.

2. First, if copy-choice were a correct model, no recombinant phage should be produced in the absence of new DNA synthesis. Second, according to that model, no recombinant DNA duplexes should contain both bromouracil and ^{32}P. However, the Holliday

model for homologous recombination accounts for how different labels from different DNA molecules could occur in the same progeny molecule.

3. Exons often encode protein domains. Genetic recombination can lead to rearrangements in the order of exons in a gene. Upon expression, such rearranged genes could give rise to proteins with new domain orders and possibly new capabilities.

4. The mutagen 5-bromouracil changes A·T pairs to G·C pairs and G·C pairs to A·T pairs. The mutation in (c) could be induced by 5-bromouracil. For example, the DNA sequence AAA, which codes for phenylalanine, could be changed to the sequence AAG, which codes for leucine. The other mutations could not arise from treatment with 5-bromouracil. Remember that the genetic code presented in the text is expressed in terms of RNA. The sequence UUU on RNA corresponds to the sequence AAA on the informational strand of DNA. Leucine is encoded by the sequence CUU on RNA, which corresponds to the sequence AAG on the informational strand of DNA. Remember also that, unless otherwise specified, nucleotide sequences are written in the 5′ → 3′ direction.

5. Hydroxylamine causes the unidirectional change of C·G pairs to T·A pairs. The mutation in (a) cannot result from the action of hydroxylamine. Those in (b), (c), and (d) might. In (b), TTC (Glu) could change to TTT (Lys). In (c), ATG (His) could be converted to ATA (Tyr). In (d), ACC (Gly) could change to ATC (Asp), or GCC (Gly) could change to GTC (Asp).

6. Because thymidylate synthase is inactivated, the supply of dTTP is insufficient to support the synthesis of DNA at normal rates. If DNA synthesis is suppressed, so too will be the rate of division of the tumor cells. This type of treatment takes advantage of the fact that tumor cells divide more rapidly than do normal cells. The dosage of the drug is adjusted so that it will primarily affect more rapidly dividing cells. However, the division of some normally rapidly dividing cells, for example, those lining the intestinal tract and blood forming cells, may be retarded as well.

7. The fibroblasts from the two patients show complementation (the defect in each is remedied by the other), so it is likely that the two patients suffer from different genetic variants of xeroderma pigmentosum. The action of several genes is likely responsible for the excision and subsequent repair of damaged DNA. One patient, for example, could have produced a normal nuclease that excises damaged DNA but have been deficient in a ligase. The other patient could have produced normal ligase but have been deficient in nuclease activity. There are at least nine different complementation groups among xeroderma patients.

8. C-5 methyl cytosine can spontaneously deaminate just as cytosine can. When C-5 methyl cytosine deaminates, it forms thymidine, not uracil. Therefore uracil N-glycosylase, a DNA repair enzyme, will not recognize this product of deamination as an inappropriate base and will not remove it from the DNA, causing a transition mutation.

RNA Synthesis and Regulation in Bacteria

In this chapter, the authors describe the biochemistry underlying several mechanisms that control gene expression in prokaryotes. They point out that control of transcription is the primary mechanism of gene regulation, and that the specific binding of proteins to particular regulatory DNA sequences is the basis of the control. The chapter begins with a discussion of the nature of the variety of RNA polymerases in *E. coli*. The next section discusses in detail the processes of initiation, elongation and termination of RNA synthesis, and the three stages of transcription. The role of promoters, the sigma submit of RNA polymerase, and the rho protein are highlighted. The lactose (lac) operon in bacteria is an example of a mechanism in which the initiation of transcription is regulated. Negative control is exerted through the binding of a repressor protein to DNA carrying the lac operator. Positive control of the lac operon is accomplished by a complex of CAP protein and cyclic AMP (cAMP). The complex binds near the lac promoter in the absence of the repressor and through protein-protein interactions stimulates the activity of RNA polymerase at the lac promoter. The authors finish this section with the introduction of biofilms, complex communities of prokaryotes that are promoted by quorum-sensing mechanisms.

LEARNING OBJECTIVES

When you have mastered this chapter, you should be able to accomplish the following objectives:

Cellular RNA Is Synthesized by RNA Polymerases (Text Section 36.1)

1. Define the term *transcription* and relate it to the flow of genetic information.

2. List the components necessary for the function of *RNA polymerases (DNA-dependent RNA polymerases)*.

3. Name the *three major classes of RNA* found in E. coli and explain their functions.

4. Name the subunits of E. coli RNA polymerases and state their relative sizes and functions.

RNA Synthesis Comprises Three Stages (Text Section 36.2)

5. Describe the *subunit structure* of *RNA polymerase* from E. coli and assign functions to the individual subunits.

6. Recognize the convention for numbering the nucleotides in the DNA template with regard to the *transcription start site*. Distinguish between the *template* (or *antisense*) *strand* and the *coding* (or *sense*) *strand* of the duplex DNA template.

7. Note the *consensus sequences* around the -35 and -10 positions and the *upstream element* of E. coli promoters. Contrast the rates of transcript initiation on *strong* and *weak promoters* in E. coli.

8. Know that RNA polymerases backtrack and correct errors.

9. Explain how the σ *factor* enables RNA polymerase to *recognize promoters*. Distinguish between the σ^{70} and σ^{32} subunits, contrast the sequences of *standard promoters* and *heat-shock promoters,* and provide examples of how σ factors can determine which genes are expressed.

10. Distinguish between *closed* and *open promoter complexes*.

11. Detail the de novo initiation of chain growth by RNA polymerase, name the usual initiating ribonucleoside, and describe the chemical nature of the 5′ end of the RNA.

12. Describe the model for the *transcription bubble*. State the *number of base pairs in the RNA–DNA hybrid*. Appreciate the *rate of RNA chain elongation* in terms of both the nucleotides added and the distance on the template traversed by RNA polymerase.

13. Contrast ρ-*dependent* and ρ-*independent* transcription termination. Outline the mechanisms of the ρ protein and explain the role of *ATP hydrolysis* in its function.

14. Describe the mechanisms of *inhibition of transcription* by *rifampicin* and *actinomycin* D.

15. Outline the processing and modification of the precursors of rRNA and tRNA in prokaryotes.

The Lac Operon Illustrates the Control of Bacterial Gene Expression (Text Section 36.3)

16. Outline the metabolism of lactose in E. coli. Draw the structure of *lactose*, describe its entry into the cell, and write the equations for the reactions catalyzed by *β-galactosidase*, providing both the substrates and the products.

17. Provide a definition of *operon*.

18. Draw the *genetic map* of the lac operon and outline the functions of the *promoter, repressor, operator,* and *inducer* in controlling the production of *polycistronic* lac *mRNA*. Distinguish between regulatory and structural genes.

19. Describe the *subunit structure* of the *lac* repressor and relate it to the *symmetrical sequence* of the *lac* operator. Describe the effect of the binding of *allolactose* by the repressor on its affinity for the operator.

20. Recognize that many other gene-regulatory networks in prokaryotes functions like the *lac* operon.

21. Explain the functions of *cyclic AMP (cAMP)* and the *catabolite activator protein (CAP)* in modulating the expression of the *lac* operon.

22. Diagram the relative positions of cAMP–CAP complex, RNA polymerase, and *lac* repressor on the DNA template. Explain their effects on one another and on the DNA structure.

23. Relate the levels of cAMP to the concentration of glucose in the cell.

24. Define the term *quorum sensing* and use the bacteria *Vibrio fisheri* as an example of it. Explain the role of *autoinducers* in the process and how they allow a bacterium to determine the density of the *V. fisheri* population in its environment.

25. Describe *biofilms* and relate the role quorum sensing plays in their formation.

SELF-TEST

Cellular RNA Is Synthesized by RNA Polymerases

1. If each of the three major classes of RNA found in a cell were hybridized to denatured DNA from the same cell and the presence of RNA-DNA hybrids were tested, which of the classes would be retained on the filter?
   - (a) mRNA
   - (b) rRNA
   - (c) tRNA

2. What are the three major classes of RNA in a cell and which are the most abundant?

3. Which of the following are required for the DNA-dependent RNA polymerase reaction to produce a unique RNA transcript?
   - (a) ATP
   - (b) CTP
   - (c) GTP
   - (d) dTTP
   - (e) UTP
   - (f) DNA
   - (g) RNA
   - (h) Mg^{2+}
   - (i) promoter sequence
   - (j) operator sequence
   - (k) terminator sequence

4. What is the sequence of the mRNA that will be synthesized from a template strand of DNA having the following sequence?

   . . .ACGTTACCTAGTTGC. . .

5. Describe the mechanism of chain growth during RNA synthesis. What is the polarity of synthesis and how is it related to the polarity of the template strand of DNA?

RNA Synthesis Comprises Three Stages

6. Give the subunit composition of the RNA polymerase of E. coli for both the holoenzyme and the core enzyme.
7. Match the subunit of the RNA polymerase of *E. coli* in the left column with its putative function during catalysis from the right column.

(a) α	(1) binds the DNA template
(b) β	(2) binds regulatory proteins and sequences
(c) β'	(3) binds NTPs and catalyzes bond formation
(d) σ^{70}	(4) recognizes the promoter and initiates synthesis

8. Which of the following statements about *E. coli* promoters are correct?
   (a) They may exhibit different transcription efficiencies.
   (b) For most genes they include variants of consensus sequences.
   (c) They specify the start sites for transcription on the DNA template.
   (d) They have identical and defining sequences.
   (e) They are activated when C or G residues are substituted into their −10 regions by mutation.
   (f) Those that have sequences that correspond closely to the consensus sequences and are separated by 17 base pairs are very efficient.
9. The sequence of a duplex DNA segment in a longer DNA molecule is

   5′-ATCGCTTGTTCGGA-3′

   3′-TAGCGAACAAGCCT-5′

   When this segment serves as a template for E. coli RNA polymerase, it gives rise to a segment of RNA with the sequence 5′-UCCGAACAAGCGAU-3′. Which of the following statements about the DNA segment are correct?
   (a) The top strand is the coding strand.
   (b) The bottom strand is the sense strand.
   (c) The top strand is the template strand.
   (d) The bottom strand is the antisense strand.
10. The text states that RNA polymerases backtrack for proofreading. Why would this be energetically unfavorable? What is the error rate of RNA synthesis?
11. Which of the following statements about the σ subunit of RNA polymerase are correct?
    (a) It enables the enzyme to transcribe asymmetrically.
    (b) It confers on the core enzyme the ability to initiate transcription at promoters.
    (c) It decreases the affinity of RNA polymerase for regions of DNA that lack promoter sequences.
    (d) It facilitates the termination of transcription by recognizing hairpins in the transcript.
12. When growing *E. coli* are subjected to a rapid increase in temperature, a new and characteristic set of genes is expressed. Explain how this alteration in gene expression occurs.

13. Match the regions of a ρ-independent transcription termination signal in a DNA template in the left column with the structures or the functions performed by the encoded transcript segments in the right column.

   (a) GC-rich palindromic region
   (b) AT-rich region

   (1) oligo(U) stretch in RNA
   (2) hairpin in RNA
   (3) promotes the dissociation of RNA–DNA hybrid helix
   (4) causes the enzyme to pause

14. Which of the following statements about the ρ protein of *E. coli* are correct?

   (a) It is an ATPase that is activated by binding to single-strand DNA.
   (b) It recognizes specific sequences in single-strand RNA.
   (c) It recognizes sequences in the DNA template strand.
   (d) It causes RNA polymerase to terminate transcription at template sites that are different from those that lead to ρ-independent termination.
   (e) It acts as a RNA–DNA helicase.

15. Match the functions in the right column with the appropriate antibiotic inhibitor of *E. coli* transcription in the left column.

   (a) rifampicin
   (b) actinomycin D

   (1) interacts with the template
   (2) interacts with nascent mRNA polymerase
   (3) prevents initiation
   (4) prevents elongation
   (5) intercalates into mRNA hairpins

16. Explain how a mutation might give rise to an *E. coli* that is resistant to the antibiotic rifampicin.

The Lac Operon Illustrates the Control of Prokaryotic Gene Expression

17. Which of the following are common mechanisms used by bacteria to regulate their metabolic pathways?

   (a) control of the expression of genes
   (b) control of enzyme activities through allosteric activators and inhibitors
   (c) formation of altered enzymes by the alternative splicing of mRNAs
   (d) deletion and elimination of genes that specify enzymes
   (e) control of enzyme activities through covalent modifications

18. Which of the following statements about β-galactosidase in *E. coli* are correct?

   (a) It is present in varying concentrations depending on the carbon source used for growth.
   (b) It is a product of a unit of gene expression called an *operon*.
   (c) It hydrolyzes the β-1,4-linked disaccharide lactose to produce galactose and glucose.
   (d) It forms the β-1,6-linked disaccharide allolactose.
   (e) Its levels rise coordinately with those of galactoside permease and thiogalactoside transacetylase.

19. Match each feature or function in the right column with the appropriate DNA sequence element of the *lac* operon in the left column.

(a) *i*
(b) *p*
(c) *o*
(d) *z*
(e) *y* and *a*
(f) CAP binding site

(1) contains a specific binding sequence for the *lac* repressor
(2) encodes a galactoside permease
(3) contains a binding sequence for the cAMP–CAP complex
(4) encodes a protein that interferes with the activation of RNA polymerase
(5) encodes a protein that binds allolactose
(6) contains a specific binding sequence for RNA polymerase
(7) encodes β-galactosidase
(8) is a regulatory gene
(9) is the *lac* promoter
(10) encodes thiogalactoside transacetylase
(11) is the *lac* operator
(12) encodes the *lac* repressor

20. When *E. coli* is added to a culture containing both lactose and glucose, which of the sugars is metabolized preferentially? What is the mechanism underlying this selectivity?

21. What happens after the first-used sugar is depleted during the experiment described in question 7?

22. Which of the following statements about the cAMP–CAP complex are correct?

(a) It protects the -87 to -49 sequence of the *lac* operon from nuclease digestion.
(b) It protects the -48 to $+5$ sequence of the *lac* operon from nuclease digestion.
(c) It protects the -3 to $+21$ sequence of the *lac* operon from nuclease digestion.
(d) It affects RNA polymerase activity in a number of operons.
(e) Upon binding to the *lac* operon, it contacts RNA polymerase.

23. Place the following steps in the order they occur in quorum sensing by *V. Fisheri*.

(a) Luciferase is produced.
(b) LuxR binds AHL.
(c) Transcription of LuxA, LuxB, and LuxI is increased.
(d) *V. Fisheri* release an autoinducer called AHL.

ANSWERS TO SELF-TEST

1. a, b, c. All cellular RNA is encoded by the DNA of the cell.

2. The three major classes are messenger RNA (mRNA), transfer RNA (tRNA) and ribosomal RNA (rRNA). Messenger RNA encodes the information for protein synthesis while tRNA and rRNA are components in protein synthesis machinery.

3. a, b, c, e, f, h, i, and k. Answer (f) is correct because DNA is needed to serve as the template. Answers (k) and (i) are correct because the promoter and terminator sequences are needed to specify the precise start and stop points, respectively, for the transcription.

4. The mRNA sequence will be ...GCAACUAGGUAACGU..., written in the 5′ to 3′ direction.

5. The 3′-hydroxyl terminus of the growing RNA chain makes a nucleophilic attack on the α-phosphate (the innermost phosphate) of the ribonucleoside triphosphate that has been selected by base pairing to the template strand of the duplex DNA. RNA polymerase catalyzes the reaction. A ribonucleoside monophosphate residue is added to the chain as a result, and the chain has grown in the 5′ to 3′ direction; that is, the chain has grown at its 3′ end. As with all Watson-Crick base pairing, the strands are antiparallel; that is, the RNA chain is assembled in the 3′ to 5′ direction with respect to the polarity of the template strand of the DNA.

6. The holoenzyme has the subunit composition $\alpha_2\beta\beta'\omega\sigma$. The core enzyme lacks the σ subunit.

7. (a) 2   (b) 3   (c) 1   (d) 4

8. a, b, c, f. The promoters of most *E. coli* genes include variants of defining consensus sequences that are centered at about the −35 and −10 positions. The nearer the sequences of a promoter are to the consensus sequence and the nearer the separation between them is to the optimal 17-bp spacing, the more efficient the promoter. The −10 consensus sequence is TATAAT. The substitution of a C or G into the sequence would likely lower the efficiency of a promoter.

9. b, c. The sense (bottom) strand of the template DNA has the same sequence as the mRNA.

10. Backtracking involves breaking hydrogen bonds between an RNA-DNA base pair, but if the base pair is incorrect there will often be fewer hydrogen bonds to break. The text states that the final error rate is between one mistake in 10^4 and one in 10^5 nucleotides added. Compare this to the DNA error rate (after various corrective processes have been applied, including mismatch repair) of one in 10^9–10^{10}.

11. a, b, c. The σ subunit recognizes promoter sites, decreases the affinity of the enzyme for regions of DNA lacking promoter sequences, and facilitates the specific, oriented initiation of transcription. Orienting the binding of the enzyme to the DNA results in only one of the two DNA strands functioning as a template for RNA transcription; that is, it gives rise to asymmetric transcription.

12. The temperature increase induces the synthesis of a new σ factor, σ^{32}, which directs RNA polymerase to promoters that have −10 and −35 sequences different from those recognized by σ^{70}. Transcription from these promoters gives rise to characteristic heat-shock proteins.

13. (a) 2, 4   (b) 1, 3

14. d, e. The ρ protein recognizes and binds stretches of RNA that are devoid of hairpins and are at least 72 nucleotides long. It acts to hydrolyze ATP and to unwind the RNA–DNA hybrid in the transcription bubble.

15. (a) 2, 3   (b) 1, 4. Actinomycin D intercalates only into duplex DNA.

16. Rifampicin must bind to the β subunit of RNA polymerase to inhibit the enzyme. A mutation in the gene encoding this subunit that would interfere with the binding of the antibiotic but not with polymerization would produce a rifampicin-resistant cell.

17. a, b, e. Answer (c) is incorrect because the splicing of mRNA is rare in bacteria.

18. All of the answers are correct.

19. (a) 4, 5, 8, 12   (b) 6, 9   (c) 1, 11   (d) 5, 7   (e) 2, 10   (f) 3. For (d), 5 is correct because allolactose is the product of a reaction catalyzed by β-galactosidase and, as a product, it binds to the enzyme.

20. Glucose is metabolized preferentially because it results in a decrease in the synthesis of cAMP by adenylate cyclase. The lack of cAMP prevents the formation of the cAMP–CAP complex, which is necessary for the efficient transcription of the *lac* operon and other catabolite-repressible operons.

21. When glucose is depleted, the concentration of cAMP rises. The cAMP–CAP complex forms and binds to the CAP binding site just upstream of the RNA polymerase binding site in the *lac* promoter. At the same time, some lactose has entered the cell, has been converted to allolactose by β-galactosidase, and is bound by the *lac* repressor so that it no longer binds to the *lac* operator. RNA polymerase now binds to the *lac* promoter even more effectively because of protein–protein interactions with the cAMP–CAP complex. The enzymes and permease of the *lac* operon are expressed fully; consequently, lactose readily enters the cell and is efficiently metabolized.

22. a, d, e. Answers (b) and (c) are incorrect because they correspond to the binding sequences for RNA polymerase and *lac* repressor, respectively.

23. The steps are d, b, c, and finally a.

PROBLEMS

1. When lactose is used as an inducer a lag occurs before the enzymes of the lactose operon are synthesized. Explain this observation.

2. Since the permease required for the entry of lactose into *E. coli* cells is itself a product of the lactose operon, how might the first lactose molecules enter uninduced cells? Explain.

3. The three enzymes of the lactose operon in *E. coli* are not produced in precisely equimolar amounts following induction. Rather, more galactosidase than permease is produced, and more permease than transacetylase is produced. Propose a mechanism to account for this that is consistent with known facts about the lactose operon.

4. The kinetics of induction of enzyme X are shown in Figure 36.1. What percentage of total cellular protein is due to enzyme X in induced cells when 60 μg of total bacterial protein has been synthesized?

FIGURE 36.1   Kinetics of induction of enzyme X.

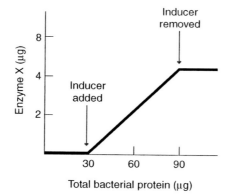

5. Assume that the dissociation constant K for the repressor-operator complex is 10^{-13} M and that the rate constant for association of operator and repressor is 10^{10} M^{-1} s^{-1}. Calculate the rate constant k_{diss} for the dissociation of the repressor–operator complex. What is the $t_{1/2}$ (half-time of dissociation, or half-life) of the repressor–operator complex?

6. In systems of genetic regulation involving positive control, a regulatory gene produces a substance that enhances rather than inhibits transcription. Are there elements of positive control in the lactose operon of *E. coli*? Explain.

7. Suppose that a system regulating the expression of a single copy DNA leads to the synthesis of an enzyme having a turnover number (k_{cat}) of 10^4 s^{-1}. Each DNA copy is transcribed into 10^3 molecules of mRNA and that each of the mRNA molecules is translated into 10^5 molecules of enzyme protein. How many molecules of substrate are converted into product per second for each wave of transcription that sweeps over the DNA?

8. All proteins that bind DNA at specific sites also show affinity for DNA at sequences other than the ones that comprise their targets. In general, what effect do you think that nonspecific DNA could have on the ability of a repressor to regulate an operon? Consider the *lac* operator-repressor system in *E. coli* in which the operator is 35 bp within 4.6×10^6 bp total DNA. What would the nonspecific DNA do to the concentration of the free repressor in the cell?

9. Antibiotic resistance occurs when bacteria that are not resistant to the antibiotic are killed, leaving behind bacteria that have developed resistance to the antibiotic. Eventually only the antibiotic-resistant bacteria are left. Speculate on how antibiotics could be developed that target quorum sensing, especially in bacteria that form biofilms.

10. On page 635 of the text, it states that RNA polymerases "detect termination signals that specify where a transcript ends." Consider the ways in which transcription terminates in bacteria, and suggest an argument that the above statement might be considered incorrect.

11. The rho protein (ρ) that is involved in termination of bacterial transcription has six subunits and rotates around the emerging RNA strand as it "climbs" it, all propelled by conformational changes due to ATP hydrolysis. What sort of proteins come to mind as possible homologues?

12. One would expect an analog of 5'-ATP that lacks an oxygen at the 3' position of its ribose (3'-deoxy-5'-ATP; see Figure 36.2) to interrupt RNA formation because it cannot form phosphodiester bonds at its 3' position. Could such a compound be used to ascertain the direction of chain growth in RNA synthesis? Explain.

FIGURE 36.2   Structure of 3'-deoxy-5'-ATP.

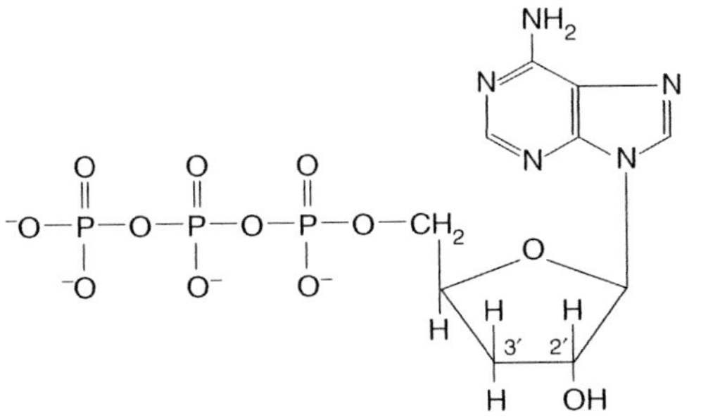

13. When mammalian genes are cloned, a strategy that is frequently followed involves the isolation of mRNA rather than DNA from a cell and the preparation of a complementary DNA (cDNA) by the enzyme reverse transcriptase. Suppose that mRNA isolated from a cell specialized for the production of protein X is used as a template for the production of cDNA. What major difference or differences would you expect to find between the structure of that cDNA and genomic DNA for protein X?

14. Rifampicin specifically inhibits the initiation of transcription in prokaryotes and may therefore be used in humans as a therapeutic antibacterial agent. Would you expect actinomycin D to be useful in antibacterial therapy? Why or why not?

15. Sketch the most stable secondary structure that could be assumed by the oligonucleotide AAGGCCCUACGGGGCCG.

16. Negative supercoiling affects transcription at many promoters in *E. coli*. In addition to facilitating the unwinding of the DNA helix necessary to form a transcription bubble, how might negative supercoiling affect transcription either positively or negatively?

ANSWERS TO PROBLEMS

1. The actual inducer of the lactose operon in vivo is 1,6-allolactose. (See page 639 of the text.) The lag represents the time it takes for lactose to be converted into 1,6-allolactose by residual β-galactosidase.

2. Very low levels of lactose operon enzymes are synthesized even in the absence of an inducer (see page 638 of the text, which indicates that few enzymes are produced in the absence of inducer).

3. Differential expression of the three structural genes in the lactose operon must be at the level of translation and not transcription since a single, polycistronic mRNA molecule is formed. Following induction, mRNA transcripts containing genetic information for all three genes are produced. Some ribosomes might drop off the messenger at the end of the structural genes, with a smaller number reading through the more distal genes.

4. From the graph in Figure 36.1, we see that 2 µg of enzyme X is present when the total bacterial protein present is equal to 60 µg. Thus, the percentage of enzyme X is 100% × 2/60 = 3.3%.

5. Remembering that the dissociation constant K is equal to the ratio of the off rate to the on rate for a reaction,

$$[RO] \rightleftharpoons [R] + [O]$$

$$\frac{[R][O]}{[RO]} = K = 10^{-13} \text{ M } \frac{k_{diss}}{10^{10} \text{ M}^{-1}\text{s}^{-1}}$$

$$k_{diss} = 10^{-3}\text{s}^{-1}$$

$$t_{\frac{1}{2}} = \frac{0.693}{k_{diss}} = \frac{0.693}{10^{-3}\text{s}^{-1}} = 693 \text{ s} \cong 11.6 \text{ min}$$

6. Catabolite activator protein (CAP) is a positive control element. When the level of glucose in cells is low, the level of cAMP is high, leading to the formation of cAMP−CAP complex. The cAMP−CAP complex binds to DNA in the promoter region, creating an entry site for RNA polymerase. The result is the transcription of the lactose operon (providing that no repressor is present). (See Figure 36.19 on page 639 of the text.)

7. Depending on the equilibrium dissociation constants of the repressor for its target and for nonspecific sequences, the number of target sequences present, and the ratio of specific to nonspecific DNA present, much of the repressor could be sequestered through binding to the nonspecific DNA. Such nonspecific binding would decrease the concentration of free repressor that could interact with the operator. Since the

DNA binding reaction depends on the concentrations of the interacting repressor and DNA, lowering the repressor's concentration would decrease the fraction of operator bound and thereby repressed. The *lac* repressor-operator system provides a good example of this situation. See Kao-Huang, Y., Revzin, A., Butler, A.P., O'Connor, P., Noble, D.W., and von Hippel, P. (1977) *Proc. Natl. Acad. Sci. USA* 74:4228-4232. These authors found that nonspecific DNA competed effectively with the specific sequence for the repressor. When one copy of *lac* operator is present in *E. coli*, ~4.6 × 10^6 different, nonspecific binding sites will be present. Think of this by considering that the repressor binds to a 35-bp-long operator site. By sliding this 35-bp-long window along the DNA, one bp at a time, there are ~4.6 × 10^6 nonspecific sites that can compete with the one correct site. The ability of the operon to be transcribed depends on the average fraction of free operator present, and nonspecific DNA significantly affected that fraction. Thus, nonspecific DNA can play an important role in the functioning of a repressor–operator interaction in the cell. See the article if you wish to see a detailed, quantitative analysis of the phenomenon.

8. Bacteria that form biofilms are of particular medical importance because organisms that form them are often resistant to the immune response as well as to antibiotics. Quorum sensing appears to play a major role in the formation of biofilms in that cells are able to sense other cells in their environments and to promote the formation of communities with particular compositions. The opportunistic bacteria *Pseudomonas aeruginosa*, for example, uses quorum sensing to coordinate the formation of biofilms. If a molecule could be designed that binds to the autoinducer receptor, but blocks dimerization, and therefore blocks activation of transcription, quorum sensing would also be blocked. This should prevent the bacteria from forming biofilms, and give the body's immune system time to remove the infection through normal immune pathways. This process is called quorum quenching. An advantage to this approach compared to traditional antibiotic design is that there would be few evolutionary forces that select for resistance. Non-resistant strains could still multiply, and resistant strains would have to compete with them. There would be no strong survival advantage to resistant mutations.

9. Negative supercoiling affects transcription at many promoters in *E. coli*. In addition to facilitating the unwinding of the DNA helix necessary to form a transcription bubble, how might negative supercoiling affect transcription either positively or negatively?

10. One method of termination is "hairpin-poly-U" (see text Fig. 36.11). When the hairpin forms, the formation stresses the weak A-U base pairs and the RNA is "yanked" from the active site of the enzyme. If formation of the hairpin is prevented then the sequence itself does not cause termination. So just what is the enzyme doing to cause termination? Arguably it is the RNA itself that is removing itself from the enzyme and causing termination. Similarly, ρ the rho protein may pull the RNA from the active site when it recognizes a target sequence.

11. The text points out that the rho protein is related to helicases, which also can have a circular hexameric structure, and can "pull the string" on a nucleic acid (Fig. 36.12). The discussion of helicases states that they are related to a large family of P-loop NTPase proteins, which include several interesting molecules. One of the most interesting connections is the relationship between the rho protein and the F1 ATPase in mitochondria, which is also a circular arrangement of six subunits and a rotary mechanism. This relationship has long been known [*J. Bacteriol.* (1994) 176:5033]. Of course F1 is forced to run "backwards," which causes ATP to be synthesized rather than broken down.

12. A 3′-deoxy analog of ATP could be used to establish the direction of chain growth. In 5′ → 3′ growth the analog would donate a nucleotide containing 3′-deoxyadenosine, and the polynucleotide chain would be terminated as a result. No additional nucleotides could be added because of the lack of a 3′-OH group on the terminal 3′-deoxyadenosine. In 5′ → 3′ growth the nucleotide could not be added to the growing polynucleotide chain because of the lack of the 3′-OH group.

13. The cDNA prepared from mRNA would have a long poly(T) tail, unlike genomic DNA. Remember that the poly(A) tail is added to the 3′ end of mammalian mRNA and that there is no counterpart on DNA. A second striking difference would be that the cDNA would contain no intervening sequences (introns) and would therefore be much shorter than the corresponding sections of genomic DNA. (Remember that most mammalian genes are mosaics of introns and exons.) A third difference would be found if any RNA editing were involved. An edited mRNA could generate a cDNA with nucleotides that did not correspond to those in genomic DNA.

14. In order to be useful as a therapeutic antibacterial agent, a compound must selectively inhibit processes in prokaryotes but leave the corresponding processes in eukaryotes (including those in mitochondria) largely unaffected. Because rifampicin selectively inhibits the initiation of transcription in prokaryotes but not in eukaryotes, it is useful as an antibacterial agent. Actinomycin D is an intercalating agent that binds to DNA duplexes and inhibits both DNA replication and transcription, although it has a greater inhibiting effect on transcription than on replication. It cannot discriminate between the duplex DNA of bacteria and that of humans, however, and will therefore bind to both. Because it disrupts eukaryotic as well as prokaryotic processes, it is not very useful as an antibacterial agent. It is sometimes used as an anticancer agent, however, because of its ability to slow the replication rate of human DNA.

15. The structure is a stem-and-loop ("lollipop") hairpin structure, as shown in Figure 36.3.

FIGURE 36.3 Stable secondary structure for the oligonucleotide in problem 8.

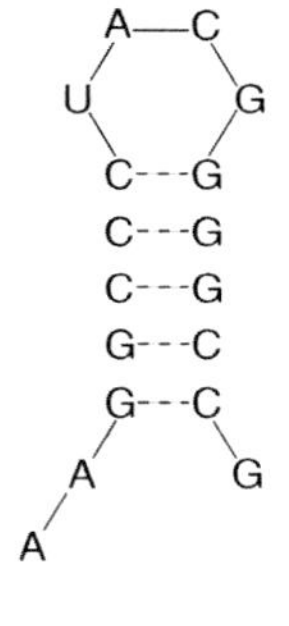

16. The interaction of the σ subunit of RNA polymerase with a promoter requires the precise positioning of the atomic determinants on the surface of the DNA at the −10 and −35 regions to which it binds. Particular hydrogen bond donors and acceptors in the grooves of the DNA in these regions must be positioned so that the amino acids on the protein can interact optimally with them. The degree of supercoiling of a DNA molecule affects the precise positioning of these groups because the base pairs are moved with respect to one another by twisting the DNA. Thus, supercoiling could either promote or hinder the interaction of the polymerase with the DNA by bringing the groups in the −10 region and in −35 regions of the DNA of particular promoters into a configuration that was better or worse for interaction. (If you are interested in this topic, see Hatfield, W.G., and Benham, C.J. (2002) *Annu. Rev. Genet.* 36:175–203.)

Gene Expression in Eurkaryotes

In this chapter, the authors describe the biochemistry underlying gene expression in eukaryotes, using the discussion of prokaryotic gene expression in Chapter 36 for comparison. They discuss how the abundance of DNA, chromosome structure, and the existence of the cellular differentiation and posttranscriptional gene regulatory mechanisms complicate the control of gene expression. After a brief discussion that provides an overview of the major differences between gene regulation and gene-regulatory proteins in prokaryotes and eukaryotes, the authors outline the three types of RNA polymerases, identifying their different locations, products, and sensitivity to modification by the toxin α-Amanitin. The authors then focus on the complex regulation involved in the action of RNA polymerase II, which synthesizes mRNA. The role of the TATA box and TATA-box-binding proteins in the binding of RNA polymerase to promoter regions are explored in depth. Enhancers are then introduced as a mechanism for control of gene expression from more than 1000 bp away from the start site of transcription. The second section ends with a brief discussion of induced pluripotent stem cells (iPS) and how they may play a role in the treatment of a variety of diseases. The authors next move on to the regulation of gene expression by steroid hormones through nuclear receptors. The role of components such as ligands, steroid hormone response elements (SRE), zinc fingers, and coactivators and corepressors are explored. The chapter ends with a discussion of the role of histone acetylation in chromatin remodeling. The structural basis for the effect that histone acetylation has on chromatin structure as well as the binding of acetylated histones to bromodomains, regions of DNA that are designed to bind to acetylated histones, are discussed. The authors present a detailed mechanism by which chromatin remodeling occurs and enhances RNA transcription and the role that deacetylases play in regulating transcription.

LEARNING OBJECTIVES

When you have mastered this chapter, you should be able to accomplish the following objectives:

Introduction

1. Discuss the characteristics of gene expression unique to eukaryotes.

2. Note the spatial and temporal differences in transcription and translation between prokaryotes and eukaryotes. Consider the regulatory implications of these differences.

Eukaryotic Cells Have Three Types of RNA Polymerases (Text Section 37.1)

3. Describe the *RNA polymerases* of eukaryotes, locate them within the cell, and list the kinds of RNA they synthesize. Account for the toxic effects of α -amanitin, and describe how it can be used to differentiate the three eukaryotic RNA polymerases.

4. Identify the unique method of regulation of *RNA polymerase II*.

5. List the classes of RNA and summarize their relative sizes and functions.

6. List the salient *sequence elements* of *eukaryotic promoters*. Contrast the nucleotide sequences and locations of the *TATA box* of eukaryotes and the −10 sequence of prokaryotes.

7. Contrast the promoter specificity of the three eukaryotic RNA polymerases.

RNA Polymerase II Requires Complex Regulation (Text Section 37.2)

8. Explain the key role of *TATA-box-binding protein (TBP)* in assembling active *TFII transcription complexes*. Describe the role of phosphorylation of the *carboxy-terminal domain (CTD)* of RNA polymerase II.

9. Outline the combinatorial activity of *transcription factors* and other DNA-binding regulatory proteins in directing RNA polymerase to specific genes. Indicate the properties of *enhancer* sequences.

10. Describe the characteristics of *induced pluripotent stem cells (iPS)* and explain how they hold promise in the treatment of a variety of diseases.

Gene Expression Is Regulated By Hormones (Text Section 37.3)

11. Contrast the mechanism of the *steroid hormones* with hormones initiating their actions through interactions with a transmembrane receptor.

12. Describe the domain structure of *nuclear hormone receptors*.

13. Describe the zinc-finger structure of nuclear hormone receptors and describe how it is involved in the interaction of the estrogen–estrogen receptor complex interaction with *estrogen response elements (ERE)*.

14. Outline the role of *coactivators* in transcription by nuclear hormone receptors.

15. Distinguish between *agonists* and *antagonists*. Characterize *anabolic steroids* as agonists of the androgen receptor. Contrast mechanisms of positive and negative gene regulation in eukaryotes.

16. Explain how *tamoxifen* and *raloxifene* serve as an anticancer agents. Recognize the origin of their characterization as *estrogen receptor modulators (SERMs)*.

Histone Acetylation Results in Chromatin Remodeling (Text Section 37.4)

17. Outline the effects of the *acetylation* and *deacetylation* of *histone tails* on chromatin structure and gene transcription.

18. Describe the mechanism by which histone acetylation recruits components of the transcription machinery.

19. Describe the reaction catalyzed by *histone acetyltransferases (HATs)* and explain the resulting effect on histone structure.

20. List the three mechanisms by which histone acetylation activates transcription.

21. Summarize the variety of histone modifications.

SELF-TEST

Introduction

1. For each of the following, identify it as a feature of eukaryotic (E) or prokaryotic (P) gene transcription.
   (a) The ends of mRNA are modified.
   (b) Transcription and translation are coupled.
   (c) There are three RNA polymerases involved.
   (d) There are three promoter elements involved.
   (e) The resulting mRNA is spliced.

Eukaryotic Cells Have Three Types of RNA Polymerases

2. Match the descriptions in the right column with the appropriate eukaryotic DNA-dependent RNA polymerase(s) in the left column.
   (a) RNA polymerase I
   (b) RNA polymerase II
   (c) RNA polymerase III

   (1) is located in the nucleolus
   (2) is located in the nucleoplasm
   (3) makes mRNA precursors
   (4) makes tRNA precursors
   (5) makes 5S rRNA
   (6) makes 18S, 5.8S, and 28S rRNA precursors
   (7) is strongly inhibited by α-amanitin
   (8) synthesizes RNA in the $5' \rightarrow 3'$ direction
   (9) is composed of several subunits
   (10) has a subunit with repeated amino acid sequences subject to phosphorylation

3. Match each type of RNA listed below with its function.
   (a) lncRNA
   (b) miRNA
   (c) piRNA
   (d) siRNA
   (e) snRNA
   (f) snoRNA

   (1) Involved in RNA splicing
   (2) Gene regulation
   (3) Helps control the use of mRNA
   (4) Involved in rRNA biogenesis and modification
   (5) Participates in antiviral defense via mRNA degradation

4. List the major sequence features of promoters for eukaryotic mRNA genes.

RNA Polymerase II Requires Complex Regulation

5. Describe the role of TATA-box-binding protein (TBP, TFIID) in forming the basal transcription apparatus. What properties does TBP confer on this apparatus?

6. Which of the following statements about enhancers are correct?

   (a) They function as promoters.
   (b) They function in either orientation in the DNA.
   (c) They function on either side of the activated promoter.
   (d) They function even when located many base pairs away from the promoter.
   (e) They function only in specific types of cells.

7. Specific combinatorial control of transcription

   (a) is enabled by specific interactions between transcription factors and specific DNA sequences.
   (b) allows a given regulatory protein to have different effects depending upon the neighboring proteins with which it is associated.
   (c) is effected by transcription factors some of which do not themselves interact with DNA.
   (d) depends upon the assembly of multicomponent nucleoprotein complexes.
   (e) results from the ability of one protein to recruit another to a complex.

8. For each of the following, indicate whether it is a feature of an activator (A), an enhancer (E), or neither (N).

   (a) They recruit other proteins to promote transcription.
   (b) They are often redundant; part of them can be deleted with little loss of function.
   (c) They are modular.
   (d) They can act synergistically.
   (e) They perturb local chromatin structure.

Gene Expression Is Regulated by Hormones

9. Which of the following statements about steroid hormones are correct?

   (a) They bind to a seven-helix transmembrane receptor to initiate a series of phosphorylations that culminate in gene transcription.
   (b) Upon binding to their specific receptor proteins, they enable the receptors to bind specific DNA sequences.
   (c) They activate specific protein kinases and protein phosphatases.
   (d) They are recognized by members of the nuclear receptor superfamily of proteins.
   (e) They require plasma membrane transporters to go from the blood to the cytosol.

10. Nuclear hormone receptors

    (a) are dimers.
    (b) bind to response elements, which are specific DNA sequences at or near the genes the hormones control.
    (c) undergo conformational changes when they bind their ligand.
    (d) contain zinc-finger domains.
    (e) interact with coactivators and corepressors in the presence of their ligands.

11. Differentiate between an antagonist and an agonist and give examples of each.

Histone Acetylation Results in Chromatin Remodeling

12. The tails of histones
    (a) when acetylated have lower affinity for DNA.
    (b) are involved in recruiting chromatin-remodeling engines that move nucleosomes.
    (c) when acetylated, serve as substrates for histone deacetylases.
    (d) have their positive charges reduced by acetylation.
    (e) when acetylated interact with the bromodomain of many eukaryotic transcription factors when that domain is brominated.

13. Place the following steps in chromatin remodeling in their correct order of occurrence.
    (a) Acetylation of lysine in the histone tail.
    (b) ATP-dependent exposure of DNA.
    (c) Binding of remodeling complex.
    (d) Binding of RNA polymerase
    (e) Recruitment of a coactivator.

ANSWERS TO SELF-TEST

1. (a) E; (b) P; (c) E; (d) P; (e) E

2. (a) 1, 6, 8, 9 (b) 2, 3, 7, 8, 9, 10 (c) 2, 4, 5, 8, 9. Both RNA polymerases I and III are involved in rRNA synthesis, with polymerase I synthesizing the 18S, 5.8S, and 28S precursor transcripts and polymerase III synthesizing the 5S rRNA.

3. (a) 2; (b) 3; (c) 2; (d) 5; (e) 1; (f) 4

4. A TATA box centered at about -25 from the start site of transcription and consisting of a variant of the consensus heptanucleotide sequence *TATAAAA* is usually essential for promoter activity. Nearby, an initiator element (Inr) defines the transcriptional start site. In promoters lacking a TATA box, a downstream promoter element is sometimes paired with the Inr site on its 3′ side. In addition, many genes have a CAAT box, GC boxes, or both elements located between -40 and -150. These sequences can function in either orientation, that is, be in either DNA strand. Genes that are expressed constitutively, as distinct from those whose expression is regulated, tend to have GC boxes. Activating sequences farther upstream of these promoter elements are necessary for the functioning of most promoters.

5. TBP serves a critical role as an enucleating center for the assembly of the minimal molecular apparatus (the basal transcription assembly) required for transcription by RNA polymerase II. After TBP binds the TATA box, other TFII proteins and RNA polymerase II join the supramolecular complex to render it transcriptionally competent. In addition to enabling the assembly of the apparatus through its ability to recognize and bind the TATA box, TBP binds this asymmetric sequence in one orientation that "points" the RNA polymerase in the right direction, thereby defining the strand of DNA that will serve as the template.

6. b, c, d, e. Answer (a) is incorrect because enhancer sequences do not serve as promoters per se. They will not by themselves enable RNA polymerase II to initiate a transcript and will function only when the basal transcription apparatus exists.

7. a, b, c, d, e. Although a critical feature of combinatorial control is mediated by protein-protein interactions, some components of the transcription complex must interact specifically with DNA in order to locate the transcriptional assemblage to the proper region on the DNA. For instance, some transcription factors bind to enhancers far from the site of transcription initiation.

8. (a) A, E; (b) A; (c) A, E; (d) E; (e) N. Answer e is not a feature of either because DNA-binding proteins that influence transcription initiation through the control of enhancers are the molecules that cause the DNA perturbation, not the enhancers themselves.

9. b, d. Answers (a) and (c) are wrong because they are properties of a class of hormones that act by initiating phosphorylation cascades within cells after binding outside the cell to a transmembrane receptor.

10. a, b, c, d, e.

11. An agonist binds to a receptor and triggers signaling pathways. Two examples of agonists in gene regulation by steroid hormones are estradiol and anabolic steroids. An antagonist, by contrast, binds to a receptor but either triggers the signaling pathway weakly or not at all. Two examples of antagonists in steroid hormone signaling are tamoxifen and raloxifene, both of which are used in treatment of cancer.

12. a, b, c, d. Answer (e) is incorrect because, although named "bromodomain," bromination has nothing to do with the action of this acetyllysine-binding protein structure. The name derives from the *brahma* gene in *Drosophila,* where the archetype bromodomain was found.

13. e, a, c, b, d. See Figure 37.14 in text for details.

PROBLEMS

1. Would you expect the interaction between protamines and DNA to be enhanced or diminished in solutions that have highly ionic strength, that is, high salt concentrations? Protamines, which are found in very high concentrations in sperm where they participate in condensation of the DNA, are low molecular weight compounds rich in groups with high pK_a values, that is, they are basic compounds. Explain the basis for your answer. Does the action of histone acetyltransferases (HATs) use a similar principle? Explain.

2. The rate constant for the binding of RNA polymerase holoenzyme to a promoter on a long DNA molecule is greater than that for the collision of two small molecules in solution. Since small molecules diffuse through solutions more rapidly than large ones, how can this be true?

3. Would you expect a zinc deficiency in eukaryotes to be associated with any sort of developmental abnormality? Explain.

4. Would you be surprised if your analysis of the gene regulatory machinery of an eukaryotic cell indicated that DNA sequences far removed (1 or more kbp) from the site of transcription initiation were involved? Explain.

5. In sex determination in humans, female is the default state. To become male, genes must be activated that lead to the development of the testes and external male genitalia and suppression of the development of what would ultimately become the female sex organs. Many of these genes are on the Y chromosome, which is absent in

genotypic (XX) females. The steroid hormone testosterone, an androgen, is involved in this process. What would you predict would happen to a genetic male (XY) fetus whose testosterone receptor had a mutation in its C-terminal domain that rendered that domain resistant to binding the androgen?

6. Unlike bacterial RNA polymerases, eukaryotic polymerases have relatively low affinity for their promoters and therefore often depend on several activator proteins for initiation of transcription. Thus, while many bacterial genes are subject to negative regulation by repressor proteins, eukaryotic genes are more likely to be under positive regulatory control. The reasons for this difference in the mode of regulation may be related to the great difference in genome sizes. For example, the human haploid genome is ~650 times larger than that of *E. coli* and may contain over 25,000 genes. What are the advantages of positive regulation in the control of gene expression in eukaryotes?

7. Describe the experiment that demonstrated that four genes in embryonic stem cells could induce pluripotency (iPS). Comment on the potential therapeutic use of iPS cells.

ANSWERS TO PROBLEMS

1. Just as histones can be dissociated from DNA with salt, the interaction between protamines and DNA is diminished in highly ionic solutions because the salt in solution disrupts the ionic interactions between the ligands and the DNA. Protamines are arginine-rich proteins whose positively charged guanidinium groups can associate with the negatively charged phophodiester bonds in a DNA helix. These electrostatic interactions bind the protamines or histones tightly to the polynucleotide. The positively and negatively charged ions that result from the addition of a salt to an aqueous solution compete with DNA-ligand interactions and, hence, weaken them. By acetylating the primary amino groups on the side chains of lysine, HATs remove their positive charges and thereby weaken the interaction between the histone and the DNA. Thus, the physicochemical principle, reduction of charge–charge interactions is the same whether accomplished through the action of HATs or the addition of salts.

2. RNA polymerase holoenzyme has lower affinity for nonspecific DNA sequences than for promoter sequences. The nonspecific affinity, however, allows the enzyme to bind to "random-sequence" DNA and then "slide" along the molecule in a unidimensional random walk until it encounters a promoter sequence for which its binding affinity is higher. Diffusion in one dimension is much faster than diffusion in three dimensions, thereby explaining the observed rapid rate constant for the binding of RNA polymerase holoenzyme to promoter sequences. If one measured the encounter of the polymerase with the nonspecific regions of the DNA rather than with promoter sequences, the value of the rate constant would be much lower and would fit our expectations for a three-dimensional, diffusion-limited reaction between macromolecules.

3. The transcription of many eukaryotic genes is activated by proteins containing from one or more zinc fingers, each of which is a ~30-residue-long amino acid sequence containing (usually) two cysteines and two histidines coordinated to a zinc ion. For example, zinc is involved in the structure of DNA-binding domains of the nuclear hormone receptors. (See page 652 of the text.) It is also involved in a large number of other enzyme-catalyzed reactions, including the conversion of acetaldehyde to ethanol, the formation of bicarbonate ion, and the cleavage of peptides by chymotrypsin. Because of its essential roles in gene expression and in cellular metabolism, it is likely that zinc deficiencies could lead to significant developmental abnormalities.

4. You would not be surprised because the distant sequences might well be enhancers that bind transcription factors that themselves associate with the core transcription machinery by looping the DNA to achieve proximity to the transcription start site.

5. The testosterone–nuclear hormone receptor complex could not form and the genes necessary to promote virilization and suppress feminization would not function properly. The outcome would be a genetic male who developed into a phenotypic female. Recall (see page 652 of the text) that the ligand binding domain of nuclear hormone receptors is near their C termini. The inability to form the testosterone–receptor complex results in a male genotype expressing a phenotype similar to one arising from a missing Y chromosome, that is, being a female—in neither case is a functional androgen receptor formed. The disorder arising from the situation described is called testicular feminization, and many other biochemical and developmental factors beyond those mentioned here are involved.

6. In bacteria, negative regulation requires synthesis of a specific repressor that blocks transcription of a gene or an operon. To carry out negative regulation of genes in a human genome, ~25,000 repressor proteins would need to be synthesized, which would be an inefficient means of controlling transcription. Because most eukaryotic genes are not in operons and are normally inactive with regard to transcription, selective activation through synthesis of a small group of activator proteins is used to promote transcription of a particular array of genes needed by the cell at a certain time. Another reason for positive control may be related to the fact that a larger genome presents the possibility that a relatively short DNA sequence for a regulatory protein would be present in multiple and possibly wrong locations, bringing about inappropriate or unneeded gene activation. This can be avoided by requiring that several positive regulatory proteins form a complex that can specifically activate a gene and promote its transcription, thereby reducing the possibility of incorrect gene activation.

7. The experiment involved introducing DNA encoding four transcription factors into fibroblasts (skin cells). Fibroblasts are cells that have differentiated from pluripotent cells into cells with fixed characteristics and function. Pluripotent cells have the ability to differentiate into many different cell types. In a differentiated cell, most of the genes in the cells are no longer actively transcribed. Until recently, this process of silencing genes during differentiation was thought to be irreversible. The four transcription factors were identified, along with dozens of others, as contributing to pluripotency of embryonic stem cells. When the four genes were introduced into the fibroblast cells, they de-differentiated into cells that appeared to have characteristics very nearly identical with those of embryonic stem cells. This result appears to have opened the way for development of a new class of therapeutic agents. In theory, a patient's fibroblast cells could be converted into iPS cells, then treated to differentiate them into the desired cell type. These new cells could be transplanted back into the patient. The book gives the example of using nerve cells to treat a neurodegenerative disease.

Chapter 38

RNA Processing in Eukaryotes

The conversion of DNA nucleotide sequences into RNA sequences is an early step in the expression of genetic information. Chapter 36 described the DNA-dependent RNA polymerases that catalyze this reaction and the mechanisms of regulation in prokaryotes, Chapter 38 discusses the various ways in eukaryotes in which the product RNA transcript must sometimes be cleaved and modified before it becomes functional.

The chapter begins with a recognition of the impossibility of coupling transcription and translation in eukaryotes as occurs in prokaryotes because of eukaryotic subcellular separation in the nucleus and cytoplasm. The three eukaryotic RNA polymerases that carry out transcription are described and related to the kinds of RNA they synthesize. The roles of the eukaryotic TATA box and the TATA-box-binding protein in forming the Transcription Factor IIFD (TFIID) complex that is active in basal transcription are explained, as are some other eukaryotic promoters and enhancers and the proteins that bind them. The reactions that modify the 5′ and 3′ ends of typical eukaryotic mRNA transcripts to cap and add a poly(A) tail are described, as are ways in which the nucleotide sequence of certain mRNAs can be modified by base alterations and insertions (a process called RNA editing). Splicing—the molecular machinery and reactions that remove introns from eukaryotic mRNA—is described along with the consequences of alternative splicing reactions. The chapter concludes with the discovery of catalytic RNA and the mechanism of RNA-catalyzed self-splicing in *Tetrahymena*.

LEARNING OBJECTIVES

When you have mastered this chapter, you should be able to accomplish the following objectives.

Introduction

1. Differentiate between *introns* and *exons* in DNA.

Mature Ribosomal RNA Is Generated by the Cleavage of a Precursor Molecule
(Text Section 38.1)

2. List the three components of ribosomal RNA that are synthesizes by *RNA polymerase I*.

3. Explain the three steps in the processing of *pre-rRNA* into *mature rRNA*.

Transfer RNA Is Extensively Processed (Text Section 38.2)

4. List the modifications that are part of processing tRNA precursors into mature tRNA molecules.

Messenger RNA Is Modified and Spliced (Text Section 38.3)

5. Draw the structure of the 5′ end of a typical *eukaryotic mRNA* and distinguish *caps 0, 1, and 2*. Outline the reactions required to cap the primary transcript.

6. Describe the events leading to the production of mRNA with a *poly(A) tail*. Relate the half-life of an mRNA molecule to its poly (A) tail

7. Describe the *splicing of eukaryotic mRNA*, give the *consensus sequences* at the *splice site junctions*, and designate the other nucleotide *sequence elements* involved in the process. List the functions of this *posttranscriptional modification*.

8. Describe the role of *transesterification reactions* in splicing, and compare the number of phosphodiester bonds broken and formed during mRNA splicing.

9. Describe the *spliceosome* and detail the structural and catalytic involvement of *small nuclear ribonucleoprotein particles* (snRNPs) in mRNA splicing.

10. Differentiate between *cis-* and *trans-acting* mutations in DNA splicing. Give an example of each as a cause of genetic diseases.

11. Explain the importance of *alternative splicing* in gene expression. Give several examples of human disorders attributed to alternative splicing.

12. List the components of the *posttranscriptional* machinery recruited through interactions with the CTP of RNA polymerase II.

13. Describe *RNA editing* and provide examples of its effects on gene expression.

RNA Can Function As a Catalyst (Text Section 38.4)

14. Outline the reactions that occur during the *self-splicing* conversion of a ribosomal RNA (rRNA) precursor from *Tetrahymena* into the mature rRNA plus other linear and circular products. Explain the role of *guanosine* or a *guanylyl nucleotide* in the self-splicing reaction.

15. Contrast the *group I* and *group II self-splicing* introns. Compare *spliceosome-catalyzed* splicing with self-splicing.

SELF-TEST

Mature Ribosomal RNA Is Generating by the Cleavage of a Precursor Molecule

1. Which of the following statements is true?
   (a) RNA polymerase I transcribes a single precursor that encodes 18S, 28S, 5.8S and 5S rRNA.
   (b) The pre-rRNA is modified by methylation, directed by snoRNAs.
   (c) Most of the processing steps take place in the nucleolus.
   (d) The pre-rRNA is cleaved before post-transcriptional modification.

Transfer RNA Is Extensively Processed

2. Identify the post-transcriptional modifications of tRNA precursor processing. What modifications are made to the bases?

Messenger RNA Is Modified and Spliced

3. Which of the following statements about the poly(A) tails that are found on most eukaryotic mRNAs are correct?
   (a) They are added as preformed polyriboadenylate segments to the 3′ ends of mRNA precursors by an RNA ligase activity.
   (b) They are encoded by stretches of polydeoxythymidylate in the template strand of the gene.
   (c) They are added by RNA polymerase II in a template-independent reaction using ATP as the sole nucleotide substrate.
   (d) They are added by poly(A) polymerase using dATP as the sole nucleotide substrate.
   (e) They are cleaved from eukaryotic mRNAs by a sequence-specific endoribonuclease that recognizes the RNA sequence AAUAAA.

4. What functions are the caps and tails of mRNAs thought to perform?

5. Which of the following statements about apolipoprotein B (apo B) are correct?
   (a) The apo B-48 form is formed by the proteolytic cleavage of the primary (apo B-100) translation product.
   (b) Apo B-48 and apo B-100 are formed in different tissues.
   (c) Apo B-48 arises from the expression of a form of the gene for apo B-100 that has been shortened by nonhomologous recombination.
   (d) The transcript of the apo B-100 gene is spliced to remove a segment and form apo B-48.
   (e) A specific nucleotide in the apo B-100 transcript is altered, thereby creating a stop codon in the mRNA.

6. Which of the following are important sequence elements in the splicing reactions that produce eukaryotic mRNAs?
   (a) exon sequences located between 20 and 50 nucleotides from the 5′ splice site
   (b) exon sequences located between 20 and 50 nucleotides from the 3′ splice site
   (c) intron sequences located between 20 and 50 nucleotides from the 5′ splice site
   (d) intron sequences located between 20 and 50 nucleotides from the 3′ splice site
   (e) intron sequences at the 5′ splice site
   (f) intron sequences at the 3′ splice site

7. Eukaryotic mRNA splicing involves which of the following?
    (a) the formation of 2′ → 5′ phosphodiester bonds
    (b) a sequence-specific endoribonuclease that hydrolyzes the phosphodiester bond at the junctions of the intron with the exon
    (c) the spliceosome
    (d) the coupling of phosphodiester bond formation to ATP hydrolysis
    (e) the formation of lariat intermediates

8. Answer the following questions about what was revealed when DNA encoding the gene for the β-chain of hemoglobin and the mRNA for the β-chain were compared.
    (a) What was the major finding when the nucleotide sequence of the gene and the amino acid sequence of the β-chain were compared?
    (b) What must happen to the primary transcript from the β-globin gene before it can serve as an mRNA for protein synthesis?

RNA Can Function As a Catalyst

9. Spliceosomes
    (a) recombine DNA sequences in a process called exon shuffling.
    (b) are composed of RNA and proteins.
    (c) recognize RNA sequences that signal for the removal of introns.
    (d) can produce different mRNA molecules by splicing at alternative sites.

10. Place the following events in the order in which they occur during the formation of mature rRNA in *Tetrahymena*.
    (a) The 3′-hydroxyl of a guanine nucleoside attacks the phosphodiester bond at the 5′ splice site leaving the 5′ (upstream) exon with a free 3′-hydroxyl and attaching the guanine nucleoside to the 5′ end of the intron.
    (b) The transcript from the rRNA gene folds into a specific structure.
    (c) The rRNA transcript specifically binds a guanine nucleoside or nucleotide.
    (d) Self-splicing occurs within the intron to form L19 RNA.
    (e) The 3′-hydroxyl of the 5′ exon attacks the bonds at the 3′ splice junction to form the spliced rRNA and eliminate the intron.

11. Identify the attacking group in group I and group II splicing.

ANSWERS TO SELF-TEST

1. Answers a and d are false; b and c are true. Answer a is false because RNA polymerase I, not RNA polymerase III, encodes 5S rRNA. Answer d is false because the pre-rRNA is modified before it is cleaved.

2. The modifications are cleavage of the 5- and 3′ ends of the tRNA, removal of a 14-nucleotide intron, and addition of a CCA to the 3′-end. The modification to the base shown on Figure 38.2 is the conversion of uracil to pseudouracil.

3. None of the statements is correct. Poly(A) polymerase uses ATP, not dATP, to add a stretch of A residues to the 3′-hydroxyl formed by the cleavage of an mRNA precursor by a specific ribonuclease that recognizes the upstream sequence AAUAAA within particular mRNA sequence contexts.

4. The 5′ caps are thought to contribute to the stability and efficiency of translation of the mRNA. The poly(A) tails probably perform the same functions, albeit by different, unknown mechanisms.

5. b, e. The apo B system illustrates one kind of RNA editing. The pre-mRNA transcript has its sequence altered—in this case, a specific cytidine is deaminated to uracil to create the stop codon. Other editing mechanisms involve the addition and removal of U residues, an A-to-G change, and an adenosine-to-inosine change.

6. d, e, f

7. a, c, e. Answers (b) and (d) are incorrect because hydrolysis of phosphodiester bonds is not involved during mRNA splicing up to the point of intron removal and lariat formation; only transesterification reactions occur. Consequently, ATP is not required for the synthesis of phosphodiester bonds.

8. (a) The number of nucleotides in the gene was significantly greater than three times the number of amino acids in the protein. There were two stretches of extra nucleotides between the exon sequences that encode the amino acids in the β-chain.

   (b) The intervening sequences (introns) in the nascent or primary transcript, which are complementary to the template strand of the DNA of the gene but do not encode amino acids in the protein, must be removed by splicing to generate the mRNA that functions in translation.

9. b, c, and d. (a) is incorrect because exon shuffling takes place at the DNA level through breakage and rejoining of DNA, not RNA.

10. b, c, a, e, d

11. Group I: the 3′-OH of guaosine. Group II: the 2′-OH of adenylate.

PROBLEMS

1. The ciliated protozoan *Tetrahymena* contains an enzyme that can synthesize 5′-pseudouridine monophosphate from a mixture of PRPP and uracil. For a time it was thought that this enzyme was instrumental in the synthesis of transfer RNAs in *Tetrahymena*. Explain why this is not the case.

2. The mRNAs produced by mammalian viruses undergo modification at the 5′ and 3′ ends in a fashion similar to that of eukaryotic mRNA. Why do you think this is the case?

3. Suppose that human DNA is cleaved into fragments approximately the size of a given mature human messenger RNA and that mRNA–DNA hybrids are then prepared. The corresponding procedure is then carried out for *E. coli*. When the mRNA–DNA hybrids from each species are examined with an electron microscope, which will show the greater degree of hybridization? Explain.

4. What are snRNPs, and how are they involved in the eukaryotic mRNA splicing reaction?

5. Figure 38.9 in the text gives an example of how a base-change mutation (A → G) within an intron in the β-globin gene can produce a 5′ splice site downstream from the normal 5′ splice site. The result is that extra amino acids not normally present in the protein are inserted into the chain before synthesis is terminated by a stop codon.

   (a) Corresponding mutants in exons are also known in which base change mutations introduce 5′ splice sites upstream from the normal 5′ sites (see Figure 38.1A; X marks the location of the new 5′ splice site). Sketch the resulting processed mRNA. What changes in amino acid sequence would you expect to result?

FIGURE 38.1A Creation of a new 5′ splice site in exon 2 of β-globin.

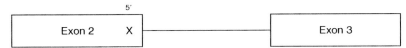

(b) In some forms of thalassemia, the creation of a new 5′ splice site within intron 2 activates a "cryptic" 3′ splice site upstream from the 5′ site (see Figure 38.1B; X marks the location of the new 5′ splice site and the cryptic 3′ side is labeled). Sketch the resulting processed mRNA. How would the resulting changes in amino acid sequence differ from those in (A)?

FIGURE 38.1B Activation of a cryptic 3′ splice site in intron 2 of β-globin.

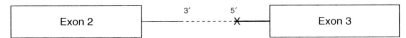

6. In an attempt to determine whether a given RNA was catalytically active in the cleavage of a synthetic oligonucleotide, the following experimental results were obtained. When the RNA and the oligonucleotide were incubated together, cleavage of the oligonucleotide occurred. When either the RNA or the oligonucleotide was incubated alone, there was no cleavage. When the RNA was incubated with higher concentrations of the oligonucleotide, saturation kinetics of the Michaelis-Menten type were observed. Do these results demonstrate that the RNA has catalytic activity? Explain.

ANSWERS TO PROBLEMS

1. Nascent polynucleotides formed by RNA polymerases contain only the four usual bases. Subsequently, some of the bases are chemically modified. Were unusual nucleotides to be incorporated into a growing RNA chain, this would in turn require the presence of unusual bases on DNA. The pseudouridine found in transfer RNAs is formed by breaking the nitrogen–carbon bond linking uracil to ribose and forming a carbon–carbon bond instead. Only certain uracils are modified in this manner, owing to their position in the three-dimensional structure of the RNA and to the specificity of the enzymes that carry out the modification.

2. Viruses use the host's enzyme system to replicate their DNA and to synthesize their proteins. Since eukaryotic translation systems must synthesize viral protein, the structure of viral mRNAs must mimic that of the host mRNA.

3. The mRNA–DNA hybrid of *E. coli* will show greater hybridization because it is produced continuously from a DNA template without processing. Because of the presence of intervening sequences in human DNA, there will be regions in the human RNA–DNA hybrids where no base pairing occurs.

4. The snRNPs are small ribonucleoprotein particles that occur in the nucleus. Each is composed of a small RNA molecule and several characteristic proteins, some of which are common to different snRNPs. Distinct snRNPs recognize and bind to splice junctions and the branch site and are involved in assembling the spliceosome in an ATP-dependent manner. They are requisite components of the splicing apparatus, and the RNA components of some of them are probably catalytically active. The RNAs of some snRNPs form hydrogen bonds with sequences within introns and exons to help to juxtapose properly the reacting splice junctions.

5. (a) The spliced gene arising from the mutation would be shorter than the correctly spliced version (see below) and some amino acids (those between the X in the figure and the right-hand edge of the box labeled "Exon 2") would be omitted from the region of the protein encoded by nucleotides between the newly introduced and normal 5′ splicing sites. Since the splicing machinery might also recognize the unchanged, normal 5′ splice site, some normal mRNA could also be formed.) Also, the introduction of a new splicing site could lead to changes in the reading frame, and therefore to gross changes in amino acid sequence, polypeptide chain length, or both.

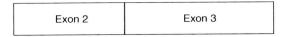

(b) The resulting processed mRNA would be longer than the normal processed β-globin gene, introducing the possibility of a misfolded or malfunctioning protein or a truncated protein if a stop codon were introduced from the intron sequence. As in (a), a change in reading frame could also result. Again, some normal mRNA might be formed by recognition of the unchanged, original 5′ splice site.

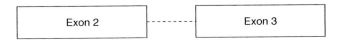

6. These results alone do not establish that the RNA has catalytic activity, because a catalyst must be regenerated. It is entirely possible that the results observed could be accounted for by a stoichiometric, as opposed to a catalytic, interaction between RNA and the oligonucleotide, in which the RNA may "commit suicide" as the oligonucleotide is cleaved. In such an interaction, a portion of the RNA would participate chemically in the cleavage of the oligonucleotide, but it would also be cleaved itself as a part of the reaction. Four reaction products would accumulate, two resulting from the cleavage of RNA and two from the cleavage of the oligonucleotide. To show that this particular RNA was catalytic, it would be necessary to demonstrate that it turns over and is regenerated in the course of the reaction. You could perform experiments in which the putative catalytic RNA was present in much lower molar concentrations than those of the substrate oligonucleotide. If more substrate oligonucleotide molecules were hydrolyzed than the total number of the presumed catalytic RNA, you would have evidence that true turnover had occurred.

Chapter 39

The Genetic Code

In Chapter 39 the components of protein synthesis, a process called translation, are examined in detail. Translation is a complicated process in which the four-letter alphabet of nucleic acids is translated into the 20-letter alphabet of proteins. The major components of translation are mRNA, tRNA, ribosomes, and aminoacyl-tRNA synthetases. The authors first introduce the genetic code, the relationship between the sequence of bases in DNA (or its RNA transcript) and the sequence of amino acids in a protein. The detailed structures and conformations of tRNAs, the adaptor molecules that recognize both the codons on the mRNAs and the enzymes that attach the corresponding amino acids, are discussed first. The wobble hypothesis is then presented to explain the lack of strict one-to-one Watson-Crick base-pairing interactions among the three nucleotides of the tRNA anticodons and the mRNA codons. The importance of accurate translation is emphasized, and the rationale for an error frequency of less than 10^{-4} is explored.

Next the authors explain how amino acids are activated for the subsequent formation of peptide bonds through their attachment to tRNAs by the two classes of aminoacyl-tRNA synthetases. The exquisite specificity of these reactions is explored, in terms of correct binding of amino acids and tRNAs to a given synthetase. Threonyl-tRNA synthetase is used as an example of specificity at the level of amino acid selection. This enzyme discriminates between threonine and the isosteric valine and the isoelectronic serine, using a combination of selective binding at the active site and proofreading after aminoacylation.

The authors next turn to the structure and composition of the ribosome, a molecular machine that coordinates charged tRNAs, mRNA, and proteins, leading to protein synthesis. The fact that the ribosome is now recognized to be a ribozyme, with the RNA components playing the major role in catalysis, is introduced. The chapter ends with a discussion of the directionality of protein synthesis and the authors point out the utility of synthesizing proteins in the same direction as transcription. The existence of polysomes, wherein a single mRNA is translated by multiple ribosomes, has been confirmed by electron microscopy.

LEARNING OBJECTIVES

When you have mastered this chapter, you should be able to accomplish the following objectives.

Introduction

1. Explain the origin of the word *translation* as it pertains to protein synthesis.

Genetic Code Links Nucleic Acid and Protein Information (Text Section 39.1)

2. Explain what the *genetic code* is and list its major characteristics. Define the terms *triplet code (codon)*, *nonoverlapping*, *degenerate*, *synonym*, *triplet*, and *reading frame* as they apply to the genetic code.

3. Identify the benefits of a *degenerate* genetic code.

4. Discuss the *universality* of the genetic code.

5. Using the genetic code, predict the sequence of amino acids in a peptide encoded by a *template DNA* or mRNA sequence. Identify the *initiation* and *termination* codons.

6. List the features common to all tRNAs.

7. Draw the *cloverleaf structure* of a *tRNA* and identify the regions containing the *anticodon* and the *amino acid attachment site*.

8. Relate the two-dimensional cloverleaf representation of the tRNA structure to its three-dimensional configuration.

9. Explain how some *codons are recognized by more than one anticodon*, that is, how they interact with more than one species of *aminoacyl-tRNA*. List the base-pairing interactions allowed according to the *wobble hypothesis*.

10. Explain the effect of error frequency on synthesis of different-size proteins.

11. Outline the purpose for using an aminoacyl-tRNA instead of a free amino acid in protein synthesis.

Amino Acids Are Activated by Attachment to Transfer RNA (Text Section 39.2)

12. Write the two-step reaction sequence of the *aminoacyl-tRNA synthetases*. Enumerate the high-energy phosphate bonds that are consumed in the overall reaction.

13. Describe the mechanisms of amino acid selection and *proofreading* that contribute to the accuracy of the attachment of the appropriate amino acid to the correct tRNA.

14. Describe the different modes of recognition of the correct tRNA molecule by aminoacyl-tRNA synthetases.

A Ribosome Is a Ribonucleoprotein Particle Made of Two Subunits
(Text Section 39.3)

15. List the kinds and numbers of macromolecular components of the prokaryotic ribosome. Give the *mass, sedimentation coefficient,* and *dimensions* of the *ribosome* of *E. coli.*

16. Outline the three-dimensional structure of a ribosome.

17. List the evidence that suggests that the RNA components of ribosomes have active roles in protein synthesis.

18. Identify the direction of protein synthesis and explain the benefits to this direction in prokaryotic protein synthesis.

SELF-TEST

The Genetic Code Links Nucleic Acid and Protein Information

1. Which of the following are characteristics or functions of tRNA?
   (a) It contains a codon.
   (b) It contains an anticodon.
   (c) It can become covalently attached to an amino acid.
   (d) It interacts with mRNA to stimulate transcription.
   (e) It can have any of a number of different sequences.
   (f) It serves as an adaptor between the information in mRNA and an individual amino acid.

2. What is the minimum number of contiguous nucleotides in mRNA that can serve as a codon? Explain.

3. What is the sequence of the polypeptide that would be encoded by the DNA sequence ACGTTACCTAGTTGC? Assume that the reading frame starts with the 5′ nucleotide given. The genetic code is given on page 677 of the text.

4. The following is a partial list of mRNA codons and the amino acids they encode:

   AGU = serine   AGC = serine
   AAU = asparagine   AAC = asparagine
   AUG = methionine   AUA = isoleucine

   From this list, which of the following statements are correct?

   (a) The genetic code is degenerate.
   (b) The alteration of a single nucleotide in the DNA directing the synthesis of these codons could lead to the substitution of a serine for an asparagine in a polypeptide.
   (c) The alteration of a single nucleotide in the DNA directing the synthesis of these codons would necessarily lead to an amino acid substitution in the encoded polypeptide.
   (d) A tRNA with the anticodon ACU would be bound by a ribosome in the presence of one of these codons.

5. Explain how mitochondria and some organisms can use a genetic code that is different from the standard code used in the nucleus.

6. Which of the following statements about functional tRNAs are correct?
   (a) They contain many modified nucleosides.
   (b) About half their nucleosides are in base-paired helical regions.
   (c) They contain fewer than 100 ribonucleosides.
   (d) Their anticodons and amino acid accepting regions are within 5 Å of each other.
   (e) They consist of two helical stems that are joined by loops to form a U-shaped structure.
   (f) They have a terminal AAC sequence at their amino acid accepting end.

7. Explain why tRNA molecules must have both unique and common structural features.

8. How many errors would be expected to occur in a 1000-amino acid protein given an error frequency of 10^{-3}?

9. Which of the following answers completes the sentence correctly? The wobble hypothesis
   (a) accounts for the conformational looseness of the amino acid acceptor stem of tRNAs that allows sufficient flexibility for the peptidyl-tRNA and aminoacyl-tRNA to be brought together for peptide-bond formation.
   (b) accounts for the ability of some anticodons to recognize more than one codon.
   (c) explains the occasional errors made by the aminoacyl-tRNA synthetases.
   (d) explains the oscillation of the peptidyl-tRNAs between the A and P sites on the ribosome.
   (e) assumes steric freedom in the pairing of the first (5′) nucleotide of the codon and the third (3′) nucleotide of the anticodon.

Amino Acids Are Activated by Attachment to Transfer RNA

10. Which of the following statements about the aminoacyl-tRNA synthetase reaction are correct?
    (a) ATP is a cofactor.
    (b) GTP is a cofactor.
    (c) The amino acid is attached to the 2′- or 3′-hydroxyl of the nucleotide cofactor (ATP).
    (d) The amino group of the amino acid is activated.
    (e) A mixed anhydride bond is formed.
    (f) An acyl ester bond is formed.
    (g) An acyl thioester bond is formed.
    (h) A phosphoamide (P–N) bond is formed.

11. The $\Delta G°'$ of the reaction catalyzed by the *aminoacyl-tRNA synthetases* is
    (a) ~0 kcal/mol.
    (b) <0 kcal/mol.
    (c) >0 kcal/mol.

12. Considering the correct answer to question 6, explain how aminoacyl-tRNAs can be produced in the cell.

13. Indicate the possible ways in which different aminoacyl-tRNA synthetases may recognize their corresponding tRNAs.
    (a) by recognizing the anticodon
    (b) by recognizing specific base pairs in the acceptor stem
    (c) by recognizing the 3′ CCA sequence of the tRNA
    (d) by recognizing both the anticodon and acceptor stem region
    (e) by recognizing extended regions of the L-shaped molecules

14. In an experiment, it was found that Cys-tRNA^{Cys} can be converted to Ala-tRNA^{Cys} and used in an in vitro system that is capable of synthesizing proteins.

    (a) If the Ala-tRNA^{Cys} were labeled with ^{14}C in the amino acid, would the labeled Ala be incorporated in the protein in the places where Ala residues are expected to occur? Explain.

    (b) What does the experiment indicate about the importance of the accuracy of the aminoacyl-tRNA synthetase reaction to the overall accuracy of protein synthesis?

A Ribosome Is a Ribonucleoprotein Particle Made of Two Subunits

15. Assuming that each nucleoside in the left column is in the first position of an anticodon, with which nucleoside or nucleosides in the right column could it pair during a codon–anticodon interaction if each of the nucleosides on the right is in the third position (3′ position) of a codon?

    (a) adenosine
    (b) cytidine
    (c) guanosine
    (d) inosine
    (e) uridine

    (1) adenosine
    (2) cytidine
    (3) guanosine
    (4) uridine

16. Which of the following statements about an *E. coli* ribosome are correct?

    (a) It is composed of two spherically symmetrical subunits.
    (b) It has a large subunit comprising 34 kinds of proteins and two different rRNA molecules.
    (c) It has a sedimentation coefficient of 70S.
    (d) It has two small subunits, one housing the A site and the other the P site.
    (e) It has an average diameter of approximately 200 Å.
    (f) It has a mass of approximately 270 kd, one-third of which is RNA.

ANSWERS TO SELF-TEST

1. b, c, e, and f. Answer (d) is incorrect because the interaction of tRNA with mRNA takes place during translation, not transcription.

2. Three contiguous nucleotides is the minimum that can serve as a codon. There are four kinds of nucleotides in mRNA. A codon consisting of only two nucleotides (either of which could be any of the four possible nucleotides) allows only 16 possible combinations ($4 \times 4 = 16$). This would not be sufficient to specify all 20 of the amino acids. A codon consisting of three nucleotides, however, allows 64 possible combinations ($4 \times 4 \times 4 = 64$), more than enough to specify the 20 amino acids.

3. The sequence of the polypeptide would be Ala-Thr-Arg. The reading frame is set by the nucleotide at the 5′ end of the mRNA transcript; the fourth codon of the mRNA transcript is UAA, which is a translation termination codon.

4. a, b, and d. Answer (a) is correct because both AGU and AGC specify serine; since more than one codon can specify the same amino acids, the genetic code is said to be degenerate. Answer (b) is correct because the alteration of a single nucleotide in the DNA could change a codon on the mRNA transcript from AGU, which specifies serine, to AAU, which specifies asparagine. Answer (d) is correct because the anticodon ACU would base-pair with the codon AGU. Answer (c) is *not* correct because the alteration of a single nucleotide in the DNA could result in another codon that specifies the same amino acid; for example, a codon changed from AGU to AGC would continue to specify serine.

5. Mitochondria and some organisms can use a genetic code that differs from the standard code because mitochondrial DNA encodes a distinct set of tRNAs that are matched to the genetic code used in their mRNAs.

6. a, b, c. The molecules consist of two helical stems, each of which is made of two stacked helical segments. However, the molecules are L-shaped, and the anticodon and amino acid accepting regions are some 80 Å from each other. Functional tRNAs have a CCA sequence, not an AAC sequence at their 3′ termini.

7. Transfer RNAs need common features for their interactions with ribosomes and elongation factors but unique features for their interactions with the activating enzymes.

8. One error would be expected. An ε value of 10^{-3} means 1 error per 1000 amino acids.

9. b

10. a, e, f. The carboxyl group of the amino acid is activated in a two-step reaction via the formation of an intermediate containing a mixed anhydride linkage to AMP. The amino acid is ultimately linked by an ester bond to the 2′- or 3′-hydroxyl of the tRNA.

11. a. Since the standard free energy of the hydrolysis of an aminoacyl-tRNA is nearly equal to that of the hydrolysis of ATP, the reaction has a $\Delta G^{\circ\prime} \sim 0$; that is, it has an equilibrium constant near 1.

12. In the cell, the hydrolysis of PP_i by pyrophosphatase shifts the equilibrium toward the formation of aminoacyl-tRNA.

13. a, b, d, e. There are many different ways in which aminoacyl-tRNA synthetases recognize their specific tRNAs. Answer (c) is incorrect because the 3′ CCA sequence is common to all tRNAs and cannot be used to distinguish among them.

14. (a) No. The tRNA, acting as an adaptor between the amino acid and mRNA, would associate with Cys codons in the mRNA through base-pairing between codon and anticodon. The labeled alanine would incorporate only at sites encoded by the Cys codons and not at those encoded by Ala codons.

    The experiment demonstrates that the tRNA and not the amino acid reads the mRNA. Thus, if the activating enzyme mistakenly attaches an incorrect amino acid to a tRNA, that amino acid will be incorporated erroneously into the protein.

    (b) Answer (e) is incorrect because the ambiguities in base-pairing occur between the third nucleotide of the codon and the first nucleotide of the anticodon.

15. (a) 4   (b) 3   (c) 2, 4   (d) 1, 2, 4   (e) 1, 3.

16. b, c, e. Answer (f) is incorrect because two-thirds of the 2700-kd mass of a ribosome is rRNA.

PROBLEMS

1. (a) The template strand of DNA known to encode the N-terminal region of an *E. coli* protein has the following nucleotide sequence: GTAGCGTTCCATCAGATTT. Give the sequence for the first four amino acids of the protein.

   (b) Suppose that the sense strand of the DNA known to encode the amino acid sequence of the N-terminal region of a mammalian protein has the following nucleotide sequence: CCTGTGGATGCTCATGTTT. Give the amino acid sequence that would result.

2. The nucleotide sequence on the sense strand of the DNA that is known to encode the carboxy terminus of a long protein of *E. coli* has the following nucleotide sequence: CCATGCAAAGTAATAGGT. Give the resulting amino acid sequence.

3. Suppose that a particular aminoacyl-tRNA synthetase has a 10% error rate in the formation of aminoacyl-adenylates and a 99% success rate in the hydrolysis of incorrect aminoacyl-adenylates. What percentage of the tRNAs produced by this aminoacyl-tRNA synthetase will be faulty?

4. Students of biochemistry are frequently distressed by "Svedberg arithmetic," that is, for instance, by the fact that the 30S and 50S ribosomal subunits form a 70S particle rather than an 80S particle. Why don't the numbers add up to 80?

5. The possible codons for valine are GUU, GUC, GUA, and GUG.

    (a) For each of these codons write down all the possible anticodons with which it might pair (use the wobble rules in Table 39.1 in the text).
    (b) How many codons could pair with anticodons having I as the first base? How many could pair with anticodons having U or G as the first base? How many could pair with anticodons beginning with A or C?

6. What amino acid will be specified by a tRNA whose anticodon sequence is IGG?

7. According to the wobble principle, what is the *minimum* number of tRNAs required to decode the six leucine codons—UUA, UUG, CUU, CUC, CUA, and CUG? Explain.

8. Coordination of the threonine hydroxyl by an active site Zn in the threonyl-tRNA synthetase allows discrimination between threonine and the isosteric valine (Sankaranarayanan et al., *Nat. Struct. Biol.* 7[2000]:461–465). Given the similarity of serine and threonine (Ser lacks only the methyl group of Thr), if this is the only mechanism for amino acid discrimination available, threonyl-tRNA synthetase mistakenly couples Ser to threonyl-tRNA at a rate several-fold higher than it does threonine. Since this would lead to unacceptably high error rates in translation, how it is it avoided?

9. Mutations from codons specifying amino acid incorporation to one of the chain-terminating codons, UAA, UAG, or UGA, so-called *nonsense* mutations, result in the synthesis of shorter, usually nonfunctional, polypeptide chains. It was discovered that some strains of bacteria can protect themselves against such mutations by having mutant tRNAs that can recognize a chain-terminating codon and insert an amino acid instead. The result would be a protein of normal length that may be functional, even though it may contain an altered amino acid residue. How can bacteria with such mutant tRNA molecules ever manage to terminate their polypeptide chains successfully?

10. Change of one base pair to another in a sense codon frequently results in an amino acid substitution. Change of a C–G to a G–U base pair at the 3:70 position of tRNA^{Cys} causes that tRNA to be recognized by alanyl-tRNA synthetase.

    (a) What amino acid substitution or substitutions would result with the mutated tRNA^{Cys} present?
    (b) How does the pattern differ from that resulting from base substitutions within a codon?

ANSWERS TO PROBLEMS

1. (a) The sequence of the first four amino acids of the protein is (formyl)Met-Glu-Arg-Tyr. As the name implies, the template (antisense) strand of DNA serves as the template for the synthesis of a complementary mRNA molecule. (Remember

that by convention nucleotide sequences are always written in the 5′ to 3′ direction unless otherwise specified.) The template strand of DNA and the mRNA synthesized are as follows:

DNA template strand: 5′-GTAGCGTTCCATCAGATTT-3′

mRNA: 3′-CAUCGCAAGGUAGUCUAAA-5′

Remember that the codons of an mRNA molecule are read in the 5′-to-3′ direction. Because this particular nucleotide sequence specifies the N-terminal region of an *E. coli* protein, the first amino acid must be (formyl)-methionine, which may be encoded by either AUG or GUG. Because there is no GUG and only a single AUG in the mRNA sequence, the location of the initiation codon can be established unambiguously. The portion of the mRNA sequence encoding protein and the first four amino acids it encodes are

mRNA: 5′-AUG-GAA-CGC-UAC-3′

Amino acid sequence: (Formyl)Met-Glu-Arg-Tyr

(b) The expected amino acid sequence is Met-Leu-Met-Phe. The nucleotide sequences on DNA and mRNA are

Sense strand of DNA: 5′-CCTGTGGATGCTCATGTTT-3′

mRNA: 5′-CCUGUGGAUGCUCAUGUUU-3′

In eukaryotes the first triplet specifying an amino acid is almost always the AUG that is closest to the 5′ end of the mRNA molecule. In this example there are two AUGs, so there will be two Met residues in the polypeptide that is produced. The reading frame and the resulting amino acids are as follows:

mRNA: 5′-CCUGUGG-AUG-CUC-AUG-UUU-3′

Amino acid sequence: Met-Leu-Met-Phe

2. The sequence is His-Ala-Lys. The DNA and mRNA sequences are

Sense strand of DNA: 5′-CCATGCAAAGTAATAGGT-3′

mRNA: 5′-CCAUGCAAAGUAAUAGGU-3′

Since this sequence specifies the carboxyl end of the peptide chain, it must contain one or more of the chain-termination codons: UAA, UAG, or UGA. UAA and UAG occur in tandem in the sequence, so we can infer the reading frame. The mapping of the amino acid residues to the mRNA is as follows:

mRNA: 5′-C-CAU-GCA-AAG-UAA-UAG-GU-3′

Amino acid sequence: His-Ala-Lys

3. The percentage of tRNAs that will be faulty is 0.11%. For every 1000 aminoacyl-adenylates that are produced, 100 are faulty and 900 are correct. The 900 correct intermediates will be converted to correct aminoacyl tRNAs because the intermediates are tightly bound to the active site of the aminoacyl-tRNA synthetase. Of the 100 incorrect aminoacyl-adenylates, 99 will be hydrolyzed and will therefore not form aminoacyl tRNAs. Only one will survive to become an incorrect aminoacyl tRNA. The fraction of incorrect aminoacyl tRNAs is therefore 1/901, or 0.11%.

4. The Svedberg unit (S) is a sedimentation coefficient, which is a measure of the velocity with which a particle moves in a centrifugal field. It represents a hydro-

dynamic property of a particle, a property that depends on, among other factors, the size and shape of the particle. When two particles come together, the sedimentation coefficient of the resulting particle should be less than the sum of the individual co-efficients because there is no frictional resistance between the contact surfaces of the particles and the centrifugal medium.

5. (a) The possible anticodons with which the codons might pair are as follows:

Codon	Possible anticodon
GUU	AAC, GAC, IAC
GUC	GAC, IAC
GUA	UAC, IAC
GUG	CAC, UAC

(b) Three codons could pair with the anticodon beginning with I; two codons could pair with an anticodon beginning with U or G; only one codon could pair with an anticodon beginning with A or C.

6. Proline. The three codons that will pair with IGG—CCU, CCC, and CCA—all specify proline.

7. A minimum of three tRNAs would be required. One tRNA having the anticodon UAA could decode both UUA and UUG. For the other four codons, which have C in the first position and U in the second, there are two different combinations of two tRNAs each that could decode them. The first combination would be two tRNAs that have anticodons with A in the second position and G in the third, one with I in the first position to decode CUU, CUC, and CUA, and the other with U or C in the first position to decode CUG. The second combination would be two tRNAs that have anticodons with A in the second position and G in the third, one with G in the first position to decode CUU and CUC, and the other with U in the first position to decode CUA and CUG.

8. Threonyl-tRNA synthetase has a proofreading mechanism. Any Ser-tRNA^{Thr} that is mistakenly formed is hydrolyzed by an editing site 20 Å from the activation site. The "decision" to hydrolyze the aminoacyl-tRNA appears to depend on the size of the amino acid substituent. If it is smaller than the correct amino acid, the amino acid fits into the hydrolytic site and is cleaved. If it is the same size as the correct amino acid, it does not fit and is not destroyed. Discrimination between amino acids that are larger than the correct one or are not isoelectronic with it occurs at the aminoacylation step.

9. If two different legitimate stop codons are present in tandem, it would be extremely improbable that mutant tRNAs would exist for both and would simultaneously bind to each of them and thereby prevent proper chain termination.

10. (a) The tRNA^{Cys} will become loaded with Ala rather than Cys, and as a result will insert Ala rather than Cys into polypeptide chains.

(b) In the case of a base change within a codon, only a single amino acid of a single polypeptide is changed. In the case of a tRNA recognition mutation, amino acid substitutions at many positions of many polypeptides would occur.

Chapter 40

The Mechanism of Protein Synthesis

In Chapter 40 the mechanism of protein synthesis, a process called translation, is examined in detail. The authors begin the chapter by discussing the initiation of translation, outlining the roles of a specialized initiator tRNA, the mRNA start codon, and 16S rRNA sequences are outlined. The spatial and functional relationships of the sites on the ribosome that bind aminoacyl-tRNAs and peptidyl-tRNAs, the peptide-bond–forming reaction, the role of GTP, and the mechanism of the translocation of the peptidyl-tRNA from site to site on the ribosome are presented in the description of the elongation stage of protein synthesis.

The critical role that protein factors play in translation is discussed next, including initiation, elongation, and release factors. The termination of translation is outlined, and the role of release factors that recognize translation stop codons is described. The chapter closes with a brief overview of translation in eukaryotes, emphasizing the major contrasting features with respect to translation in prokaryotes. Differences in the initiator tRNA, the selection mechanism of the initiator codon, the ribosomes, and the overall complexity of the process are highlighted. Next, the mechanisms of several potent inhibitors of translation and the mechanism of the bacterial toxin that causes diphtheria is presented. The chapter ends with a discussion of how proteins are targeted to different cellular destinations. The role of signal sequences and signal-recognition particle are discussed as are transport vesicles.

LEARNING OBJECTIVES

When you have mastered this chapter, you should be able to accomplish the following objectives.

Protein Synthesis Decodes the Information in Messenger RNA (Text Section 40.1)

1. Name and describe the functions of the three tRNA binding sites on the *70S ribosome*.

2. Name the major *initiator codon* and the amino acid it encodes. Explain the roles of the nucleotide sequences in *16S rRNA*, mRNA, and tRNA in *selecting the initiation codon* rather than the identical codon that encodes an internal amino acid. Recognize characterists of the *Shine-Delgarno* sequence.

3. Distinguish between the *initiator tRNA* ($tRNA_i$) and $tRNA_m$ and outline the conversion of methionine into *formylmethionyl-tRNA_f*.

4. List the components of the *70S initiation complex* and indicate the roles of the *initiation factors (IF)* and GTP in its formation.

5. Account for the fact that internal AUG codons are not read by the initiator tRNA.

6. Describe how the GTP–GDP cycle of *EF-Tu* controls its affinity for its reaction partners. Relate the GTP-GDP cycle of EF-Tu with that of G proteins (Chapter 13).

7. Explain the role of EF-Tu in determining the accuracy and timing of protein synthesis.

Peptidyl Transferase Catalyzes Peptide-Bond Synthesis (Text Section 40.2)

8 Outline the elongation stage of protein synthesis and describe the roles of the *elongation factors (EFs)* and GTP in the process. Locate the *aminoacyl-tRNAs* and *peptidyl-tRNAs* in the *A or P sites of the ribosome* during one cycle of elongation.

9. Describe the mechanism of peptide bond formation in the *peptidyl transferase center.*

10. Outline the *translocation* steps that occur after the formation of a peptide bond and describe the roles of *EF-G* and GTP.

11. Name the *translation stop codons*, describe the termination of translation, and explain the roles of the *release factors (RFs)* in the process.

Bacteria and Eukaryotes Differ in the Initiation of Protein Synthesis
(Text Section 40.3)

12. Contrast eukaryotic and prokaryotic ribosomes with respect to composition and size.

13. Contrast the mechanisms of translation initiation in prokaryotes and eukaryotes. Note the different initiator tRNAs, AUG codon selection mechanisms, and numbers of IFs and RFs.

14. Discuss the structure of eukaryotic mRNA including a possible advantage in such a structure

15. Compare prokaryotic and eukaryotic elongation and termination.

16. Describe the physiological consequences of defects in *eIF2*.

A Variety of Biomolecules Can Inhibit Protein Synthesis (Text Section 40.4)

17. Provide examples of *antibiotics that inhibit translation*, and describe their mechanisms of action.

18. Describe the mechanisms by which *diphtheria toxin* and ricin inhibit protein synthesis in eukaryotes.

Ribosomes Bound to the Endoplasmic Reticulum Manufacture Secretory and Membrane Proteins. (Text Section 40.5)

19. Discuss sorting of proteins into different cellular locations.

20. Describe the translocation of proteins across the ER, highlighting the four components involved.

Protein Synthesis Is Regulated by a Number of Mechanisms (Text Section 40.6)

21. Outline the role of RNA secondary structure in the regulation of iron metabolism in animals. Describe the roles of *transferrin, transferrin receptor, ferritin*, the *iron-response element* (IRE), and the *IRE-binding protein*.

22. Relate the IRE-binding protein to *aconitase* and *iron sensing*.

23. Define *microRNAs (miRNA)* and describe the discovery of the first microRNA.

24. Relate the mechanism of microRNAs to that of *RNA interference (RNAi)*. Distinguish between the RNA sources in the two types of posttranscriptional regulation.

SELF-TEST

Protein Synthesis Decodes the Information In Messenger RNA

1. What is the significance of the reconstitution of a functional ribosome from its separated components?

2. Which of the following statements about translation are correct?
   (a) Amino acids are added to the amino terminus of the growing polypeptide chain.
   (b) Amino acids are activated by attachment to tRNA molecules.
   (c) A specific initiator tRNA along with specific sequences of the mRNA ensures that translation begins at the correct codon.
   (d) Peptide bonds form between an aminoacyl-tRNA and a peptidyl-tRNA positioned in the A and P sites, respectively, of the ribosome.
   (e) Termination involves the binding of a terminator tRNA to a stop codon on the mRNA.

3. An experiment is carried out in which labeled amino acids are added to an in vitro translation system under the direction of a single mRNA species. Samples are withdrawn at different times, and the labeling patterns below are observed in the *completed* polypeptide chains. The dashes (-) represent unlabeled amino acids, X represents labeled amino acids, and A and B represent the ends of the intact protein.

```
Time 1 (early)    A - - - - - - - - - - - - - - XXB
Time 2            A - - - - - - - - - - - XXXXB
Time 3            A - - - - - - - XXXXXXB
Time 4 (late)     A - - - - XXXXXXXXB
```

Which of the following statements about these proteins are correct?

(a) The labeled amino acids are added in the B-to-A direction.
(b) The labeled amino acids are added in the A-to-B direction.
(c) A is the amino terminus of the protein.
(d) B is the amino terminus of the protein.

4. Given an in vitro system that allows protein synthesis to start and stop at the ends of any RNA sequence, answer the following questions:

(a) What peptide would be produced by the polyribonucleotide 5'-UUUGUUUUUGUU-3'? (See the table with the genetic code in your textbook.)
(b) For this peptide, which is the N-terminal amino acid and which is the C-terminal amino acid?

5. What sequence on the 16s rRNA binds to the Shine-Delgarno sequence on mRNA?

(a) CCUCC
(b) CAGGU
(c) GGAGG
(d) There is no specific sequence, it is merely a purine-rich region of the 16s rRNA.

6. What is the role of the vitamin folate in prokaryotic translation?

Peptidyl Transferase Catalyzes Peptide-Bond Synthesis

7. Match the functions or characteristics of prokaryotic translation in the right column with the appropriate translation components in the left column.

(a) IF1
(b) IF2
(c) IF3
(d) EF-Tu
(e) EF-Ts
(f) EF-G
(g) peptidyl transferase
(h) RF1
(i) RF2

(1) moves the peptidyl-tRNA from the A to the P site
(2) delivers aminoacyl-tRNA to the A site
(3) binds to the 30S ribosomal subunit
(4) recognizes stop codons
(5) forms the peptide bond
(6) delivers fMet-tRNA$_f^{Met}$ to the P site
(7) cycles on and off the ribosome
(8) binds GTP
(9) prevents the combination of the 50S and 30S subunits
(10) is involved in the hydrolysis of GTP to GDP
(11) associates with EF-Tu to release a bound nucleoside diphosphate
(12) hydrolyzes peptidyl-tRNA
(13) modifies the peptidyl transferase reaction

8. Which of the following statements about occurrences during translation are correct?

(a) The carboxyl group of the growing polypeptide chain is transferred to the amino group of an aminoacyl-tRNA.

    (b) The carboxyl group of the amino acid on the aminoacyl-tRNA is transferred to the amino group of a peptidyl-tRNA.

    (c) Peptidyl-tRNA may reside in either the A or the P site.

    (d) Aminoacyl-tRNAs are shuttled from the A to the P site by EF-G.

9. About 5% of the total bacterial protein is EF-Tu. Explain why this protein is so abundant.

10. For each of the following steps of translation, give the nucleotide cofactor involved and the number of high-energy phosphate bonds consumed.

    (a) amino acid activation

    (b) formation of the 70S initiation complex

    (c) delivery of aminoacyl-tRNA to the ribosome

    (d) formation of a peptide bond

    (e) translocation

11. Which of the following statements about release factors are correct?

    (a) They recognize terminator tRNAs.

    (b) They recognize translation stop codons.

    (c) They cause peptidyl transferase to use H_2O as a substrate.

    (d) They are two proteins in *E. coli,* each of which recognizes two mRNA triplet sequences.

Bacteria and Eukaryotes Differ in the Initiation of Protein Synthesis

12. Which of the following statements about eukaryotic translation are correct?

    (a) A formylmethionyl-tRNA initiates each protein chain.

    (b) It occurs on ribosomes containing one copy each of the 5S, 5.8S, 18S, and 28S rRNA molecules.

    (c) The correct AUG codon for initiation is selected by the base-pairing of a region on the rRNA of the small ribosomal subunit with an mRNA sequence upstream from the translation start site.

    (d) It is terminated by a release factor that recognizes stop codons and hydrolyzes GTP.

    (e) It involves proteins that bind to the 5′ ends of mRNAs.

    (f) It can be regulated by protein kinases.

13. Which of the following is a correct statement regarding the disease vanishing white matter (VWM)?

    (a) It is caused by a mutation in eIF4-G.

    (b) It is caused by a mutation in eIF2.

    (c) The mutation is found in all cells in the body but the effects are limited to brain tissue.

    (d) The mutation occurs only in cells in the brain.

A Variety of Antibiotics and Toxins Can Inhibit Protein Synthesis

14. Many antibiotics act by inhibiting protein synthesis. How can some of these be used in humans to counteract microbial infections without causing toxic side effects due to the inhibition of eukaryotic protein synthesis?

15. Increasing the concentration of which of the following would most effectively antagonize the inhibition of protein synthesis by puromycin?

    (a) ATP   (d) peptidyl-tRNAs

    (b) GTP   (e) eIF3

    (c) aminoacyl-tRNAs

16. Which of the following statements about the diphtheria toxin are correct?

    (a) It is cleaved on the surface of susceptible eukaryotic cells into two fragments, one of which enters the cytosol.
    (b) It binds to peptidyl transferase and inhibits protein synthesis.
    (c) It reacts with ATP to phosphorylate eIF2 and prevent the insertion of the Met-tRNA$_i$ into the P site.
    (d) It reacts with NAD$^+$ to add ADP-ribose to eEF2 and prevent movement of the peptidyl-tRNA from the A to the P site.
    (e) One toxin molecule is required for each translation factor inactivated, that is, it acts stoichiometrically.

Ribosomes Bound to the Endoplasmic Reticulum Manufacture Secretory and Membrane Proteins

17. Which of the following proteins are usually synthesized by free ribosomes?

    (a) lysosomal proteins
    (b) cytoplasmic proteins
    (c) secretory proteins
    (d) integral membrane proteins

18. Place the following in the order in which a newly synthesized protein is transported out of the lumen of the ER.

    (a) Cis-Golgi
    (b) Secretory granules
    (c) Trans-Golgi
    (d) Transport vesicles

Eukaryotic Gene Expression Can Be Controlled at Posttranscriptional Levels

19. What are the biochemical similarities and differences between an iron-response element (IRE) and an estrogen-response element (ERE) (Chapter 37)?

20. Describe the mechanism of action of the IRE-BP.

21. Which of the following is involved in the mechanism of microRNA posttranslational regulation?

    (a) miRNAs bind to complementary mRNA sequences and prevent them from being translated.
    (b) Double-stranded RNAs are cleaved into 21-nucleotide fragments, the single-stranded components of which form RISC complexes that cleave complementary mRNAs.
    (c) The Argonaute family of proteins are RNases that cleave sequences complementary to the microRNA.
    (d) The single-stranded miRNAs are generated from larger genetically encoded precursors.

ANSWERS TO SELF-TEST

1. It shows that the components themselves contain all the information necessary to form the structure and that neither a template nor any other factors are involved. Thus, the ribosome serves as model from which we might learn the general principles

involved in self-assembly. Reassembly allows systematic study of the roles of the individual components through the determination of the effects of substitutions of mutant or altered individual proteins or rRNAs.

2. b, c, d. Answer (a) is incorrect because the incoming activated aminoacyl-tRNA, in the A site of the ribosome, adds its free amino group to the activated carboxyl of the growing polypeptide on a peptidyl-tRNA in the P site. Answer (e) is incorrect because termination does not involve tRNAs that recognize translation stop codons but rather protein release factors that recognize these and cause peptidyl transferase to donate the growing polypeptide chain to H_2O rather than to another aminoacyl-tRNA.

3. b, c. Although longer incubation times result in completed proteins that have labeled polypeptides closer to their amino terminus, the chains actually grow in the amino-to-carboxyl direction. When the labeled amino acid is introduced into the system, it begins adding to the carboxyl ends of the growing chains that are already present in all stages of completion. The completed chains in samples withdrawn after a short time will have labeled polypeptides only near their carboxyl end. As time passes, more and more polypeptides that began adding labeled polypeptides near their amino terminals will become complete chains.

4. (a) Phenylalanylvalylphenylalanylvaline
   (b) Phe is the N-terminal amino acid and Val is the C-terminal amino acid.

5. a. Answers b and c are actual Shine-Delgarno sequences or parts of one.

6. After folic acid is converted to N^{10}-formyltetrahydrofolate, it acts as a carrier of formyl groups and is a substrate for a transformylase reaction that converts Met-tRNA_f to fMet-tRNA_f—the initiator tRNA.

7. (a) 3, 7, 9 (b) 3, 6, 7, 8, 10 (c) 3, 7, 9 (d) 2, 7, 8, 10 (e) 11 (f) 1, 7, 8, 10 (g) 5, 12 (h) 4, 7, 13 (i) 4, 7, 13

8. a, c. The aminoacyl-tRNA in the A site becomes a peptidyl-tRNA when it receives the carboxyl group of the growing polypeptide chain from the peptidyl-tRNA in the P site. After the free tRNA leaves, the extended polypeptide on its new tRNA is then moved to the P site by EF-G. Answer (d) is incorrect because transfer RNAs bearing aminoacyl derivatives with free amino groups are never found in the P site.

9. The large amounts of EF-Tu in the cell bind essentially all of the aminoacyl-tRNAs and protect these activated complexes from hydrolysis.

10. (a) ATP, 2 (b) GTP, 1 (c) GTP, 1 (d) none (e) GTP, 1. With regard to the answer for (d), the formation of a peptide bond per se does not require a cofactor. The energy for the exergonic reaction is supplied by the activated aminoacyl-tRNA.

11. b, c, d. Each of the two release factors of E. coli recognizes two of the three translation stop codons and interacts with the synthesis machinery such that peptidyl transferase donates the polypeptide chain to H_2O and thus terminates synthesis by hydrolyzing the ester linkage of the protein to the tRNA.

12. b, d, e, f. Eukaryotic ribosomes usually scan the mRNA from the 5′ end for the first AUG codon, which then serves to initiate the synthesis. Answer (e) is correct because proteins that bind to the cap of the mRNA are involved in the association of the ribosome with the mRNA.

13. b, c. Answer a is incorrect because defective eIF4-G has been implicated in fragile-X syndrome not VWM.

14. The inhibition of the prokaryotic translation and not that of the eukaryote can result from differences between their respective ribosomes. Some antibiotics interact with the RNA components that are unique to bacterial ribosomes and, consequently, can inhibit bacterial growth without affecting the human cells.

15. c. Puromycin is an analog of aminoacyl-tRNA. It inhibits protein synthesis by binding to the A site of the ribosome and accepting the growing polypeptide chain from the peptidyl-tRNA in the P site and thus terminating polymer growth. Because aminoacyl-tRNAs compete with the puromycin for the A site, increasing their concentration would lessen the extent of inhibition.

16. d. Answer (e) is incorrect because the toxin acts catalytically and is thus extremely deadly; one toxin molecule can inactivate many translocase molecules by modifying them covalently.

17. b. Free ribosomes synthesize proteins that remain in the cell, either in the cytoplasm or in organelles such as the nucleus or mitochondria.

18. d, a, c, b

19. The IRE is a sequence in the 5′-untranslated region of the mRNA that encodes the ferritin molecule.

20. The IRE-binding protein (IRE-BP) binds to the IRE and blocks translation. The ERE is a DNA sequence to which the estrogen receptor-estrogen complex binds to facilitate transcription. The iron-sulfur cluster at the center of the IRP is unstable, and under conditions of low iron dissociates from the protein, allowing binding of the IRE.

21. c, d. Answer b is incorrect. This is part of the mechanism of RNAi.

PROBLEMS

1. The methionine codon AUG functions both to initiate a polypeptide chain and to direct methionine incorporation into internal positions in a protein. By what mechanisms are the AUG start codons selected in prokaryotes?

2. Laboratory studies of protein synthesis usually involve the addition of a radioactively labeled amino acid and either natural or synthetic mRNAs to systems containing the other components. To observe the formation of protein, advantage is taken of the fact that proteins, but not amino acids, can be precipitated by solutions of trichloroacetic acid. Thus, one can observe the extent to which radioactivity has been incorporated into "acid-precipitable material" as a function of time to estimate the rate of formation of protein. In one such experiment, poly(U) is used as a synthetic mRNA in an in vitro system derived from wheat germ (a eukaryote).

   (a) What labeled amino acid would you add to the reaction mixture?
   (b) What product will be formed?

   For each of the following procedures, explain the results observed. Assume that in a complete system 3000 cpm (counts per minute) are found in acid-precipitable material at the end of 30 minutes and that values below 150 cpm are not significantly above the background level.

   (c) 85 cpm is recovered when RNase A is added to the complete system.
   (d) 2900 cpm is recovered when chloramphenicol is added to the complete system.
   (e) 300 cpm is recovered when cyclohexamide is added to the complete system.
   (f) 640 cpm is recovered when puromycin is added to the complete system.

(g) 1518 cpm is recovered when puromycin and extra wheat germ tRNA are added to the complete system.

(h) 120 cpm is recovered when poly(A) is used instead of poly(U).

3. For each of the following antibiotics, indicate the difference in prokaryotic and eukaryotic translation that enables them to act as effective antibiotics.

(a) Streptomycin
(b) Neomycin
(c) Chloramphenicol
(d) Erythromycin

ANSWERS TO PROBLEMS

1. A purine-rich mRNA sequence, three to nine nucleotides long (called the Shine-Dalgarno sequence), which is centered about 10 nucleotides upstream of (to the 5′ side of) the start codon, base-pairs with a sequence of complementary nucleotides near the 3′ end of the 16S rRNA of the 30S ribosomal subunit. This interaction plus the association of fMet-tRNA$_f$ with the AUG in the P site of the ribosome sets the mRNA reading frame.

2. (a) Poly(U) codes for the incorporation of phenylalanine. Therefore, labeled phenylalanine must be added to the reaction mixture.

(b) Polyphenylalanine will be formed.

(c) RNase A will digest poly(U) almost completely to 3′-UMP, thus destroying the template for polyphenylalanine synthesis. Also the tRNA will be digested and the ribosomes damaged. No protein synthesis will take place.

(d) Chloramphenicol inhibits the peptidyl transferase activity of the 50S ribosomal subunit in prokaryotes but has no effect on eukaryotes so synthesis in a eukaryote is unaffected.

(e) Cyclohexamide inhibits the peptidyl transferase activity of the 60S ribosomal subunit in eukaryotes so synthesis is largely blocked.

(f) Puromycin mimics an aminoacyl-tRNA and causes premature polypeptide chain termination leading to a low level of protein synthesis.

(g) The addition of extra wheat germ tRNA reduces the inhibiting effect of puromycin, since they both compete for the A site on ribosomes. Therefore synthesis is increased over that in experiment (f).

(h) Poly(A) directs the synthesis of polylysine; since there is no lysine (either labeled or unlabeled) in the system, no product can be detected.

3. (a) Streptomycin interferes with the binding of formylmethionyl-tRNA to ribosomes, preventing the initiation of protein synthesis. Since eukaryotes use Met-tRNAi instead, the antibiotic does not interfere with eukaryotic protein synthesis.

(b) Neomycin interferes with the interaction between tRNA and the 16S rRNA of the 30S subunit. Eukaryotes have different rRNA components in their ribosomes and the antibiotic is not able to bind to the 18S subunit.

(c) Chloramphenicol inhibits the peptidyl transferase activity of the 50S subunit. As with Neomycin, the difference in components of the ribosomes results in the antibiotic having minimal effects on eukaryotic protein synthesis.

(d) Erythromycin binds to the 50S subunit and blocks translocation. The specificity for binding to the eukaryotic ribosome is not great enough to disrupt synthesis in eukaryotes.

Recombinant DNA Techniques

In this chapter, the authors present the methods and techniques used to analyze and manipulate DNA. They begin with an overview of recombinant DNA technology and the tools that make it possible. Of particular importance are the specificity of base pairing between nucleic acids and the enzymes that act on nucleic acids. Restriction endonucleases, the ability to immobilize nucleic acids onto solid supports, DNA sequencing, and chemical synthesis of oligodeoxyribonucleotides, plus the polymerase chain reaction (PCR) are introduced. A more detailed description of restriction enzymes and the joining of their products, specific DNA restriction fragments, by DNA ligase are described. They next present the major method of determining the sequence of DNA and an automated method for synthesizing oligodeoxyribonucleotides by chemical means. The authors then describe how specific fragments of genes can be amplified by PCR, a process that depends on specific hybridization of short oligodeoxyribonucleotide primers to a template strand followed by polymerase-catalyzed synthesis of DNA. A more detailed description of restriction enzymes and DNA ligase follows; these enzymes make possible the precise production and joining of DNA fragments. Next, various vectors, the self-replicating carriers of the target genes, are discussed and their roles in the cloning and expression of genes is described. The special role in recombinant DNA technology of complementary DNA (cDNA), which is produced from mRNA, is discussed. The authors describe how DNA chips can be used to monitor the pattern and level of gene expression in an organism. The methods for creating transgenic animals and plants are presented, and the information that can be obtained from them outlined. The authors describe how site-specific mutagenesis can be used with cloned genes to produce proteins having any desired amino acid at any position. An overview is provided to explain how the methods described allow the information in either protein or DNA to be manipulated. The authors then turn to describing the sequencing of entire genomes, including that of man, and to how such massive amounts of sequence information can be organized, analyzed, and exploited.

The problems of locating specific genes in the genome and of inserting and expressing foreign genes in eukaryotes are also considered. The chapter closes with a description of RNA interference, introducing genes into plants, and the potential for gene therapy in medicine. Throughout the chapter, the authors use the example of amyotropic lateral sclerosis (ALS) to illustrate the effect that recombinant DNA technology has had on our knowledge of disease mechanisms.

LEARNING OBJECTIVES

When you have mastered this chapter, you should be able to accomplish the following objectives.

Reverse Genetics Allows the Synthesis of Nucleic Acids from a Protein Sequence (Text Section 41.1)

1. Explain how *cDNA* and *cDNA libraries* are created.

2. Describe what a *probe* is and explain the biochemical basis of its specificity. Describe how probes are obtained.

3. Explain how to design a probe by converting an amino acid sequence into nucleotide sequences using the genetic code.

4. Describe how *oligodeoxyribonucleotides* are synthesized chemically. Indicate the roles of activated precursors, coupling, protecting groups, oxidation, and differential deprotection in the process. List some common experimental uses of oligonucleotides.

Recombinant DNA Technology Has Revolutionized All Aspects of Biology (Text Section 41.2)

5. Describe the reaction catalyzed by *restriction enzymes* and the characteristics of the *restriction sites* they recognize.

6. Explain why *gel electrophoresis* of DNA is essential to recombinant DNA technology. Describe how DNA *restriction fragments* can be detected in gels.

7. Contrast the *Southern, Northern, Western,* and *protein blotting techniques.*

8. Outline how restriction enzymes and *DNA ligase* have enabled recombinant DNA technology.

9. List the desired characteristics of a *vector.* Distinguish *plasmids* and *viruses.*

10. Draw the termini of the DNA fragments joined by DNA ligase. Distinguish between sticky and blunt ends of dsDNA.

Eukaryotic Genes Can Be Manipulated with Considerable Precision (Text Section 41.3)

11. Outline the major steps in *cloning* a DNA molecule.

12. Explain the roles of oligonucleotide *linkers* and *polynucleotide kinase* in creating recombinant molecules.

13. Describe the reactions catalyzed by *reverse transcriptase* and *terminal transferase.*

14. Distinguish between *screening* and *selection*.

15. Explain the function of *expression vectors* and the use of *immunochemical screening* in isolating genes.

16. Explain the process of expression cloning. Give an example of a eukaryotic protein expressed in bacteria.

17. Outline how specific genes can be cloned from a digest of an organism to form a *genomic library*. Define genomic library.

18. Explain how the presence of *introns* in some eukaryotic genes complicates the expression of these genes in prokaryotes.

19. Explain the process of *DNA sequencing* by controlled termination of DNA synthesis *in vitro* (Sanger dideoxy method), including the role for *fluorescence* in this process.

20. List some of the discoveries arising from *comparative genomics*.

21. Describe the *polymerase chain reaction*. Explain the roles of the *primer* and *thermostable DNA polymerase* in amplifying the *target* DNA sequence.

22. Give examples of practical applications of PCR.

23. Outline five noteworthy features of the PCR technique.

24. Explain how qPCR is used to determine copy number in cells.

25. Outline how *DNA microarrays (gene chips)* are used to monitor patterns of gene expression.

SELF-TEST

Reverse Genetics Allows the Synthesis of Nucleic Acids from a Protein Sequence

1. Which of the following statements are correct? Chemically synthesized oligonucleotides can be used
   (a) to synthesize genes.
   (b) to construct linkers.
   (c) to introduce mutations into cloned DNA.
   (d) as primers for sequencing DNA.
   (e) as probes for hybridization.

2. Which of the following statements are correct? The efficient, successful chemical synthesis of oligonucleotides requires
   (a) high yields at each condensation step.
   (b) the protection of groups not intended for reaction.
   (c) a single treatment for the removal of all blocking groups.
   (d) methods for the removal of the blocking groups that do not rupture phosphodiester bonds.
   (e) a computer-controlled, automated "gene machine."

3. Which of the following partial amino acid sequences from a protein whose gene you wish to clone would be most useful in designing an oligonucleotide probe to screen a cDNA library?
   (a) Met-Leu-Arg-Leu
   (b) Met-Trp-Cys-Trp
   Explain why.

4. Outline the steps necessary to synthesize a gene. Be explicit about the information and reagents, including enzymes, that you would need.

Recombinant DNA Technology Has Revolutionized All Aspects of Biology

5. Which of the following portions of a longer duplex DNA segment are likely to be recognition sequences of a restriction enzyme?

   (a) 5'-AGTC-3'
        3'-TCAG-5'
   (b) 5'-ATCG-3'
        3'-TAGC-5'
   (c) 5'-ACCT-3'
        3'-TGGA-5'
   (d) 5'-ACGT-3'
        3'-TGCA-5'

6. Which of the following reagents would be useful for visualizing DNA restriction fragments that have been separated by electrophoresis in an agarose gel and remain in the wet gel?

   (a) ^{32}Pi
   (b) $[\alpha$-^{32}P]ATP
   (c) diphenylamine
   (d) ethidium bromide
   (e) DNA polymerase
   (f) polynucleotide kinase

7. Which blotting technique is used for the detection of DNA that has been separated from a mixture of DNA restriction fragments by electrophoresis through an agarose gel and then transferred onto a nitrocellulose sheet?

   (a) Eastern blotting
   (b) Northern blotting
   (c) Southern blotting
   (d) Western blotting

Eukaryotic Genes Can Be Manipulated with Considerable Precision

8. Complete the following statements about the Sanger dideoxy method of DNA sequencing.

   (a) The incorporation of a ddNMP onto a growing DNA chain stops the reaction because
   (b) The sequence of the DNA fragments emerging from the capillary is determined by
   (c) A sequencing primer does not have to anneal directly to the gene to be sequenced if
   (d) It is preferable to label the oligonucleotide primer with a fluorescent rather than a radioactive group because

9. Match the conditions of the PCR reaction, in the left column, with the appropriate reaction in the right column.

   (a) cooling abruptly to 54°C
   (b) heating to 72°C, 30 s
   (c) heating to 95°C, 15 s

   (1) DNA synthesis by Taq DNA polymerase
   (2) hybridization of primers
   (3) strand separation

10. Using the information in Question 9, give the sequence of the PCR reaction steps, and explain the rationale for each step.

11. Which of the following are possible applications of the PCR technique?

    (a) detection of very small amounts of bacteria and viruses
    (b) introduction of a normal gene into animals containing the corresponding defective gene
    (c) amplification of DNA in archaeological samples

(d) monitoring of certain types of cancer chemotherapy

(e) identification of matching DNA samples in forensic specimens

12. You have been supplied with the linker oligonucleotide d(GGAATTCC) and an isolated and purified DNA restriction fragment that has been excised from a longer DNA molecule with a restriction endonuclease that produces blunt ends. Which of the following reagents would you need to tailor the ends of the fragment so it could be inserted into an expression vector at a unique EcoRI cloning site?

(a) DNA polymerase

(b) all four dNTPs

(c) EcoRI restriction endonuclease

(d) ATP

(e) DNA ligase

(f) polynucleotide kinase

What would happen if the restriction fragment had an internal EcoRI site?

13. Briefly describe genomic and cDNA libraries. Which library, from a given organism, has more clones?

14. Explain how the presence of introns in eukaryotic genes complicates the production of the protein products they encode when expression is attempted in bacteria. How can this problem be circumvented?

15. Which of these reagents would be required to perform an immuno-chemical screen of a population of bacteria for the presence of a particular cloned gene if you have the pure protein encoded by the gene?

(a) $[\gamma$ -^{32}P]ATP

(b) polynucleotide kinase

(c) DNA polymerase

(d) all four dNTPs

(e) a radioactive antibody to the protein encoded by the cloned gene

16. Reverse transcriptase requires the following for the conversion of a single-strand RNA into a double-strand DNA.

(a) all four NTPs

(b) all four dNTPs

(c) a DNA template

(d) an RNA template

(e) a primer

17. Give an example of a result of comparative genomics

18. The gene for a eukaryotic polypeptide hormone was isolated, cloned, sequenced, and overexpressed in a bacterium. After the polypeptide was purified from the bacterium, it failed to function when it was subjected to a bioassay in the organism from which the gene was isolated. Speculate why the recombinant DNA product was inactive.

19. Which of the following is true of C_T in qPCR?

(a) It is cycle number at which the fluorescence becomes detectable.

(b) It is directly proportional to the number of copies of the original template.

(c) It is the fluorescence detection threshold.

(d) All of the above are true.

20. Which of the following treatments of a yeast cell results in the largest changes in gene expression as monitored by microarry analysis?

(a) A heat shock treatment at 37°C

(b) Nitrogen depletion

(c) Amino acid starvation

(d) All three affect gene expression equally.

ANSWERS TO SELF-TEST

1. All are correct.

2. a, b, d, and e. Answer (c) is not correct, because the blocking groups must be removed differentially; for example, the dimethoxytrityl group must be removed from the 5'-hydroxyl (so that the next condensation with an incoming nucleotide can occur) without removing the blocking groups on the exocyclic amines of the bases. Answer (e) is correct because, although the synthesis can be carried out manually, it is slow and laborious.

3. b. This amino acid sequence is the better choice for reverse translation into a DNA sequence because it contains fewer amino acid residues having multiple codons; Trp and Met have one codon each and Cys has two. Thus, for the (b) sequence, Met-Trp-Cys-Trp, there are $1 \times 1 \times 2 \times 1 = 2$ different dodecameric oligonucleotide coding sequences. In contrast, Leu and Arg each have six codons, so for the (a) sequence, Met-Leu-Arg-Leu, there are $1 \times 6 \times 6 \times 6 = 216$ different coding sequences. Therefore, the probe for (b) would be simpler to construct and would be more likely to give unambiguous hybridization results.

4. You would need to know the sequence of the gene you wish to synthesize. This could be derived from the amino acid sequence of the protein the gene encodes by reverse translation using the genetic code. You would also need to know what restriction sites you wish to build into the synthetic sequence for cloning the synthetic product. You would have to decide on the individual sequences of the different oligonucleotides that compose both strands of the gene. These sequences would be determined by the final desired sequence, the individual lengths (30 to 80 nucleotides long) that can be easily synthesized and purified, and the requirement for overlapping ends that will be necessary to allow unique joinings of the cohesive ends of the partially duplex segments. Self-complementary oligomers would be mixed together to form duplex fragments with cohesive ends. DNA ligase and ATP would be added to join these together to form the complete duplex. If appropriate ends have been designed into the synthesis, the product can then be ligated into a vector for cloning.

5. d. It has two-fold rotational symmetry; that is, the top strand, 5'-ACGT-3', has the same sequence as the bottom strand. Many restriction enzymes recognize and cut such palindromic sequences.

6. d. Ethidium bromide intercalates into the DNA double strand, and its quantum yield of fluorescence consequently increases. Upon uv irradiation, it fluoresces with an intense orange color wherever DNA is present in the gel.

7. c

8. (a) . . .the newly synthesized ddNMP terminus lacks the requisite 3'-hydroxyl onto which the next dNMP residue would add.
   (b) . . .the colors of the fluorescence tags on the chain terminators.
   (c) . . .it anneals to the vector that the gene has been cloned into.
   (d) . . .it avoids the use of radioisotopes and allows the automated detection of the terminated primers.

9. (a) 2   (b) 1   (c) 3

10. The sequence of steps is 3, 2, and 1. Heating to 95°C completely separates all the double-strand DNA molecules. The subsequent rapid cooling to 54°C causes the excess primers to hybridize to the complementary parent DNA strands. Then at 72°C the Taq DNA polymerase (which retains its activity after the 95°C step) carries out DNA

synthesis using the four dNTPs. Amplification of DNA is achieved by repeating these steps many times.

11. a, c, d, e.

12. c, d, e, f. The oligonucleotide must have a 5'-phosphate group to serve as a substrate for DNA ligase. Therefore, ATP and polynucleotide kinase would be used, as would bacteriophage T4 DNA ligase and ATP, to join the duplex form of the palindromic (self-complementary) oligonucleotide to the blunt-end fragment. Finally, the fragment with the linker covalently joined to it would be cut with *Eco*RI endonuclease to produce cohesive ends that match those of the cut vector. It is assumed that the fragment itself lacks *Eco*RI sites because, if one or more internal *Eco*RI sites were present, the fragment would be cut when it is treated with the enzyme to generate the cohesive ends. Such fragmentation of the DNA would complicate the joining reaction by forming product with various combinations of *Eco*RI-joined ends.

13. A genomic library is composed of a collection of clones, each of which contains a fragment of DNA from the target organism. The entire collection should contain all the sequences present in the genome of the target organism. A cDNA library is composed of a collection of clones that contain the sequences present in the mRNA of the target organism from which the mRNA was isolated. A cDNA library contains far fewer clones than does a genomic library because only a small fraction of the genome is being transcribed into mRNA at any given time. The content of a cDNA library depends on the cells from which the mRNA was isolated. The type of cell, its state of development, and environmental factors influence the identity and quantity of its mRNA population.

14. In eukaryotes the introns are removed from the primary transcript by processing, to produce the mRNA that is translated. Prokaryotes lack the machinery to perform this processing; consequently, the translation product of the primary transcript would not be functional because it would encode amino acid sequences that are specified by the intron sequences. The problem can be circumvented by using cDNA prepared from the mRNA from the gene encoding the protein; the cDNA will contain only the sequences present in the processed RNA; that is, the intron sequences will have been removed.

15. e. An immunochemical screen could be performed by adding the radioactive antibody to lysed bacterial colonies and examining the population by autoradiography to see which colonies contain the antigen (protein) produced by the cloned gene.

16. b, d, e. Since reverse transcriptase makes DNA, it requires dNTPs not NTPs. RNA is required as a template to direct the synthesis of a complementary DNA strand. That DNA strand itself then serves as a template for the synthesis of its complement to form the duplex DNA product. All polymerases that form DNA need a primer to start the synthesis of a new DNA chain.

17. Comparison of the genomes of two species of pufferfish with that of the human genome resulted in the identification of more than 1000 formerly unrecognized human genes.

18. Omitting such an obvious explanation as the destruction of the polypeptide during the bioassay, it is possible that the polypeptide might not have undergone some post-translational modification that is needed for it to function. For example, the polypeptide might need to be acetylated, methylated, or trimmed at the N- or C-terminus, or it might need to have a carbohydrate or lipid group attached to it. The bacterium in which it was produced would be unlikely to contain the enzymatic machinery necessary to carry out these modifications, or if it did, it might lack the ability to recognize

the eukaryotic signals that direct these modifications. It is also possible that the bacterium might have contained a peptidase or protease that inactivated the peptide without destroying its antigenic properties.

19. a. C_T is determined by amplfying a standard and is the cycle number in which the fluorescence threshold is reached. It is inversely proportional to the number of copies of the original cDNA template.

20. b. In a microarray analysis, each gene in the sample is represented by an individual square. A black color indicates that expression of the gene was not affected by the conditions of the study relative to the control. Red indicates induction, or an increase in gene's expression relative to the control and green indicates repression, or a decrease. A large number of squares that are either red or green indicates a large number of genes have had their expression perturbed by the stressor. Using Figure 5.21 in the text, you can see that nitrogen depletion in yeast results in widespread increases (red) and decreases (green) in gene expression. Although there are some changes in the heat shock and amino acid starvation arrays, there are fewer colored squares in both relative to the nitrogen depletion sample.

PROBLEMS

1. Before the development of modern methods for the analysis and manipulation of genes, many attempts were made to transform both prokaryotic and eukaryotic cells with DNA. Most of these experiments were unsuccessful. Suggest why these early efforts to transform cells largely failed.

2. Pseudogenes are composed of nonfunctional (unexpressed) DNA sequences that are related by sequence similarity to actively expressed genes. Some researchers have proposed that pseudogenes are copies of functional genes that have been inactivated during genome evolution. Suggest several ways that such genes could have become nonfunctional. Suppose you clone a number of closely related sequences, any of which may code for a particular protein. How can you tell which of the sequences is the functional gene, that is, which of the sequences codes for the protein?

3. The Sanger dideoxy method for determining DNA sequence is limited in that a stretch of only 1000 or fewer bases can be analyzed in one reaction. Suppose you wish to sequence a newly isolated double-strand DNA tumor virus that contains ~5000 base pairs. You decide to use the Sanger method on restriction fragments of the DNA for sequencing. You use an enzyme that makes a significant number of cuts to give, on average, fragments of ~275 nucleotides or less. Why might it be a good idea also to sequence a second set of fragments cleaved by another restriction enzyme?

4. You wish to clone a yeast gene in λ phage. Why is it desirable to cleave both the yeast DNA and the λ-phage DNA with the same restriction enzyme?

5. Cleavage of a double-strand DNA fragment that contains 500 bases with restriction enzyme A yields two unique fragments, one 100 bases and the other 400 bases in length. Cleavage of the DNA fragment with restriction enzyme B yields three fragments, two containing 150 nucleotides and one containing 200 nucleotides. When the 500-base fragment is incubated with both enzymes (this is called a double-digest), two fragments 100 bases in length and two 150 bases in length are found. Diagram the 500-base fragment, showing the cleavage sites of both enzymes. Now suppose you also have a double-strand DNA fragment that is identical with the original fragment,

except that the first 75 base pairs at the left end are deleted. How can this fragment help you construct a cleavage map for the two enzymes?

6. You wish to express a eukaryotic gene—chicken ovalbumin—in *E. coli.* To avoid transcribing and translating intron sequences, you should use cDNA for protein expression. However, if you introduce only the chicken ovalbumin cDNA into bacteria, the level of expression of functional protein will likely be low. What other sequences are necessary in order to ensure optimal expression?

7. Because PCR can amplify DNA templates one millionfold or more, contaminating DNA must not be present in the sample to be used for amplification. To see why, consider a PCR procedure that begins with 1 μg DNA (about 10^6 templates) in a reaction mixture of 100 μL. This sample can be easily amplified about one millionfold in 20 cycles (an amplification of 2^{20}). Suppose that 0.1 μL of DNA from the initial amplification cycle is inadvertently introduced into another reaction mixture containing 1 μg of a different DNA. Could the contaminant cause problems with PCR analysis of the second sample? Why?

8. One method of analysis of evidence from cases of sexual assault often includes histocompatability locus antigen (HLA) type analysis using PCR. Samples collected from a victim may contain not only sperm but also epithelial cells from the victim. Such samples are first incubated in a protease-detergent mixture. The epithelial cells are lysed, while the sperm heads are not. The sperm heads are collected by centrifugation and then washed several times. They are then lysed in the presence of a reducing agent such as dithiothreitol, which makes sperm heads sensitive to the protease-detergent mixture. Lysis products are then used for PCR analysis. Why is it necessary to carry out separation of sperm and epithelial cells? Why are cells and sperm heads lysed before PCR analysis? Suppose that blood and hair samples are also found as evidence at the scene of the alleged crime. Why should precautions be taken to keep these samples isolated from each other?

9. Unlike DNA polymerase I from *E. coli,* DNA polymerase I from the bacterium *T. aquaticus* has no proofreading activity and is therefore unable to remove mismatched bases that are randomly incorporated into newly synthesized DNA strands. Under standard conditions used for the polymerase chain reaction, misincorporation of nucleotides occurs at a frequency of approximately 1 per 900 nucleotide residues in DNA.

   (a) Suppose that you are using PCR to detect copies of an oncogene in a tissue sample. You will challenge the amplified sample with a radioactive probe containing the oncogene sequence, using Southern blot analysis. Will low-frequency, random misincorporation of bases during amplification of the oncogene interfere with your analysis?

   (b) Suppose you are using PCR with a mutant primer, that is, a primer with a sequence differing from the wild-type sequence, to introduce a deliberate alteration in a eukaryotic gene. You plan to use the amplified mutant gene for cloning and expression in *E. coli* to determine how the directed change affects the expressed protein. How might misincorporation level in the amplification procedure interfere with your cloning and expression experiments? What could you do to solve the problem?

10. *E. coli* DNA polymerase I has a $5' \rightarrow 3'$ polymerase activity and also two other catalytic activities. One is a $3' \rightarrow 5'$ exonuclease activity whose function is to remove from the growing $3'$ end of the chain those mismatched bases occasionally incorporated erroneously by the polymerase activity. The other catalytic activity is a $5' \rightarrow 3'$ exonuclease, which removes both paired and mispaired DNA stretches ahead of the polymerase. If the $5' \rightarrow 3'$ exonuclease acts concomitantly with the polymerase in the same enzyme, new nucleotides are incorporated by the polymerase in place of the ones

removed by the nuclease, and the nick is essentially "translated," that is, moved, in the 5′→3′ direction. This nick-translating ability of DNA polymerase I has been exploited to create radioactive DNA probes for use in Southern blots and other techniques. Describe how nick translation could be used for such purposes.

11. Patients with a particular form of hemophilia (a deficiency in blood clotting) have a loss of an EcoRI restriction site within the gene for a coagulation factor protein. In one family with an affected son, PCR analysis was carried out on 200 μL blood samples from a male fetus and from several family members to determine whether the fetus also carried the mutation. Using appropriate primer oligonucleotides, DNA fragments 150 bp in length and spanning the EcoRI polymorphic site in intron 10 were synthesized. These fragments were incubated with EcoRI, and the resulting cleavage fragments were then separated by electrophoresis on a gel and stained with ethidium bromide. A diagram of the gel is shown in Figure 41.1, along with the source of the blood sample for each lane. Note that any 150-bp fragment that contains the EcoRI site will be cut by the enzyme into two fragments, 100 bp and 50 bp in length.

FIGURE 41.1

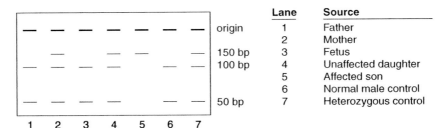

Lane	Source
1	Father
2	Mother
3	Fetus
4	Unaffected daughter
5	Affected son
6	Normal male control
7	Heterozygous control

(a) Specify the genotype for each member of the family and for the controls. Does the fetus carry the mutation?

(b) This analysis can also be done by using Southern blotting to detect single-copy sequences in genomic DNA. Why is the PCR analysis preferable?

12. Base pairing by hydrogen bond formation between complementary bases is a fundamental feature in interactions of nucleic acids. Discuss the role of base pairing in the context of each of the following:

(a) the fidelity of messenger RNA synthesis
(b) synthesis of cDNA by reverse transcriptase
(c) the use of primers in the polymerase chain reaction (PCR)
(d) identifying a desired clone using a radioactive DNA probe
(e) measuring the relatedness of two DNA species without sequencing them

13. DNA microarray or chip technology allows one to monitor simultaneously the level of mRNA production from every gene in a bacterium. Why might such an analysis of a microbe not give an accurate estimate of the levels of the proteins in the microbe?

14. The plasmid pBR322, a double-strand circular DNA molecule containing ~4.4 kilobase pairs, is commonly used in cloning experiments. A technician in a molecular biology laboratory needs to prepare a large quantity of pBR322 by growing a liter culture of E. coli containing the plasmid and then isolating the pBR322 DNA.

(a) How many milligrams of plasmid DNA can be prepared from a liter of bacterial cells growing at a density of 10^8 cells per ml? Assume that each cell contains 100 plasmid molecules and that the molecular weight of the average base pair in the plasmid is ~660.

(b) If the technician decides to use a nanogram of pBR322 as the template in a PCR experiment, how many templates will be present in the reaction mixture?

15. You have isolated cDNAs containing the genes encoding malarial proteins with the aim of developing an anti-malarial vaccine. How could you use these cDNAs to direct the efficient synthesis of their encoded proteins in an *in vitro* translation system in order to study their antigenic properties? Be sure to consider the entire information flow pathway.

16. You wish to use the restriction enzyme HhaI, which hydrolyzes the duplex sequence GCGC between the last G and C, to cut a large double-strand plasmid DNA (several kbp) at the single site operator site where a repressor protein binds very tightly to it. You know the site contains one HhaI site. Unfortunately, the rest of the DNA contains 31 HhaI site in its sequence. Considering what you learned about restriction endonucleases and modification methyl transferases (methylases), can you devise a method that would allow you to achieve the desired, unique cut in the DNA without fragmenting it elsewhere? You have at your disposal the DNA, repressor protein, and the HhaI restriction and modification enzymes. The HhaI DNA methylase adds a methyl group to the second C of the GCGC recognition sequence.

17. If you have access to the genomic library of an unkown eukaryote and you know the sequence from a segment of its genomic DNA, devise a method to determine the sequences of the adjacent genes.

18. If you wanted to make a human DNA library with the minimum number of clones required for complete coverage, why wouldn't you insert random human DNA fragments into the vector bacteriophage λ?

19. You have sequenced the genome of a new, previously unknown, bacterium. How might you go about identifying the function of a particular open reading frame encoded by a gene in your bacterium? Reminder: an open reading frame is a gene sequence that contains an initiator codon and a terminator codon and likely encodes a protein product.

ANSWERS TO PROBLEMS

1. During the early years of such experiments, few ways were available to determine what happened to the DNA during transformation attempts, so specific remedies could not be sought. Consequently, the fate of the test DNA could not be determined. Among the reasons that these transformation attempts were not successful were the failure of the cells to take up the DNA, the rapid degradation of the DNA inside the cell (restriction enzymes in bacteria are a good example of a cause of this particular problem), the lack of accurate transcription or translation, and the inability of the host cells to replicate and maintain the foreign DNA as they divided.

2. Among the ways that a gene could be inactivated are the insertion of a stop codon in the sequence, which would prevent the complete translation of the protein; a mutation in the promoter region of the gene, which would prevent proper transcription; and other mutations that could prevent proper splicing or processing. To distinguish a functional gene from a pseudogene, you would have to determine the sequence of the protein and then compare it with the coding sequence for each of the gene sequences. These types of analyses remind us that protein sequencing remains a very necessary tool in molecular biology.

3. Whenever one attempts, using gel electrophoresis, to locate all the fragments produced by a particular enzyme, a chance exists that very small fragments generated by the cleavages may not be detected. Determining the sequences of a second set of fragments whose sequences extend across the junctions of the original set of fragments serves as a check on the overall assignment of sequence.

4. To insert the yeast gene into the λ-phage vector, you must have complementary base pairs on the ends of each duplex in order for them to be joined efficiently by DNA ligase. Because each restriction enzyme cleaves at a unique sequence, the yeast and λ-phage molecules will have complementary ends if both have been cleaved with the same enzyme. Of course, you must also make sure that the sites of cleavage are in appropriate places so that the gene to be cloned is intact, and that the vector or fragment has not been fragmented by multiple cleavages.

5. The 500-base fragment has one site that is cleaved by enzyme A. This cleavage yields two fragments with two possible sets of products:

FIGURE 41.2

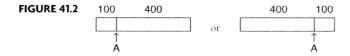

Enzyme B cleaves the 500-base molecule twice, so there are three possible cleavage patterns:

FIGURE 41.3

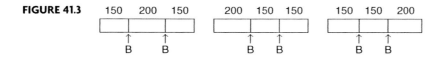

Since we cannot distinguish between ends of the molecule by this type of analysis, let us arbitrarily assume that enzyme A cuts the molecule of 100 nucleotides from the left end. We can then superimpose the possible cleavage patterns for enzyme B:

FIGURE 41.4

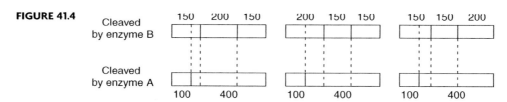

Only one of the patterns for enzyme B, that in which a cut occurs 200 bases from the left end, yields the results obtained when the fragment is incubated with both enzymes. The other patterns would yield at least one 50-base fragment. The correct pattern is therefore:

FIGURE 41.5

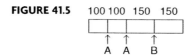

Because we still cannot distinguish between the right- and left-hand ends of the molecule, an alternative cleavage pattern can also be constructed from the analysis outlined above:

FIGURE 41.6

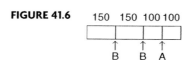

The deletion fragment serves as a marker for the left-hand end of the molecule, and using both enzymes in the double-digest technique allows us to establish which cleavage pattern is correct. For example, if the cleavage pattern shown below (Figure 41.7) on the left is correct, the cleaved deletion molecule will yield four fragments, including one only 25 nucleotides in length. Alternatively, the pattern shown below on the right means that double digestion of the deletion fragment will again yield four fragments, but the smallest will have a length of 75 nucleotides.

FIGURE 41.7

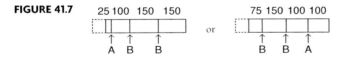

The complexity of cleavage patterns (known as restriction maps) increases greatly when additional cleavages are involved. Often the best way to use the double-digest technique is to isolate the fragments generated by one enzyme and then digest each of them with the other. This allows you to determine the location of different cleavage sites within a particular fragment. In restriction mapping, as in genetic mapping, it is important to remember that the sum of the fragment lengths generated by one enzyme must equal the sum of the fragment lengths generated by the other.

6. In order to obtain optimal expression in *E. coli*, you should have prokaryotic DNA sequences that include the appropriate transcriptional and translational signal elements. For example, in Chapter 4 of the text, promoter sites that determine where transcription begins are mentioned; these include the Pribnow box and the −35 region, both of which would be required to initiate efficient transcription of your cDNA clone by the bacterial RNA polymerase. You may also need the stem-loop and GC-rich terminator sequence at the 3′-end of your cDNA, in order to cause the nascent messenger RNA to terminate at the correct site. In addition, you should see that the Shine-Dalgarno ribosome recognition sequence and the proper start and stop signals for translation are also present, so that the mRNA code is read in the proper frame and that proper termination occurs. These signals ensure that the expressed protein has the proper amino acid sequence and is the correct length. The desired bacterial signals can be built into a vector so that only the cDNA itself need be cloned.

7. It is indeed possible that the contaminant could complicate the analysis of the second sample. If the 10^6 templates in the original sample are amplified one millionfold, then the concentration of templates at the completion of 20 cycles is 10^{12}/100 μL, or 10^{10} templates per μL. A contaminating volume of 0.1 μL will therefore contain 10^9 templates, compared with about 10^6 templates in the second sample. Such contamination could mask the identity of the DNA in the analyte sample. In practice, a number of precautions are taken to avoid introduction of foreign DNA into PCR reaction mixtures. These include use of sterile containers and reaction solutions; disposable gloves; laminar flow hoods; and separate work areas for preparing reaction mixtures, pipetting template samples, and analyzing the products. For the PCR reaction itself, it is important to run reactions that contain no added DNA in order to check for contamination with DNA from sources other than the solution containing the analyte.

8. In forensic PCR analysis, it is common to use cells from the victim as well as sperm from the alleged rapist to generate DNA templates for amplification and analysis. The differential lysis procedure allows the two to be efficiently separated, to avoid cross-contamination of DNA samples. Lysis is necessary so that the DNA templates will be accessible to DNA polymerase and substrates for amplification. During the gathering of evidence from crime scenes, it is necessary to keep samples that could contain large

amounts of DNA, such as bloodstains, separate from those that contain little DNA, like a single shed hair. As noted in Problem 11, the presence of contaminating DNA can confound PCR analyses.

9. (a) There should be little interference if you utilize amplified sequences with some misincorporated bases in Southern blot experiments. The results of the experiments depend on the complementarity of relatively long sequences of DNA, and occasional mismatches should not interfere with the ability of the amplified templates and the probe to anneal with each other. Remember that the primers, which are present in excess during the initial cycles of amplification, continue to initiate the synthesis of new DNA strands. If the incorporation of mismatches is random, the chances are that any particular strand will have few base changes and that it could still form complementary base pairs with the radioactive probe.

(b) In these experiments, the low frequency of base misincorporation could interfere with your analysis, because each of your clones to be used for expression experiments will be derived from a single DNA molecule obtained in the amplification process. Cloning therefore amplifies any error introduced by the polymerase in the chain reaction, and random errors could alter the expressed protein in a non-controlled way. There are two ways to deal with this problem. You can use a thermostable DNA polymerase that has a proofreading activity and improved fidelity; several of these are commercially available. On the other hand, you can also prepare a number of clones and sequence them. Such a procedure will ensure that the clone you want to examine for altered expression has the sequence you wanted to generate during the amplification process. Even if you use the proofreading polymerase, you should sequence the product to see that no unintended changes were introduced.

10. Nick translation can be used with labeled nucleoside triphosphates to generate highly radioactive probes for use in Southern blot analysis as well as for other techniques that require such labeled DNA samples. The usual procedure includes isolating the DNA you wish to use for the probe, treating it with a nuclease that will create a small number of nicks or single-strand breaks per molecule, and then incubating the DNA with DNA polymerase I and α-^{32}P-labeled deoxyribonucleoside triphosphates (the α-phosphate is labeled because it is incorporated along with the deoxynucleoside when the DNA chain is extended by DNA polymerase). The DNA molecules then will contain stretches of radioactive sequences, and they can then be used for autoradiography in Southern or Northern blot experiments.

11. (a) Treatment of an organism with a chemical or radiation-inducing mutagen does not allow you to make changes soley in a particular region of a gene and its encoded protein because the changes occur at random. Much work would be required to find a mutant organism that had the desired alteration in a protein and to characterize that alteration. Treating a purified protein with a chemical agent may modify other amino acid residues in addition to the one or more specific residues of interest. Both the older approaches are relatively nonspecific, compared with the ability of site-specific mutagenesis to target a specific region of a particular gene.

(b) One should have at a minimum the amino acid sequence for the protein and the exact DNA sequence coding for it. More information about the protein of interest would allow for more selective mutagenesis. Examples include the location of residues involved with the active site, with allosteric interactions, or with membrane association or those involved in protein-lipid or protein-nucleic acid interactions.

12. (a) The father and the normal male control have the EcoRI site, so that their amplified DNAs are cut into two fragments. The affected son has lost the site, and his DNA is not cut. The mother, daughter, and a heterozygous control have one copy of the normal gene (giving two fragments) and one copy of the mutant gene (giving one larger fragment). The amplified fetal DNA is cleaved completely by the enzyme, which shows that the male fetus is normal.

   (b) Southern blotting, used to detect single-copy sequences in genomic DNA, requires relatively large amounts of material from which DNA is isolated, and it requires a highly radioactive probe to detect a particular sequence. Autoradiography, which is often used to detect annealing of the probe to the genomic sequence, can take a long time if the signal is weak. Analysis by PCR requires only nanogram amounts of DNA from very small amounts of tissue or blood, with minimal sample preparation. In addition, one can dispense altogether with radioactive probes, instead using a DNA staining reagent such as ethidium bromide to detect amplified sequences.

13. (a) Guided by a DNA template, hydrogen bonding mediates proper insertion of mononucleotides into the growing RNA chain, in the reaction catalyzed by RNA polymerase. Complementary base pairing is the guiding principle in determining the order of ribonucleotide assembly.

   (b) Guided by an RNA template, hydrogen bonding mediates proper insertion of deoxymononucleotides into the growing DNA chain, in the reaction catalyzed by reverse transcriptase. Complementary base pairing guides the order of deoxyribonucleotide assembly. Reverse transcriptase can also use cDNA as a template for the creation of a duplex DNA molecule; again, hydrogen bonding of complementary base pairs establishes the order of deoxynucleotide addition.

   (c) The PCR technique requires that DNA is denatured (breaking hydrogen bonds) and then annealed to a pair of primers, whose sequences are complementary to those flanking the target sequence in DNA. DNA polymerase then carries out chain extension by adding deoxynucleotides to those primers. After denaturation of the newly formed duplexes, the strands are reannealed with the excess primers. The process is carried out as many as 30 times. For each reaction sequence, specificity of the chain reaction for a particular DNA segment is mediated by specific base pairing between primers and templates.

   (d) Radioactively labeled DNA probes are denatured and allowed to anneal to a mixture of DNA molecules. The extent of hydrogen bonding determines the homology between probe and DNA. Southern blotting uses this hybridization technique for DNAs resolved by gel electrophoresis. Location of a specific DNA is visualized by autoradiography, which locates the radioactive band in the gel.

   (e) The two species are denatured and reannealed together. The more duplex DNA formed upon annealing, the greater the degree of relatedness. The extent of duplex DNA formation is determined by measuring the melting temperature of the DNA, which is a reflection of the number of hydrogen bonds between strands.

14. Levels of mRNA are not necessarily correlated with protein production. For instance, translational control might not allow an abundant mRNA to direct the synthesis of the protein it encodes. If one is interested in proteins, they have to be measured directly. Proteomics is the science of examining protein levels on a global level in an organism.

15. (a) First determine how many plasmid molecules are present in the bacterial cell culture: 10^8 cells/ml = 10^{11} cells/L, and 10^{11} cells/L × 100 plasmids = 10^{13} plasmid

molecules in the culture. Then use the molecular weight of a base pair (~660 g/mol bp) in the plasmid, the length of the plasmid in base pairs (4.4×10^3 bp), and Avogadro's number to determine the mass of 10^{13} plasmid molecules.

$$\frac{10^{13}\,\text{plasmids} \times 4.4 \times 10^3\,\text{bp}/\text{plasmid} \times 6.6 \times 10^2\,\text{g}/\text{mol bp}}{6.023 \times 10^{23}\,\text{bp}/\text{mol}} = 4.8 \times 10^{-5}\,\text{g},$$

or 0.048 mg pBR322 DNA

(b) A nanogram of DNA equals 10^{-9} g. Divide this quantity by the molecular weight of a base pair to obtain the number of moles of DNA base pairs, and then multiply by Avogadro's number to determine how many molecules are present in the reaction mixture.

$$10^{-9} \text{ g DNA}/6.6 \times 10^2 \text{ g/mol bp} = 1.51 \times 10^{-12} \text{ mol DNA bp}$$

1.51×10^{-12} mol bp $\times$ 6.023×10^{23} molecules/mol = 9.1×10^{11} bp in the reaction mixture

$$\frac{9.1 \times 10^{11}\,\text{bp}}{4.4 \times 10^3\,\text{bp}/\text{plasmid}} = 2.1 \times 10^8 \text{ plasmids}$$

16. You could use PCR to isolate the DNA from the plasmids in which it had been cloned (or from the genome itself). To obtain maximal amounts of mRNA and optimal *in vitro* translation, you could design oligodeoxyribonucleotide primers (universal promoter primers) containing the signals necessary for efficient transcription and translation. Transcription of the amplified product would yield large amounts of mRNA customized for the chosen translation system. The primers could contain a promoter for bacteriophage T7 RNA polymerase, for which conditions have been developed that allow production of large amounts of transcript. In addition, an optimized upstream, untranslated region could be designed into the primers to produce an mRNA that contained optimal sequences for *in vitro* translation in the system of choice. Factors to consider would be the potential secondary structure of the mRNA (stem-loops inhibit translation), sequences preferred by the ribosomes, and the spacings between the various elements including the location of the start codon itself. This problem was derived from K. C. Kain, D. E. Lanar, and P. A. Orlandi. Universal promoter for gene expression without cloning. *Biotechniques* 10(1991):366–374.

17. You could take advantage of the fact that the tight binding of the repressor molecule to its operator DNA sequence prevents the action of enzymes at the sequence covered by the protein. Since two proteins cannot be in the same place on the DNA at the same time, one tightly bound protein prevents the binding of the other. Repressor binding thus would prevent HhaI endonuclease cleavage or methylase methylation. You could exploit this effect by binding the repressor to the DNA, treating the specific protein-DNA complex with HhaI methylase to methylate all the 30 remaining, uncovered GCGC sites. Then you would remove the repressor and treat the naked DNA with the endonuclease. The site covered by the repressor would be unmethylated and subject to cleavage. The result would be that the DNA would be cleaved uniquely at the one HhaI site that had been protected from methylation by having the repressor bound to it. This problem was based on M. Koob, E. Grimes, and W. Szybalski. Conferring operator specificity on restriction endonucleases. *Science* 241(1988):1084–1086.

18. You could synthesize oligodeoxyribonucleotide primers that were complementary to the sequences at the 3'-ends of the two strands of the known DNA. These could then be used as sequencing primers with subcloned pieces of DNA from a DNA library of the organism. Using the Sanger sequencing technique you could sequence the DNA that was downstream, in other words, 3' to each of the strands of known sequence. You could repeat this procedure with new sequencing primers based on the newly determined sequence, and in that way, "walk" along the chomosome determining more and more sequence that was adjacent to the original DNA.

19. Bacteriophage λ, even those strains constructed especially to carry large amounts of DNA, can accept foreign DNA fragments of only ~45 kb in length. A YAC vector could take fragments ~1000 kb in length and thus ~20X fewer clones would be required to carry the human DNA. Furthermore, because of sampling problems and overlap, the actual number of clones required to have a >99% chance of covering the entire genome is much larger than the number derived by dividing the genome size by the fragment size carried by the vector.

20. You would use a computer and readily available software to compare the sequence of your gene to the known sequences from all genes from all the organisms and genes sequenced and placed into the sequence database. You might find that many organisms have sequences that are more or less similar to your new sequence. If you were lucky, earlier studies with one of the related organisms will have assigned a function to one of these evolutionary gene relatives by showing that it encodes a particular protein with a particular activity. You could then assay for the protein in your organism to see if the activity was present. If so, you could knock out the gene, and see if the activity was absent to further show that your gene encoded that protein. If you are unlucky, you face the arduous task of identifying the function of your gene. Consider how you might do this. How might doing a gene knockout help?

Expanded Solutions to Text Problems

CHAPTER 1

1. The phrase refers to the fact that all organisms are remarkably similar at a biochemical level. This strongly suggests that all organisms on Earth are derived from a common ancestor.

2. DNA is double stranded and its sugar is deoxyribose. DNA contains the base thymine. RNA is usually single stranded and its sugar is ribose. RNA uses uracil in place of thymine.

3. Proteins are linear polymers composed from 20 different amino acids. Glycogen is a branched polymer composed only of glucose.

4. The central dogma describes the fundamental information flow in biological systems. DNA is replicated to form new DNA, which is then transcribed into RNA. The RNA is translated into protein.

5. Replication is the generation of two daughter double helices from a single parent double helix. The process is catalyzed by DNA polymerase. Transcription is the process of copying DNA information into RNA and is catalyzed by RNA polymerase. Translation converts the sequence information of RNA into proteins, and occurs on ribosomes.

6. An enzyme is a catalyst, usually a protein, although some types of RNA also function as catalysts. A catalyst enhances the rate of a chemical reaction without itself being permanently altered by the reaction.

7. Eukaryotic cells contain a nucleus and a complex of membrane-bounded internal structures called organelles. Prokaryotic cells do not have a nucleus and lack the complex internal organization of eukaryotic cells.

8. An organelle can be any of a number of membrane-bounded structures inside eukaryotic cells.

9. Mitochondria, chloroplasts, and nuclei.

10. The nuclear membrane is not continuous. It is a set of closed membranes that comes together at pores.

11. The gene is transcribed into RNA, which is translated into the protein on ribosomes bound to the endoplasmic reticulum. The protein enters the lumen of the endoplasmic reticulum, is sequestered into transport vesicles, and moves to the Golgi complex, where the protein is modified. The protein is packaged into secretory vesicles that fuse with the plasma membrane, resulting in the exocytosis of the protein.

12. a. 9; b. 12; c. 5; d. 10; e. 11; f. 8; g. 4; h. 7; i. 2; j. 6; k. l; l. 3.

CHAPTER 2

1. Brownian motion is the random movement of molecules in a fluid or gas powered by the background thermal energy.

2. Water is polar in that the hydrogen atoms bear a partial positive charge while the oxygen atom has a partial negative charge due to the greater electronegativity of the oxygen atom. However, the total charge on the molecule is zero; that is, the sum of the partial positive charges is equal to the partial negative charge.

3. Many weak bonds allow for highly specific yet transient interactions.

4. Ionic bonds, hydrogen bonds, and van der Waals interactions. Water disrupts ionic bonds and hydrogen bonds. Because van der Waals interactions are most common between hydrophobic groups, water can be said to strengthen these bonds by facilitating their formation via the hydrophobic effect.

5. Lowering the temperature would reduce the motion of the water molecules and allow the formation of more hydrogen bonds. This is indeed the case, as each molecule of water in ice is hydrogen-bonded to approximately 3.7 molecules of water. The opposite occurs as the water is heated, and one would expect fewer hydrogen bonds to form. At 100°C, a molecule of water is hydrogen-bonded to 3.2 water molecules.

6. Electrostatic interactions would be stronger in an organic solvent relative to a polar solvent because there would be no competition from the solvent for the components of the electrostatic interaction.

7. An electronegative atom is one that has a high affinity for electrons. Consequently, when bonded to a hydrogen atom, the electronegative atom assumes a partial negative charge and the hydrogen a partial positive charge. Such polarity allows the formation of hydrogen bonds.

8. The hydrophobic effect is the tendency of nonpolar molecules to interact with one another in the presence of water. The interaction is powered by the increase in entropy of water molecules when the nonpolar molecules are removed from the watery environment.

9. The second law of thermodynamics states that the entropy of a system and its surroundings always increase in a spontaneous process. When hydrophobic molecules are

sequestered away from water, the entropy of the water increases. Such sequestration, called the hydrophobic effect, also leads to the formation of biochemical structures.

10. $[H^+] * [OH^-] = 10^{-14}$ M.

    $[OH^-] = (10^{-14}$ M$) / [H^+]$.

    $[OH^-] = (10^{-14}$ M$) / (10^{-5}$ M$)$.

    $[OH^-] = (10^{-(14 + 5)}$ M$) = 10^{-9}$ M.

11. $[H^+] * [OH^-] = 10^{-14}$ M.

    $[H^+] = (10^{-14}$ M$) / [OH^-]$.

    $[H^+] = (10^{-14}$ M$) / (10^{-2}$ M$)$.

    $[H^+] = (10^{-(14+2)}$ M$) = 10^{-12}$ M.

12. The Henderson–Hasselbalch equation is $pH = pK_a + \log[A^-]/[HA]$. If $[A^-] = [HA]$, then the equation becomes $pH = pK_a + \log 1$. But the $\log 1 = 0$. Thus, $pH = pK_a$ under the conditions stated.

13. Because the pK_a calculation involves the negative logarithm, the lower the pKa, the higher the value of K_a, and the stronger the acid.

14. $pH = pK_a + \log([A^-]/[HA])$.

    Solve for $pK_a = pH - \log([A^-]/[HA])$.

    Substituting the given values, $pK_a = 6.0 - \log(0.025/0.075)$.

    $pK_a = 6.0 - \log(1/3)$

    $pK_a = 6.0 - (-0.48)$.

    $pK_a = 6.48$.

15. $pH = pK_a + \log([A^-]/[HA])$.

    $[HA] = 0.0002$ M.

    $[A^-] = 0.0008$ M.

    $pH = 7.2 + \log(0.0008/0.0002)$.

    $pH = 7.2 + \log(4)$.

    $pH = 7.2 + 0.6$.

    $pH = 7.8$.

16. $pH = pK_a + \log([A^-]/[HA])$.

    Solve for $\log([A^-]/[HA]) = pH - pK_a$.

    $\log([A^-]/[HA]) = 6.0 - 8.0$.

    $\log([A^-]/[HA]) = -2.0$.

    Therefore, using the inverse ratio, $\log([HA]/[A^-]) = +2.0$.

    $([HA]/[A^-]) = 10^2 = 100$.

17. For those cases where the added [HCl] is less than the initial [acetate ion], one uses the HCl to titrate a portion of the acetate ion to give acetic acid (HA). Then the final [HA] is equal to the concentration of HCl that is added. Since the HA is formed from the acetate, the final [acetate ion] is equal to the difference between the initial [acetate ion] and the amount of [HA] that is formed. One enters the molar

concentrations into a table, and then calculates the logarithms and applies the Henderson–Hasselbalch equation, entering a pK_a of 4.76, to calculate the pH:

Initial [acetate]	Added [H+]	Final [acetate]	Final [HA]	Ratio [A−]/[HA]	log (A−)/[HA])	pK_a	pH
0.1	0.0025	0.0975	0.0025	39	1.59	4.76	6.35
0.1	0.005	0.095	0.005	19	1.28	4.76	6.04
0.1	0.01	0.09	0.01	9	0.95	4.76	5.71
0.1	0.05	0.05	0.05	1	0.00	4.76	4.76
0.01	0.0025	0.0075	0.0025	3	0.48	4.76	5.24
0.01	0.005	0.005	0.005	1	0.48	4.76	4.76

When the concentration of added HCl approaches or exceeds the initial [acetate ion], so that (almost) all of the acetate ion *is* depleted, the buffering capacity indeed is exhausted, and a different approach is needed.

For cases of buffer depletion, let x = [HA].

Then $[H^+]$ = [HCl] − x, and

$[A^-]$ = (initial [acetate ion]) − x.

Use the equation: K_a = ($[H^+]$ * $[A^-]$)/ [HA].

Use K_a = $10^{-4.76}$ for the ionization of acetic acid.

When the added [HCl] is 0.01 M and the initial [acetate ion] is 0.01 M,

K_a = (0.01 − x)(0.01 − x)/x = $10^{-4.76}$.

Group terms to express a quadratic equation:

x^2 − 0.02x + 0.0001 = 0. (Note that the 0.02 is rounded.)

Apply the quadratic formula, x = (−b $\sqrt{}$(b^2 − 4ac))/2a,

in which a = 1, b = −0.02 and c = 0.0001.

Solving gives x = 0.0096, so that $[H^+]$ = 0.0004.

Since log(0.0004) is −3.39, **the pH is about 3.4.**

(when 0.01 M HCl is added to 0.01 M acetate).

Finally, when the added [HCl] is very high, one may assume that essentially "all" of the acetate ion is neutralized (although the concentration does **not** go to zero, which would cause some methods of calculation to fail), and that the pH is determined by the "left over" HCl after the neutralization is complete.

Therefore, when the added [HCl] is 0.05 M and the initial [acetate ion] is 0.01 M, the final $[H^+]$ is approximately 0.04 M. Since log(0.04) is −1.39, **the pH is about 1.4** (when 0.05 M HCl is added to 0.01 M acetate).

Comparing all of the results illustrates that the buffer capacity for neutralizing added HCl is significantly higher for 0.1 M acetate ion than for 0.01 M acetate ion.

18. Let x = [A−].

Then [HA] = (0.2 M − x).

pH = pK_a + log([A−]/[HA]).

5.0 = 4.76 + log(x/(0.2 M − x)).

log(x/(0.2 M − x)) = 0.24.

$(x/(0.2\ M - x)) = 10^{0.24.}$

$(x/(0.2\ M - x)) = 1.74.$

Solving, $x = 1.74 * (0.2\ M - x).$

$x = 0.35\ M - 1.74\ x.$

Grouping, $2.74\ x = 0.35\ M.$

$x = (0.35/2.74)\ M.$

But x is $[A^-] = 0.128\ M = $ [acetate ion].

$[HA] = 0.2\ M - 0.128\ M = 0.072\ M = $ [acetic acid].

CHAPTER 3

1. ELVISISLIVINGINLASVEGAS
2. (A) Proline, Pro, P; (B) tyrosine, Tyr, Y; (C) leucine, Leu, L; (D) lysine, Lys, K.
3. (a) C, A; (b) D; (c) B, D; (d) B, D; (e) B.
4. (a) 6; (b) 2; (c) 3; (d) 1; (e) 4; (f) 5.
5. (a) Ala is more soluble in water because it has the smaller hydrocarbon side chain.
   (b) Tyr is more soluble in water because it has the polar hydroxyl group.
   (c) Ser is more soluble in water because it has the polar hydroxyl group.
   (d) His is more soluble in water because it has the smaller aromatic side chain and because the side chain titrates with a pK_a of about 6.0. When the pH is below the pK_a value, a majority of the His side chains carry a positive charge.
6. At pH 7, the glycine amino group charge of +1 is balanced by the charge of −1 on the glycine carboxyl group. The overall net charge is zero. This form of glycine at pH 7 is called the zwitterionic form.
   At pH 12, the glycine amino group charge is zero, and the glycine carboxyl group charge is −1. The net charge on glycine at pH 12 is −1.
7. The pI is calculated by taking the average of the two pK_as. Thus, pI $= (pK_a^{acid} + pK_a^{amino})/2 = (2.72 + 9.60)/2 = 6.16.$
8. At pH 7, the side chains of lysine and arginine will have full positive charges of +1. At pH 7, the side chain of histidine will have a positive charge about 9% of the time (if the pK_a is 6.0). The net charge on the histidine side chain will be about +0.1 at pH 7. (The pK_a value may vary somewhat depending on the histidine environment in a particular protein. 6.0 is a typical value.)
9. Nonessential amino acids can be synthesized from other molecules in the body. Essential amino acids cannot, and thus must be consumed in the diet.
10. Phenylalanine, tyrosine, and tryptophan.
11. Aspartate, glutamate, histidine, cysteine, tyrosine, lysine, and arginine.
12. Tyrosine.
13. The −OH groups of the side chains of Ser, Thr, and Tyr have hydrogen-bonding potential. The carboxyl group of Glu also has hydrogen-bonding potential. The hydrocarbon side chains of Ala, Phe, and Leu and the hydrogen side chain of Gly do not have hydrogen-bonding potential.

14. Use the Henderson–Hasselbalch equation, $pH = pK_a + \log([A^-]/[HA])$.

For the amino group, $pH = pK_a + \log([NH_2]/[NH_3^+])$.

With $pH = 7$ and $pK_a = 8$, $\log([NH_2]/[NH_3^+]) = (7 - 8)$.

$([NH_2]/[NH_3^+]) = 10^{-1}$.

For the carboxyl group, $pH = pK_a + \log([COO^-]/[COOH])$.

With $pH = 7$ and $pK_a = 3$, $\log([COO^-]/[COOH]) = (7 - 3)$.

$([COO^-]/[COOH]) = 10^4$,

so that $([COOH]/[COO^-]) = 10^{-4}$.

Multiply to get the overall ratio:

$([NH^2] * [COOH]) / ([COO^-] * [NH_3^+]) = (10^{-1})(10^{-4}) = \underline{10^{-5}}$.

15. Recall that the pK_a is the pH at which the concentration of the unionized form of a molecule is equal to the ionized form. The carboxylic acid group in Figure 3.2 has a pK_a of a bit greater than 2, while the amino groups shows a pK_a of 9.

CHAPTER 4

1. The energy barrier that must be crossed to go from the polymerized state to the hydrolyzed state is large even though the reaction is thermodynamically favorable.

2. (a) Alanine-glycine-serine; (b) Alanine;

(c and d):

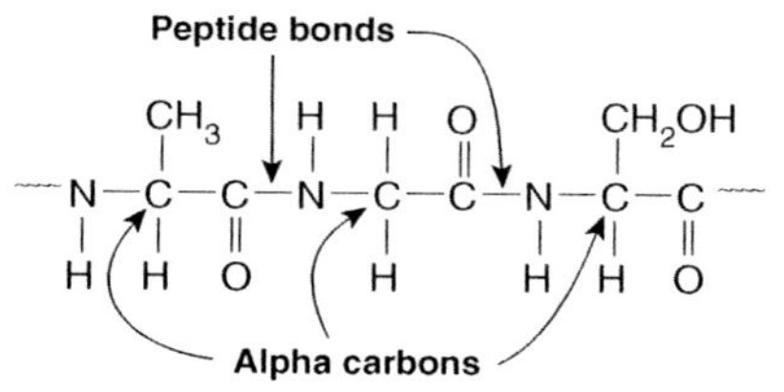

4. 3. TEPIVAPMEYGK

At pH 7, these groups will have +1 charge: amino terminus, K. Total, +2.

At pH 7, these groups will have −1 charge: carboxyl terminus, E, E. Total −3.

Net charge at pH 7 = (+2 − 3) = −1.

At pH 12, these groups will have +1 charge: (none).

At pH 12, these groups will have −1 charge: carboxyl terminus, E, E Y. Total −4.

Net charge at pH 12 = (0 − 4) = −4.

5. 4. This observation demonstrates that the pK_a values are affected by the environment. A given amino acid residue can have a variety of pK_a values, depending on the chemical environment in the vicinity of the particular side chain inside the protein.

6. 5. This observation demonstrates that the pK_a values are affected by the environment. A given amino acid can have a variety of pK_a values, depending on the chemical environment inside the protein.

6. The peptide bond has partial double bond character, which prevents rotation. This lack of rotation constrains the conformation of the peptide backbone, and limits possible structures.

7. a. 8: b. 7; c. 1; d. 3; e. 9; f. 10; g. 2; h. 5; i. 4; j. 6.

8. There are 20 choices for each of the 50 amino acids: 20^{50} or 1.13×10^{65}, a very large number.

9.

$$\text{}^+\text{H}_3\text{N}-\text{CH}-\overset{\overset{\text{O}}{\|}}{\text{C}}-\text{N}-\text{CH}-\overset{\overset{\text{O}}{\|}}{\text{C}}-\text{O}-\text{CH}_3$$

with side chains $CH_2-C(=O)-O^-$ and CH_2 (benzyl, H on N)

Aspartame at pH 7

10. The (nitrogen-α carbon-carbonyl carbon) repeating unit.

11. Side chain is the functional group attached to the α-carbon atom of an amino acid.

12. The amino acid composition refers simply to the amino acids that make up the protein. The order is not specified. Amino acid sequence is the same as the primary structure—the sequence of amino acids from the amino terminal to the carboxyl terminal of the protein. Different proteins may have the same amino acid composition, but amino acid sequence identifies a unique protein.

13. The primary structure determines the tertiary structure. Knowing the primary structure helps to elucidate the function of the protein. Knowledge of the primary structure of mutated proteins allows the understanding of the biochemical basis of some diseases. Primary structure can reveal the evolutionary history of the protein.

14. Protein primary structure is characterized by covalent amide bonds (peptide bonds) that link the successive amino acid residues in sequence.

    Secondary structure describes the spatial arrangement of amino acid residues that are near to each other in the primary sequence. Regular secondary structures are characterized by patterns of hydrogen bonds that link backbone NH and carbonyl groups that may be relatively close in sequence (α-helix) or quite distant from each other in the primary sequence (β-sheet).

    Tertiary structure is characterized by noncovalent interactions between side-chain R groups that are far apart in the primary structure.

    Quaternary structure is characterized by noncovalent interactions between different subunits that are not covalently linked to each other.

15. Primary structure—peptide bond; secondary structure—local hydrogen bonds between components of the polypeptide backbone; tertiary structure-various types of noncovalent bonds between R groups that are far apart in the primary structure; quaternary structure—various noncovalent bonds between R groups on the surface of subunits.

16. a. 5; b. 10; c. 7; d. 1; e. 8; f. 2; g. 3; h. 6; i. 4; j. 9.

17. No, the Pro–X bond would have the characteristics of any other peptide bond. The steric hindrance in X–Pro arises because the R group of Pro is bonded to the amino group. Hence, in X–Pro, the proline R group is near the R group of X, which would not be the case in Pro–X.

18. The methyl group attached to the β-carbon atom of isoleucine sterically interferes with α-helix formation. In leucine, this methyl group is attached to the γ-carbon atom, which is farther from the main chain and hence does not interfere.

19. The first mutation destroys activity because valine has two additional carbons and occupies more space than does alanine, and so the protein must take a different shape, assuming that this residue lies in the closely packed interior. The second mutation restores activity because of a compensatory reduction of volume; glycine is three carbons smaller than isoleucine.

20. Loops invariably are on the surface of proteins, exposed to the environment. Because many proteins exist in aqueous environments, the exposed loops will be hydrophilic to interact with water.

21. (a) Heat will increase the thermal energy of the chain. The weak bonds holding the chain in its correct three-dimensional structure will not be able to withstand the increased wiggling of the backbone, and the tertiary structure will be lost. Often, the denatured chains will interact with each other to form large complexes that precipitate out of solution.

    (b) Detergents will denature the protein essentially by turning it inside out. The hydrophobic residues from the interior of the protein will interact with the detergent, while the hydrophilic residues will interact with one another and not with the environment.

    (c) The ionic interactions and hydrogen bonds of titratable groups will be disrupted when the pH is either raised or lowered by a large amount. The result will be protein denaturation.

22. Glycine has the smallest side chain of any amino acid. Its small size is often critical in allowing the polypeptide chains to make tight turns or to approach one another closely. Therefore, it is often detrimental to replace glycine with a larger amino acid.

23. Glutamate, aspartate, and the terminal carboxylate group of a protein can form salt bridges with the guanidinium group of arginine. In addition, the guanidinium can be a hydrogen-bond donor to the side chains of glutamine, asparagine, serine, threonine, aspartate, glutamate and tyrosine, and to the main-chain carbonyl group. At pH 7, histidine can hydrogen bond with arginine also.

24. Disulfide bonds in hair can be broken by use of a thiol-containing reagent and application of gentle heat. Then after the hair is mechanically curled, an oxidizing agent is added to re-form disulfide bonds to stabilize the curls in the desired shape. The resulting cross-linked curls will be "permanent" for several weeks until there is substantial growth of new hair.

25. Some proteins that span biological membranes are "the exceptions that prove the rule" because they have the reverse distribution of hydrophobic and hydrophilic amino acids. For example, consider *porins*, proteins found in the outer membranes of many bacteria. Membrane proteins are built largely of hydrophobic chains. Thus, porins are covered on the outside largely with hydrophobic residues that interact with the neighboring hydrophobic lipid molecules. In contrast, the center of a porin protein contains many charged and polar amino acids that surround a water-filled channel that extends through the middle of the protein. Thus, because porins function in hydrophobic environments, they are "inside out" relative to proteins that function in aqueous solution.

26. The amino acids that compose a membrane-spanning helix would be hydrophobic in nature. Furthermore, an α helix is especially suitable for crossing a membrane because all of the polar amide hydrogen atoms and carbonyl oxygen atoms of the peptide

backbone take part in intra-chain hydrogen bonds. Thereby these polar atoms are stabilized in the hydrophobic environment of the lipid bilayer.

27. Recall that hemoglobin exists as a tetramer while myoglobin is a monomer. While the entire surface of a myoglobin monomer is exposed to water, the hydrophobic residues on the surface of hemoglobin subunits are probably involved in van der Waals interactions with similar regions on the neighboring subunits. These subunit interactions in hemoglobin will shield some of the hydrophobic residues from the aqueous environment.

28. A possible explanation is that the severity of the symptoms corresponds to the degree of structural disruption of the collagen triple helix. Hence, a substitution of alanine for glycine, for example, might result in mild symptoms, but substitution of a much larger side chain such as tryptophan might prevent or seriously inhibit formation of the collagen triple helix.

29. The added β-mercaptoethanol allowed disulfide bonds transiently to break and re-form, thereby catalyzing the rearrangement of the disulfide pairings until the native structure with four correct disulfide bands was regained. The process was driven by the decrease in free energy as the scrambled conformations were converted into the stable, native conformation of the enzyme. The native disulfide pairings of ribonuclease thus contribute to the stabilization of the thermodynamically preferred structure.

30. The native conformation of insulin is not the thermodynamically most stable form because it contains two separate chains linked by disulfide bonds. The effect of the PDI is to break the covalent bonds that hold the two different insulin a and b subunits together. The released subunits diffuse apart and then can no longer "find" each other to form new disulfide bonds. (The native insulin is formed originally from proinsulin, a single-chain precursor within which the correct disulfide bonds are formed, after which the proinsulin is cleaved to form the shorter insulin, which has 51 residues in two linked subunits.)

31. A segment of the main chain of the protease could hydrogen bond to the main chain of the target protein to induce an extended parallel or antiparallel pair of β strands, in which one stand from the protease would pair with one strand from the target.

32. As the size of the protein increases, the surface-to-volume ratio decreases. Consequently, relatively fewer surface residues are needed, and the ratio of hydrophilic amino acids to hydrophobic amino acids also will decrease.

33. Each strand is 35 kd and hence has about 318 residues (because the mean residue mass is 110 daltons, and 35,000/110 = 318). Because the rise per residue in an α helix is 1.5 Å, the length is (318 * 1.5) = 477 Å. More precisely, for an α-helical coiled coil, the rise per residue is reduced slightly to about 1.46 Å; so the revised length will be about (318 * 1.46) = 464 Å.

34. The reason is that the cysteines pair randomly to form all of the possible combinations of disulfides in urea. Most of these combinations are wrong. There are 105 different ways of pairing eight cysteine residues to form four disulfides; only one of these combinations is enzymatically active. The 104 wrong pairings have been picturesquely termed "scrambled" ribonuclease. The number 105 derives from the formula (7 * 5 * 3 * 1) = 105. (If one arbitrarily picks one Cys residue at random, it can pair with any of the seven other Cys residues. Then once the first such disulfide bond is formed, pick one of the remaining Cys residues, and it can pair with any of five cysteines. Therefore, there are (7 * 5) ways of forming the first two disulfide bonds. Extrapolation of this method to the 3rd and 4th disulfides leads to the formula noted above.)

CHAPTER 5

1. An assay usually identifies the functional activity of the desired protein. A functional assay is important for monitoring the biological activity and for determining whether particular purification steps are effective in isolating the protein from other cellular material. (If a functional assay is not available, another type of assay may be required, such as specific antibody binding.)

2. a. 10; b. 1; c. 6; d. 9; e. 2; f. 8; g. 5; h. 7; i. 3; j. 4.

3. The salt ions compete with charged groups on the protein for interactions with the solvent water molecules. If the salt concentration becomes too high, eventually, there are not enough water molecules to interact with the protein, and the protein precipitates.

4. If there is a lack of salt in a protein solution, the proteins may interact with one another, such that the positive charges on one protein are attracted to the negative charges on another protein, or several other protein molecules. Such an aggregate eventually becomes too large to be solubilized by water alone. If salt is added, it will neutralize the charges on the protein molecules and prevent protein-protein interactions.

5. Charged and polar R groups on the surface of the enzyme, namely the charged groups of Asp, Glu, Lys, Arg and sometimes His; and the polar groups of Ser, Thr, Tyr, Trp, Asn, Gln, or Cys.

6. (a) Trypsin cleaves after arginine (R) and lysine (K), generating AVGWR, VK, and S. Because they differ in size, these products could be separated by molecular exclusion chromatography.

   (b) Chymotrypsin, which cleaves after large aliphatic or aromatic R groups, generates two peptides of equal size (AVGW) and (RVKS). Separation based on size would not be effective. The peptide RVKS has two positive charges (R and K), whereas the other peptide is neutral. Therefore, the two products could be separated by ion-exchange chromatography.

7. The long hydrophobic tail on the SDS molecule (p. 73) disrupts the hydrophobic interactions in the interior of the protein. The protein unfolds, with the hydrophobic R groups now interacting with the SDS rather than with one another.

8. An inhibitor of the enzyme being purified might have been present and subsequently removed by a purification step. This removal would lead to an apparent increase in the total amount of enzyme present.

9. To calculate the specific activity, divide: (total activity units)/(mg protein).

   To obtain the purification level, divide the current level of specific activity (following each step of the purification) by the original <u>specific</u> activity of the "crude" sample, 200 units mg^{-1}.

   To obtain the % yield, divide the current level of total activity by the original <u>total</u> activity of the "crude" sample, 4,000,000 units (and multiply by 100%).

   The calculations will give these results:

Purification procedure	Total protein (mg)	Total activity (units)	Specific activity (units mg^{-1})	Purification level	Yield (%)
Crude extract	20,000	4,000,000	200	1.0	100
$(NH_4)_2SO_4$ precipitation	5,000	3,000,000	600	3.0	75
DEAE-cellulose chromatography	1,500	1,000,000	667	3.3	25
Size-exclusion chromatography	500	750,000	1,500	7.5	19
Affinity chromatography	45	675,000	15,000	75.0	17

10. (a) Because one SDS molecule binds to a protein for every two amino acids in the protein, in principle, all proteins will have the same charge-to-mass ratio. For instance, a protein consisting of 200 amino acids will bind 100 SDS molecules, whereas a protein consisting of 400 amino acids will bind 200 SDS molecules. The average mass of an amino acid is 110, and there is one negative charge conferred by each bound dodecyl sulfate ion. (We ignore the mass of the bound SDS.) Thus, the charge-to-mass ratio (considering the protein mass only) of each protein is about −1 for each two amino acids $(-1/220) = (-0.0045)$.

(b) The statement might be incorrect if the protein contains many charged amino acids, particularly if there is a large imbalance between the positive and negative charges on the protein. The calculation in part (a) considers only the charge on the dodecyl sulfate and not the charges on the protein itself. For many proteins—when there are relatively few charges on the protein, and/or approximately equal numbers of + and − charges—this is not a problem.

(c) The protein may be modified. For instance, some serine, threonine, and tyrosine side chains may have phosphoryl groups attached. Some side chains (such as Asn, Gln, Ser or Thr) may have carbohydrate groups attached.

11. The estrogen receptor has a unique, high-affinity binding site for estradiol. This property can be exploited as a basis for a binding assay to detect the presence of the receptor protein, and for affinity chromatography to purify the receptor.

12. Polyclonal antibodies are a collection of antibodies that recognize the same antigen, yet have different primary sequences and bind to multiple epitopes on the antigen. A monoclonal antibody is a single protein with a unique primary structure that recognizes a single epitope on an antigen. Different monoclonal antibodies, nevertheless, may recognize the same epitope on a particular antigen.

13. If an antibody to a protein of interest exists, the antibody can be attached to an insoluble bead of some sort. A mixture of proteins that includes the protein of interest is mixed with the beads that have the antibody attached. Only the protein of interest will bind to the antibody. The mixture is then centrifuged, and the supernatant is discarded. The protein of interest can then be released from the antibody beads, by interfering with the antigen/antibody binding. Because the binding is often quite tight, a protein denaturant may be needed to unfold the protein (and the antibody) in order to disrupt the binding. (Then a protein refolding procedure would be needed to recover the functionally active protein of interest.)

14. An enzyme-linked immunoabsorbant assay, ELISA, is used as a sensitive method for quantitating the presence of an antigen by using an enzyme linked to an antibody. The presence of the enzyme serves to amplify the detection of possibly small numbers of antigen/antibody binding events. Following the antigen/antibody binding, an assay of the enzyme activity will yield many copies of the enzyme reaction product for each individual binding event that has taken place.

15. The Western blotting is an immunological technique used to detect a specific protein in a cell or in a body fluid. A sample is subjected to SDS-polyacrylamide electrophoresis. The resolved proteins are transferred, or blotted, to a polymer sheet, and then an antibody specific for the protein of interest is incubated with the blotted sample. Other, enzyme-linked antibodies can then be used to visualize the desired antigen-antibody complex.

16. Because the Edman reaction is not quite 100%, cleavage of the N-terminal residue is slightly incomplete, namely does not occur on exactly every cycle for exactly every peptide in the sample being sequenced. For example, if each sequencing cycle is 99% efficient, the yield of correct product on the 50th cycle will be 0.99^{50}, or 60%. If each

sequencing cycle is 98% efficient, the yield of correct product on the 50th cycle is 0.98^{50}, or 36%. Consequently, after many repetitions, a number of different peptides are releasing different amino acids at the same time, so that mixtures are detected and, eventually, the major product for a particular sequencing cycle becomes obscured.

17. Treatment with urea disrupts noncovalent bonds. Thus, the original 60-kd protein must be made of two 30-kd subunits. When these subunits are treated with urea and β-mercaptoethanol, a single 15-kd species results, suggesting that one or more disulfide bonds link two individual 15-kd subunits to form the 30-kd subunit, two of which then associate to form the 60-kd protein.

18. Treatment with urea disrupts noncovalent bonds. Thus, the original 60-kd protein must be made of two 30-kd subunits. When these subunits are treated with urea and β-mercaptoethanol, a single 15-kd species results, suggesting that disulfide bonds link the 30-kd subunits.

19. N terminal: A

    Trypsin digestion: Cleaves at R. Only two peptides are produced. Therefore, one R must be internal and the other must be the C-terminal amino acid. Because A is N terminal, the sequence of one of the peptides is AVR.

    Carboxypeptidase digestion: No digestion confirms that R is the C-terminal amino acid.

    Chymotrypsin digestion: Cleaves only at Y. Combined with the preceding information, chymotrypsin digestion tells us that the sequences of the two peptides are AVRY and SR.

    Thus the complete peptide is AVRYSR.

20. First amino acid: S

    Last amino acid: L

    Cyanogen bromide cleavage: M in 10th position, C-terminal residues are: (2S,L,W)

    N-terminal residues: (G,K,S,Y), tryptic peptide, ends in K

    N-terminal sequence: SYGK

    Chymotryptic peptide order: (S,Y), (G,K,L), (F,I,S), (M,T), (S,W), (S,L)

    Sequence: SYGKLSIFTMSWSL

CHAPTER 6

1. Rate enhancement and substrate specificity.

2. The active site is three-dimensional crevice or cleft; it makes up only a small part of the total volume of the enzyme; active sites have unique microenvironments; substrates bind to the active site with multiple weak interactions; the specificity of the active site depends on the precise three-dimensional structure of the active site.

3. A cofactor.

4. Coenzymes and metals.

5. Vitamins are converted into coenzymes.

6. Enzymes facilitate the formation of the transition state.

7. The intricate three-dimensional structure of proteins allows the construction of active sites that will recognize only specific substrates.

8. Binding energy is the free energy released when two molecules bind together, as when an enzyme and substrate interact.

9. The binding energy is maximized when the enzyme interacts with the transition state, thereby facilitating the formation of the transition state and enhancing the rate of the reaction.

10. There would be no catalytic activity. If the enzyme-substrate complex is more stable than the enzyme-transition state complex, the transition state would not form and catalysis would not occur.

11. a. 4; b. 7; c. 8; d. 3; e. 9; f. 10; g. 5; h. 1; i. 2; j. 6.

12. The energy required to reach the transition state (the activation energy) is returned when the transition state proceeds to product.

13. In each graph, the transition state occurs at the point of maximum free energy along the path of "reaction progress." The activation energy is (transition state free energy) minus (substrate free energy). As diagrammed, the activation energy is lower for reaction A than for reaction B.

    The ΔG for each reaction is (product free energy) minus (substrate free energy). The product is more stable than the substrate in A, so the ΔG change is negative and the reaction is exergonic. In B, the product has more energy than the substrate and the ΔG change is positive, meaning the reaction is endergonic.

14. Proteins can be quite stable because the hydrolysis of proteins has a large activation energy. The ultimate thermodynamic instability of proteins indicates that protein synthesis must require energy to proceed.

15. Lysozyme and other enzymes help protect the fluid that surrounds eyes from bacterial infection.

16. Transition states are very unstable. Consequently, molecules that resemble transition states are themselves likely to be unstable and, hence, difficult to synthesize.

17. With T = 298 K, and R = 8.315×10^{-3} kJ/mol, $\Delta G^{\circ\prime} = -RT(\ln K'_{eq})$, we fill in the table below:

	K'_{eq}	$\ln K'_{eq}$	$G^{\circ\prime}$ (kJ mol)
a	1	0.00	0.0
b	10^{-3}	-11.51	28.53
c	10^4	9.21	-22.82
d	10^2	4.61	-11.41
e	10^{-1}	-2.30	5.71

18. $K'_{eq} = 19$.

    $\Delta G^{\circ\prime} = -RT(\ln K'_{eq}) = -2.94$ RT $= -7.3$ kJ mol^{-1} (-1.74 kcal mol^{-1}).

19. This reaction takes place in glycolysis (p. 104). At equilibrium, the ratio of GAP to DHAP is 0.0475 at 25°C (298 K) and pH 7. Hence, $K'_{eq} = 0.0475$. The standard free-energy change for this reaction is then calculated from equation 5:

    $\Delta G^{\circ\prime} = -\Delta G^{\circ\prime} = -RT \ln K'_{eq}$

    $= -8.315 \times 10^{-3} \times 298 \times \ln (0.0475)$

    $= +7.53$ kJ mol^{-1} ($+1.80$ kcal mol^{-1})

    Under these conditions, the reaction is endergonic. DHAP will not spontaneously convert into GAP.

Substituting these values into equation 1 gives

$$\Delta G = 7.53 \text{ kJ mol}^{-1} + RT \ln \frac{3 \times 10^{-6} \text{ M}}{2 \times 10^{-4} \text{ M}}$$

$$= 7.53 \text{ kJ mol}^{-1} - 10.42 \text{ kJ mol}^{-1}$$

$$= -2.89 \text{ kJ mol}^{-1} \, (-0.69 \text{ kcal mol}^{-1})$$

This negative value for the ΔG indicates that the isomerization of DHAP to GAP is exergonic and can take place spontaneously when these species are present at the above concentrations. Note that ΔG for this reaction is negative, although $\Delta G^{\circ\prime}$ is positive.

20. The mutation slows the reaction by a factor of 100.

The activation-free energy is increased $RT[\ln(100)] = 11.4 \text{ kJ mol}^{-1}$ (2.73 kcal mol^{-1}). Strong binding of the substrate relative to the transition state slows catalysis.

21. (a) Incubating the enzyme at 37°C leads to the denaturation of enzyme structure and a loss of activity. For this reason, most enzymes must be kept cool if they are not actively catalyzing their reactions.

(b) The coenzyme apparently helps to stabilize the enzyme's structure, because enzyme from PLP-deficient cells denatures faster. Cofactors often help to stabilize enzyme structure.

22. (a) $\Delta G^{\circ\prime} = -RT \ln K'_{eq}$

$+7.3 \text{ kJ mol}^{-1} = -(8.315 \times 10^{-3} \text{ K}^{-1} \text{ deg}^{-1} \text{ mol}^{-1})(298 \text{ K})(\ln [\text{G1P}]/[\text{G6P}])$

$-2.94 = \ln [\text{G1P}]/[\text{G6P}]$

$+2.94 = \ln [\text{G6P}]/[\text{G1P}]$

$K'^{-1}_{eq} = 19 \text{ or } K'_{eq} = 5.3 \times 10^{-2}$

Because [G6P]/[G1P] = 19, there is 1 molecule of G1P for every 19 molecules of G6P. Because we started with 0.1 M, the [G1P] is 1/20(0.1 M) = 0.005 M and [G6P] must be 19/20(0.1 M) or 0.095 M. The reaction does not proceed to a significant extent as written.

(b) Supply G6P at a high rate and remove G1P at a high rate by other reactions. In other words, make sure that the [G6P]/[G1P] is kept large.

23. Potential hydrogen-bond donors at pH 7 are the side chains of the following residues: arginine, asparagine, glutamine, histidine, lysine, serine, threonine, tryptophan, and tyrosine.

CHAPTER 7

1. A first-order rate constant relates the rate of a reaction to the concentration of only one reactant and has the unit of s^{-1} (per second). Usually the one reactant is the sole reactant in the reaction. A second-order rate relates the rate of a reaction to the concentrations of two reactants and has the units M^{-1}s^{-1}.

2. A pseudo-first-order reaction is actually a second-order reaction that nevertheless appears to be first order. If the concentration of one reactant is much greater than that of the second reactant, the velocity will appear to depend only on the concentration of the "limiting" reactant that is present in the lower concentration. In other words, the reaction will *appear* to be first order with respect to reactant that is present in the lower concentration.

3. (a) 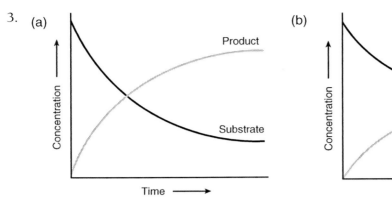 (b)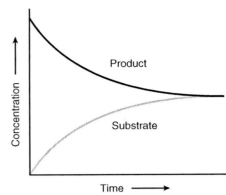

4. K_M is equal to the substrate concentration that yields half of the maximal velocity for the enzyme-catalyzed reaction. Therefore, when the substrate concentration is near the K_M, the enzyme displays significant catalysis yet at the same time is sensitive to changes in the substrate concentration.

5. Sequential reactions are characterized by the formation of a ternary complex consisting of the enzyme and both of the substrates (after the substrates bind in sequence). Double-displacement reactions involve first the formation of a substituted enzyme intermediate involving one of the substrates, followed by a reaction of the intermediate with a second reactant.

6. No, K_M is not equal to the dissociation constant because the numerator also contains k_2, the rate constant for conversion of the enzyme-substrate complex into enzyme and product. If, however, k_2 is much smaller than k_{-1}, $K_M \approx K_D$.

7. The graphs and analysis below indicate that, *yes*, penicillinase appears to obey Michaelis–Menten kinetics.

    Data:

µM	nmol min^{-1}		
[S]	v_0	1/[S]	1/v
1	0.11	1.00	9.09
3	0.25	.033	4.00
5	0.34	0.20	2.94
10	0.45	0.10	2.22
30	0.58	0.03	1.72
50	0.61	0.02	1.64

    Graphs:

    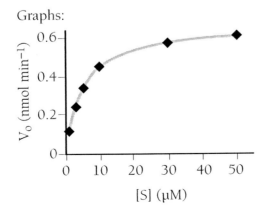

    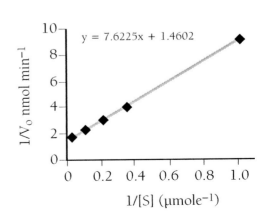

Analysis (from the double-reciprocal plot):

intercept	slope		
1/Vmax	Km/Vmax	Vmax	Km
1.46E+09	7.62E+03	6.85E−10	5.22E−06

(a) From the above analysis, $K_M = 5.22 \times 10^{-6}$ M.

(b) From the above analysis, $V_{max} = 6.85 \times 10^{-10}$ mol min^{-1}.

(c) Turnover = (mol S s^{-1})/(mol E) =
$(6.85 \times 10^{-10}$ mol min$^{-1})/[(60$ s min$^{-1}) \times (10^{-9}$ g/29,600 g mol$^{-1})] = 337$ s^{-1}.

8. (a) One unit of enzyme hydrolyzes $10 \times 2,800$ mol substrate in 15 min, or 900 seconds. (28,000 mol)/(900 s) = 31.1 μmol s^{-1}.

(b) Each subunit has a mass of 20,000 g mol^{-1}. For a sample size of 1 mg, therefore, $(10^{-3}$ g)/(20,000 g mol$^{-1}) = 5.0 \times 10^{-8}$ mol, or 0.05 μmol.

(c) Dividing the answers from parts (a) and (b), (31.1 μmol s^{-1}) / (0.05 μmol) gives a turnover number of 622 s^{-1}. This is a midrange value for enzymes (see Table 6.2).

9. (a) $(1/V_o) = (K_M/V_{max}) \times (1/[S]) + (1/V_{max})$.

Multiply both sides by $(V_o) \times (V_{max})$ to get: $V_{max} = (K_M) \times (V_o/[S]) + V_o$.

Rearrange to: $V_o = V_{max} - (V_o/[S]) K_M$.

(b) From the equation in (a), the slope is $-K_M$, the y intercept is V_{max}, and the x intercept is V_{max} / K_M.

10. Use the Michaelis–Menten equation: $V_o = V_{max}([S])/([S] + K_M)$. Solve for V_{max}:

$V_{max} = V_o([S] + K_M)/[S]$. Substitute the given information:

$V_{max} = (1$ μmol min$^{-1}) \times (1.1 K_M)/(0.1 K_M) = $ **11 μmol min^{-1}**.

11. a. 7; b. 4; c. 5; d. 1; e. 8; f. 2; g. 9; h. 6; i. 10; j. 3.

12.

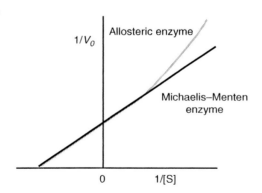

13. Use the relation:

$$V_0 = \frac{V_{max} [S]}{K_M + [S]} \qquad \text{giving:} \qquad \frac{V_0}{V_{max}} = \frac{[S]}{K_M + [S]}$$

When $[S] = K_M$, $(V_0 / V_{max}) = 0.50$.

When $[S] = 10 K_M$, $(V_0 / V_{max}) = 0.91$.

When $[S] = 20 K_M$, $(V_0 / V_{max}) = 0.95$.

The ratio (V_0 / V_{max}) is approaching 1.0, but it never reaches 1.0.

14. The inhibition of an allosteric enzyme by the end-product of the pathway controlled by the enzyme. It prevents the production of too much end-product and the consumption of substrates when product is not required.

15. The enzyme would show simple Michaelis–Menten kinetics because it is essentially always in the R state.

16. Homotropic effectors are the substrates of allosteric enzymes. Heterotropic effectors are the regulators of allosteric enzymes. Homotropic effectors account for the sigmoidal nature of the velocity versus substrate concentration curve, whereas heterotropic effectors alter the midpoint of K_M of the curve. Ultimately, both types of effectors work by altering the T/R ratio.

17. The reconstitution shows that the complex quaternary structure and the resulting catalytic and regulatory properties are ultimately encoded in the primary structures of the individual components.

18. The sequential model more readily accounts for negative cooperativity than does the concerted model. The concerted model would dictate that substrate binding to one active site should (always) enhance the substrate affinity of the other sites; namely positive cooperativity is operating. By contrast, with the sequential model, a local change in conformation of one subunit, due to substrate binding at one active site, could *either* increase or decrease the binding affinities of other active sites in neighboring subunits; namely, negative cooperativity is possible in this case.

19. (a) K_M is a measure of affinity **only** if is rate-limiting. The condition is satisfied here. Therefore the lower K_M means higher affinity. The mutant enzyme has higher affinity for substrate.

    (b) When $[S] = K_M$, as is the case here, $V_o = 1/2\ V_{max}$. V_{max} is 100 μmol/min, so 1/2 V_{max} is 50 μmol/min.

    (c) Enzymes do not alter the equilibrium of the reaction.

20. Enzyme 2. Despite the fact that enzyme 1 has a higher Vmax than enzyme 2, enzyme 2 shows greater activity for the concentration of substrate that typically is found in the environment. At that relatively low concentration, enzyme 2 displays greater activity because enzyme 2 has a lower K_M for the substrate.

21. If the total amount of enzyme (E_T) is increased, V_{max} will increase, because $V_{max} = k_2[E_T]$. By contrast, $K_M = (k_{-1} + k_2)/k_1$ and is independent of enzyme concentration. The middle graph describes this situation.

22. The first step will be the rate-limiting step. Enzymes E_B and E_C are operating at 1/2 V_{max}, whereas the K_M for enzyme E_A is much greater than the substrate concentration. E_A would therefore be operating at approximately 10^{-2} Vmax.

23. (a) The most effective means of measuring the efficiency of an enzyme-substrate complex is to determine the k_{cat}/K_M value. For the three substrates in question, the respective values of k_{cat}/K_M are: 6, 20, and 36. Thus, the substrate EMTAF is cleaved most rapidly, and the substrate EMTAG is cleaved most slowly. The enzyme exhibits a preference for cleaving peptide bonds in which the nitrogen of the second residue is contributed by a large hydrophobic amino acid.

    (b) The value of k_{cat}/K_M for the substrate EMTIF is only 2, therefore not very effective. The poor result when isoleucine precedes the peptide bond suggests that the enzyme prefers to cleave peptide bonds for which a small R group is followed by a large hydrophobic R group.

24. The rates of utilization of substrates A and B are given by

$$V_A = \left(\frac{k_2}{K_M}\right)_A [E][A]$$

and

$$V_B = \left(\frac{k_2}{K_M}\right)_B [E][B]$$

Hence, the ratio of these rates is

$$\frac{V_A}{V_B} = \frac{\left(\dfrac{k_2}{K_M}\right)_A [A]}{\left(\dfrac{k_2}{K_M}\right)_B [B]}$$

Thus, an enzyme discriminates between competing substrates on the basis of their values of k_2/K_M rather than that of K_M alone.

25. The fluorescence spectroscopy reveals the existence of an enzyme-serine complex that has unique spectral properties (high quantum yield for PLP fluorescence). The existence of a second unique complex, enzyme-serine-indole, is also demonstrated by not only the reversal but also the further decrease in the intensity of the fluorescence emission.

26. (a)

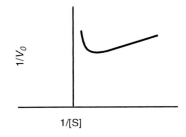

(b) This behavior is substrate inhibition: at high concentrations, the substrate forms unproductive complexes at the active site. The adjoining drawing shows what might happen. Substrate normally binds in a defined orientation, shown in the drawing as red to red and blue to blue. At high concentrations, the substrate may bind at the active site such that the proper orientation is met for each end of the molecule, but two different substrate molecules are binding. For more information, please refer to the answer provided in the main text on page C6 of the Answers Section. For more information, please refer to the answer provided in the main text on page C6 of the Answers Section.

27. The binding of PALA switches ATCase from the T to the R state because PALA acts as a substrate analog. An enzyme molecule containing bound PALA has fewer free catalytic sites than does an unoccupied enzyme molecule. Therefore, high concentrations of PALA will inhibit the enzyme, slowing the reaction rate. However, the PALA-containing enzyme will be in the R state and hence have higher affinity for the substrates, such that low concentrations of PALA will activate the enzyme. The dependence of the degree of activation on the concentration of PALA is a complex function of the allosteric constant L_0 and of the binding affinities of the R and T states for the analog and the substrates. For an account of this experiment, see J. Foote and H. K. Schachman, *J. Mol. Biol.* 186(1985):175.

28. The simple sequential model predicts that the fraction of catalytic chains in the R state, f_R, is equal to the fraction containing bound substrate, Y. The concerted model, in contrast, predicts that f_R increases more rapidly than Y as the substrate concentration is increased. The change in f_R leads to the change in Y on addition of substrate, as predicted by the concerted model.

29. As in problem 27, this experiment also supports a concerted mechanism. The binding of succinate to the functional catalytic sites of the native catalytic trimer changes the visible absorption spectrum of nitrotyrosine residues in the *other*, modified trimer of the hybrid enzyme. (Substrate is prevented from binding to the same trimer that reports the 430 nm absorbance change.) Thus, the binding of substrate analog to the active sites of a native trimer alters the structure of a different trimer (that carries the reporter nitrotyrosine group).

30. According to the concerted model, an allosteric activator shifts the conformational equilibrium of all subunits toward the R state, whereas an allosteric inhibitor shifts it toward the T state. Thus, ATP (an allosteric activator) shifted the equilibrium to the R form, resulting in an absorption change similar to that obtained when substrate is bound. CTP had a different effect. Hence, this allosteric inhibitor shifted the equilibrium to the T form. Thus, the concerted model accounts for the ATP-induced and CTP-induced (heterotropic), as well as for the substrate-induced (homotropic), allosteric interactions of ATCase.

CHAPTER 8

1. Covalent catalysis; general acid-base catalysis; metal ion catalysis; catalysis by approximation and orientation.

2. The three-dimensional structure of an enzyme is stabilized by interactions with the substrate, reaction intermediates, and products. This stabilization minimizes thermal denaturation.

3. (a) This piece of information is necessary for determining the correct dosage of succinylcholine to administer. The length of time for the paralysis to persist can be controlled by balancing the serum cholinesterase activity and the amount of succinylcholine administered.

   (b) The duration of the paralysis depends on the ability of the serum cholinesterase to clear the drug. If there were one-eighth the amount of enzyme activity, paralysis could last eight times as long, which is undesirable for a number of reasons, including stress on the patient.

   (c) K_M is the substrate concentration needed for the enzyme to perform catalysis at a rate that is $1/2\ V_{max}$. Consequently, for a given concentration of substrate, the reaction rate will be lower when K_M is higher. The patient having the mutant enzyme with the higher K_M will therefore clear the drug at a much lower rate, thereby causing the paralysis to last longer for a given dose of succinylcholine.

4. If a particular amino acid side chain is suspected of participating in a catalytic mechanism, covalent modification of the residue by a group specific reagent may alter it sufficiently that the enzyme activity is altered or inhibited.

5. Competitive inhibition: 2, 3, 9; Uncompetitive: 4, 5, 6; Noncompetitive: 1, 7, 8.

6. First, construct a double-reciprocal plot:

μM	μmol min^{-1}	inhibited			
[S]	v_o	1/[S]	$1/v_o$	v_o'	$1/v_o'$
3	10.4	0.33	0.10	4.1	0.24
5	14.5	0.20	0.07	6.4	0.16
10	22.5	0.10	0.04	11.3	0.09
30	33.8	0.03	0.03	22.6	0.04
90	40.5	0.01	0.02	33.8	0.03

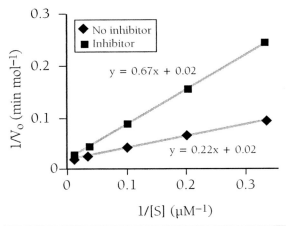

	intercept	slope		
	$1/V_{max}$	K_M/V_{max}	V_{max}	K_M
not inhibited	0.021	0.22	47.6	10.5
inhibited	0.021	0.67	47.6	31.9
	min μmol^{-1}		μmol min^{-1}	μM

(a) From the above analysis, in the absence of inhibitor, V_{max} is about 47.6 μmol min^{-1} and K_M is about 10.5 μM. In the presence of inhibitor, V_{max} is the same and the apparent K_M is about 31.9 μM.

(b) Because K_M increases and V_{max} remains the same, the inhibition is **competitive**.

7. First, construct a double-reciprocal plot:

μM	μmol min^{-1}	inhibited			
[S]	v_o	1/[S]	$1/v$	v_o'	$1/v_o'$
3	10.4	0.33	0.10	2.1	0.48
5	14.5	0.20	0.07	2.9	0.34
10	22.5	0.10	0.04	4.5	0.22
30	33.8	0.03	0.03	6.8	0.15
90	40.5	0.01	0.02	8.1	0.12

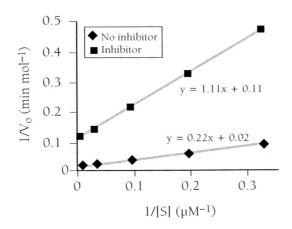

	intercept	slope		
	$1/V_{max}$	K_M/V_{max}	V_{max}	K_M
not inhibited	0.021	0.22	47.6	10.5
inhibited	0.11	1.11	9.1	10.1
	min μmol^{-1}		μmol min^{-1}	μM

(a) From the above analysis, in the absence of inhibitor, the new V_{max} is reduced to about 9.1 μmol minute^{-1}, whereas K_M remains about the same as when no inhibitor was present.

(b) Because V_{max} decreases and K_M remains the same, the inhibition is **noncompetitive**.

8. Group specific inhibitors; affinity analogs; suicide inhibitors; transition state analogs.

9. The lactam ring of penicillin reacts with a serine residue at the active site of glyco-peptide transpeptidase, an enzyme that stabilizes the bacterial cell wall. If the lactam were to be destroyed, penicillin would be ineffective. Indeed, the presence of β-lactamase confers resistance to penicillin.

10. The catalytic triad, composed of Ser 195, His 57, and Asp 102, are amino acid residues at the active site of chymotrypsin. The serine attacks the carbonyl group of the target peptide bond to form the acyl-enzyme intermediate. The histidine residue serves to position the serine side-chain and to polarize its hydroxyl group so that it is poised for deprotonation. In the presence of the substrate, His 57 accepts the proton from the serine-195 hydroxyl group. The aspartate residue helps orient the histidine residue and make it a better proton acceptor through hydrogen bonding and electrostatic effects.

11. The oxyanion hole is a structure at the active site of chymotrypsin that stabilizes the tetrahedral intermediate by binding to the inherently unstable negative charge on the oxygen atom that derives from the susceptible carbonyl group during the proteolysis reaction. The oxyanion hole thereby facilitates the formation of the acyl-enzyme intermediate.

12. Chymotrypsin cleaves peptide bonds in a two-step reaction. For model ester substrates, the first step, formation of the acyl enzyme intermediate, is much faster than the second step, hydrolysis of the intermediate to release product and the free enzyme. In such cases, a fast "burst" of activity is observed during which each enzyme molecule is converted to an acyl enzyme intermediate, followed by a much slower

turnover of enzyme in a steady-state phase of the reaction. With amide substrates, nevertheless, the rates of the two steps are more nearly equal, and the initial "burst" of activity generally is not observed. (See problem 16.)

13. Chymotrypsin recognizes large hydrophobic groups, which are usually buried in the enzyme's core owing to the hydrophobic effect.

14. The mechanism suggests that H^+ is behaving as a competitive inhibitor. Therefore, at sufficiently high substrate concentration, the substrate will overcome the inhibition, and the velocity, v_o, will equal V_{max}, independent of pH (part a). At a low (constant) substrate concentration, the observed v_o will follow a titration curve with a pK of 6.0 (parts b, c).

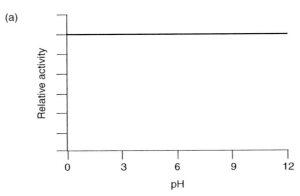

(a)

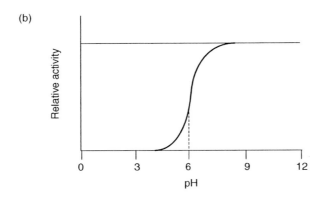

(b)

15. The negative charge on the aspartic acid helps to orient histidine 57 so that it acts as a general base catalyst to assist nucleophilic serine in its reaction with the target carbonyl group to form the tetrahedral intermediate. Asparagine, lacking a charge, is less effective at orienting the imidazole ring of histidine 57, and furthermore has been observed to repel the ring somewhat toward an unfavorable orientation for catalysis. Indeed, chymotrypsin with this mutation has 10,000-fold lower activity than the wild-type enzyme.

16. The formation of the acyl-enzyme intermediate is slower than the hydrolysis of this amide substrate, and so no burst is observed. For ester substrates, the formation of the acyl-enzyme intermediate is faster.

17. (a) Tosyl-L-lysine chloromethyl ketone (TLCK). (b) Determine whether substrates protect trypsin from inactivation by TLCK. Ascertain whether the D isomer of TLCK is an effective inhibitor.

CHAPTER 9

1. a. 6; b. 10; c. 5; d. 7; e. 9; f. 3; g. 4; h. 2; i.1; j. 8

2. (a) Convert μm^3 to cm^3 because $1 \ cm^3$ is 1 mL. $1 \ \mu m = 10^{-4} \ cm$. $1 \ \mu m^3$ is $10^{-12} \ cm^3$. $87 \ \mu m^3 = 87 * 10^{-12} \ cm^3$. $0.34 \ g \ mL^{-1} * 8.7 * 10^{-11} \ mL = \underline{\mathbf{2.96 * 10^{-11} \ g}}$.

   (b) Using molecular weight of about 65,000 g mol^{-1} for hemoglobin, the number of moles of hemoglobin is about $(2.96 * 10^{-11} \ g)/(65,000 \ g \ mol^{-1}) = 4.55 * 10^{-16} \ mol$.

   Multiplying by Avogadro's number gives

   $(4.55 * 10^{-16} \ mol) * (6.02 * 10^{23} \ \text{molecules} \ mol^{-1}) = \underline{\mathbf{2.74 * 10^8 \ molecules}}$.

   (c) 65 Å is $65 * 10^{-8} \ cm$, or $6.5 * 10^{-7} \ cm$.

   The volume of a cube that is $(65 \ Å)^3$ is $(6.5 * 10^{-7} \ cm)^3 = 2.75 * 10^{-19} \ cm^{-3}$.

   The number of these cubes that could fit into a cell volume of $8.7 * 10^{-11} \ cm^3$ (see part a, above) is about $(8.7 * 10^{-11} \ cm^3)/(2.75 * 10^{-19} \ cm^3) = 3.17 * 10^8$, which is only slightly greater than the number of molecules in the answer to part b, above. The hemoglobin concentration in red cells could <u>not</u> be much higher.

3. The total blood volume is about $(70 \ kg)(70 \ mL \ kg^{-1}) = 4900 \ mL$.

   The total hemoglobin is about $(0.16 \ g \ mL^{-1})(4900 \ mL) = 784 \ g$.

   One mole of hemoglobin ($\sim 65,000 \ g \ mol^{-1}$) contains $(4 \ mol)(55.8 \ g \ mol^{-1})$ iron, or about 223 g iron. The mass % iron in hemoglobin is therefore about $100\% * (223 \ g)/(65000 \ g) = 0.34\%$ iron.

   So the total iron in the 70-kg adult is about $(0.0034)(784 \ g) = \underline{\mathbf{2.7 \ g}}$.

4. (a) The molecular weight of myoglobin is about 17,800 g mol^{-1}. Each myoglobin molecule binds one O_2 molecule. Therefore, the number of moles of myoglobin or O_2 per kg is:

   $(8 \ g)/(17,800 \ g \ mol^{-1}) = \underline{\mathbf{4.49 * 10^{-4} \ mol \ of \ O_2}}$ per kg of human muscle. In grams, the answer is $(16 \ g \ mol^{-1})(4.49 * 10^{-4} \ mol) = \underline{\mathbf{1.44 * 10^{-2} \ g \ O_2}}$ per kg human muscle.

   The sperm whale muscle has 10-fold more oxygen, namely $\underline{\mathbf{4.49 * 10^{-3}}}$ mol or $\underline{\mathbf{1.44 * 10^{-1} \ g \ O_2}}$ per kg whale muscle.

   (b) The units of (mol kg^{-1}) are approximately equal to (mol L^{-1}) (or molar). Therefore, the ratio of bound to free oxygen is about $(4.49 * 10^{-3} \ mol$ bound $O_2)/(3.5 * 10^{-5} \ mol$ free $O_2) = \underline{\mathbf{128}}$.

5. The cooperativity allows hemoglobin to become saturated in the lungs, where oxygen pressure is high. When the hemoglobin moves to tissues, the lower oxygen pressure induces it to release oxygen and thus deliver oxygen where it is needed. Thus, the cooperative release favors a more-complete unloading of oxygen in the tissues.

6. Deoxyhemoglobin is in the T-state. The presence of oxygen disrupts the R:T equilibrium in favor of the R-state. The structural changes are significant enough to cause the crystal to come apart.

7. Hemoglobin with oxygen bound to only one of four sites remains primarily in the T-state quaternary structure, an observation consistent with the sequential model. On the other hand, hemoglobin behavior is concerted in that hemoglobin with three sites occupied by oxygen is almost always in the quaternary structure associated with the R state.

8. Fetal hemoglobin does not bind 2,3-BPG as well as maternal hemoglobin. Recall that tight binding of 2, 3-BPG by hemoglobin reduces the oxygen affinity of hemoglobin.

9. HbS molecules bind together to form large fibrous aggregates that extend across the cell, deforming the red cells and giving them their sickle shape. This occurs predominantly in the deoxygenated form of HbS. Blockage of the small blood vessel occurs because of the deformed cells, which creates a local region of low oxygen concentration. Hence, more hemoglobin changes into the deoxy form and so more sickling occurs. Sickled red cells become trapped in the small blood vessels, impairing circulation and leading to the damage of many tissues. Sickled cells, which are more fragile than normal red blood cells, rupture (hemolyze) readily to produce severe anemia.

10. Deoxy Hb A contains a complementary site, and so it can add on to a fiber of deoxy Hb S. The fiber cannot then grow further, because the terminal deoxy Hb A molecule lacks a sticky patch. The text answer is sufficient.

11. The whale swims long distances between breaths. A high concentration of myoglobin in the whale muscle maintains a ready supply of oxygen for the muscle between breathing episodes.

12. The presence of 2,3-BPG shifts the equilibrium toward the T-state. 2,3-BPG only binds to the center cavity of deoxyhemoglobin (T-state). The size of the center cavity decreases upon the change to the R-form, so that the 2, 3-BPG is expelled, facilitating the formation of the R-state.

13. A higher concentration of BPG would shift the oxygen-binding curve to the right. The right-ward shift of the oxygen-binding curve would promote the dissociation of oxygen in the tissues and would thereby increase the percentage of oxygen delivered to the tissues. The text answer is sufficient.

14. The Bohr effect, not to be confused with the boring effect of a monotonous lecture, is the regulation of hemoglobin oxygen binding by hydrogen ions and carbon dioxide. Deoxyhemoglobin is stabilized by ionic bonds that stabilize the T-state. One of these is formed between the C-terminal His $\beta146$ and an Asp ($\beta94$). As the pH increases, this stabilizing salt bridge is broken because His becomes deprotonated and loses its positive charge, facilitating the formation of the R state. At lower pH values, this His is positively charged. The formation of the ionic bonds shifts the equilibrium from the R-state to the T-state, thus releasing oxygen.

15. Oxygen binding appears to cause the copper ions, along with their associated histidine ligands, to move closer to each other, thereby also moving the helices to which the histidines are attached (in similar fashion to the conformational change in hemoglobin).

16. Inositol pentaphosphate in part c. Inositol pentaphosphate has negative charges, similarly to 2,3-BPG.

17. (a) Curve 2, because increasing concentrations of carbon dioxide decrease the oxygen affinity, whereas decreasing concentrations of carbon dioxide increase the oxygen affinity (see the Bohr effect). (The O_2 binding remains somewhat cooperative, so curve 2 is favored over curve 1 for this answer.)

   (b) Curve 4, because BPG decreases the oxygen affinity.

   (c) Curve 2, noting that increasing the pH will <u>decrease</u> the concentration of H^+ and increase the oxygen affinity. The effects of CO_2 and H^+ are similar (see the Bohr effect).

(d) Curve 1, because loss of quaternary structure will remove the cooperative behavior and cause the binding curve to resemble that of myoglobin.

18. The electrostatic interactions between 2,3-BPG and hemoglobin would be weakened by competition with water molecules. The T state would not be stabilized.

19. (a) $K = (k_{off}/k_{on}) = 10^{-6}$ M (given).

$k_{on} = 2 \times 10^7$ M^{-1} s^{-1} (given).

$k_{off} = k_{on} \times K = 20$ s^{-1}.

(b) The mean duration is $(1/k_{off}) = 0.05$ s.

20. (a) The nearby positive charge on the lysine side chain will <u>favor</u> the negatively charged COO$^-$ state for the Glu side chain, so the pKa of the Glu will be lowered.

(b) The presence of the nearby negatively charged carboxyl group will <u>disfavor</u> the negatively charged COO$^-$ state for the Glu side chain, so the pK_a of the Glu will be raised.

(c) The nonpolar environment in the protein interior will <u>disfavor</u> any charged groups, such as the charged COO$^-$ state for the Glu side chain, so the pK_a of the Glu will be raised (favoring the neutral COOH state for the side chain).

21. Carbon monoxide bound to one heme alters the oxygen affinity of the other hemes in the same hemoglobin molecule. The tight binding of CO forces the tetramer into the quaternary structure characteristic of oxyhemoglobin (R state), even when the oxygen pressure is low. Specifically, CO increases the oxygen affinity of hemoglobin and thereby decreases the amount of O_2 released in actively metabolizing tissues. In essence, the bound CO shifts the oxygen saturation curve to the left and inhibits the release of oxygen.

22. $Y = pO_2{}^n / (pO_2{}^n + P_{50}{}^n)$. $P_{50} = 26$ torr. $n = 2.8$

$Y_{lung} =$ when $pO_2 = 75$ torr is 95.1%.

$Y_{tissue} =$ when $pO_2 = 20$ torr is 32.4%

$Y_{lung} - Y_{tissue} = $ <u>**62.7%**</u> oxygen-carrying capacity.

23. The modified hemoglobin should not show cooperativity. Although the imidazole in solution will bind to the heme iron atom (in place of histidine) and will facilitate oxygen binding, the imidazole lacks the crucial connection to the particular α-helix that must move in order to transmit the change in conformation.

24. Release of acid will lower the pH. At lower pH, oxygen dissociation in the tissues is promoted. The influence of low pH on oxygen dissociation is more pronounced than the rather small effect on oxygen binding in the lungs, such that the oxygen-carrying capacity of the red blood cells will increase. However, the enhanced release of oxygen in the tissues will increase the concentration of deoxy-Hb, thereby increasing the likelihood that the cells will sickle.

CHAPTER 10

1. Carbohydrates were originally regarded as hydrates of carbon because the empirical formula of many of them is $(CH_2O)_n$.

2. Three different amino acids can be linked by peptide bonds in only $(3)(2)(1) = 6$ different ordered sequences.

   However, three different monosaccharides can be linked in a plethora of ways. The monosaccharides can be linked in a linear or branched manner, with α or β linkages, with bonds between C-1 and C-3, between C-1 and C-4, between C-1 and C-6, and so forth. If each ordered sequence of monosaccharides can be linked in 11 different ways, then there are $6 \times 2^{11} = 12{,}288$ possible trisaccharides but, as noted, only six different tripeptides.

3. a. 10; b. 6; c. 8; d. 9; e. 2; f. 4; g. 1; h. 5; i. 7; j. 3.

4. (a) aldose-ketose; (b) epimers; (c) aldose-ketose; (d) anomers; (e) aldose-ketose; (f) epimers.

5. Erythrose: tetrose aldose; Ribose: pentose aldose; Glyceraldehyde: triose aldose; Dihydroxyacetone: triose ketose; Erythrulose: tetrose ketose; Ribulose: pentose ketose; Fructose: hexose ketose

6. Lipids are primarily hydrophobic molecules. For instance, triacylglycerols have three fatty acid side chains. This predominately hydrophobic nature accounts for their solubility in organic solvents and their lack of solubility in aqueous solvents.

7. Glucose is reactive because of the presence of an aldehyde group in its open-chain form. The aldehyde group slowly condenses with amino groups to form an amino ketone.

8. No, sucrose is not a reducing sugar. The anomeric carbon atoms of glucose and fructose act as reducing agents but, in sucrose, the anomeric carbon atom of glucose is joined by a covalent bond to the anomeric carbon of fructose, and thus neither of them is available to react.

9. The formation of acetals (such as methylglucoside) is acid-catalyzed. In a mechanism similar to that of the esterification of carboxylic acids (shown in most organic chemistry texts), the anomeric hydroxyl group is replaced. The resulting carbocation is susceptible to attack by the nucleophilic oxygen of methanol, leading to the incorporation of this oxygen into the methylglucoside molecule.

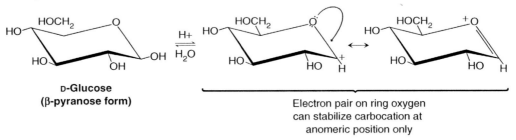

D-Glucose
(β-pyranose form)

Electron pair on ring oxygen
can stabilize carbocation at
anomeric position only

10. (a) β-D-Mannose; (b) β-D-galactose; (c) β-D-fructose; (d) β-D-glucosamine.

11. The trisaccharide itself should be a competitive inhibitor of cell adhesion if the trisaccharide unit of the glycoprotein is critical for the interaction.

12. (a) No, raffinose is not a reducing sugar. There is no hemiacetal linkage in raffinose, but rather two acetal linkages.
    (b) D-galactose, D-glucose, and D-fructose.
    (c) D-galactose and sucrose.

13. (a) No. There is no hemiacetal linkage in raffinose, but rather two acetal linkages.
(b) galactose, glucose, and fructose.
(c) Galactose and sucrose. (After digestion, the released galactose—in water solution—will establish an equilibrium among the α, β, and open-chain forms. See also the answer to problem 14, below.)

14. The sweeter β-D-pyranose form of fructose will convert via an open-chain form to the more stable α-D-furanose form in water solution. This process will be accelerated by heat. (The β-D-furanose and α-D-pyranose forms are also accessible from the open-chain molecule.)

β-D-fructopyranose (sweeter form)   Open-chain (rotameric) forms   α-D-fructofuranose (more stable form)

15. (a) Regardless of its length or the number of branches, a glycogen molecule will have only one reducing end. (All of the glycosidic—acetal—linkages are either 1 → 4 or 1 → 6; therefore, only one C-1 hydroxyl group will not be involved in a glycosidic linkage to either C-4 or C-6.) By contrast, each branch of a glycogen molecule will terminate with a nonreducing end. The number of nonreducing ends, therefore, will be one more than the number of branch points.

(b) For rapid mobilization of glucose monomers, most metabolism should be predicted to take place at the nonreducing ends.

16. Glycogen is a polymer of glucose linked by β-1,4-glycosidic bonds with branches formed approximately every 10 glucose units by β-1,6-glycosidic bonds. Starch consists of two polymers of glucose. Amylose is a straight-chain polymer formed by β-1,4-glycosidic bonds. Amylopectin is similar to glycogen but amylopectin has fewer branches, one branch per 30 or so glucose units.

17. Cellulose is a linear polymer of glucose joined by β-1,4 linkages. Glycogen is a branched polymer with the main chain being formed by α-1,4-glycosidic bonds. The β-1,4 linkages allow the formation of a linear polymer ideal for structural roles. The α-1,4 linkages of glycogen form a helical structure, which allows the storage of many glucose moieties in a small space. Furthermore, different enzymes are required to digest the α-1,4- and β-1,4-glycosidic bonds.

18. Simple glycoproteins are often secreted proteins and thus play a variety of roles. Usually, the protein component constitutes the bulk of the glycoprotein by mass. In contrast, proteoglycans and mucoproteins are predominantly carbohydrates. Proteoglycans have glycosaminoglycans attached, and play structural roles as in cartilage and the extracellular matrix. Mucoproteins often serve as lubricants and have multiple carbohydrates attached through an N-acetylgalactosamine moiety.

19. The attached carbohydrate moiety extends the lifetime of EPO in circulation and thus enables the EPO to function for longer periods of time than would be possible with an equivalent carbohydrate-free protein.

20. A glycoprotein is a protein that is decorated with carbohydrates. A lectin is a protein that specifically recognizes carbohydrates. A particular lectin may in some cases also be a glycoprotein.

21. The heavily charged glycosaminoglycan binds many water molecules. When cartilage is stressed, such as when a human heel hits the ground while a person is walking, the water is released, thus cushioning the impact. The water binds again when the heel is lifted.

22. The universal observation of lectins in all organisms suggests that carbohydrates are found on the cell surfaces of all organisms for the purpose of recognition by other organisms or by the environment.

23. The lectin receptor that binds the mannose 6-phosphate might be defective. The receptor would then not recognize a correctly addressed protein.

24. Each of six sites has two choices: to be glycosylated, or not. The number of possible proteins with different extents of glycosylation is therefore $2^6 = 64$. (Diversity within each carbohydrate chain would further increase this number.)

25. The wide array of possible linkages between carbohydrates in concert with the wide variety of monosaccharides and their many isomeric forms makes complex carbohydrates information-rich molecules.

26. As discussed in Section 3, many enzymes display stereochemical specificity. Clearly, the enzymes of sucrose synthesis are able to distinguish among the isomers of the substrates and link only the correct pair. Furthermore, as the particular substrate anomers are drawn from the solution, Le Chatelier's principle dictates that they will be replenished from the supply of other anomers and open forms that are also present in the solution, based on equilibrium thermodynamics.

27. (a) Aggrecan is heavily decorated with glycosaminoglycans. If glycosaminoglycans are released into the media, aggrecan must be undergoing degradation.
    (b) Another enzyme might cleave glycosaminoglycans from aggrecan without degrading it.
    (c) The control provides a baseline to indicate whether inherent "background" degradation is taking place when no enzymes or factors are added.
    (d) Aggrecan degradation is greatly enhanced.
    (e) Aggrecan degradation is reduced to the background level.
    (f) Not all factors that contribute to cartilage stabilization in vivo are present in the in vitro system that is used for the assay.

28. The reason the specific rotation of α-D-glucopyranose changes after it is dissolved in water is that the ring form is in equilibrium with a small amount of the straight-chain form of glucose. The straight-chain form then converts to either α-D-glucopyranose or β-D-glucopyranose. This process, called *mutarotation*, continues until after 1–2 hours a thermodynamically stable mixture of the α and β anomers is obtained. Its specific rotation is 52.7°. The difference in the specific rotations of the two anomers is 93.3° (112° − 18.7°), and the difference between the equilibrium value and that of the β anomer is 34° (52.7° − 18.7°). Since the optical rotation of the equilibrium mixture is closer to that of the β anomer than it is to that of the α anomer, obviously more than half the equilibrium mixture is in the β configuration. The fraction present in the α configuration is 34° ÷ 93.3° = 0.36. The fraction in the β configuration is 1 − 0.36 = 0.64.

29. Whereas pyranosides have a series of three adjacent hydroxyls, furanosides have only two. Therefore, oxidation of pyranosides uses *two* equivalents of periodate and yields *one* mole of formic acid, whereas oxidation of furanosides uses only *one* equivalent of periodate and yields *no* formic acid.

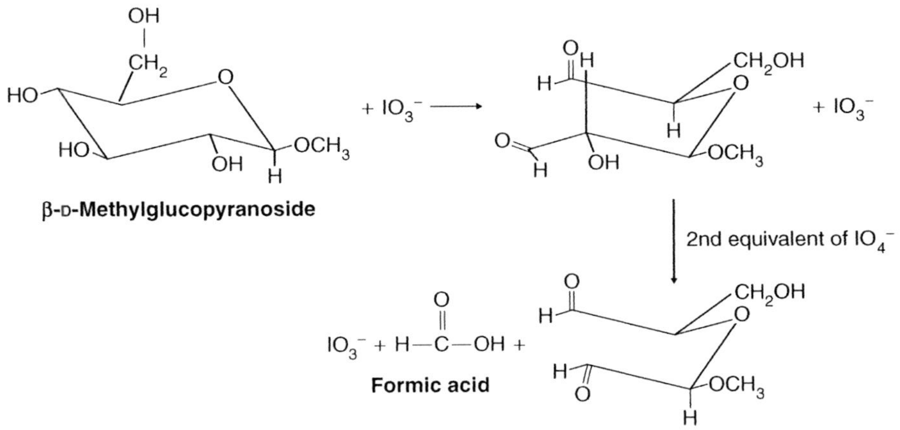

β-D-Methylglucopyranoside

2nd equivalent of IO_4^-

IO_3^- + H—C—OH + **Formic acid**

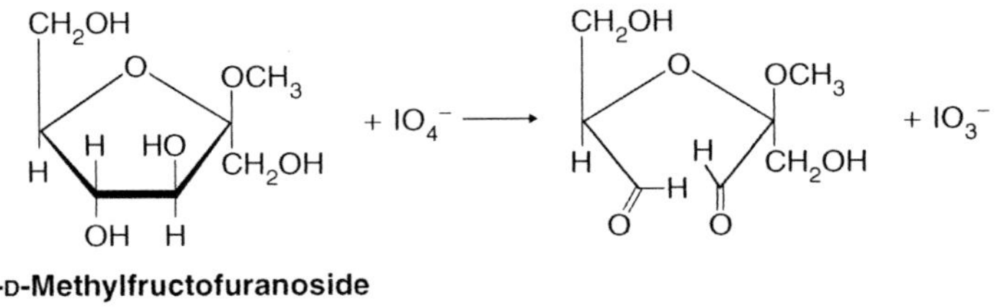

β-D-Methylfructofuranoside

30. The nonreducing carbon-1 oxygens cannot be methylated, whereas the carbon-1 hydroxyls at the reducing ends can be methylated. Conversely, most of the carbon-6 hydroxyls can be methylated, but not at the branch points. Therefore, the ratio of methylated to nonmethylated C-1 hydroxyls in the final digestion mixture will indicate the relative proportion of reducing ends. Likewise, the ratio of nonmethylated to methylated C-6 hydroxyls in the digestion mixture will indicate the relative proportion of branch points.

CHAPTER 11

1. Lipids are water-insoluble molecules that are highly soluble in organic solvents.

2. a. 5; b.10; c. 8; d. 7; e. 1; f. 2; g. 4; h. 3; i. 6; j. 9

3. Refer to the answer provided in the main text on page C9 of the Answers Section.

4. Triacylglycerols from plants may have many cis double bonds or have shorter fatty acid chains than those from animals.

5. Triacylglycerols consist of three fatty acid chains attached to a glycerol backbone. Triacylglycerols are a storage form of fuel. Phosphoglycerides consist of two fatty acid chains attached to a glycerol backbone. The remaining alcohol of the glycerol is bonded to a phosphate, which is in turn bonded to an alcohol. Phosphoglycerides are membrane components.

6. The backbone in phosphoglycerides is glycerol, whereas that in sphingolipids is sphingosine. In sphingolipids, one of the fatty acids is linked to the sphingosine by an amide bond.

7. The examples of head groups include serine, ethanolamine, choline, glycerol, and inositol.

8. Refer to the answer provided in the main text on page C10 of the Answers Section.

9. Lipids are primarily hydrophobic molecules. For instance, triacylglycerols have three fatty acid side chains. This predominately hydrophobic nature accounts for their solubility in organic solvents and their lack of solubility in aqueous solvents.

10. The hydrophobic chains would shun the water, interacting with similar chains in other molecules. Meanwhile, the hydrophilic head groups would readily interact with the water, resulting in the formation of a bilayer membrane or a small membrane vesicle called a liposome. The major driving force for bilayer or vesicle formation comes from the hydrophobic effect, namely the tendency of the lipid hydrocarbon chains to sequester themselves away from water.

11. Steroids are cyclical rather than linear. The main steroid framework consists of a fused tetracyclic ring system in which three cyclohexane rings and a cyclopentane ring are joined together.

12. The glycerol and phosphocholine groups of PAF are similar to those of phospholipids. However, there are notable differences: (a) The C_{16} fatty acid is attached to carbon 1 of glycerol by an ether linkage instead of an ester linkage. (b) The C-2 carbon atom of glycerol in PAF furthermore has only an acetyl group attached by an ester linkage, instead of a long fatty acid.

13. The sodium stearate will form a micelle, with the hydrophilic head groups exposed to water and the fatty acid chains in the interior. When the sodium stearate is worked into the clothes by agitation or onto the skin by rubbing in the presence of water, the grease, which is hydrophobic, will localize in the hydrophobic interior of the micelle and be washed down the drain with rinsing. For more information, refer to the answer provided in the main text on page C10 of the Answers Section.

14. Instead of forming a soluble micelle that will be washed down the drain, the magnesium or calcium salts will precipitate, forming a scum-like bathtub ring. You should clean the bathtub immediately because once the scum dries it is more difficult to remove.

15. Lipids are more reduced than glycogen and they are stored in anhydrous form.

16. Hibernators selectively feed on plants that have a high proportion of polyunsaturated fatty acids, which will incorporate into the body fat and confer a lower melting temperature.

17. Molecules (a), (b), and (c) are saturated fatty acids and will have the highest melting points, which will decrease as the saturated chain becomes shorter. Therefore, the longest saturated chain (a) will melt at the highest listed temperature of 76 °C. The intermediate saturated chain (b) will melt at the next lower temperature of 63 °C. The shortest of the saturated chains (c) will melt at the next lower temperature of 45 °C. Next, the monounsaturated fatty acids of different lengths will have the next two lower melting points from the list, 13 °C for the longer (d) and 0 °C for the shorter (e) monounsaturated fatty acid. Next will come the fatty acid with two double bonds (f) at –5 °C, and finally the fatty acid with four double bonds (g) will display lowest melting temperature in the list, –49 °C.

18. The single cis double bond causes the dramatically lower melting point for oleic acid, compared to the fully saturated stearic acid. The presence of the cis double bond introduces a kink in the fatty acid chain that prevents tight packing and reduces the number of atoms in van der Waals contact. The kink feature lowers the melting point compared with that of a saturated fatty acid. Trans fatty acids do not have the kink, and so their melting temperatures will be higher, more similar to those of saturated fatty acids.

19. Palmitic acid is two carbons shorter than stearic acid. Thus, when the chains pack together, there are somewhat fewer atoms in van der Waals contact and the melting point of the shorter chain fatty acid is thereby marginally lower. The effect of chain length is nevertheless not as dramatic as the influence of just one cis double bond (see problem 18).

CHAPTER 12

1. 1) Bilayer membranes are sheet-like structures, two molecules thick. 2) Membranes are composed of lipids and proteins, both of which may be decorated by carbohydrates. 3) Membrane lipids are amphipathic molecules, composed of hydrophilic and hydrophobic components that spontaneously form closed bimolecular sheets in aqueous solution. 4) Proteins, unique to each membrane, mediate transfer of molecules and information across the membrane. 5) Membranes are noncovalent assemblies. 6) The monolayer leaflets of a bilayer membrane are different. That is, membranes are asymmetric. 7) Membranes are fluid, rather than rigid structures. 8) Cell membranes are electrically polarized, with the inner monolayer surface, facing the cytoplasm, negative with respect to the surface of the outer leaflet.

2. First, the molecule must be lipophilic and second, the concentration of the molecule must be greater on one side of the membrane than the other.

3. a. 3 ; b. 5; c. 6 ; d. 1; e. 7 ; f. 10; g. 2; h. 4; i. 8 ; j. 9.

4. Among those on the list, chloride (c) will display the lowest permeable through lipid bilayers because Cl^- is charged and has no hydrophobic component.

   Glucose (a) is next least permeable because its numerous polar, hydrogen-bonding OH groups make it quite incompatible with the interior of the bilayer.

   Tryptophan (e) overall is hydrophobic and has no net charge, but the individual NH_3^+ and COO^- charges of the zwitterion will lower its membrane permeability.

   Glycerol (b) is quite membrane permeable because it is small and uncharged. Its three OH groups make it somewhat polar and therefore not the most permeable molecule in the list.

   Indole (d) will be most permeable among this set because it is significantly hydrophobic and has only one hydrogen-bonding NH group.

5. In simple diffusion, the molecule in question can diffuse down its concentration gradient through the membrane. In facilitated diffusion, the molecule is not lipophilic and cannot directly diffuse through the membrane. A channel or carrier is required to facilitate movement down the gradient.

6. In passive transport (facilitated diffusion), a substance moves down its concentration gradient through a channel or transporter. In active transport, a concentration gradient of the transported substance is generated at the expense of another source of energy, such as the hydrolysis of ATP. The energy source is thereby used to drive the transport and further accumulation of the substance against its concentration gradient.

7. Most proteins are not static structures, but require conformational changes to perform their biochemical tasks. If the membrane were to become too rigid, the required structural changes could not occur. On the other hand, if the membrane were too fluid, the folded structure of the protein might be unstable because some of the interactions with the hydrophobic core of the membrane that the protein needs to maintain its structure would be disrupted.

8. The heart contraction (heart beat) is initiated by the release of calcium from calcium stores. The contraction is terminated by removing calcium from the cytoplasm. This is accomplished, in part, by a sodium-calcium antiporter, which moves calcium out of the cell, against its concentration gradient, by allowing sodium to flow into the cell down its concentration gradient. The sodium gradient is established by the $Na^+ - K^+$ ATPase. Therefore, the necessary sodium gradient constitutes the link between the activity of $Na^+ - K^+$ ATPase and the strength of a heartbeat. The primary transport component sodium drives the active transport of the secondary component, calcium.

   Cardiotonic steroids function by inhibiting the $Na^+ - K^+$ ATPase, which in turn lowers the sodium gradient and inhibits the sodium-calcium antiporter. As a result, calcium, the signal for contraction, remains in the heart cell longer and the heartbeat is stronger.

9. Ouabain, like digitalis, inhibits the $Na^+ - K^+$ ATPase. The $Na^+ - K^+$ ATPase is crucial to maintaining the sodium gradient that renders neurons and muscle cells electrically excitable. Inhibition of the enzyme would shut down a host of biochemical process required for life, such as cardiac and respiratory function.

10. Inhibition of the symporter would eventually lead to the inhibition of the ATPase. Because the sodium gradient is not being dissipated by the symporter, the sodium concentration outside the cell would become so great that the hydrolysis of ATP by the ATPase would no longer provide sufficient energy to pump against such a large gradient.

11. Selectivity and the rapid transport of ions.

12. Ligand-gated channels open in response to the binding of a molecule by the channel, whereas voltage-gated channels open in response to changes in the membrane potential.

13. False. Although the cotransporter does not directly depend on ATP, the formation of the Na^+ gradient that powers glucose uptake depends on ATP hydrolysis.

14. The two forms are (1) ATP hydrolysis and (2) the movement of one molecule down its concentration gradient coupled with the movement of another molecule up its concentration gradient.

15. Databases could be searched for proteins with stretches of 20 hydrophobic amino acids.

16. The hydrophobic effect. If there is a hole, the hydrophobic tails of the phospholipids will come together, freeing any associated water.

17. Peripheral proteins can be solubilized by relatively mild means, such as extraction by a solution of high ionic strength. Integral membrane proteins can be solubilized only by using a detergent or an organic solvent that disrupts the membrane.

18. Generating the membrane asymmetry involves complex features of pathways for membrane biosynthesis. But maintaining the asymmetry is easy because there is a large energetic barrier for moving charged or polar hydrophilic groups through the membrane interior. For both sides of an asymmetric membrane to become identical, the hydrophilic parts of the lipids, proteins, and carbohydrates would need to pass through the hydrophobic interior of the membrane. Such movement is energetically unfavorable.

19. Establish a glucose gradient across vesicle membranes that contain properly oriented Na^+-glucose cotransporter protein molecules. Initially, the Na^+ concentration should be the same on both sides of the vesicle membranes. As the glucose flows "in reverse" through the cotransporter, down its concentration gradient, a sodium concentration gradient will become established, even as the glucose gradient is being dissipated.

20. The direction of passive transport of ions depends on the ion concentration gradient, not the orientation of the specific ion channel in the membrane. Indeed, an ion channel must transport ions in either direction at the same rate, passively, by means of facilitated diffusion. The net flow of Na^+ or K^+ ions is determined only by the relative concentrations of the ions in the solutions on either side of the membrane.

21. In an alpha-helical segment of a protein, all of the backbone amide hydrogen atoms and carbonyl oxygen atoms are stabilized in the hydrophobic environment by intrachain hydrogen bonds. If the R groups of the side chains are hydrophobic, they will interact with the hydrophobic interior of the membrane.

22. The catalytic prowess of acetylcholinesterase ensures that the duration of the nerve stimulus will be short, and the corresponding signal transmission through the nervous system will be fast.

23. It is reasonable that ibuprofen might be a competitive inhibitor of the synthase.

24. (a) The graph shows that, as temperature increases, the phospholipid bilayer becomes more fluid, with a sharp transition near Tm, the midpoint temperature of the transition from the predominantly less fluid state to the predominantly more fluid state. Cholesterol broadens the transition from the less fluid to the more fluid state. In essence, cholesterol makes membrane fluidity less sensitive to temperature changes.

    (b) The effect is important because the presence of cholesterol tends to stabilize membrane fluidity by preventing sharp transitions. Because protein function depends on the proper fluidity of the membrane, the influence of cholesterol is critical. Cholesterol maintains the proper environment for membrane-protein function.

25. Glucose displays a transport curve that suggests the participation of a carrier, because the initial rate is high but then levels off at higher concentrations, consistent with saturation of the carrier, which is reminiscent of Michaelis-Menten kinetics for an enzyme. Indole shows no such saturation phenomenon, which implies that the molecule simply diffuses across the membrane spontaneously. Ouabain is a specific inhibitor of the $Na^+ - K^+$ pump. If ouabain were to inhibit glucose transport, then a Na^+-glucose cotransporter would be assisting in the transport of glucose.

26. The membrane lipid composition may adjust to help the organism adapt to the environmental temperature. During the day, the membrane lipids of the desert fish are likely to be long saturated hydrocarbon chains which can maintain stable bilayers at high temperature. With the onset of the cooler night temperature, the chains may be shorter or contain cis double bonds, or both.

27. Cells may be exposed to many environmental chemicals, called xenobiotics, some of which are likely to be toxic. The multi-drug resistance protein could help cells remove such chemicals in order to survive longer.

28. Essentially an inverted micelle would form in the organic solvent. The hydrophilic groups would come together on the interior of the structure, away from the solvent, while the hydrocarbon chains on the outside of the lipid aggregate would interact with the solvent.

29. (a) Only ASIC1a is inhibited by the toxin.

    (b) Yes, when the toxin is removed, the activity of the acid-sensing channel is restored over time.

    (c) In the graph in part B, the peak current level is 50% when the toxin concentration is about <u>0.9 nM</u>.

30. This mutation results in slow channel syndrome, a defect in channel closing that causes the channel to remain open for prolonged periods. Either the mutant channel is intrinsically slower to close or, alternatively, the mutant channel may have a higher affinity for acetylcholine that in turn causes the slow closing, compared to the control channel.

31. The mutation may increase the rate of dissociation of acetylcholine from the receptor, thereby reducing the average time period for acetylcholine to be bound to the receptor (reducing the mean channel open time). The recordings would show only brief channel openings.

32. The blockage of ion channels by toxin molecules inhibits action potentials, leading to a dangerous loss of nervous system function. These toxin molecules are useful for isolating, inhibiting, and probing the mechanism of action of particular ion channels.

33. For either a sodium ion or a potassium ion to pass through the channel, the ion must shed the water of solvation. This is an endergonic process. In the case of potassium, the energy to compensate for the loss of water is provided by interaction between the ion and the selectivity filter of the channel. Because sodium is smaller than potassium, the water of hydration is held more tightly, such that the energetic compensation between the ion and the selectivity filter is too small to compensate the sodium ions for the loss of the water of solvation. Thus, sodium cannot pass through the potassium channel.

CHAPTER 13

1. a. 7; b. 13; c. 6; d. 1; e. 10; f. 2; g. 14; h. 3; i. 12; j. 8; k. 4; l. 9; m. 11; n. 5.

2. G-protein coupled (seven transmembrane-helix) receptors; receptors that dimerize upon ligand binding and recruit tyrosine kinases; receptors that dimerize on ligand binding that are tyrosine kinases (receptor tyrosine kinases (RTK)).

3. The initial signal-the binding of the hormone by a receptor-is amplified by enzymes that may generate second messengers, and by channels. When there is a series of sequential steps, amplification is possible at each stage.

4. The receptor must have a site on the extracellular side of the membrane to which the signal molecule can bind, and must have an intracellular domain. Binding of the signal to the receptor must induce structural changes on the intracellular domain, so the signal can be transmitted.

5. The GTPase activity terminates the signal. Without such activity, after a pathway has been activated, it remains activated and is unresponsive to changes in the initial signal.

6. The presence of the appropriate receptor governs the specificity of hormone action.

7. a. 7; b. 3; c. 1; d. 10; e. 3; f. 9; g. 4; h. 6; i. 5; j. 8.

8. The insulin receptor and the EGF receptor employ a common mechanism of signal transmission across the plasma membrane.

9. Growth-factor receptors can be activated by dimerization. If an antibody causes a receptor to dimerize, the signal-transduction pathway in a cell will be activated.

10. Heterotrimeric G proteins are composed of αβγ subunits. The α subunit contains the GTP binding site. Upon activation by the signal-receptor event, the GDP is exchanged with a GTP, and the βγ subunits dissociate from the α bound with GTP, which then activates adenylate cyclase. Small G proteins, such as ras, are single subunit proteins.

They are activated by proteins such as Sos in the EGF signal pathway. The activation causes the exchange of GDP for GTP to activate ras, which in turn, actives specific kinases.

11. The mutated α subunit would always be in the active GTP form. Hence, the mutated subunit would stimulate its signaling pathway all the time.

12. Calcium ions diffuse slowly because they bind to many protein surfaces within a cell. The binding to proteins impedes the free motion of Ca^{+2}. Cyclic AMP does not bind as frequently; as a free molecule the cyclic AMP diffuses more rapidly.

13. Gαs stimulates adenylate cyclase, leading to the generation of cAMP. The cAMP in turn is a signal (second messenger) that leads to glucose mobilization. If cAMP phosphodiesterase were inhibited, then cAMP levels would remain high even after the termination of the epinephrine signal, and glucose mobilization would continue for a longer period of time.

14. The extensive network of pathways initiated by insulin includes a large number of proteins. Furthermore, many additional proteins take part in the termination of insulin signaling. A defect in any of the proteins in the insulin signaling pathways, or in the subsequent termination of the insulin response, could potentially cause problems. Therefore, it is not surprising that many different gene defects can cause type 2 diabetes.

15. As stated, the binding of growth hormone causes its monomeric receptor to dimerize. The dimeric receptor could then bind to a separate tyrosine kinase and activate the kinase. The signaling pathway could then continue in similar fashion to the pathways that are activated by the insulin receptor or other mammalian EGF receptors.

16. Proto-oncogenes usually are genes that encode proteins that regulate cell growth and are themselves subject to normal expression and regulation. Oncogenes are proto-oncogenes that have become either mutated or overexpressed to the extent that the encoded protein provides constitutive or too much enhancement of growth. Tumor-suppressor genes encode proteins that inhibit cell growth or induce death of tumor cells.

17. Proto-oncogenes often initiate or advance pathways that lead to cell growth and cell division in response to some sort of signal. If only one copy of such a gene is mutated, the cell could be stimulated to grow continuously, even though the other gene is functioning normally. On the other hand, tumor-suppressor genes inhibit the growth signals in some fashion. Thus, even if one gene is non-functional, the remaining normal gene will inhibit unrestricted growth and usually is sufficient.

18. Other potential drug targets within the EGF signaling cascade could include, for example, the kinase active sites of the EGF receptor, Raf, MEK, or ERK; or downstream signaling elements.

19. Like the receptors discussed in this chapter, a ligand-gated channel binds a signal molecule, and the binding in turn serves to open the channel and thereby propagate a signal. For example, the IP_3-activated calcium channel is closed until it binds IP_3.

20. Recall that hydrophobic residues are rarely exposed to the aqueous environment of the cells. The exposure of such residues allows calmodulin to bind to other proteins. The new protein-protein interactions will propagate the signal.

21. A reasonable conclusion is that the G protein is a component of the signal transduction pathway. The terminal sulfate must not be an effective substrate for the GTPase activity of the G protein. With the terminal sulfate moiety of the GTP analog not being cleaved, the response to the hormone will persist.

22. The hormone itself is not symmetric. Therefore, the two identical receptors must recognize different aspects of the same signal molecule.

23. Apparently, the negatively charged glutamate residues can mimic the negatively charged phosphoserine or phosphothreonine residues and stabilize the active conformation of the enzyme. The negative charge must be the important feature.

24. Calcium ion levels are kept low by energy-requiring active transport systems that extrude Ca^{2+} from the cell. The cell takes advantage of the difference in intracellular and extracellular Ca^{2+} concentrations by means of gated Ca^{2+} channels that respond to signaling events and allow a small influx of Ca^{2+}. Small changes in the intracellular concentration of Ca^{2+} can be readily sensed.

25. The truncated receptor will dimerize with the full-length monomers on EGF-binding, but cross-phosphorylation cannot take place because the truncated receptor possesses neither the substrate for the neighboring kinase domain nor its own kinase domain to phosphorylate the C-terminal tail of the other monomer. Hence, these mutant receptors will block normal EGF signaling.

26. The level of amplification is multiplied at each stage. Therefore: $(100) \times (1000) = 100,000$; or 10^5 molecules of cAMP per second.

27. (a) From the graphs, the concentrations that yield 50% of maximal binding to the receptor are $\approx 10^{-7}$ M for hormone X; $\approx 5 \times 10^{-6}$ M for hormone Y; and $\approx 10^{-3}$ M for hormone Z.
   (b) Because much less X is required to fill half of the sites, X displays the highest affinity.
   (c) The binding affinity almost perfectly matches the ability to stimulate adenylate cyclase, suggesting that the hormone–receptor complex leads to the stimulation of adenylate cyclase.
   (d) Try performing the experiment in the presence of antibodies to $G_{\alpha s}$.

28. (a) The total binding does not distinguish binding to a specific receptor from binding to other different receptors, or from nonspecific binding to the membrane as a whole.
   (b) The rationale is that the true receptor will have a high affinity for the ligand. Thus, in the presence of a very large excess of nonradioactive ligand, the receptor will bind to nonradioactive ligand, essentially exclusively. Therefore, any residual binding of the radioactive ligand must be nonspecific.
   (c) The plateau suggests that the number of receptor-binding sites in the cell membrane is limited, such that the binding sites become saturated with the ligand.

29. The number of receptors per cell can be calculated as:

$$\frac{10^4 \text{ cpm}}{\text{mg of membrane protein}} \times \frac{\text{mg of membrane protein}}{10^{10} \text{ cells}} \times \frac{\text{mmol}}{10^{12} \text{ cpm}} \times \frac{6.023 \times 10^{20} \text{ molecules}}{\text{mmol}} = 600$$

CHAPTER 14

1. a. 6; b. 4; c. 1; d. 9; e. 2; f. 10; g. 5; h. 3; i. 12; j. 11; k. 7; l. 8.

2. In stage 1, large molecules such as proteins and complex carbohydrates, are broken down into smaller units. Stage 2 consists of converting the numerous small molecules

resulting from stage 1 into a few molecules that are central to oxidative metabolism, most importantly, acetyl CoA. In Stage 3, ATP is produced when acetyl CoA is oxidized to CO_2 and H_2O.

3. Our most important foods—lipids, complex carbohydrates, and proteins—are large macromolecules that cannot be taken up by cells of the intestine. They must be converted into small molecules—such as amino acids, monosaccharides, and fatty acids—for which we have transport systems that enable them to enter into the cells of the intestine.

4. Chewing well efficiently homogenizes the food, rendering it more accessible to the digestive enzymes.

5. Denaturation unfolds the protein's three-dimensional structure. The denatured, extended protein is more open, more accessible, and is a much more efficient substrate for digestion by the proteases.

6. For digestion of both starch and glycogen, alpha-amylase hydrolyzes the α-(1, 4) bonds, generating limit dextrin, maltotriose, maltose, and glucose. Maltase then digests the maltose, while α-glucosidase digests maltotriose along with other oligosaccharides that might have been generated by the α-amylase. Dextrinase digests the limit dextrin. The simple sugars resulting from these enzyme activities are absorbed by the intestine.

7. If a small amount of trypsinogen were inappropriately activated in the pancreas or the pancreatic ducts, trypsin could activate other zymogens and lead to the destructive digestion of the pancreas itself. Therefore, pancreatic trypsin inhibitor serves a highly useful role.

8. Macaroni is starch. Hydrating the starch enables α-amylase to bind more effectively to the starch molecules and degrade them.

9. Unlike proteins and carbohydrates, neither lipids nor fatty acids (the products of lipid digestion) are water-soluble. The lipids are made accessible for digestion by means of their conversion into mixtures of lipid droplets and water (emulsions), a process that is enhanced by the bile salts. The emulsions are then accessible to lipases. The fatty acids generated by the lipases are carried in micelles to the intestinal membrane.

10. The formation of emulsions allows aqueous lipase to gain access to the ester linkages of the lipids in the lipid droplets.

11. Due to solubility problems, lipid digestion and absorption would be hindered in the absence of bile salts, and much lipid would be excreted in the feces.

12. Secretion of the digestive enzymes as precursors reduces the likelihood that the secretory tissue itself will be damaged by its own secretory products.

13. Caloric homeostasis is the condition of energy balance, such that the energy expenditure of an organism is equal to the energy intake.

14. CCK produces the satisfaction of feeling full, without hunger, and stimulates the secretion of digestive enzymes by the pancreas and the secretion of bile salts by the gall bladder. GLP-1 also produces a feeling of satiety, and, in addition, potentiates the glucose-induced secretion of insulin by the β cells of the pancreas.

15. Activation is independent of zymogen concentration because the reaction is unimolecular.

16. (a) Over the 40 years under consideration, the individual will have consumed

$$40 \text{ years} \times 365 \text{ days year}^{-1} \times 2000 \text{ kcal day}^{-1} = 2.92 \times 10^7 \text{ kcal.}$$

(b) Thus, over the 40-year span, our subject will have ingested about

$$2.92 \times 10^7 \text{ kcal} / (9 \text{ kcal g}^{-1}) = 3.24 \times 10^6 \text{ g} = 3,240 \text{ kg of food},$$

which is equivalent to more than 6 tons of food! Yet, remarkably, the body weight has remained constant without a need to accurately and constantly calibrate and equalize the energy intake and energy output. Although willpower, exercise, and a bathroom scale often play a role in this homeostasis, some biochemical signaling also must be taking place to help with the energy regulation.

17. (a) $12 \text{ pounds} \times 0.454 \text{ kg pound}^{-1} = 5.45 \text{ kg} = 5.45 \times 10^3 \text{ g} = $ total weight gain. $5.45 \times 10^3 \text{ g}/40 \text{ years}/365 \text{ days year}^{-1} = 0.373 \text{ g day}^{-1}$.

Thus, to gain 12 pounds in 40 years, our subject needed to eat only 373 mg more food per day than needed to meet the body's biochemical needs.

(b) Many examples are possible. Consider butter. Because butter is essentially pure fat, 0.38 g of butter or approximately one-quarter of a pat daily will provide the weight gain. In other words, the simple excess of the equivalent of one-quarter pat of butter per day will lead to a (modest) weight gain of 12 pounds over 40 years-a startling if depressing fact.

CHAPTER 15

1. Intermediary metabolism consists of the highly integrated biochemical reactions that occur inside a living cell.

2. Anabolism is the set of biochemical reactions that use energy to build new molecules and ultimately new cells. Catabolism is the set of biochemical reactions that extract energy from fuel sources by the breakdown of biomolecules.

3. • Cellular movements and the performance of mechanical work
   • Active transport
   • Biosynthetic reactions

4. a. 6; b. 8; c. 9; d. 1: e. 7; f. 2; g. 3; h. 5; i. 10; j. 4.

5. The hydrolysis of the triphosphate group relieves charge repulsion. The products of the reaction are furthermore stabilized by resonance and by hydration. Each of these factors contributes to the high transfer potential of the phosphoryl group.

6. Having only one primary source of chemical energy allows the cell to better monitor its energy status.

7. The divalent Mg^{2+} or Mn^{2+} ions complex with the negatively charged oxygens on the phosphate groups of the ATP. The ionic interactions help stabilize the charges on the ATP.

8. The standard free energy of hydrolysis applies under standard conditions, including 1 M concentrations of reactants and products. Changing the concentrations of reactants or products will alter the reaction free energy under actual conditions. Therefore, increasing the concentration of ATP or decreasing the concentration cellular ADP or P_i (by rapid removal by means of other reactions, for instance) would make the intracellular reaction more exergonic.

9. (a) $\Delta G^{\circ\prime} = -30.5 - (-43.1) \text{ kJ mol}^{-1} = +12.6 \text{ kJ mol}^{-1}$. Reverse reaction (left) is favored.

(b) $\Delta G^{o\prime} = -30.5 - (-9.2)$ kJ mol^{-1} = -21.3 kJ mol^{-1}. Forward reaction (right) is favored.

(c) $\Delta G^{o\prime} = -30.5 - (-61.9)$ kJ mol^{-1} = $+31.4$ kJ mol^{-1}. Reverse reaction (left) is favored.

(d) $\Delta G^{o\prime} = -30.5 - (-13.8)$ kJ mol^{-1} = -16.7 kJ mol^{-1}. Forward reaction (right) is favored.

10. None whatsoever. The standard free energies provide thermodynamic information about the reactant and products, but no information about the reaction kinetics (rates).

11. (Note: Use use RT = 2.478 kJ mol^{-1}.)

(a) $\Delta G^{o\prime} = -30.5 - (-61.9)$ kJ mol^{-1} = 31.4 kJ mol^{-1} (7.5 kcal mol^{-1}).

$K'_{eq} = e^{(\Delta G^{o\prime}/RT)} = 3.1 \times 10^{-6}$.

(b) $K'_{eq} = ([phosphoenolpyruvate]/[pyruvate]) \times ([ADP]/[ATP]) = 3.1 \times 10^{-6}$.

Solve: $([phosphoenolpyruvate]/[pyruvate]) = 10 \times K'_{eq} = 3.1 \times 10^{-5}$.

Take the reciprocal to get:

$([pyruvate]/[phosphoenolpyruvate]) = 1/(3.1 \times 10^{-5}) = $ (b) 3.2×10^4.

12. (Note: Use use RT = 2.478 kJ mol^{-1}.)

Reaction 1: G-6-P + $H_2O \rightarrow$ glucose + P_i. $\Delta G^{o\prime}$ = 13.8 kJ mol^{-1}.

Reaction 2: G-1-P + $H_2O \rightarrow$ glucose + P_i. $\Delta G^{o\prime}$ = 20.9 kJ mol^{-1}.

Subtract reaction 2 from reaction 1 to get the net reaction: G-6-P $\rightarrow$ G-1-P.

For the net reaction, $\Delta G^{o\prime} = -13.8 \ (-20.9)$ kJ mol^{-1} = **+7.1 kJ mol^{-1}** (1.7 kcal mol^{-1}).

Reverse of the net reaction is favored. (Forming G-6-P is favored.)

The equilibrium ratio [G-6-P]/[G-1-P] is $e^{(7.1/RT)}$ = **17.6**.

13. (a) Acetate + CoA + H$^+$ $\rightarrow$ acetyl CoA + H_2O, $\Delta G^{o\prime}$ = +31.4 kJ mol^{-1}.

For ATP hydrolysis, $\Delta G^{o\prime}$ = -30.5 kJ mol^{-1}.

Overall reaction, $\Delta G^{o\prime}$ = $(-30.5$ kJ + 31.4$)$ mol^{-1} = +0.9 kJ mol^{-1}.

(b) With pyrophosphate hydrolysis, $\Delta G^{o\prime} = (0.9 - 19.2)$ kJ mol^{-1} = -18.3 kJ mol^{-1}. Pyrophosphate hydrolysis makes the overall reaction exergonic.

14. The free-energy changes of the individual steps in a pathway are summed to determine the overall free-energy change of the entire pathway. Consequently, a reaction with a positive free-energy value can be powered to take place if coupled to a sufficiently exergonic reaction. Furthermore, physiological conditions may differ from standard conditions. High concentrations of reactants and low concentrations of products will make a particular reaction more favorable (comparing ΔG under actual conditions versus $\Delta G^{o\prime}$). See also problem 19, below.

15. An ADP unit is common to ATP, coenzyme A, and the adenine dinucleotides: FAD and NAD$^+$.

16. NADH and FADH$_2$ are electron carriers for catabolism. NADPH is the electron carrier for anabolism.

17. The electrons in the π bond of the C$=$O double bond form less stable resonance structures with the C$-$S bond of the thioester than with the C$-$O bond of the ester. Thus, the thioester is not stabilized by resonance to the same extent as an oxygen ester.

18. Metabolic reactions are regulated by controlling the amounts of available enzymes, the activities of available enzymes, and the availability of substrates.

19. Recall that $\Delta G = \Delta G^{o\prime} + RT \ln$ [products]/[reactants]. Altering the ratio of products to reactants will cause ΔG to vary under actual intracellular conditions. In glycolysis, the intracellular concentrations of the components of the pathway result in a value of ΔG whose absolute value is greater than that of $\Delta G^{o\prime}$. (See also problem 14, above.)

20. (a) Ethanol is more reduced because it has more C—H bonds and fewer carbon-oxygen bonds.
    (b) Lactate is more reduced, also because it has more C—H bonds and fewer carbon-oxygen bonds.
    (c) Succinate is more reduced because it has more C—H bonds and lacks the C=C double bond.
    (d) Isocitrate is more reduced because it has more C—H bonds and fewer carbon-oxygen bonds.
    (e) Once again, malate is more reduced because it has more C—H bonds and fewer carbon-oxygen bonds. (The pattern described in part a, above, holds.)

21. Unless the ingested food is converted into molecules capable of being absorbed by the intestine, no energy can ever be extracted by the body.

22. Reaction kinetics and reaction thermodynamics are separate properties. Although a reaction is thermodynamically favorable, it may nevertheless take place slowly if there is a large activation energy barrier between the reactants and a transition state. Enzymes serve to lower the activation energy barrier so that a reaction may take place within a time scale required for cell function.

23. (a) For an acid AH,

$$AH \rightleftharpoons A^- + H^+ \qquad K = \frac{[A^-] + [H^+]}{[AH]}.$$

The pK_a is $-\log_{10} K$, and $\Delta G^{o\prime}$ is the standard free-energy change at pH 7.

We make use of the relation, $\Delta G^{o\prime} = -RT \ln K$. Converting ln to $\log_{10}$ gives:

$\Delta G^{o\prime} = -2.303 \, RT \log_{10} K$. Substituting give $\Delta G^{o\prime} = +2.303 \, RT \, pK_a$.

   (b) $\Delta G^{o\prime} = 2.303 \times 2.478$ kJ mol$^{-1} \times 4.8 = $ __27.4 kJ mol^{-1}__ (6.5 kcal mol^{-1}).

24. The activated form of sulfate in most organisms is 3′-phosphoadenosine-5′-phosphosulfate.

25. (a) As the Mg^{2+} concentration falls, the ΔG of hydrolysis rises. Note that pMg is a negative logarithmic plot, and so each increment on the x-axis represents a 10-fold decrease in $[Mg^{2+}]$.
    (b) Mg^{2+} binds to the phosphoryl groups of ATP and helps to mitigate charge repulsion. As the $[Mg^{2+}]$ falls, charge the stabilization of ATP would be less, leading to greater charge repulsion and a more negative ΔG of hydrolysis (making hydrolysis more favorable).

26. Arginine phosphate in invertebrate muscle, like creatine phosphate in vertebrate muscle, can serve as a reservoir of high-potential phosphoryl groups. Arginine phosphate thereby could function to maintain a high level of ATP during muscular exertion.

27. (a) The rationale behind creatine supplementation is that it would be converted into creatine phosphate and thus could serve as a rapid means of replenishing ATP after muscle contraction.
    (b) If creatine supplementation were beneficial, it would most benefit exercises that depend on short bursts of activity. More sustained activity would require ATP generation by fuel metabolism, which requires more time.

28. Under standard conditions, $\Delta G^{\circ\prime} = -RT \ln$ [products]/[reactants].

Substituting 23.8 kJ mol^{-1} for $\Delta G^{\circ\prime}$ and solving yields

[products]/[reactants] $= e^{-(\Delta G^{\circ\prime}/RT)} = e^{-(23.8/2.478)} = 7 \times 10^{-5}$.

In other words, the forward reaction does not take place to a significant extent.

Under intracellular conditions, ΔG is -1.3 kJ mol^{-1}.

Note the equation $\Delta G = \Delta G^{\circ\prime} + RT \ln$ [products]/[reactants].

To achieve ΔG of -1.3 kJ mol^{-1}, $RT \ln$ [products]/[reactants] must $= -25.1$ kJ mol^{-1}, and [products]/[reactants] $= e^{-(25.1/2.478)} = 4 \times 10^{-5}$.

Thus, a reaction that is endergonic under standard conditions can be converted into an exergonic reaction by maintaining the [products]/[reactants] ratio below the equilibrium value. This situation is usually achieved by removing the products as soon as they are formed in another coupled reaction.

29. Under standard conditions

$$K'_{eq} = \frac{[B]_{eq}}{[A]_{eq}} \times \frac{[ADP]_{eq}\,[P_i]_{eq}}{[ATP]_{eq}} = 10^{3.3/1.36} = 2.67 \times 10^2$$

At equilibrium, the ratio of [B] to [A] is given by

$$\frac{[B]_{eq}}{[A]_{eq}} = K'_{eq}\,\frac{[ATP]_{eq}}{[ADP]_{eq}\,[P_i]_{eq}}$$

The ATP-generating system of cells maintains the [ATP]/[ADP][P$_i$] ratio at a high level, typically of the order of 500 M^{-1} given. For this ratio,

$$\frac{[B]_{eq}}{[A]_{eq}} = 2.67 \times 10^2 \times 500 = 1.34 \times 10^5$$

This equilibrium ratio is strikingly different from the value of 1.15×10^{-3} for the reaction A ⟶ B in the absence of ATP hydrolysis. In other words, coupling the hydrolysis of ATP with the conversion of A into B has changed the equilibrium ratio of B to A by a factor of about 10^8.

30. Use the equation: $\Delta G = \Delta G^{\circ\prime} + RT \ln ([ADP] \times [P_i]/[ATP])$.

Note that __molar__ concentrations must be used.

In the table below "ratio" refers to $([ADP] \times [P_i]/[ATP])$. ΔG is obtained as the sum of $\Delta G^{\circ\prime}$ plus $RT \ln(\text{ratio})$.

[ATP], Molar	[ADP]	[P$_i$]	Ratio	$RT \ln$ (ratio)	$\Delta G_0{}'$	ΔG	
3.5E–03	1.8E–03	5.0E–03	2.57E–03	–14.78	–30.5	–45.3	kJ/mol
8.0E–03	9.0E–04	8.0E–03	9.00E–04	–17.38	–30.5	–47.9	kJ/mol
2.6E–03	7.0E–04	2.7E–03	7.27E–03	–17.91	–30.5	–48.4	kJ/mol

Summarizing the values from the table yields the values of ΔG for hydrolysis of ATP in each organ:

- liver: -45.3 kJ mol^{-1} (-10.8 kcal mol^{-1})
- muscle: -47.9 kJ mol^{-1} (-11.5 kcal mol^{-1})
- brain: -48.4 kJ mol^{-1} (-11.6 kcal mol^{-1})

The free energy of ATP hydrolysis is most negative in the brain.

CHAPTER 16

1. a. 4; b. 3; c. 1; d. 6; e. 8; f. 2; g. 10; h. 9; i. 7; j. 5.

2. In both cases, the ultimate electron donor is glyceraldehydes 3-phosphate. In lactic acid fermentation, the electron acceptor is pyruvate, which is converted into lactate. In alcoholic fermentation, acetaldehyde is the electron acceptor, which is converted into ethanol. During intermediate steps, the electrons are passed temporarily to NAD^+ (forming NADH) before they are returned to the ultimate acceptor, either pyruvate or acetaldehyde, respectively.

3. Glucose or fructose requires "investment" of 2 ATP to form fructose 1,6-bisphosphate. Fructose 1,6-bisphosphate is then split to form dihydroxyacetone phosphate and glyceraldehyde 3-phosphate, each of which returns 2 ATP. So the net answer would be 4 ATP from fructose 1,6-bisphosphate, and the other answers are:

    (a) Glucose 6-phosphate requires "investment" of only 1 ATP to form the fructose 1,6-bisphosphate and hence yields a net of 3 ATP.

    (b) Dihydroxyacetone yields 2 ATP.

    (c) Glyceraldehyde 3-phosphate yields 2 ATP.

    (d) Fructose yields 2 ATP.

    (e) Sucrose yields 1 glucose and 1 fructose, each of which yields 2 ATP, so the net yield from sucrose is 4 ATP.

4. Glucokinase enables the liver to remove glucose from the blood when hexokinase is saturated, ensuring that glucose is captured and stored for later use.

5. Glucokinase has a higher K_M, which keeps its activity low when the glucose concentration is low. Higher glucose concentrations, conditions that may saturate hexokinase, enable glucokinase to become more active.

6. Glucose cannot be cleaved into three-carbon fragments, whereas fructose can be cleaved into the three-carbon molecules that are metabolized in the third stage of glycolysis. The further phosphorylation of fructose 6-phosphate to form fructose 1,6-bisphosphate prevents the conversion back to the glucose isomer.

7. Once formed, the GAP is immediately removed by subsequent reactions, a process sometimes known as "product removal." Because the intracellular conditions do not constitute equilibrium, the conversion of DHAP into GAP by the enzyme can proceed.

8. A thioester couples the oxidation of glyceraldehyde 3-phosphate to 3 phosphoglycerate with the formation of 1,3-bisphosphoglycerate. In turn, the 1,3-bisphosphoglycerate can subsequently power the formation of ATP.

9. Glycolysis is a component of alcoholic fermentation, the pathway that produces alcohol for beer and wine. The belief was that understanding the biochemical basis of alcohol production might lead to more efficient means of producing beer.

10. Niacin deficiency could lead to a shortage of NAD^+. The conversion of glyceraldehyde 3-phosphate into 1,3-bisphosphoglycerate would be impaired. Glycolysis would be less effective.

11. Glucose 6-phosphate must have other uses in addition to its role in glycolysis. Indeed, glucose 6-phosphate can be converted into glycogen or can be processed to yield reducing power for biosynthesis. Therefore, it is appropriate that hexokinase is not the

pacemaker of glycolysis. The pacemaker step should not only be irreversible but also should be a step that is required for only one pathway.

12. The energy needs of a muscle cell vary widely, from rest to intense exercise.

   Consequently, the regulation of phosphofructokinase by energy charge is vital for muscle function. In other tissues, such as the liver, the energy needs are much less variable, the ATP concentration is less likely to fluctuate, and there is therefore no need for the ATP concentration to be a key regulator of phosphofructokinase.

13.

$$
\begin{array}{ccc}
\text{CH}_2\text{OH} & \xrightarrow[\text{Glycerol kinase}]{\text{ATP} \quad \text{ADP}} & \text{CH}_2\text{OH} \\
\mid & & \mid \\
\text{HO}-\text{C}-\text{H} & & \text{HO}-\text{C}-\text{H} \\
\mid & & \mid \\
\text{CH}_2\text{OH} & & \text{CH}_2\text{OPO}_3^{-2} \\
\text{glycerol} & & \text{glycerol phosphate}
\end{array}
$$

$$
\xrightarrow[\text{Glycerol phosphate dehydrogenase}]{\text{NAD}^+ \quad \text{NADH} \quad \text{H}^+}
\begin{array}{c}
\text{CH}_2\text{OH} \\
\mid \\
\text{O}=\text{C} \\
\mid \\
\text{CH}_2\text{OPO}_3^{-2} \\
\text{dihydroxyacetone phosphate}
\end{array}
$$

After the glycerol is converted into DHAP, it is isomerized into GAP, which can then proceed down the glycolysis pathway to pyruvate.

14. The $\Delta G°'$ for the reverse of glycolysis is $+96$ kJ mol^{-1} ($+23$ kcal mol^{-1}) far too endergonic for a direct reversal of the pathway. Instead, key steps that are energetically unfavorable in the reverse pathway must be bypassed through the use of alternate reaction steps.

15. Pyruvate can be completely oxidized to CO_2 and H_2O in cellular respiration. Under anaerobic or low-oxygen conditions, complete oxidation will not be possible and the result will be fermentation. Under low-oxygen conditions, therefore, pyruvate will be metabolized either to ethanol by means of alcoholic fermentation, or to lactate in the lactic acid fermentation pathway.

16. Three steps are not readily reversible: the conversion of glucose into glucose 6-phosphate by hexokinase; the conversion of fructose 6-phosphate into fructose 1,6 bisphosphate by phosphofructokinase; and the formation of pyruvate from phosphoenolpyruvate by pyruvate kinase.

17. Lactic acid is a strong acid. If it would remain in a muscle cell, the pH of the cell would fall, which could lead to the denaturation of muscle proteins and result in muscle damage.

18. In tissues other than liver, fructose is converted into fructose 6-phosphate by hexokinase. In liver, a more specialized pathway is used, beginning with fructokinase converting fructose into fructose 1-phosphate. Fructose 1-phosphate then is cleaved by a specific aldolase to yield glyceraldehyde and dihydroxyacetone phosphate, which enters the glycolytic pathway directly. The glyceraldehyde so produced is converted into the glycolytic intermediate glyceraldehyde 3-phosphate by triose kinase.

19. Without triose phosphate isomerase, only the glyceraldehyde 3-phosphate and not the dihydroxyacetone phosphate generated by aldolase could be used to generate ATP.

   Therefore, the yield of ATP from the metabolism of fructose 1,6-bisphosphate would be only two molecules of ATP. But two molecules of ATP would still be required to form fructose 1,6-bisphosphate during the early steps of glycolysis. Therefore, the net yield of ATP from fermentation of glucose would be zero, a yield incompatible with life. The organism would not survive.

20.
$$-31.4 = -2.47 \ln \frac{[\text{Pyr}][\text{ATP}]}{[\text{PEP}][\text{ADP}]}$$

$$12.7 = \ln \frac{[\text{Pyr}]}{[\text{PEP}]} + \ln 10$$

$$\frac{[\text{Pyr}]}{[\text{PEP}]} = e^{(12.7-2.3)}$$

$$\frac{[\text{PEP}]}{[\text{Pyr}]} = e^{-10.4} = 3.06 \times 10^{-5}$$

21. Since $\Delta G^{\circ\prime}$ for the aldolase reaction is $+23.8$ kJ/mol (page 281), $K_{eq} = e^{-23.8/2.47} = 6.5 \times 10^{-5}$. If we let the concentration of each of the trioses (DHAP and G-3P) formed during the reaction be X, then the concentration of F-1,6-BP is $(10^{-3}$ M $- X)$ at equilibrium because we started with millimolar F-1,6-BP. Then,

$$\frac{X^2}{10^{-3} - X} = 6.5 \times 10^{-5}$$

Solving this quadratic equation leads to the answer of 2.24×10^{-4} M for X (DHAP and G-3P). Subtracting this from 10^{-3} gives the F-1,6-BP concentration of 7.76×10^{-4} M.

22. (a) The fructose 1-phosphate pathway forms glyceraldehyde 3-phosphate. Phosphofructokinase, a key control enzyme, is bypassed. Furthermore, fructose 1-phosphate stimulates pyruvate kinase.

(b) The rapid, unregulated production of lactate can lead to metabolic acidosis.

23. Energy generation will be inhibited because arsenate will uncouple oxidation and phosphorylation. The arsenate will establish a small futile cycle that will shuttle between 3-phosphoglycerate and 1-arseno-3-phosphoglycerate. If the conditions also are anaerobic, NADH will accumulate, and NAD⁺ will become unavailable for the continuation of sustained glycolysis.

24. The synthesis of lactate is an emergency stop-gap measure that is undertaken because of (a) a local shortage of oxygen in a tissue, and (b) an immediate need for energy. A "quick fix" for the situation is to regenerate NAD⁺ from NADH using lactic acid dehydrogenase so that glycolysis can continue. When the emergency passes and oxygen is more plentiful, then the lactate can be reoxidized.

New synthesis of NAD⁺ would be too slow to provide the necessary rapid response. Furthermore, the cell would waste energy in accumulating larger pools of pyridine nucleotides than are needed. Catalytic enzymes, by contrast, are needed in only small molar amounts.

25. (a) 4; (b) 10; (c) 1; (d) 5; (e) 7; (f) 8; (g) 9; (h) 2; (i) 3; (j) 6.

26. Fructose 2,6-bisphosphate stabilizes the active R state of phosphofructokinase.

27. Several plausible answers may be possible here. There could likely be alternative nondietary sources of galactose that pose problems. For example, galactose derivatives may arise from epimerization of the equivalent glucose derivatives. Subsequent metabolic breakdown of one such derivative conceivably could produce free galactose in the galactosemic patient and lead to peripheral damage (e.g., in the nervous system).

28. A potassium channel is inhibited by binding ATP. This alters the voltage across the plasma membrane, which activates a calcium channel, allowing an influx of calcium

ions. The calcium ions stimulate the fusion of insulin containing granules with the plasma membrane, resulting in the secretion of insulin.

29. (a) The graph suggests that ADP rather that ATP is the phosphate donor for *P. furiosus* phosphofructokinase. Furthermore, AMP and ATP have similar regulatory effects on this enzyme, rather than the opposing effects discussed in the chapter. (See the legend to Figure 16.15.)

   (b) AMP and ATP are both inhibitors. They both convert the hyperbolic binding curve of ADP into a sigmoidal one, probably by allosterically decreasing the affinity of the enzyme for ADP.

30. ATP initially stimulates PFK activity, as would be expected for a substrate. Higher concentrations of ATP, however, inhibit the enzyme. Although this seems to be a counterintuitive effect for a substrate, recall that the function of glycolysis in muscle is to generate ATP. Consequently, high concentrations of ATP signal that the ATP needs are met and glycolysis should stop. In addition to being a substrate, ATP is an allosteric inhibitor of PFK.

31. (a) Carbon dioxide is a good indicator of the rate of alcoholic fermentation because it is, along with ethanol, a product of alcoholic fermentation.

   (b) Phosphate is a required substrate for the reaction catalyzed by glyceraldehyde 3-phosphate dehydrogenase. The phosphate is incorporated into 1,3-bisphosphoglycerate.

   (c) The result indicates that the amount of free phosphate must have been limiting.

   (d) The ratio should be 1. One phosphate would be consumed for every pyruvate that is decarboxylated.

   (e) Lack of phosphate would inhibit glyceraldehyde 3-phosphate dehydrogenase. This would "back-up" glycolysis, resulting in the accumulation of fructose 1,6-bisphosphate.

32. D-glucopyranose is a cyclic hemiacetal, which is in equilibrium with its open-chain form that contains an active aldehyde group. In contrast, the anomeric carbon atoms of glucose and fructose are joined in an α-glycosidic linkage in sucrose. Hence sucrose is not in equilibrium with an active aldehyde or ketone form.

33. (a) The key is the aldolase reaction. Note that the carbons attached to the phosphate in glyceraldehyde 3-phosphate and dihydroxyacetone phosphate are interconverted by triose phosphate isomerase and *both* become the terminal carbon of the glyceric acids. Hence, the label is in the methyl carbon of pyruvate.

   (b) By definition, specific activity is radioactivity/mol (or mmol). In this case the specific activity is halved (to 5 mCi/mmol) because the number of moles of product (pyruvate) is twice that of the labeled substrate (glucose).

34. (a) Glucose $+ 2\,P_i + 2\,ADP \longrightarrow 2$ lactate $+ 2\,ATP$

   (b) To obtain the overall $\Delta G^{\circ\prime}$, -123 kJ/mol (-29.4 kcal/mol), you add the $\Delta G^{\circ\prime}$ values given in Table 16.1 in the text and the value given for the reduction of pyruvate to lactate. Remember that the values for the three carbon molecules must be doubled, since each hexose yields two trioses.

$$\Delta G' = -123.1 + RT \ln \frac{(5 \times 10^{-5})^2 (2 \times 10^{-3})}{(5 \times 10^{-3})(10^{-3})^2 (2 \times 10^{-4})}$$

$$= -123.1 + 2.47 \ln 50$$

$$= -114 \text{ kJ mol}^{-1} \ (-27.2 \text{ kcal / mol}).$$

The concentrations of ATP, ADP, P_i, and lactate are squared because, in reactions such as A $\longrightarrow$ 2 B, the K_{eq} = $[B]^2/[A]$.

35. GLUT2 will transport glucose only when the blood concentration of glucose is high, which is precisely the condition in which the β cells of the pancreas should secrete insulin.

36. The conversion would involve steps catalyzed by three enzymes: fructokinase, fructose 1-phosphate aldolase, and triose kinase. These are the steps:

    • Fructose + ATP $\longrightarrow$ fructose 1-phosphate + ADP (fructokinase).
    • Fructose 1-phosphate $\longrightarrow$ dihydroxyacetone phosphate + glyceraldehyde (fructose 1-phosphate aldolase).
    • Glyceraldehyde + ATP $\longrightarrow$ glyceraldehyde 3-phosphate + ADP (triose kinase).

    The primary controlling step of glycolysis catalyzed by phosphofructokinase is bypassed by the set of three reactions. Glycolysis will therefore proceed in an unregulated fashion under conditions where energy and ATP synthesis are not needed.

37. Hexokinase has a low ATPase activity in the absence of a sugar because it is in a catalytically inactive conformation. The addition of xylose closes the cleft between the two lobes of the enzyme. However, the xylose hydroxymethyl group (at C-5) cannot be phosphorylated. Instead, a water molecule at the site normally occupied by the C-6 hydroxymethyl group of glucose acts as the phosphoryl acceptor from ATP.

38. The equilibrium constant K_{eq}, [ATP].[AMP]/([ADP].[ADP]), is directly proportional to both the ATP and AMP concentrations. However, the intracellular concentration of AMP is much smaller than the intracellular concentration of ATP. Therefore, the same absolute changes in the ATP and AMP concentrations (due to adenylate kinase activity) will result in much larger percentage changes for the level of AMP. The [AMP] is therefore a more sensitive signal. As an example, let us consider an ATP concentration of 1 mM and an AMP concentration of 0.1 mM. Let us then assume that [ATP] decreases transiently to 0.95 mM, a 5% drop due to metabolic activity. This difference could be compensated by adenylate kinase activity (with a constant pool of total adenylate, i.e., [ATP] + [ADP] + [AMP] constant). Then adenylate kinase activity to make up the 0.05 mM of spent ATP would also produce an additional 0.05 mM of AMP, or a 50% increase in the level of AMP, from 0.10 mM to 0.15 mM. This increase in [AMP] would signal a low-energy state for the cell. The small change in [ATP] (e.g., 5%) therefore is magnified into a much larger signal, namely a 50% change in [AMP] in this hypothetical example.

CHAPTER 17

1. The reverse of glycolysis is highly endergonic under cellular conditions. In particular, the three reactions catalyzed by hexokinase, phosphofructokinase and pyruvate kinase exhibit large energy barriers for the reverse pathway. The expenditure of six NTP molecules in gluconeogenesis overcomes these barriers and renders gluconeogenesis exergonic.

2. a. 6; b. 1; c. 7; d, 3; e. 2; f. 5; g. 4.

3. Three reactions of glycolysis follow different scenarios in gluconeogenesis.

    i. The formation of pyruvate and ATP by pyruvate kinase is irreversible. This step is bypassed by two reactions in gluconeogenesis: (1) the formation of oxaloacetate from pyruvate and CO_2 by pyruvate carboxylase and (2) the formation of phosphoenolpyruvate from oxaloacetate and GTP by phosphoenolpyruvate carboxykinase.

ii. The formation of fructose 1,6-bisphosphate at the expense of ATP by phospho-fructokinase also is not reversible. Rather, the reaction is bypassed by fructose 1,6-bisphosphatase in gluconeogenesis, which catalyzes the conversion of fructose 1,6-bisphosphate into fructose 6-phosphate, without forming any ATP.

iii. Likewise, the hexokinase-catalyzed formation of glucose 6-phosphate, at the expense of ATP in glycolysis, is bypassed by glucose 6-phosphatase, without formation of ATP, but only in the liver.

4. Biotin is a cofactor for the synthesis of oxaloacetate from pyruvate by pyruvate carboxylase. Therefore, metabolic conversions, which require pyruvate carboxylase, will be inhibited. These will include only reaction (e) pyruvate → oxaloacetate, and conversion (b) pyruvate → glucose (which must begin with the pyruvate → oxaloacetate reaction). The other listed conversions (a, c, d, f) are independent of pyruvate carboxylase and independent of biotin.

5. The sites of glucose synthesis and glucose breakdown are different. During intense exercise, glycolysis proceeds to lactate in active skeletal muscle, with insufficient oxygen for the complete oxidation, as well as in erythrocytes. Meanwhile, gluconeogenesis proceeds in the liver, using the major raw materials of lactate and alanine produced by the active skeletal muscle and erythrocytes. The glucose that is produced by the liver enters the bloodstream and becomes available to the muscles for continued exercise. The advantages to the organism are to buy time and to shift part of the metabolic burden from muscle to liver.

6. Muscle is likely to produce lactic acid during contraction. Lactic acid is a strong acid and would be detrimental if allowed to accumulate in muscle or blood. Liver takes care of the problem by removing the lactic acid from the blood and converting it into glucose. The glucose can then either be released into the bloodstream or stored as glycogen for later use.

7. Glucose 6-phosphate produced in the liver could not be converted to glucose for release into the bloodstream. The glucose 6-phosphate would be trapped in the liver. Tissues that rely on glucose as an energy source would not function well, unless a sufficient and relatively constant supply of glucose was provided in the diet.

8. Glucose is an important energy source for both muscle and brain, and is essentially the only source of energy for the brain. Consequently, these tissues should never release glucose. The release of glucose is prevented by the absence of glucose 6-phosphatase.

9. In gluconeogenesis, lactate dehydrogenase synthesizes pyruvate from lactate. In lactic acid fermentation, the enzyme synthesizes lactate from pyruvate. The role of the enzyme is reversed when comparing the two pathways.

10. (a) A, B; (b) C, D; (c) D; (d) A; (e) B; (f) C; (g) A; (h) D; (i) none; (j) A; (k) A.

11. Some of the amino acids from the protein degradation will be released into the bloodstream. The liver will take up the amino acids and convert the carbon skeletons into glucose by means of gluconeogenesis.

12. A total of 6 NTP molecules are required. Two ATP and two GTP are required to synthesize two molecules of phosphoenolpyruvate from two pyruvate molecules. Two additional ATP are required to synthesize two 1,3-bisphosphoglycerate from two molecules of 3-phosphoglycerate during gluconeogenesis. Two molecules of NADH are required to produce two molecules of glyceraldehyde 3-phosphate from two molecules of 1,3-bisphosphoglycerate.

13. (a) None. Glucose 6-phosphatase will remove the phosphate from glucose-6-phosphate, yielding glucose with no involvement of NTP.

(b) None. Fructose 1,6-bisphosphatase and glucose 6-phosphatase together will sequentially remove the two phosphate groups from fructose 1,6-bisphosphate, yielding glucose with no involvement of NTP.

(c) Four NTP molecules. Two GTP are required to synthesize two molecules of phosphoenolpyruvate from two oxaloacetate molecules. In a later step, two ATP molecules are required to synthesize two 1,3-bisphosphoglycerate from two molecules of 3-phosphoglycerate.

(d) None.

14. One substrate cycle would consist of the glycolytic enzyme phosphofructokinase and the gluconeogenic enzyme fructose 1,6-bisphosphatase. The other substrate cycle involves pyruvate kinase from glycolysis together with the combination of pyruvate carboxylase with phosphoenolpyruvate carboxykinase from gluconeogenesis.

15. The substrate cycles may regulate flux on one pathway or the other by amplifying metabolic signals. In some cases, these cycles may generate body heat from the hydrolysis of ATP, which is the only net reaction of such a cycle.

16. The enzymes involved in two substrate cycles are control points. The glycolytic pathway is activated by F-2,6-BP, AMP, and F-1,6-BP; whereas ATP, alanine, citrate, and protons inhibit glycolysis. Conversely, gluconeogenesis is activated by citrate and acetyl-CoA and inhibited by F-2,6-BP, AMP, and ADP.

17. (a) 2, 3, 6, 9; (b) 1, 4, 5, 7, 8.

18. The ketoacid pyruvate is produced by removal of the amino group from alanine. The ketoacid oxaloacetate is produced by removal of the amino group from aspartate. Both pyruvate and oxaloacetate are components of the gluconeogenic pathway.

19. (a) Glycolysis increases because ATP can no longer inhibit PFK, phosphofructokinase.

(b) Glycolysis increases because citrate can no longer inhibit PFK.

(c) Glycolysis will increase because in the absence of fructose 2,6-bisphosphatase, the level of fructose 2,6-bisphosphate will increase, resulting in activation of PFK.

(d) Glycolysis will decrease because fructose 1,6-bisphosphate can no longer activate pyruvate kinase.

20. (a) If both enzymes operated simultaneously, the following reactions would take place:

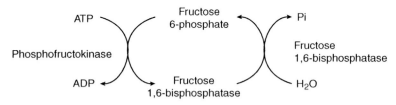

The net result would be hydrolysis of ATP:

(b) Not really. For the cycle to generate (only) heat, both enzymes must be functional (to the same extent) at the same time in the same cell.

(c) The species *B. terrestris* and *B. rufocinctus* might show some futile cycling because both enzymes are active to a substantial degree.

(d) No. These results simply suggest that simultaneous activity of phosphofructokinase and fructose 1,6-bisphosphatase is unlikely to be employed to generate heat in the species shown.

21. Lactic acid is capable of being further oxidized and thus represents useful energy. The conversion of this acid into glucose saves the carbon atoms for future combustion.

22. Fructose 2,6-bisphosphate, present at high concentration when glucose is abundant, normally inhibits gluconeogenesis by blocking fructose 1,6-bisphosphatase. In this genetic disorder, the phosphatase will be active irrespective of the glucose level. Hence, substrate cycling will be increased, and the level of fructose 1,6-bisphosphate will consequently be lower than normal. Less pyruvate will be formed and thus less ATP generated.

23. The glucose will *not* be labeled. After lactate is oxidized to pyruvate and the resulting pyruvate is carboxylated with labeled CO_2 by pyruvate carboxylase to yield oxaloacetate, then the same CO_2 will be released during the phosphorylation and decarboxylation of oxaloacetate by phosphoenolpyruvate carboxykinase. (The CO_2 serves to make the phosphorylation reaction energetically feasible, but the CO_2 does not remain in the final product.)

24. Glycolysis yields two net molecules of ATP, whereas gluconeogenesis hydrolyzes four molecules of ATP and two molecules of GTP. The sum of gluconeogenesis plus glycolysis therefore is: $2 \text{ ATP} + 2 \text{ GTP} + 4 \text{ H}_2\text{O} \rightarrow 2 \text{ ADP} + 2 \text{ GDP} + 4 \text{ P}_i$. The effects of the additional high phosphoryl-transfer equivalents multiply together to alter the equilibrium constant by a factor of $(10^8)^4 = 10^{32}$.

CHAPTER 18

1. The pyruvate dehydrogenase complex catalyzes the following reaction that links glycolysis to the citric acid cycle:

   Pyruvate + CoA + $NAD^+ \rightarrow$ acetyl-CoA + NADH + H^++ CO_2

   The pyruvate is the end product of glycolysis. The acetyl-CoA condenses with oxaloacetate to begin the citric acid cycle.

2. (a) Pyruvate dehydrogenase catalyzes the decarboxylation of pyruvate and the formation of acetyllipoamide.

   (b) Dihydrolipoyl transacetylase catalyzes the formation of acetyl-CoA.

   (c) Dihydrolipoyl dehydrogenase catalyzes the reduction of the oxidized lipoic acid.

   (d) The kinase associated with the complex phosphorylates and inactivates the complex.

   (e) The phosphatase associated with the complex dephosphorylates and activates the complex.

3. The remaining steps in the pyruvate dehydrogenase reaction cycle serve to regenerate oxidized lipoamide, which is required to begin another reaction cycle. Moreover, this regeneration results in the production of high-energy electrons in the form of NADH.

4. The three steps in the conversion of pyruvate are decarboxylation, oxidation, and finally transfer of the resulting acetyl group to CoA.

5. The principal fates of acetyl-CoA are oxidation to CO_2 by the citric acid cycle or incorporation into lipids. The carbon atoms of acetyl-CoA cannot be used for gluconeogenesis in animal cells.

6. (a) To achieve the decarboxylation of pyruvate, thiamine pyrophosphate becomes covalently bound to pyruvate and then releases carbon dioxide and the acetyl group.

(b) Lipoic acid (as lipoamide) transfers the acetyl group.

(c) Coenzyme A accepts the acetyl group from lipoic acid to form acetyl-CoA.

(d) FAD accepts the electrons and hydrogen ions when oxidized lipoic acid is reduced.

(e) NAD^+ accepts electrons from $FADH_2$.

7. The catalytic coenzymes, thiamine pyrophosphate, lipoic acid, and FAD, are modified and then regenerated in each reaction cycle. Thus, they can play a role in the processing of many molecules of pyruvate. The stoichiometric coenzymes, coenzyme A and NAD^+, are components of products of the reaction and therefore can participate in the processing of only one molecule of pyruvate. New stoichiometric coenzyme molecules must be provided in each reaction cycle.

8. The electrons from reduced lipoamide are transferred to FAD initially, and then to NAD^+. This transfer sequence is unusual because the electrons are passed to the NAD^+ from the $FADH_2$, which usually is considered uphill in terms of the respective reducing potentials. The electron transfer is usually in the other direction.

9. a. 6; b. 10; c. 1; d. 7; e. 2; f. 8; g. 3; h. 4; i. 5; j. 9.

10. In muscle, the acetyl-CoA generated by the complex is used for energy generation. Consequently, signals that indicate an energy-rich state (high ratios of ATP/ADP and $NADH/NAD^+$) inhibit the complex, whereas the reverse conditions stimulate the enzyme. Calcium as the signal for muscle contraction (and, hence, energy need) also stimulates the enzyme. In liver, the acetyl-CoA derived from pyruvate is used for biosynthetic purposes, such as fatty acid synthesis. In this case, insulin, the hormone denoting the fed state, stimulates the complex.

11. (a) Enhanced kinase activity will decrease the activity of the PDH complex because phosphorylation by the kinase inhibits the complex.

(b) Phosphatase activates the complex by removing a phosphate. If the phosphatase activity is diminished, the activity of the PDH complex also will decrease.

12. She might have been ingesting, in some fashion, the arsenite from the peeling paint or the wallpaper. Also, she might have been breathing arsine gas from the wallpaper, which would be oxidized to arsenite in her body. In any of these circumstances, the ingested arsenite would inhibit enzymes that require lipoic acid—notably, the PDH complex.

13. First, acetyllipoamide, and then acetyl-CoA.

14. As a product of the pyruvate dehydrogenase complex, acetyl-CoA from other sources will inhibit the complex. Glucose metabolism to pyruvate also will be slowed because acetyl-CoA is being derived from an alternative source.

15. A thioester is a key intermediate in the formation of 1,3-bisphosphoglycerate from glyceraldehyde 3-phosphate in the reaction catalyzed by glyceraldehyde 3-phosphate dehydrogenase. 1,3-Bisphosphoglycerate is subsequently metabolized to pyruvate.

16. Without O_2 as a terminal acceptor for electrons from NADH, the citric acid cycle cannot operate in a sustained manner. Rather, the pyruvate that is produced by glycolysis must be reduced to lactate (in muscle; or ethanol in yeast) so that the NADH produced in glycolysis can be oxidized to NAD^+. Oxygen deficiency is made worse by the presence of carbon dioxide, which, along with acetyl-CoA, is a product of the pyruvate dehydrogenase complex. Therefore, inhibiting pyruvate dehydrogenase will decrease the production of CO_2 and lessen the severity of the shock.

17. Pyruvate dehydrogenase kinase phosphorylates and inhibits the pyruvate dehydrogenase component of the pyruvate dehydrogenase complex. Inhibiting pyruvate

dehydrogenase kinase could therefore be an effective mechanism to promote the utilization of glucose and thereby lower the blood glucose level. Moreover, increasing the oxidation of pyruvate may contribute to further lowering of glucose level by decreasing the available supply of gluconeogenic substrates.

18. Thiamine thiazolone pyrophosphate is a transition state analog. The sulfur-containing ring of this analog is uncharged, and so it closely resembles the transition state of the normal coenzyme in thiamine-catalyzed reactions. See J. A. Gutowski and G. E. Lienhard, *J. Biol. Chem.* 251(1976):2863, for a discussion of this analog.

CHAPTER 19

1. The eight reactions in Table 19.1 can be added to give the net result shown at the bottom of page 335:

   Acetyl-CoA + 3 NAD^+ + FAD + ADP + P_i →

        2 CO_2 + 3 NADH + 3 H^+ + $FADH_2$ + ATP + CoA

2. The TCA cycle depends on a steady supply of NAD^+, which is typically generated from the reaction of NADH with oxygen. If there is no oxygen to accept the electrons, NADH will accumulate. The citric acid cycle will cease to operate because there will be a shortage of NAD^+.

3. In stage 1, two carbon atoms are introduced into the cycle by reaction with oxaloacetate and then oxidized to produce two molecules of CO_2. In stage 2, the resulting four-carbon molecule, succinate, is metabolized to regenerate oxaloacetate. High-energy electrons are generated in both stages.

4. a. 5; b. 7; c. 1; d. 10; e. 2; f. 4; g. 9; h. 3; i. 8; j. 6.

5. The reaction includes the formation of a new carbon-carbon bond and is powered by the hydrolysis of a thioester. Acetyl-CoA provides the thioester that is converted initially into citryl-CoA. When this thioester is hydrolyzed, citrate is formed in an irreversible reaction.

6. Two important factors prevent the wasteful hydrolysis. First, acetyl-CoA does not bind to citrate synthase unless oxaloacetate is already bound and ready for the synthesis of citryl-CoA. Second, the catalytic groups required for hydrolysis of the thioester are not positioned properly for catalysis until the citryl-CoA is formed.

7. (a) Isocitrate lyase and malate synthase are required in addition to the enzymes of the citric acid cycle.

   (b) 2 Acetyl-CoA + 2 NAD^+ + FAD + 3 H_2O →

        oxaloacetate + 2 CoA + 2 NADH + $FADH_2$ + 3 H^+

   (c) No. Hence, mammals cannot carry out the net synthesis of oxaloacetate from acetyl-CoA.

8. Summing the values of $\Delta G°$ for the reactions listed in Table 19.1 gives a value of −41.0 kJ mol^{-1} (or −9.8 kcal mol^{-1}) for the net reaction shown in the answer for problem 1, above.

9. Enzymes or enzyme complexes are biological catalysts. Recall that a catalyst facilitates a chemical reaction without the catalyst itself being permanently altered. The citric acid cycle intermediates and enzymes, and indeed the entire cycle as a whole, can be

thought of as a supramolecular catalyst because the ensemble takes in an acetyl group and catalyzes the oxidative decarboxylation of the two carbon atoms. All cycle intermediates as well as the enzymes are regenerated during the course of each turn of the cycle. At the completion of a cycle, the set of intermediates is unchanged from the initial state before the entry of acetyl-CoA. In essence, the entire cycle acts as a catalyst.

10. Due to the inhibition, succinate will increase in concentration, followed by α-ketoglutarate and then the other intermediates "upstream" of the site of inhibition. Succinate has two methylene groups that are required for the dehydrogenation, whereas malonate has only one.

11. Succinate dehydrogenase is the only enzyme in the citric acid cycle that is embedded in the mitochondrial membrane, which makes it associated with the electron-transport chain.

12. Inorganic phosphate is required for the reaction catalyzed by succinyl-CoA synthetase: Succinyl-CoA + P_i + ADP → succinate + CoA + ATP.

13. Both α-ketoglutarate and pyruvate are α-ketoacids that are decarboxylated to form thioesters of CoA. Moreover, the dihydrolipoyl dehydrogenase components of the respective enzyme complexes are identical. The other enzymes of each complex are similar. Finally, the reaction mechanisms are the same.

14. The reaction catalyzed succinyl-CoA synthetase: leads to direct formation of ATP:

Succinyl-CoA + ADP + Pi → succinate + ATP + CoA Q.

15. Isocitrate dehydrogenase and α-ketoglutarate dehydrogenase are key regulatory enzymes for the citric acid cycle.

16. The glyoxalate cycle enables organisms such as plants and bacteria to convert acetyl-CoA into glucose. Since fats can be broken down to acetyl-CoA, the glyoxalate cycle enables the organism to convert fats into glucose.

17. We cannot get the net conversion of fats into glucose because the only means to get the carbons from fats into oxaloacetate, the precursor to glucose, is through the citric acid cycle. However, although two carbon atoms enter the cycle as acetyl-CoA, two carbon atoms are lost as CO_2 before the oxaloacetate is formed. Thus, although some carbon atoms from fats may end up as carbon atoms in glucose, we cannot obtain a net synthesis of glucose from fats.

18. When "extra" acetyl-CoA is present in a cell, there is a need to produce more oxaloacetate for the running of the citric acid cycle. Pyruvate carboxylase fulfills that need.

19. The labeled carbon will be incorporated into citrate at carbon 5 (only):

*citrate labeled at carbon 5

In the drawing, carbons 1 and 2 of citrate come from acetyl-CoA. Carbon 6 is lost in the formation of α-ketoglutarate, so none of the label from carbon 5 is lost in that step. Early investigators (until Ogston in 1948; see next problem) thought that carbons 1 and 5 of citrate were indistinguishable and so were surprised when *all* of carbon 5 and *none* of carbon 1 was lost in the decarboxylation of α-ketoglutarate. In fact, citrate is *prochiral* and so the two ends are distinguishable (see next problem).

20. The enzyme can provide a "3-point landing" at sites X', Y', and H', to bind groups X, Y, and always the lower H (never the upper H on the small molecule). The two hydrogens on the tetrahedral carbon atom in the drawing are therefore distinguishable based on their relative orientations with respect to X and Y. The molecule $CXYH_2$ is "prochiral."

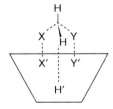

21. (a) A balanced equation for the oxidation of citrate would be

$$C_6H_8O_7 + 4.5\ O_2 \longrightarrow 4\ H_2O + 6\ CO_2$$

From the stoichiometry of the balanced equation, 4.5 moles of O_2 would be consumed per mole of citrate, corresponding to 13.5 μmol O_2 per 3 μmol citrate.

(b) The consumption of oxygen is *higher* than a stoichiometric oxidation of citrate would suggest. The result could suggest that the citrate is not being consumed, but rather is acting "catalytically" or is being regenerated in a cycle (as Krebs correctly hypothesized).

22. (a) The presence of arsenite correlates with the disappearance of citrate.

(b) When more citrate is present, a smaller fraction of the total citrate disappears (38% of 90 μmol disappears, whereas 95% of 22 μmol disappears).

(c) A site subsequent to citrate (and more than one step removed) in the citric acid cycle is inhibited by arsenite. (If the immediate step citrate ⟷ isocitrate step were inhibited, then citrate would accumulate, but this is not observed.) At low citrate concentrations, the citrate disappears almost completely because its regeneration is blocked (as some "downstream" step of the cycle is blocked by arsenite). At higher citrate concentrations, some steps between citrate and the block may reversibly approach equilibrium; in this case not all citrate would be depleted.

23. (a) The number of bacterial colony-forming units is much lower in the absence of the gene for isocitrate lyase. (After 15 weeks, the difference is a factor of 100, i.e., fewer than 10^5 cfu without the gene, compared to $>10^7$ cfu when the gene is present.)

(b) Yes. When the isocitrate lyase gene is restored, then the number of cfu also is restored.

(c) The experiment in part b confirms the direct influence of the gene for isocitrate lyase. (Because replacing the gene restores the number of CFU, other possible indirect factors or unexpected side-effects of removing the gene can be excluded.)

(d) The glyoxalate cycle will allow the bacteria to subsist on acetate from the breakdown of fatty acids from the lipid-rich environment. Without the glyoxalate cycle, the synthesis of carbohydrates from lipids is not possible. One can speculate that without the glyoxalate cycle, the bacteria will lack carbohydrates or other key metabolic intermediates.

24. To answer this problem one must follow carbon atoms around the citric acid. Remember that the randomization of carbon occurs at succinate, a truly symmetrical molecule. Also, this problem (and the answers given) assumes that all pyruvate goes to acetyl-CoA. In fact, this is not necessarily true because pyruvate can also enter the cycle at oxaloacetate.

(a) After one round of the citric acid cycle, the label emerges in C-2 and C-3 of oxaloacetate.

(b) The label emerges in CO_2 in the formation of acetyl-CoA from pyruvate.

(c) After one round of the citric acid cycle, the label emerges in C-1 and C-4 of oxaloacetate.

(d) The fate is the same as in (a).

(e) C-1 of G-6-P becomes the methyl carbon of pyruvate and hence has the same fate as in (a).

25. (a) Isocitrate lyase and malate synthase are required in addition to the enzymes of the citric acid cycle.

(b) 2 Acetyl-CoA + 2 NAD^+ + FAD + 3 H_2O → oxaloacetate + 2 CoA + 2 NADH + $FADH_2$ + $3H^+$

(c) No, because they lack these two enzymes and hence cannot carry out the glyoxylate cycle.

26. The energy released when succinate is reduced to fumarate is not sufficient to power the synthesis of NADH but is sufficient for synthesis of $FADH_2$ from FAD.

27. Citrate is a tertiary alcohol that cannot be oxidized because oxidation requires a hydrogen atom to be removed from the carbon atom bonded to the OH group. No such hydrogen exists in citrate. The isomerization converts the tertiary alcohol into isocitrate, which is a secondary alcohol that can be oxidized.

28. We need a scheme for the *net* synthesis of α-ketoglutarate from pyruvate, that is, we seek reactions that will allow all of the carbons in α-ketoglutarate to come from pyruvate. This will be possible *only* if half of the available pyruvate is converted to oxaloacetate by the anaplerotic reaction (pyruvate carboxylase), while the other half is converted to acetyl-CoA by pyruvate dehydrogenase. Here is the set of reactions that must be summed:

Pyruvate + CO_2 + ATP + H_2O → oxaloacetate + ADP + P_i + $2H^+$

Pyruvate + CoA + NAD^+ → acetyl-CoA + CO_2 + NADH

Acetyl-CoA + oxaloacetate + H_2O → citrate + CoA + H^+

Citrate → isocitrate

Isocitrate + NAD^+ → α-ketoglutarate + CO_2 + NADH

Sum: 2 Pyruvate + ATP + 2 NAD^+ + 2 H_2O →
α-ketoglutarate + CO_2 + ADP + P_i + 2 NADH + $3H^+$

CHAPTER 20

1. An oxidizing agent, or oxidant, accepts electrons in an oxidation-reduction reaction. The oxidant itself becomes reduced as a consequence of the reaction. A reducing reagent, or reductant, on the other hand, donates electrons in such a reaction, thereby becoming oxidized.

2. a. 4; b. 5; c. 2; d. 10; e. 3; f. 8; g. 9; h. 7; i. 1; j. 6

3. Biochemists use E'_0, the value at pH 7, whereas chemists use E_0, the value in 1 M H^+ (when the pH is 0). The prime denotes that pH 7 is designated as the standard state for biochemistry.

4. For succinate + FAD $\rightarrow$ fumarate + $FADH_2$, $\Delta E'_0$ is ~ 0.00 V $-(0.03)$ V $= -0.03$ V, and $\Delta G^{o\prime}$ is $\sim(-2)(96.48$ kJ mol^{-1} V^{-1} $(-0.03$ V$) = +5.8$ kJ mol^{-1}.

   For succinate + NAD^+ $\rightarrow$ fumarate + NADH + H^+, $\Delta E'_0 = -0.32$ V $- (0.03)$ V $= -0.35$ V,
   and $\Delta G^{o\prime}$ is $= (-2)(96.48$ kJ mol^{-1} $V^{-1})(-0.35$ V$) = \underline{+67.5$ kJ $mol^{-1}}$.

   The oxidation of succinate by NAD^+ is not thermodynamically feasible; the energy cost is too high. When E'_0 is assumed to be nearly 0 V for the FAD-$FADH_2$ redox couple, then the value of $\Delta G^{o\prime}$ is only mildly positive (slightly unfavorable yet still feasible).

5. The most bacteria-like mitochondrial genome, that of the protozoan *Reclinomonas Americana,* consists of 97 genes, of which 62 genes encode proteins. The protein-encoding genes in the bacterium *E. coli* include all of the protein-coding genes found in all of the sequenced mitochondrial genomes, even though they comprise only 2% of the protein-coding genes of *E. coli*. Thus, 2% of bacterial genes are found in all examined mitochondria. It seems unlikely that mitochondrial genomes resulting from several endosymbiotic events could have been independently reduced to the same set of genes found in *R. americana*. The simplest explanation is that the endosymbiotic event took place just once and that all existing mitochondria are descendants of that ancestor.

6. Pyruvate accepts electrons and is thus the oxidant.

   NADH gives up electrons and is the reductant.

7. The $\Delta E'_0$ value can be altered by changing the environment around the iron ion.

8. $\Delta G^{o\prime} = -nF\Delta E'_0$

9. The ten isoprene units render coenzyme Q soluble in the hydrophobic environment of the inner mitochondrial membrane. The two oxygen atoms of coenzyme Q can reversibly bind two electrons and two protons as the molecule transitions between the quinone form and the quinol form.

10. Based on the E'_0 values and the role of ubiquinone, the order is:

    (c) NADH-Q reductase ($E'_0 = -0.32$ V).

    (e) Ubiquinone carries electrons from NADH-Q reductase to Q-cytochrome *c* oxidoreductase.

    (b) Q-cytochrome *c* oxidoreductase ($E'_0 = +0.04$ V).

    (a) cytochrome *c* ($E'_0 = +0.22$ V).

    (d) cytochrome *c* oxidase(/O_2) ($E'_0 = +0.82$ V).

11. (a) Complex I is NADH-Q oxidoreductase (answer 4).

    (b) Complex II is succinate-Q reductase (answer 3).

    (c) Complex III is Q-cytochrome *c* oxidoreductase (answer 1).

    (d) Complex IV is cytochrome *c* oxidase (answer 5).

    (e) Ubiquinone is a mobile electron carrier, coenzyme Q (answer 2).

12. Hydroxyl radical, (OH•) hydrogen peroxide (H_2O_2), superoxide ion (O_2^-) , and peroxide (O_2^{2-}) are small molecules that react with a host of macromolecules—

including proteins, nucleotides, and lipids. The reactions damage the respective macromolecules and disrupt cell structure and function.

13. The results with each inhibitor follow the order of components in the electron-transport chain. Components before the block point will be reduced, whereas components after the block point will be oxidized. Therefore:

    - with rotenone, NADH and NADH-Q oxidoreductase will be reduced; and the remainder will be oxidized.
    - with antimycin A, NADH, NADH-Q oxidoreductase and coenzyme Q will be reduced; and the remainder will be oxidized.
    - with cyanide, all will be reduced.

14. The respirasome is yet another example illustrating the advantages of using supramolecular complexes in biochemistry. Having the three complexes that are proton pumps associated with one another will enhance the efficiency of electron flow from complex to complex, which in turn will cause more-efficient proton pumping.

15. Recall that during the cleavage of fructose 1,6-bisphosphate, glyceraldehyde 3-phosphate and dihydroxyacetone phosphate are formed. Only glyceraldehyde 3-phosphate can proceed through glycolysis to pyruvate. Although it can be converted to glycerol by some cells, dihydroxyacetone phosphate is a dead-end in glycolysis; to proceed further it must be converted to glyceraldehyde 3-phosphate by triose phosphate isomerase.

16. (a) Vitamins C and E.
    (b) Exercise induces superoxide dismutase, which converts ROS into hydrogen peroxide and oxygen.
    (c) The answer to this question is not fully established. Two possibilities are (1) the suppression of ROS by vitamins may prevent the expression of more superoxide dismutase, or (2) some ROS may be signal molecules that could be required to stimulate insulin-sensitivity pathways.

17. Succinate dehydrogenase is a component of both the citric acid cycle and Complex II of the electron-transport chain.

18. In fermentations, organic compounds are both the donors and the acceptors of electrons. In respiration, the electron donor is usually an organic compound, whereas the electron acceptor is an inorganic molecule, such as oxygen.

19. The reduction potential of $FADH_2$ is less than that of NADH. Consequently, when those electrons are passed along to oxygen, less energy is released. The consequence of the difference is that electron flow from $FADH_2$ to O_2 pumps fewer protons than do the electrons from NADH.

20. Inhibitors of electron transport cause the electron carriers between the source of electrons (e.g., NADH, $FADH_2$) and the point of inhibition to become more reduced while the electron carriers between the point of inhibition and O_2 become more oxidized.

    Thus there is a "crossover point" from reduced carriers to oxidized carriers. Therefore, from the information given we conclude that the inhibitor acts somewhere between QH_2 and cytochrome c; it prevents the reduction of cytochrome c by QH_2.

CHAPTER 21

1. The ATP is recycled by processes that generate ATP, most notably oxidative phosphorylation.

2. a. 4; b. 6; c. 8; d.1; e. 10; f. 9; g. 2; h. 3; i. 5; j 7.

3. (a) 12.5 (b) 15 (c) 32 (d) 13.5 (e) 30 (f) 16

These answers are readily obtained if one remembers the ATP yields from the various parts of glycolysis and remembers that (1) cytoplasmic NADH yields only 1.5 ATP, (2) pyruvate → acetyl CoA + 1 NADH yields 2.5 ATPs, (3) each acetyl CoA traversing the citric acid cycle yields 10 ATP (7.5 from 3 NADH, 1.5 from 1 $FADH_2$, and 1 from GTP), and (4) galactose requires 1 ATP for activation, just as glucose does.

4. (a) Blocks electron transport and proton pumping at site 3.

   (b) Blocks electron transport and ATP synthesis by inhibiting the exchange of ATP and ADP across the inner mitochondrial membrane.

   (c) Blocks electron transport and proton pumping at site 1.

   (d) Blocks ATP synthesis without inhibiting electron transport by dissipating the proton gradient.

   (e) Blocks electron transport and proton pumping at site 3.

   (f) Blocks electron transport and proton pumping at site 2.

5. The electron-transport chain and the ATP synthase are coupled because both involve a proton gradient across a membrane. The electron-transport chain established the proton gradient, while the ATP synthase dissipates the proton gradient. If the ATP synthease is inhibited, the proton gradient will remain large, the barrier to further proton pumping will be high, and consequently electron transport will cease.

6. Initially, the mitochondrial suspension (if fresh) will be respiring at a slow rate. The rate of oxygen consumption (and electron transport) will increase when glucose is added, increase further when ADP and P_i are added, and increase still further when citrate is added. Then the addition of oligomycin will stop ATP synthesis, electron transport, and the uptake of oxygen. The subsequent additions will have no effect because the system already is inhibited by oligomycin. The graph below summarizes these effects.

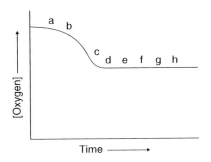

7. Such a defect (called *Luft's syndrome*) was found in a 38-year-old woman who was incapable of performing prolonged physical work. Her basal metabolic rate was more than twice normal, but her thyroid function was normal. A muscle biopsy showed that her mitochondria were highly variable and atypical in structure. Biochemical studies then revealed that oxidation and phosphorylation were not tightly coupled in these mitochondria. In this patient, much of the energy of fuel molecules was converted into heat rather than ATP. The development of mitochondrial medicine is lucidly reviewed in R. Luft. *Proc. Nat. Acad. Sci.* 91(1994):8731.

8. Dicyclohexylcarbodiimide reacts readily with carboxyl groups. Hence, the most likely targets are aspartate and glutamate side chains. In fact, Asp 61 of subunit c of *E. coli* F_0 is specifically modified by this reagent. Site-specific mutagenesis of Asp 61 to a related residue such as asparagine could be used to test whether the presence of Asp 61 is essential for proton conduction.

9. Uncouplers allow food energy to be wasted. Glucose is oxidized and electrons flow to oxygen, but ATP is not synthesized, and the energy is not available for biosynthesis. The problem is that the energy will appear as heat. Producers of antiperspirants may like this effect, but the difficulty in controlling body temperature will cause the uncouplers to be toxic.

10. If the proton gradient cannot be dissipated by flow through the ATP synthase, the proton gradient will eventually become so large that the energy released by the electron-transport chain will not be sufficient to pump protons against the larger-than-normal gradient.

11. The proton gradient drives ATP synthesis by means of proton flow through the enzyme. The flow of protons causes conformational changes that convert a T subunit into an O subunit with the subsequent release of ATP. The role of the proton gradient is not to form ATP *per se*, but rather to release the newly formed ATP from the synthase.

12. The arginine, with its positive charge, will facilitate proton release from aspartic acid by stabilizing the negatively charged aspartate.

13. Twelve protons per 3 ATP would be $12/3 = 4$ protons per ATP.

    Fourteen protons per 3 ATP would be $14/3 = 4.7$ protons per ATP.

14. Presumably, the muscle requires more ATP because it has greater energy needs, especially during exercise. This requirement for ATP means that more sites of oxidative phosphorylation are needed, and these sites can be provided by an increase in the number of cristae.

15. If the proton gradient cannot be dissipated by flow through the ATP synthase, the proton gradient will eventually become so large that the energy released by the electron-transport chain will not be sufficient to pump protons against the larger-than-normal gradient.

16. Remember that the extra negative charge on ATP relative to ADP accounts for its more rapid translocation out of the mitochondrial matrix. If the charge differences between ATP and ADP were lessened by the binding of the Mg^{2+}, ADP might more readily compete with ATP for transport to the cytoplasm.

17. The subunits are jostled by background thermal energy (Brownian motion). The proton gradient makes clockwise rotation more likely because that direction results in protons flowing down their concentration gradient.

18. The proton-motive force can be used to drive other transport processes, for example, ATP export from the matrix, or phosphate import into the matrix.

19. If ADP cannot get into mitochondria, the electron-transport chain will cease to function because there will be no acceptor for the energy. A corollary is that NADH will build up in the mitochondrial matrix. Recall that NADH inhibits some citric acid cycle enzymes and that NAD^+ is required by several citric acid cycle enzymes. Therefore, the citric acid cycle will cease operation. Furthermore, glycolysis will stop functioning aerobically but will switch to anaerobic glycolysis so that the NADH can be reoxidized to NAD^+ by lactate dehydrogenase.

20. When all of the available ADP has been converted into ATP, the ATP synthase lacks a necessary substrate and can no longer function. The proton gradient becomes so large that the energy of the electron-transport chain is no longer sufficient to pump against the gradient. Therefore, electron-transport activity decreases and, as a consequence, oxygen consumption falls.

21. Because of the H^+/OH^- equilibrium, the effect on the proton gradient is the same in each case.

22. In reverse, the ATP synthase would pump protons at the expense of ATP hydrolysis, thus maintaining the proton-motive force. The synthase would function as an ATPase. There is some evidence that damaged mitochondria actually use this tactic to maintain the proton-motive force, at least temporarily.

23. Several lines of evidence support the chemiosmotic hypothesis: 1. A closed compartment, intrinsically impermeable to protons, is required to obtain ATP synthesis. 2. Electron transport indeed generates a proton gradient across the inner mitochondrial membrane. 3. Perhaps most impressive is that an artificial system constructed according to principles of the chemiosmotic hypothesis will synthesize ATP. When synthetic vesicles containing bacteriorhodopsin and mitochondrial ATP synthase are illuminated, the light-activated bacteriorhodopsin pumps protons and ATP is synthesized.

24. Yes, the conditions would be appropriate for ATP synthesis, as the inside of the mitoplasts would be more basic (pH 7) than the outside (pH 4). The artificial pH gradient would support ATP synthesis.

25. Recall that enzymes catalyze reactions in both directions. The hydrolysis of ATP is exergonic. Consequently, ATP synthase will catalyze the conversion of ATP into its more stable products. The energy of the proton gradient is needed and is employed *in vivo* to drive the reaction in the direction of ATP synthesis and overcome the tendency toward ATP hydrolysis.

26. The finding with regard to rotenone suggests that malfunctioning mitochondria may play a role in the development of Parkinson's disease. Specifically, it implicates Complex I.

27. The cytoplasmic kinases thereby obtain preferential access to the ATP that is exported by VDAC.

28. Much of the ATP will be trapped inside mitochondria because ATP/ADP exchange is not facilitated in the absence of the translocase. Electron transport will stop because of low levels of ADP and high levels of ATP in the mitochondria (and due to coupling; see problem 4, above). With electron transport slowed, NADH and $FADH_2$ will be in excess, and dehydrogenases such as pyruvate dehydrogenase and succinate dehydrogenase will be inhibited. The low dehydrogenase activity will cause products such as lactate and alanine (from pyruvate, by reduction or transamination, respectively) as well as succinate to accumulate. Furthermore, with electron transport to oxygen incomplete, intermediate oxidation states of oxygen such as H_2O_2 also will accumulate.

29. If the mitochondria function poorly, the only means of generating ATP is by anaerobic glycolysis, which will lead to an accumulation of lactic acid in blood.

30. (a) Vitamins C and E.

    (b) Exercise induces superoxide dismutase, which converts ROS into hydrogen peroxide and oxygen.

    (c) The answer to this question is not fully established. Two possibilities are (1) the suppression of ROS by vitamins may prevent the expression of more superoxide dismutase, or (2) some ROS may be signal molecules that could be required to stimulate insulin-sensitivity pathways.

31. (a) Since P:O is the number of high-energy phosphate bonds formed per atom of oxygen and oxygen accepts two electrons, P/O = ~P/O = ATP/O = $ATP/2e^-$. The amount of ATP synthesized is directly proportional to the number of protons

pumped (H^+_{pu}) and inversely proportional to the number of protons required for ATP synthesis (H^+_{re}). Hence ATP synthesized = H^+_{pu}/H^+_{re}.

(b) Since NADH donates two electrons to one atom of oxygen, the P/O = ATP formed = $10H^+_{pu}/4H^+_{re}$ = 2.5. For succinate ($FADH_2$) oxidation the P/O = $6H^+_{pu}/4H^+_{re}$ = 1.5.

32. Cyanide can be lethal because it binds to the ferric form of cytochrome oxidase and thereby inhibits oxidative phosphorylation. Nitrite converts ferrohemoglobin to ferrihemoglobin, which also binds cyanide. Thus, ferrihemoglobin competes with cytochrome oxidase for cyanide. This competition is therapeutically effective because the amount of ferrihemoglobin that can be formed without impairing oxygen transport is much greater than the amount of cytochrome oxidase.

33. Use the relation $\Delta G^{o'} = -nF\Delta E^{o'}$. Negative values of will be favorable. The cost of ATP synthesis (under standard conditions) is 30.5 kJ/mol, so add this value to $-nF\Delta E^{o'}$, calculated for each number of protons transferred. The result will be the net excess free energy that can support the ratio of [products]/[reactants], using $\Delta G^{o'} = -RT \ln(K_{eq}')$; such that $K_{eq}' = \exp(\Delta G^{o'}/RT)$.

Using, F (Faraday's constant) = 96.5 kJ volt^{-1} mol^{-1}, R (gas constant) = 8.315 × 10^{-3} kJ mol^{-1} °K^{-1}, and temperature T = 298 °K, here is a working table:

n (# of protons)	$-nF\Delta E_0'$	$\Delta G_0'$ to make ATP	Excess $\Delta G_0'$ (residual)	K_{eq}'
1	−19.3 kJ/mol	30.5 kJ/mol	11.2 kJ/mol	(not favorable)
2	−38.6 kJ/mol	30.5 kJ/mol	−8.1 kJ/mol	26.2
3	−57.9 kJ/mol	30.5 kJ/mol	−27.4 kJ/mol	6.3 × 10^4
4	−77.2 kJ/mol	30.5 kJ/mol	−46.7 kJ/mol	1.5 × 10^8

Hence, the translocation of two, three or four protons can drive the synthesis of ATP until the [ATP]/[ADP][P_i] ratio is 26.2, 6.3 × 10^4, or 1.5 × 10^8, respectively. Suspensions of isolated mitochondria synthesize ATP until this ratio is greater than 10^4, which shows that the number of protons translocated per ATP synthesized is at least three.

34. Add the chemical with and without an uncoupler, and monitor the rate of O_2 consumption. If the O_2 consumption increases in the presence of inhibitor and uncoupler, the chemical must be inhibiting ATP synthase. If the uncoupler has no effect on the inhibition, the chemical is inhibiting the electron-transport chain.

CHAPTER 22

1. The energy captured by means of photosynthesis supports all life on the planet. All of the carbons in the complex biomolecules of which we are made enter the biosphere through the process of photosynthesis. Moreover, the oxygen that we require also is produced by photosynthesis.

2. Energy + 6 H_2O + 6 CO_2 → $C_6H_{12}O_6$ + 6 O_2.

Note: The overall stoichiometry for the light reactions is:

2 $NADP^+$ + 3 ADP^{3-} +3 P_i^{2-} + H^+ → O_2 + 2 NADPH + 3 ATP^{4-} + H_2O .

(The ATP and NADPH produced by the light reactions are then used to drive the dark reactions for the synthesis of carbohydrates to give the net result in the equation above.)

3. a. 7; b. 5; c. 4; d. 10; e. 1; f. 2; g. 9; h. 3; i. 8; j. 6.

4. Photosystem II, in conjunction with the oxygen-generating complex, powers oxygen release. The reaction center of photosystem II absorbs light maximally at 680 nm. Light of 700 nm wavelength has lower energy than 680 nm light and does not efficiently drive photosystem II. Photosystem I can be powered by 700 nm light but does not generate oxygen.

5. Maximal oxygen consumption will occur when photosystems I and II are operating cooperatively. Photosystems I and II absorb light maximally at 700 nm and 680 nm, respectively. Oxygen will be efficiently generated when not only the reaction centers of photosystem II are illuminated by 680 nm light but also electrons from photosystem II fill the electron holes in photosystem I, which are generated when the reaction centers of photosystem I are illuminated by light of 700 nm.

6. The light reactions take place on thylakoid membranes. Increasing the available thylakoid membrane surface area increases the number of ATP- and NADH-generating sites.

7. Photoinduced separation of charge is a fundamental step in photosynthesis. The charge separation takes place when a high-energy electron generated by light absorption moves to a lower excited state in a neighboring acceptor molecule. As a result, the negatively charged acceptor molecule possesses a high-energy electron that can be used to generate a proton gradient or biosynthetic reducing power.

8. The idea is to capture more photons. The light-harvesting complexes work with the reaction centers to absorb more light than would be absorbed by the reaction centers alone. The light-harvesting complexes funnel light to the reaction centers.

9. $NADP^+$ is the ultimate electron acceptor, and H_2O is the ultimate electron donor. Light energy powers the electron flow between the donor and the acceptor.

10. A greater pH gradient is required because the charge gradient, a component of the proton-motive force, is less in chloroplasts than in mitochondria. In chloroplasts, the charge gradient is neutralized by the influx of Mg^{2+} into the lumen of the thylakoid membranes.

11. Because chlorophyll is a hydrophobic molecule, it is readily inserted into the hydrophobic interior of the thylakoid membranes.

12. Chlorophyll contains networks of alternating single and double bonds, also known as conjugated double-bond networks. These networks allow the ¿ electrons in the double bonds to be shared extensively instead of each one being held tightly by a particular atom. This situation allows excitation of the electrons by visible light, instead of requiring higher-energy electromagnetic radiation.

13. Protons for the proton gradient in chloroplasts arise from several sources, including (a) those released during the oxidation of water, (b) those pumped into the lumen by the cytochrome *bf* complex, and (c) protons removed from the stroma during the reduction of $NADP^+$ and plastoquinone.

14. The electron flow from PS II to PS I is uphill, or endergonic. For this uphill flow, ATP would need to be consumed, thereby detracting from the ATP yield and working against the purpose of photosynthesis.

15. $\Delta E'_0 = -0.32 - (-0.43) = +0.11$ V. $\Delta G^{o'}$ (to reduce 1 mol of $NADP^+$) = $-2 \times 96.5 \times 0.11 = -21.2$ kJ/mol^{-1} (-5.1 kcal mol^{-1}).

16. (a) Some process for trapping energy from an external source is necessary for life as we know it. Because radiation is an efficient mechanism for transferring the energy, it is likely that photons would be involved in bringing the energy to the places where life exists. (Alternatively, a local and stable long-term source of energy would be needed. Nevertheless, *time* as well as energy is a critical factor because the evolution of life is a slow process. Therefore, the hypothetical energy source would need to be reliable for a long time.)

    (b) No. Electron donors other than water can be used for photosynthesis, for example, H_2, H_2S, or other small organic molecules.

17. DCMU inhibits electron transfer between Q and plastoquinone in the link between photosystems II and I. O_2 evolution can occur in the presence of DCMU if an artificial electron acceptor such as ferricyanide can accept electrons from Q.

18. Cyclic photophosphorylation could occur. Electrons would go from P700* to ferrodoxin to cytochrome $b6/f$ (generating a proton gradient for ATP synthesis), and finally to plastocyanin and back to P700. The site of DCMU inhibition (Q to plastoquinone) is outside this cycle.

19. Exposure to light allowed the generation of a proton gradient, but the absence of ADP and P_i prevented the synthesis of ATP. Therefore, when the chloroplasts were placed in a dark environment with ADP and P_i, ATP synthesis could occur until the proton gradient was depleted.

20. Oxygen generation would stop. The proton-gradient generated by photosystem II would not be dissipated. Soon the gradient would become so great that energy of electron flow in photosystem II would be incapable of pumping more protons. Oxygen generation would halt, and photosystem I also would halt due to a lack of electrons coming from photosystem II.

21. An uncoupler, such as dinitrophenol, would dissipate the proton gradient and allow photosystems I and II to continue cycling electrons, with oxygen evolution, in the absence of a proton gradient or ATP synthesis.

22. The cristae.

23. There are a number of similarities. Both processes take place in membranes. In eukaryotes, these membranes reside inside specialized organelles. Both processes depend on high-energy electrons to generate ATP. Photosynthesis and oxidative phosphorylation both use redox reactions to generate a proton gradient, and the enzymes that convert the proton gradient into ATP are very similar in both processes. The differences concern the sources of the high-energy electrons. In oxidative phosphorylation, the high-energy electrons originate in fuels and are extracted as reducing power in the form of NADH. In photosynthesis, the high-energy electrons are generated by light and are captured as reducing power in the form of NADPH.

24. Both enzymes transfer electrons from $FADH_2$ to a nicotinamide nucleotide: $NADP^+$ in the case of the reductase or NAD^+ in the pyruvate dehydrogenase complex. Such direction of electron flow is uncommon. Usually, electrons flow from reduced NADH or NADPH to FAD.

25. Both photosynthesis and cellular respiration are powered by high-energy electrons that flow toward more-stable states. In cellular respiration, the high-energy electrons are derived from the oxidation of carbon fuels as NADH and $FADH_2$. These electrons release their energy as they reduce oxygen, and they find stability in the water molecules that are formed. In photosynthesis, high-energy electrons are generated when the photopigments absorb light energy, and they find stability in photosystem I and ferredoxin.

26. (a) Thioredoxin is the natural regulator in vivo.

(b) There is no effect on the control mitochondrial enzyme, but increasing the reducing power increases the activity of the modified (chimeric) enzyme.

(c) Thioredoxin enhances the effect of DTT on the modified enzyme by an additional factor of approximately two. Since the DTT alone, especially at the higher concentrations, should provide sufficient reducing power, the additional enhancement with thioredoxin could be due to another effect. For example, thioredoxin could bind to the enzyme and induce a conformational change to a more active state. (In vivo—without DTT—the thioredoxin also would serve a reducing role.)

(d) Yes. The segment that was removed and replaced is responsible for the redox regulation that is observed in chloroplasts but not in mitochondria.

(e) For chloroplasts, the redox potential of the stroma provides a way to link the activities of key enzymes to the level of illumination. Enzymes that do not respond to light directly are thereby able to respond to the levels of reducing agents and have their activities coordinated with the extent of ongoing photosynthesis.

(f) The sulfhydryl groups of Cys are likely to be influenced. The Cys side chains can exist in -SH (reduced) and disulfide (-S-S-; oxidized) forms.

(g) Directed mutagenesis experiments to change selected cysteines to alanine or serine could confirm their importance in the regulatory mechanism.

27. The energy of 1 mol of 700-nm photons is Avodagro's number times hc/λ, with h being Planck's constant, c the speed of light, and $\lambda = 700$ nm. Substituting yields:

$$(6.022 * 10^{23})(6.626 * 10^{-34} \text{ J s})(2.998 * 10^{8} \text{ m s}^{-1})/(700 * 10^{-9} \text{ m}) =$$

$$(0.171 * 10^{6}) \text{ J mol}^{-1} = 171 \text{ kJ mol}^{-1}.$$

The absorption of light by photosystem I results in $\Delta E'_0$ of about -1.0 V.

Recall that $\Delta G^{o'} = -nF\Delta E'_0$, where $F = 96.48$ kJ mol^{-1} V^{-1} (or 23.06 kcal mol^{-1} V^{-1}).

Under standard conditions, the energy change for one mol of electrons is therefore about 96.5 kJ (or 23.1 kcal). Thus, the efficiency is about 96.5/171 = **56.4%**.

28. (a) The energy of photons is inversely proportional to the wavelength. Since 600-nm photons have an energy content of 47.6 kcal/einstein, 1000-nm light will have an energy content of 600/1000 × 47.6 kcal/einstein. Since 1 cal = 4.184 joule, 28.7 kcal × 4.184 = 120 kJ/einstein.

(b) -120 kJ/mol ($\Delta G^{o'}$) $= -1 \times 96.5 \times$ V. Therefore, V $= -120/-96.5 = 1.24$ volts.

(c) If 1000-nm photons have a free-energy content of 120 kJ/einstein and ATP has a free-energy content of 50 kJ/mol, then 1000-nm photon has the free-energy content of 120/50, or 2.4 ATP. Therefore, a minimum of 0.42 (1/2.4) photon is needed to drive the synthesis of an ATP.

29. The Hill reaction uses photosystem I. Electrons from P680 are excited and are replenished by electrons from water (leading to evolution of O_2). The excited electrons in P680* pass to pheophytin and then to Q and finally to the artificial acceptor such as ferricyanide.

30. One needs to factor in the NADPH from photosynthesis because it is an energy-rich molecule. Recall that NADH is worth 2.5 ATP if oxidized by the electron-transport chain. Therefore, 12 molecules of NADPH represent the energetic equivalent of 30 ATP molecules. The synthesis of glucose requires 18 molecules of ATP (directly) and 12 molecules of NADPH (representing 30 additional molecules of ATP; indirectly). In summary, the equivalent of 48 molecules of ATP is required for the synthesis of glucose.

CHAPTER 23

1. Autotrophs can use the energy of sunlight, carbon dioxide, and water to synthesize carbohydrates, which can subsequently be used to provide energy by means of catabolic processes, or to enable anabolic synthesis of required biomolecules. Heterotrophs require chemical fuels and thus are ultimately dependent on autotrophs.

2. There is nothing grim or secret about these reactions. They take place during both day and night. They are sometimes called the dark reactions because they are not directly dependent on light.

3. Stage 1 is the fixation of CO_2 with ribulose 1,5-bisphosphate and the subsequent formation of 3-phosphoglycerate.

   Stage 2 involves the conversion of some of the 3-phosphoglycerate into hexose.

   Stage 3 is the regeneration of ribulose 1,5-bisphosphate, so that a new cycle can begin.

4. a. 5; b. 1; c. 7; d. 2; e. 10; f. 3; g. 6; h. 4; i. 8; j. 9.

5. Rubisco catalyzes a crucial reaction that is widely needed, and the enzyme is highly inefficient. Consequently, it is required in large amounts to overcome its slow catalysis.

6. In the absence of CO_2, the carbamate cannot be formed on lysine 201 of rubisco. Therefore, rubisco is prevented from catalyzing the oxygenase reaction when CO_2 is absent.

7. NADPH is available in the chloroplasts because it is generated by the light reactions of photosynthesis. Therefore it is advantageous for the chloroplast isozyme of glyceraldehyde-3-phosphate dehydrogenase to make use of NADPH as a cofactor.

8. The conversion of ribulose 1,5-bisphosphate to 3-phosphoglycerate does not require ATP, so it will continue until the ribulose 1,5-bisphosphate is largely depleted.

9. The stroma will accumulate Mg^{2+} and become alkaline when protons move out of the stroma and into the thylakoid space. As a consequence, rubisco becomes primed for activity precisely when the light reactions are providing the ATP and NADPH that are required for carbon fixation and glucose synthesis.

10. The light reactions lead to increased stromal concentrations of NADPH, reduced ferredoxin, and Mg^{2+}. By pumping protons out of the stroma, the light reactions also increase the pH.

11. The ATP that is consumed when forming oxaloacetate is converted into AMP. To convert this AMP back into ATP, two molecules of ATP must be used: one to add a phosphate to form ADP from AMP, and then another to add the terminal phosphate to form ATP from ADP.

12. The crabgrass adapts better to the hot and dry conditions. One could speculate that crabgrass may close the stomata of their leaves during the day and use CO_2 that has been stored as malate in vacuoles the previous night (*Crassulacean* acid metabolism).

13. Photorespiration is the consumption of oxygen by plants with the production of CO_2, but it does not generate energy. Photorespiration is due to the oxygenase activity of rubisco. It is wasteful because, instead of fixing CO_2 for conversion into hexoses, rubisco is generating CO_2.

14. High concentrations of CO_2 inhibit photorespiration by competitive binding, thereby preventing O_2 from entering the active site of rubisco.

15. C4 plants have the advantage in hotter environments and so may become more prominent at higher latitudes as well as lower latitudes under the influence of global warming. C3 plants will retreat to cooler regions.

16. C_4 metabolism allows rubisco to function efficiently even under conditions of high temperature that favor the oxygenase activity. Moreover, C_4 metabolism allows desert plants to accumulate CO_2 at night when the temperatures are cooler and water evaporation is not a problem.

17. • The Calvin cycle takes place in the stroma of chloroplasts, whereas the Krebs cycle takes place in the matrix of mitochondria.
    • The Calvin cycle involves anabolic carbon chemistry for photosynthesis, whereas the Krebs cycle involves catabolic carbon chemistry for oxidative phosphorylation.
    • The Calvin cycle fixes CO_2, whereas the Krebs cycle releases CO_2.
    • The Calvin cycle requires high-energy electrons (NADPH), whereas the Krebs cycle generates high-energy electrons in the form of NADH.
    • The Calvin cycle requires ATP, whereas the Krebs cycle generates ATP and GTP.
    • The Calvin cycle embodies a complex stoichiometry, whereas the Krebs cycle utilizes a straightforward stoichiometry.
    • Both cycles regenerate a crucial starting compound, namely ribulose 1,5-bisphosphate for the Calvin cycle, and oxaloacetate for the Krebs cycle.

18. From the stoichiometry of the Calvin cycle, two moles of NADPH are needed for every mole of CO_2 that is incorporated into glucose:

$$6\ CO_2 + 18\ ATP + 12\ NADPH + 12\ H_2O \rightarrow$$
$$C_6H_{12}O_6 + 18\ ADP + 18\ P_i + 12\ NADP^+ + 6\ H^+$$

The production of each molecule of NADPH requires illumination from four photons (to activate photosystems I and II, which also produce the necessary ATP). Therefore, the energy of eight photons is needed for every CO_2 that is reduced to the level of hexose. The efficiency is: $(477\ kJ)/(8 * 199\ kJ) = 30\%$.

19. (a) The C_4 plant is more efficient at higher temperature. Therefore, the curve (on the right) that peaks sharply at about 39°C represents the C_4 plant.

    (b) The oxygenase activity of rubisco increases with temperature. Other key enzymes may become inactive at high temperature.

    (c) C_4 plants are able to accumulate high concentrations of CO_2 in their bundle-sheath cells.

    (d) The C_3 activity depends on passive diffusion of CO_2, whereas the C_4 activity depends on the active transport of CO_2 into the bundle-sheath cells. Once the transport system is saturated (working at maximum rate), then no further increase in photosynthetic activity is possible. By contrast, higher CO_2 concentrations continue to enhance the rate of diffusion and cause increased availability of CO_2 for the C_3 plants.

20. (a) Initially, ribulose 1,5-bisphosphate reacts with CO_2 to form two molecules of 3-phosphoglycerate. Within the first few seconds of the experiments, only 3-phosphoglycerate will be labeled.

    (b) As time passes, the ^{14}C label from CO_2 is distributed around the Calvin cycle, and the other molecules in the Calvin cycle become labeled.

21. The conversion of ribulose 1,5-bisphosphate to 3-phosphoglycerate does not require ATP, so it will continue until the ribulose 1,5-bisphosphate is largely depleted.

22. When the concentration of CO_2 is drastically decreased, the rate of conversion of ribulose 1,5-bisphosphate to 3-phosphoglycerate will greatly decrease, whereas the rate of utilization of 3-phosphoglycerate will not be diminished.

23. (a) CABP resembles the addition compound that is formed when CO_2 reacts with ribulose 1,5-bisphosphate. (b) CABP is expected to be a potent competitive inhibitor of rubisco.

CHAPTER 24

1. Step 1 of glycogen degradation is the release of glucose 1-phosphate from glycogen by glycogen phosphorylase.

   Step 2 is the conversion of the glucose 1-phosphate into glucose 6-phosphate, a reaction catalyzed by phosphoglucomutase.

   Because phosphorylase stops at branch points, debranching enzymes are also needed. Step 3 therefore involves the remodeling of the glycogen branch points and requires two additional enzymes: transferase and α-glucosidase, also known as "debranching enzyme."

2. a. 8; b. 3; c. 6; d. 5; e. 9; f. 2; g. 10; h. 1; i. 4; j. 7.

3. The regulation of glycogen metabolism is different in liver and muscle because while the muscle maintains glucose only for its own use, the liver has a larger role to maintain glucose homeostasis for the whole organism.

4. The active site of phosphorylase kinase is partially blocked in the T state. A structural change in the R state unblocks the active site and leads to the enhanced activity.

5. Two conditions must be satisfied. Phosphorylase kinase is maximally active when it is phosphorylated and when calcium is bound.

6. The enzymatic defect in von Gierke's disease is the absence of liver glucose 6-phosphatase. The resulting high concentrations of glucose 6-phosphate allosterically activate the inactive glycogen synthase b, causing a net increase in liver glycogen.

7. The difference corresponds to the difference in the metabolic role of glycogen in each tissue. Muscle uses glycogen as a fuel for contraction, so when AMP accumulates, the muscle isozyme (the b form of phosphorylase) is activated by AMP, signaling a need for more energy and hence more glucose. Liver uses glycogen to maintain blood-glucose levels, such that the liver isozyme (the a form of phosphorylase) is inhibited by glucose, signaling that the blood-glucose level is sufficient and breakdown of glycogen should cease.

8. Although glucose 1-phosphate is the actual product of the phosphorylase reaction, glucose 6-phosphate is a more versatile molecule with respect to metabolism. Among other fates, glucose-6-phosphate can be processed to yield energy or building blocks. In the liver, glucose 6-phosphate can be converted into glucose and released into the blood. Therefore, the metabolic needs are better reflected by the level of glucose-6-phosphate.

9. The predominant form of glycogen phosphorylase in resting muscle is phosphorylase b in the less active T state. When the muscle is active, the resulting AMP, from hydrolysis of ATP, acts as an allosteric activator to stabilize the more active R state of glycogen phosphorylase b.

10. Epinephrine binds to its G-protein-coupled receptor. The resulting structural changes activate a $G\alpha$ protein, which in turn activates adenyl cyclase. Adenyl cyclase synthesizes cAMP, which activates protein kinase A. Protein kinase A partially activates phosphoryl kinase, which phosphorylates and activates glycogen phosphorylase. The calcium released during muscle contraction further activates the phosphorylase kinase, leading to further stimulation of glycogen phosphorylase.

11. In the liver, in addition to the glucagon-stimulated cAMP-dependent pathway that activates protein kinase A, epinephrine binds to an α-adrenergic receptor that is present in the liver plasma membrane. The receptor in turn activates phospholipase C and the phosphoinositide cascade. The cascade causes calcium ions to be released from the endoplasmic reticulum. The Ca^{2+} ions bind to calmodulin and further stimulate phosphorylase kinase and glycogen breakdown.

12. Glycogen breakdown is inhibited in several ways. First, the signal-transduction pathway stops when the initiating hormone is no longer present. Second, the inherent GTPase activity of the G protein converts the bound GTP into inactive GDP. Third, the level of cyclic AMP becomes depleted as phosphodiesterases convert cyclic AMP into AMP. Fourth, the enzyme PP1 removes a phosphoryl group from glycogen phosphorylase, converting the enzyme into the usually inactive *b* form.

13. Glycogen is an important fuel reserve for several reasons. Glucose can be more readily mobilized as a quick energy source from glycogen than from fatty acids to satisfy the energy needs during sudden, strenuous activity. Unlike fatty acid metabolism, the release of glucose from glycogen can provide energy in the absence of oxygen and thus can supply energy for anaerobic activity. Moreover, the controlled breakdown of glycogen maintains a readily available supply of glucose between meals. Hence, glycogen serves as a buffer to maintain blood-glucose levels. Glycogen's role in maintaining blood-glucose levels is especially important because glucose is virtually the only fuel used by the brain, except during prolonged starvation.

14. The symptoms suggest central nervous system issues. If exercise is exhaustive enough or the athlete has not prepared well enough, or both, liver glycogen in addition to muscle glycogen can be depleted. The brain depends on glucose derived from liver glycogen. The symptoms suggest that the brain is not getting enough fuel.

15. Glucose 1-arsenate would be formed by the phosphorylase. This product would spontaneously hydrolyze to glucose and arsenate. Glucose liberated by phosphorylase in the presence of arsenate would therefore have to be phosphorylated by hexokinase at the expense of an ATP, in order for to the glucose to enter glycolysis.

16. Phosphorylase, transferase, glucosidase, phosphoglucomutase, and glucose 6-phosphatase working together will carry out the job of releasing glucose into the bloodstream when the organism is asleep and fasting.

17. Liver phosphorylase *a* is inhibited by glucose, which facilitates the R → T transition for the enzyme. This transition releases protein phosphatase 1, which inactivates glycogen breakdown and stimulates glycogen synthesis. Muscle phosphorylase is not sensitive to glucose.

18. As an unbranched polymer, α-amylose has only one nonreducing end. Therefore, only one glycogen phosphorylase molecule at a time is able to work on the degradation of each α-amylose molecule. With glycogen being highly branched, there are many nonreducing ends per molecule. Consequently, many phosphorylase molecules can simultaneously release many glucose molecules per glycogen molecule. The mobilization of glucose from glycogen is therefore much more efficient and more rapid than from ±-amylose.

19. a. B and D, the R states of phosphorylases *a* and *b*, are most active.

    b. Phosphorylase kinase catalyzes the C-to-A conversion.

    c. In muscle, AMP causes a transition of phosphorylase *b* from the T state (C) to the R state (D).

    d. In liver, glucose stimulates a transition of phosphorylase *a* from the R state (B) to the less active T state (A).

e. In muscle, glucose-6-phosphate stimulates a transition of phosphorylase *a* from the R state (B) to the less active T state (A).

f. Protein phosphatase 1 catalyzes the A-to-C conversion.

20. When two soluble enzymes catalyze consecutive reactions, the product formed by the first enzyme must leave and diffuse to the second enzyme. Catalytic efficiency is substantially increased if both active sites are in close proximity in the same enzyme molecule. A similar advantage is obtained when consecutive enzymes are held close to each other in multienzyme complexes.

21. The mice will be unable to generate phosphorylase *a* from phosphorylase *b*, but phosphorylase *b* will still have a low level of activity and will degrade glycogen, especially during exercise. Although the T state of phosphorylase *b* is favored, accumulation of AMP during exercise will convert some of the phosphorylase *b* to the active R state.

22. Glucose is an allosteric inhibitor of phosphorylase *a*. Hence, crystals grown in its presence are in the T state. The addition of glucose 1-phosphate, a substrate, shifts the R-to-T equilibrium toward the R state. The conformational differences between these states are sufficiently large that the crystal shatters unless it is stabilized by chemical cross-links.

23. Gluconeogenesis as well as glycogen breakdown is stimulated by glucagon in liver.

24. Insulin binds to its receptor and activates the tyrosine kinase activity of the receptor, which in turn triggers a pathway that activates protein kinases. The kinases phosphorylate and inactivate glycogen synthase kinase. Protein phosphatase 1 then removes the phosphate from glycogen synthase and thereby activates the synthase.

25. By altering the ratio of substrate and product, a cell can alter the net free-energy change in order to favor either a forward or reverse reaction. Typically, cells maintain the $[P_i]/[$glucose 1-phosphate$]$ ratio at greater than 100, thereby substantially favoring the phosphorolysis.

26. Water is excluded from the active site to prevent hydrolysis. The entry of water could lead to the formation of glucose rather than glucose 1-phosphate. A site-specific mutagenesis experiment is revealing in this regard. In phosphorylase, Tyr 573 is hydrogen-bonded to the 2′-OH of a glucose residue. The ratio of glucose 1-phosphate to glucose product is 9000:1 for the wild-type enzyme, and 500:1 for the Phe 573 mutant. Model building suggests that a water molecule occupies the site normally filled by the phenolic OH of tyrosine and occasionally attacks the oxocarbonium ion intermediate to form glucose. See D. Palm, H. W. Klein, R. Schinzel, M. Buehner, and E. J. M. Helmreich, *Biochemistry* 29(1990):1099.

27. One of the consequences of insulin resistance is failure to appropriately inhibit gluconeogenesis and glycogen breakdown, both of which lead to excess glucose. Consequently, inhibition of liver glycogen phosphorylase would help to ameliorate the high levels of blood glucose. The danger is that muscle phosphorylase, which does not contribute glucose to the blood, would also be inhibited.

CHAPTER 25

1. a. 4; b. 1; c. 5; d. 10; e. 7; f. 2; g. 8; h. 9; i. 6; j. 3.

2. Phosphoglucomutase, glycogenin, glycogen synthase, UDP-glucose pyrophosphorylase, pyrophosphatase, and branching enzyme are required for synthesis of glycogen from glucose-6-phosphate.

3. Glucose 6-phosphate $\longrightarrow$ Glucose 6-phosphate   (1)

    Glucose 1-phosphate + UTP $\longrightarrow$ UDP-glucose + PP_i (2)

    $PP_i + H_2O \longrightarrow 2\ P_i$ (3)

    UDP-glucose + $glycogen_n \longrightarrow glycogen_{n+1}$ + UDP   (4)

    UDP + ATP $\longrightarrow glycogen_n + H_2O$ (5)

    ───────────────────────────────

    Sum: Glucose 6-phosphate + ATP + $H_2O \longrightarrow glycogen_{n+1}$ + ATP + $2P_i$

    Thus one sees that the net reaction requires ATP.

4. The enzyme pyrophosphatase converts the pyrophosphate into two molecules of inorganic phosphate, thereby rendering the overall reaction irreversible.

5. The presence of high concentrations of glucose 6-phosphate indicates that glucose is abundant and that it is not being used by glycolysis. Therefore, it makes sense that glycogen synthase should be activated in order that the valuable resource of glucose 6-phosphate be saved by incorporation into glycogen.

6. Glycogenin catalyzes the addition of a carbohydrate chain, consisting of eight glucosyl units linked by α-1, 4 bonds, to each of two subunits in the glycogenin dimer. The modified glycogenin then serves as a primer for glycogen synthase, which extends the glycogen chains with the formation of more α-1,4 linkages.

7. Free glucose must be phosphorylated at the expense of one molecule of ATP. Glucose 6-phosphate derived from glycogen, by contrast, is formed by phosphorolytic cleavage, thus sparing one molecule of ATP. Therefore, the net yield of ATP when glycogen-derived glucose is processed to pyruvate is three molecules of ATP compared with two molecules of ATP from free glucose.

8. During glycogen breakdown, phosphoglucomutase converts glucose 1-phosphate, liberated from the glycogen, into glucose 6-phosphate, which can be either released as free glucose (liver) or processed in glycolysis (muscle and liver). During glycogen synthesis, phosphoglucomutase converts glucose 6-phosphate into glucose 1-phosphate, which reacts with UTP to form UDP-glucose, the substrate for glycogen synthase.

9. $Glycogen_n + P_i \longrightarrow glycogen_{n-1}$ + glucose 6-phosphate

    Glucose 6-phosphate $\longrightarrow$ glucose 1-phosphate

    UTP + glucose 1-phosphate $\longrightarrow$ UDP-glucose + $2\ P_i$

    $Glycogen_{n-1}$ + UDP-glucose $\longrightarrow glycogen_n$ + UDP

    ───────────────────────────────

    Sum: UTP $\longrightarrow$ UDP + P_i

10. In principle, having glycogen be the only primer for the further synthesis of glycogen should be a successful strategy. However, if the glycogen granules were not evenly divided between daughter cells, glycogen stores for future generations of cells might be compromised. To avoid this possibility, it is important that glycogenin synthesizes the primer for glycogen synthase.

11. Insulin binds to its receptor and activates the tyrosine kinase activity of the receptor, which in turn triggers a pathway that activates protein kinases. The kinases phosphorylate and inactivate glycogen synthase kinase. Protein phosphatase 1 then remove the phosphate from glycogen synthase and thereby activates the synthase.

12. The enzymatic defect in von Gierke's disease is the absence of liver glucose 6-phosphatase. The resulting high concentrations of glucose 6-phosphate allosterically activate the inactive glycogen synthase b, causing a net increase in liver glycogen.

13. (a) Allosteric regulation by AMP will be lost, such that muscle phosphorylase *b* will remain inactive even when the AMP concentration is high. Hence, glycogen will not be degraded unless phosphorylase is converted into the *a* form by hormone-induced or Ca^{2+}-induced phosphorylation.

   (b) Phosphorylase *b* cannot be phosphorylated and thus cannot be converted into the much more active *a* form. Hence, the mobilization of liver glycogen will be markedly impaired.

   (c) The elevated level of the kinase will lead to the phosphorylation and activation of glycogen phosphorylase. Glycogen will be persistently degraded, causing little glycogen to be present in the liver.

   (d) Protein phosphatase 1 will be continually active. Hence, the level of the less active phosphorylase *b* will be higher than normal, and glycogen will be less readily degraded.

   (e) Protein phosphatase 1 will be much less effective in dephosphorylating glycogen synthase and glycogen phosphorylase. Consequently, the synthase will stay in the less-active *b* form, and the phosphorylase will stay in the more-active *a* form. Both changes will lead to increased degradation of glycogen.

   (f) The absence of glycogenin will block the initiation of glycogen synthesis. Very little glycogen will be synthesized.

14. (a) With loss of GTPase activity, the α subunit will always be active, so cyclic AMP will always be produced. As a consequence, glycogen will always be degraded and glycogen synthesis will always be inhibited. Little or no glycogen will accumulate.

   (b) Phosphodiesterase destroys cAMP. Therefore, without phosphodiesterase activity, cAMP will always be present. Once again, glycogen degradation will always be active, glycogen synthesis will always be inhibited, and little or no glycogen will accumulate.

15. Similar symptoms could also be produced by a mutation in the gene that encodes the glucose 6-phosphate transporter. Recall that glucose 6-phosphate must be transported into the lumen of the endoplasmic reticulum to be hydrolyzed by phosphatase. Mutations in any of the other three essential proteins of this system can likewise lead to von Gierke disease.

16. Glucagon stimulates glycogen breakdown, and the immediate product of debranching enzyme is free glucose, which is released into the bloodstream. (Note that ~10% of available glucose in glycogen is contained in the α-1,6 branch points.)

17. In similar fashion, galactose is converted into UDP-galactose to eventually form glucose 6-phosphate.

18. Recall that galactose enters metabolism by reacting with ATP in the presence of galactokinase to yield galactose 1-phosphate and subsequently glucose 1-phosphate. On the way to glycogen the latter reacts with UTP to give UDP–glucose. Hence:

   Galactose + ATP + UTP + H_2O + (glycogen)$_n$ → (glycogen)$_{n+1}$ + ADP + UDP + 2 P$_i$ + H$^+$

19. Glycogenin performs the priming function for glycogen synthesis. Without α-amylase to degrade pre-existing chains, the glycogenin activity would be masked by the more prominent activity of glycogen synthase. The α-amylase treatment halts the activity of glycogen synthase by shortening existing glucose chains below the threshold size required for them to be substrates of glycogen synthase.

20. In normal glycogen, branches occur about once in 10 units. Therefore, degradation of this glycogen is expected to give a ratio of glucose 1-phosphate to glucose of about 10:1. An increased ratio (100:1) indicates that the glycogen has a much lower degree of branching, suggesting a deficiency of the branching enzyme.

21. (a) The antibodies will detect only glycogenin, and the glycogenin will be bound to glycogen. Without α-amylase treatment, the glycogen will have a high molecular weight and will remain at the top of the gel.

    (b) The glycogen is digested into small pieces that remain bound to the glycogenin. The glycogenin migration distance now will reflect approximately its true molecular weight plus that of a small bound carbohydrate oligomer.

    (c) Proteins such as glycogen phosphorylase, synthase, or debranching enzymes could also be present, but they were not stained with specific antibodies in the Western blot.

22. (a) The pattern reflects glycogenin bound to carbohydrate chains of varying sizes.

    (b) When starved for glucose, the cells use most of their glycogen and the supply is depleted.

    (c) When the cells are given glucose again, the supply of glycogen is replenished, so that lane 3 resembles lane 1.

    (d) The glycogen supply is replenished within one hour and does not further increase in three hours.

    (e) Amylase digests the glycogen in all samples to small fragments that are bound to the glycogenin, whose size is ~66 kD.

CHAPTER 26

1. a. C; b. BF; c. G; d. F; e. E; f. H; g. I; h. D; i. A; j. F; k. B.

2. The oxidative phase generates NADPH and is irreversible. The nonoxidative phase allows for the interconversion of phosphorylated sugars.

3. Glucose 6-phosphate dehydrogenase activity is regulated primarily by the level of $NADP^+$.

4. When much NADPH is required, the oxidative phase of the pentose phosphate pathway will be followed by the nonoxidative phase. The resulting fructose 6-phosphate and glyceraldehyde 3-phosphate are used to generate glucose 6-phosphate through gluconeogenesis, and the cycle is repeated until the equivalent of one glucose molecule is oxidized to CO_2.

5. Fava beans contain pamaquine, a purine glycoside that can lead to the generation of peroxides—reactive oxygen species (ROS) that can damage membranes as well as other biomolecules. Glutathione is used to detoxify the ROS. The regeneration of glutathione, however, depends on an adequate supply of NADPH, which is synthesized by the oxidative phase of the pentose phosphate pathway. People with low levels of glucose 6-phosphate dehydrogenase will be susceptible to pamaquine toxicity.

6. The nonoxidative phase of the pentose phosphate pathway can be used to convert three molecules of ribose 5-phosphate into two molecules of fructose 6-phosphate and one molecule of glyceraldehyde 3-phosphate. These molecules are components of the glycolytic pathway.

7. The conversion of fructose 6-phosphate into fructose 1,6-bisphosphate by phospho-fructokinase requires ATP.

8. Since the C-1 of glucose is lost during the conversion to pentose, carbon atoms 2 through 6 of glucose become carbon atoms 1 through 5 of the pentose. That is, each pentose carbon is numerically 1 less than its counterpart in glucose.

9. The deficiency appears to be anemia because red blood cells do not have mitochondria, and the only means for them to obtain NADPH is through the pentose phosphate pathway. Other cells will seem unsusceptible because they have mitochondrial NADH, which can be converted by indirect means into cytoplasmic NADPH.

10. The Calvin cycle begins with the fixation of CO_2 and proceeds to use NADPH in the synthesis of glucose. The pentose phosphate pathway begins with the oxidation of a glucose-derived carbon atom to CO_2 and concomitantly generates NADPH. Furthermore, the regeneration phase of the Calvin cycle converts C_6 and C_3 molecules back into the starting material—the C_5 molecule ribulose 1,5 bisphosphate. The pentose phosphate pathway converts a C_5 molecule, ribose 5 phosphate, into C_6 and C_3 intermediates of the glycolytic pathway.

11. Note that in the oxidative decarboxylation of 6-phosphogluconate, oxidation occurs at the carbon β to the carboxyl group. A similar β-oxidation occurs during the decarboxylation of isocitrate in the citric acid cycle. In both cases a β-keto acid intermediate is formed. Since β-keto acids are relatively unstable, they are easily decarboxylated.

12. Lacking mitochondria, red blood cells metabolize glucose to lactate to obtain energy in the form of ATP. The CO_2 results from extensive use of the pentose pathway coupled with gluconeogenesis. This coupling allows the generation of much NADPH with the complete oxidation of glucose by the oxidative branch of the pentose phosphate pathway.

13. Refer to Figure 26.1. Xylulose-5-P with label on C1 will be formed from some of the ribose-5-P molecules. The label on C1 of ribose-5-P will appear in C3 of sedoheptulose-7-P and then in C3 of fructose-6-P. The label on C1 of xylulose-5-P will appear in C1 of sedoheptulose-7-P and in C1 of fructose-6-P. Therefore C-1 and C-3 of fructose 6-phosphate will be labeled, whereas erythrose 4-phosphate will not be labeled.

14. (a) To make six pentoses, four glucose 6-phosphates must be converted to fructose 6-phosphate (no ATP required), and one glucose 6-phosphate must be converted to two molecules of glyceraldehyde 3-phosphate (this requires one ATP). These are converted to pentoses by the following reactions.

    2 Fructose 6-phosphate + 2 glyceraldehyde 3-phosphate → 2 erythrose 4-phosphate *+ 2 xylulose 5-phosphate*

    2 Fructose 6-phosphate + 2 erythrose 4-phosphate → 2 glyceraldehyde 3-phosphate *+ 2 sedoheptulose 7-phosphate*

    2 Glyceraldehyde 3-phosphate + 2 sedoheptulose 7-phosphate → *2 xylulose 5-phosphate + 2 ribose 5-phosphate*

    (b) What really happens is that six molecules of glucose 6-phosphate are converted to 6 CO_2 + 6 ribulose 5-phosphates + 12 NADPH + 12 H^+. The ribulose phosphates are then converted back to five molecules of glucose 6-phosphate by the action of transketolase and transaldolase. By these reactions three pentoses are converted to two hexoses and one triose. Thus six pentoses can be converted to four hexoses plus two trioses, and the latter can be converted to the fifth hexose.

15. The $\Delta E'_0$ for the reduction of glutathione by NADPH is $+\ 0.09$ V. Then $\Delta G^{o\prime} = -nF\Delta E'_0 = -2 \times 96.5 \times 0.09 = -17.5$ kJ/mol^{-1} (-4.15 kcal/mol). Also, $K'_{eq} = e^{-\Delta G^{o\prime}/RT} = e^{17.5/2.47} = 1.126 \times 10^3$. Thus,

$$K_{eq} = \frac{[GSH]^2[NADP^+]}{[GSSG][NADPH]} = 1126$$

After substituting the given concentrations for GSH and GSSG,

$$\frac{[0.01M]^2[NADP^+]}{[0.001M][NADPH]} = 1.126 \times 10^3$$

Therefore,

$$\frac{[NADP^+]}{[NADPH]} = 1.126 \times 10^4$$

and

$$\frac{[NADPH]}{[NADP^+]} = \frac{1}{1.126 \times 10^4} = 8.9 \times 10^{-5}.$$

Remember, in equilibrium constants the molar concentrations of the reactants are raised to a power equal to the number of moles taking part in the reaction. Therefore, in this problem the [GSH] is squared because, for each mole of GSSG, NADP$^+$, and NADPH, two moles of GSH are involved.

16. Labels at C-1 and C-6 of glucose will behave identically in glycolysis (both emerging at C-3 of pyruvate) and the citric acid cycle. Both labels will transfer to acetyl-CoA (methyl group) and will remain in the citric acid cycle for two rounds. Only with the third turn of the cycle will the C-1 and C-6 labels from glucose finally begin to be released as CO_2 (50% of remaining C-1 and C-6 during the third and each subsequent turn). It is important to note that none of the C-1 or C-6 label will be released in the early stages of glycolysis or the citric acid cycle. By contrast, in the pentose phosphate pathway, *all* of the C-1 label (and *none* of the C-6 label) will be released very quickly as CO_2 at the step where ribulose-5-phosphate is formed. We can put all of these facts together to propose our experiment: incubate a portion of each tissue with each labeled glucose sample, and measure the specific activity of CO_2 that is released as a function of time in each experiment. The extent by which release of C-1 label precedes the release of C-6 label will reflect the level of activity of the pentose phosphate pathway. If both labels are released at the same rate by a particular tissue, then the dominant pathway follows glycolysis and the citric acid cycle.

CHAPTER 27

1. First, the triacylglycerols are degraded to fatty acids and glycerol, which are released from the adipose tissue and transported to the energy-requiring tissues. In stage 2, the fatty acids are activated and transported into mitochondria for degradation. In stage 3, the fatty acids are broken down in a step-by-step fashion into acetyl-CoA, which is then processed in the citric acid cycle.

2. For control of triacylglycerol mobilization, glucagon and epinephrine trigger 7TM receptors in adipose tissue that activate adenylate cyclase to produce cAMP. The increased level of cyclic AMP then stimulates protein kinase A, which phosphorylates two key proteins: *perilipin*, a fat-droplet-associated protein, and a hormone-sensitive lipase. The phosphorylation of perilipin (i) restructures the fat droplet so that the triacylglycerols are more readily mobilized and (ii) triggers release of a coactivator for the adipose triglyceride lipase (ATGL). ATGL initiates the mobilization of triacylglycerols by releasing a fatty acid from triacylglycerol, forming diacylglycerol, which then is converted into a second free fatty acid and monoacylglycerol by the hormone-sensitive lipase. Monoacylglycerol lipase completes the mobilization of fatty acids with the production of yet another free fatty acid along with glycerol itself.

3. The ready reversibility is due to the high-energy nature of the thioester in the acyl-CoA. In effect, a high-energy bond in ATP is traded for a high-energy bond in acyl-CoA.

4. $RCOO^- + CoA + ATP + H_2O \rightarrow RCO\text{-}CoA + AMP + 2P_i$.

5. To return the AMP to a form that can be phosphorylated by oxidative phosphorylation or substrate-level phosphorylation, another molecule of ATP must be expended in the reaction:

$$ATP + AMP \rightarrow 2\ ADP.$$

6. There are four recurring reactions for oxidation of saturated fatty acids:
   • oxidation by flavin adenine dinucleotide (FAD)
   • hydration
   • oxidation by nicotinamide adenine dinucleotide (NAD^+)
   • thiolysis by coenzyme A

7. a. 5; b. 11; c. 1; d. 10; e. 2; f. 6; g. 9; h. 3; i. 4; j. 7; k. 8.

8. The order of events for β-oxidation of fatty acids is:
   (b) fatty acid in the cytoplasm
   (c) activation of fatty acid by joining to CoA
   (a) reaction with carnitine
   (g) acyl-CoA in mitochondrion
   (h) FAD-linked oxidation
   (d) hydration
   (e) NAD^+-linked oxidation
   (f) thiolysis

9. Fatty acids cannot be transported into the mitochondria for oxidation. Therefore, the muscles cannot use fats as a fuel; hence the muscle weakness. The muscles can use glucose derived from glycogen. However, when glycogen stores are depleted, for example after a fast, the effect of the carnitine acyltransferase deficiency will be especially apparent.

10. The eighth CoA moiety comes from the palmitoyl-CoA itself. The next-to-last degradation product, acetoacetyl-CoA, yields two molecules of acetyl-CoA by means of the thiolysis reaction with input of only one molecule of CoA.

11. Palmitic acid yields 106 molecules of ATP. This number is derived as follows. The activation of palmitic acid to palmitoyl-CoA requires the equivalent of two molecules of ATP, as ATP is split into AMP and two molecules of orthophosphate. The oxidation of palmitoyl-CoA then yields seven $FADH_2$, seven NADH, and eight acetyl-CoA molecules. The ATP yield in the subsequent respiratory chain is 10.5 from the seven $FADH_2$ and 17.5 from the seven NADH. The oxidation of eight acetyl-CoA molecules by the citric acid cycle yields the equivalent of 80 molecules of ATP. Thus, the

complete oxidation of a molecule of palmitate yields $(-2 + 10.5 + 17.5 + 80) = 106$ molecules of ATP. Palmitoleic acid has a double bond between carbons C-9 and C-10. When palmitoleic acid is processed in oxidation, one of the oxidation steps (to introduce a double bond before the addition of water) will not take place because a double bond already exists. Thus, one of the $FADH_2$ molecules will not be generated, and palmitoleic acid will yield 1.5 fewer molecules of ATP than palmitic acid, for a total of 104.5 molecules of ATP.

12. Consider the balance sheet below.

Activation to form heptadecanoyl CoA	-2 ATP
Seven rounds of β-oxidation:	
7 acetyl CoA at 10 ATP/acetyl CoA	$+70$ ATP
7 NADH at 2.5 ATP/NADH	$+17.5$ ATP
7 $FADH_2$ at 1.5 ATP/$FADH_2$	$+10.5$ ATP
Propionyl CoA, which requires an ATP to be	
converted into succinyl CoA	-1 ATP
Succinyl CoA $\longrightarrow$ succinate	$+1$ ATP (GTP)
Succinate $\longrightarrow$ fumarate + $FADH_2$ (at 1.5 ATP/$FADH_2$)	$+1.5$ ATP
Fumarate $\longrightarrow$ malate	
Malate $\longrightarrow$ oxaloacetate + NADH (at 2.5 ATP/NADH)	$+2.5$ ATP
Total	100 ATP

13. To form stearoyl CoA requires the equivalent of two molecules of ATP. Then

Stearoyl CoA + 8 FAD + 8 NAD^+ + 8 CoA + 8 H_2O $\longrightarrow$
$$9 \text{ acetyl CoA} + 8\, FADH_2 + 8 \text{ NADH} + 8\, H^+.$$

9 acetyl CoA at 10 ATP/acetyl CoA	$+90$ ATP
8 NADH at 2.5 ATP/NADH	$+20$ ATP
8 $FADH_2$ at 1.5 ATP/$FADH_2$	$+12$ ATP
Activation to form stearoyl CoA	-2.0
Total	120 ATP

14. After a night's sleep, glycogen stores will be low, but fats plentiful. Muscles will burn fat as a fuel. Why the caffeine? Lipid mobilization is stimulated by glucagon and epinephrine, both of which work through the cAMP cascade. cAMP stimulates protein kinase A, which stimulates breakdown of triacylglycerols in the adipose tissue. If cAMP hydrolysis to AMP is inhibited (by the caffeine), then protein kinase A will be maximally stimulated and fat will be maximally mobilized.

15. Fats are more highly reduced than carbohydrates and yield more energy per gram and per carbon atom. First, consider the glucose. Two molecules of ATP are produced when glucose is converted to two molecules of pyruvate during glycolysis. Two molecules of NADH also are produced, but the electrons are transferred to $FADH_2$ for entry into the mitochondria. Each molecule of pyruvate will produce one molecule of NADH and one molecule of acetyl-CoA. Each acetyl-CoA generates three molecules of NADH, one molecule of $FADH_2$, and one molecule of ATP. Recall that each molecule of $FADH_2$ can generate 1.5 ATP, while each molecule of NADH can generate 2.5 ATP. So, we have a total of 12.5 ATP per pyruvate, or 25 for the two molecules of pyruvate. The production of pyruvate during glycolysis (above) netted two ATP directly plus three more from the two molecules of $FADH_2$. The total ATP yield per molecule of glucose is therefore $(5 + 25) = 30$ ATP. (Recall furthermore that the net result

of the citric acid cycle is that one molecule of acetyl-CoA yields 10 ATP [from 2 GTP, 2 NADH, and 2 FADH$_2$].) Now, consider the hexanoic acid. Caprioic acid is activated to caprioyl-CoA at the expense of 2 ATP, and so we begin the accounting with −2 ATP. The first cycle of β oxidation generates 1 FADH$_2$, 1 NADH, and 1 acetyl-CoA; leading to $(1.5 + 2.5 + 10) = 14$ ATP. The second cycle of β oxidation generates 1 FADH2 and 1 NADH but 2 acetyl-CoA; leading to $(1.5 + 2.5 + 20) = 24$ ATP. The total yield is therefore $(2 + 14 + 24) = 36$ ATP. Thus, the foul-smelling caprioic acid has a net yield of 36 ATP. So on a per-carbon basis, this fat yields 20% more ATP than does glucose, a manifestation of the fact that fats are more reduced than carbohydrates.

16. Stearate + ATP + 13½ H$_2$O + 8 FAD + 8 NAD$^+$ →
    4½ acetoacetate + 14½ H$^+$ + 8 FADH$_2$ + 8 NADH + AMP + 2 P$_i$

    Note that this equation is the sum of the following three equations:

    (1) Stearate + CoA + ATP + H$_2$O → stearoyl CoA + AMP + 2 P$_i$ + 2H$^+$

    (2) Stearoyl CoA + 8 FAD + 8 NAD$^+$ + 3½ CoA + 8 H$_2$O →
         4½ acetoacetyl CoA + 8 FADH$_2$ + 8 NADH$^+$ + 8 H$^+$

    (3) 4½ acetoacetyl CoA + 4½ H$_2$O → 4½ acetoacetate + 4½ H$^+$ + 4½ CoA

17. Palmitate is activated and then processed by β oxidation according to the following reactions.

    Palmitate + CoA + ATP → palmitoyl CoA + AMP + 2 P$_i$.

    Palmitoyl CoA + 7 FAD + 7 NAD + 7 CoASH + H$_2$O →
    $\qquad\qquad\qquad$ 8 acetyl CoA + 7 FADH$_2$ + 7 NADH + 7H$^+$.

    The eight molecules of acetyl CoA combine to form four molecules of acetoacetate for release into the blood, and so they do not contribute to the energy yield in the liver. However, the FADH$_2$ and NADH generated in the preparation of acetyl CoA can be processed by oxidative phosphorylation to yield ATP.

    1.5 ATP/FADH$_2$ × 7 FADH$_2$ = 10.5 ATP.

    2.5 ATP/NADH × 7 NADH = 17.5 ATP.

    The equivalent of 2 ATP were used to form palmitoyl CoA. Thus, 26 ATP were generated for use by the liver.

18. NADH is produced along with the oxidation of 3-hydroxybutyrate to acetoacetate, and the NADH yields 2.5 ATP molecules. Meanwhile, the acetoacetate is converted into acetoacetyl-CoA, which is hydrolyzed to produce two molecules of acetyl-CoA, each of which is worth 10 ATP when processed by the citric acid cycle. Therefore, the total ATP yield is $(2.5 + 10 + 10) = 22.5$ ATP.

19. It is costly to produce acetoacetyl-CoA because a molecule of succinyl-CoA must be used to form the acetoacetyl-CoA. The succinyl-CoA could otherwise be used to generate one equivalent of ATP (as GTP), and so someone could argue that the yield is reduced by one.

20. For the combustion of fats, not only must they be converted into acetyl-CoA, but the acetyl-CoA must be processed by the citric acid cycle. In order for acetyl-CoA to enter the citric acid cycle, there must be a supply of oxaloacetate. Oxaloacetate can be formed from carbohydrate sources, for example the metabolism of glucose to pyruvate and the subsequent carboxylation of pyruvate to form oxaloacetate.

21. The person will be unable to oxidize fatty acids to begin their degradation. With acetyl-CoA not available from fatty acid degradation, available glucose (and ketogenic amino acids) will be used to produce acetyl-CoA for the citric acid cycle. Therefore, glucose

will be in short supply. Ketone bodies will not form because acetyl-CoA also will be in short supply (as there is an "energy crisis" with energy from fatty acids not available).

22. Liver cells lack the specific CoA transferase that converts acetoacetate into acetoacetyl-CoA, which subsequently would be cleaved into two molecules of acetyl-CoA. The lack of the particular transferase means that the ketone bodies produced by the liver cannot be used by the liver.

23. In the absence of insulin, lipid mobilization will take place to an extent that it overwhelms the ability of the liver to convert the lipids into ketone bodies. When this happens, triacylglycerols will accumulate.

24. Two carbon atoms enter the citric acid cycle as the acetyl group of acetyl-CoA, but two carbons leave the cycle as CO_2 before oxaloacetate is generated. Consequently, no net synthesis of oxaloacetate is possible using the citric acid cycle. Furthermore, the pyruvate dehydrogenase reaction is irreversible, such that pyruvate cannot be synthesized from acetyl-CoA. In contrast, plants have two additional enzymes that enable them to convert the carbon atoms of acetyl-CoA into oxaloacetate by means of the glyoxylate cycle.

25. During starvation, the carbon skeletons of amino acids released from proteins are used to synthesize glucose for use by the brain and the red blood cells.

26. To prevent undue loss of muscle protein during starvation, the muscles themselves shift from glucose to fatty acids for their energy source. This switch lessens the need to degrade protein for formation of glucose. The degradation of fatty acids by muscle furthermore halts the conversion of pyruvate into acetyl-CoA, because acetyl-CoA derived from fatty acids inhibits pyruvate dehydrogenase, the enzyme that converts pyruvate into acetyl-CoA.

27. $Glycerol + 2 NAD^+ + P_i + ADP \longrightarrow pyruvate + ATP + H_2O + 2 NADH + H^+$
Glycerol kinase and glycerol phosphate dehydrogenase are required. Remember, glycerol enters glycolysis as dihydroxyacetone phosphate; hence, the need for a kinase and a dehydrogenase.

28. The reactions of the citric acid cycle that take succinate to oxaloacetate, or the reverse, are similar to those of fatty acid metabolism.

29. (a) The entry of acetyl-CoA into the citric acid cycle will be inefficient because fat and carbohydrate degradation will not be appropriately balanced. The shortage of pyruvate, oxaloacetate, and cycle intermediates cannot be compensated by fats because mammals are unable to accomplish net synthesis of cycle intermediates from fats. The ability to derive energy from fats therefore will be impaired.
    (b) Acetyl-CoA will be converted to ketone bodies in the blood, and the breath will smell of acetone, from the decarboxylation of acetoacetate.
    (c) Yes. The activated three-carbon units from odd-chain fatty acids can be converted to succinyl-CoA and enter the citric acid cycle to allow some net synthesis of cycle intermediates.

30. (a) We can use the data in the figure to construct a double-reciprocal plot (see below). From the slope and intercept of each line (see Chapter 7), we can estimate that K_M is about 45 μM and V_{max} about 13 nmol/(mg-min) for the wild-type enzyme. For the mutant enzyme, K_M is about 75 μM and V_{max} about 8 nmol/(mg-min). The respective values are comparable, and the mutation has little effect on the enzyme activity when the concentration of carnitine is varied.

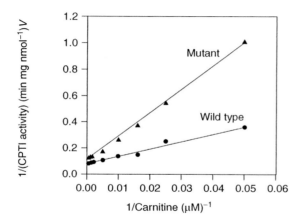

(b) In similar fashion to part (a), we use a double-reciprocal plot to estimate K_M of about 105 μM and V_{max} about 41 nmol/(mg-min) for the wild-type enzyme, and K_M of about 70 μM and V_{max} about 23 nmol/(mg-min) for the mutant enzyme. Once again, the respective values are similar (of the same order of magnitude).

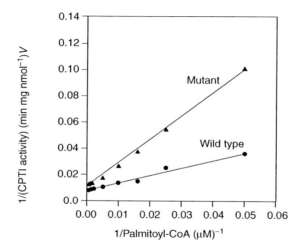

(c) The wild-type enzyme is much more sensitive to inhibition by malonyl CoA.

(d) The mutant enzyme will be more active under these conditions because it retains more than 90% of the activity that it has in the absence of malonyl-CoA. Although the wild-type enzyme is more active without malonyl-CoA, its activity is reduced to about 20% of normal when 10 μM malonyl CoA is present.

(e) Glutamate 3 probably participates in the binding of malonyl-CoA and enables malonyl CoA to be an inhibitor, but glutamate 3 is not necessary for catalysis.

31. (a) The methyl groups on the phytanic acid will block β oxidation. Because the β oxidation cannot take place, phytanic acid accumulates.

(b) How to solve the problem? One strategy would be to remove the methyl groups. Our livers use a different strategy, α oxidation, in which the OH and carbonyl groups are introduced by oxidizing the carbon. One round of oxidation releases CO_2 and converts phytanic acid into a β-oxidation substrate for the next round.

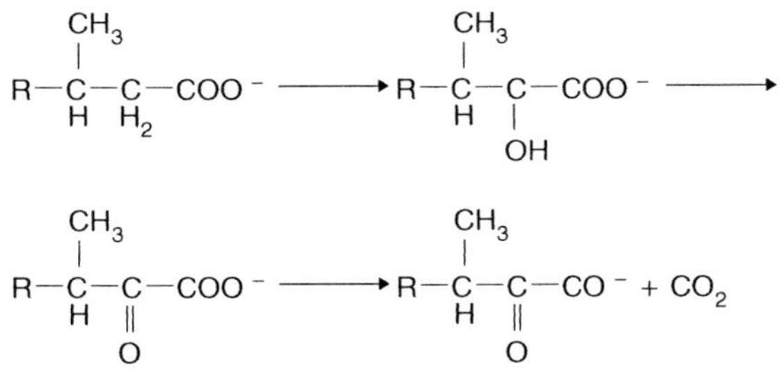

$$CH_3 \qquad\qquad CH_3$$
$$R-\underset{H}{\overset{|}{C}}-\underset{H_2}{\overset{|}{C}}-COO^- \longrightarrow R-\underset{H}{\overset{|}{C}}-\underset{OH}{\overset{|}{C}}-COO^- \longrightarrow$$

$$CH_3 \qquad\qquad CH_3$$
$$R-\underset{H}{\overset{|}{C}}-\underset{\underset{O}{\|}}{\overset{|}{C}}-COO^- \longrightarrow R-\underset{H}{\overset{|}{C}}-\underset{\underset{O}{\|}}{\overset{|}{C}}-CO^- + CO_2$$

When the next methyl group is encountered, another round of α oxidation can be implemented.

32. Radioactive lipids are combusted to acetyl-CoA, which is metabolized by the citric acid cycle. The two carbon atoms that enter the cycle as acetyl-CoA are *not* the same two carbon atoms that leave the cycle as CO_2. Consequently, some ^{14}C will appear in oxaloacetate, which can then be converted into glucose by means of gluconeogenesis, and then into glycogen. While there is no *net* synthesis of oxaloacetate, glucose or glycogen from fatty acids, labeled carbon atoms from the fatty acids can nevertheless appear in oxaloacetate, glucose, and glycogen.

33. There could be a shortage of free coenzyme A. Eventually all of the CoA would be in the form of acetyl-CoA, there would be no acceptor for additional carbons from fatty acids, and no energy could be produced. Moreover, the high concentrations of acetyl-CoA would eventually inhibit fatty acid oxidation (not to mention glucose oxidation). Getting rid of the acetyl-CoA (by generating ketone bodies) solves these problems and allows for the generation of high-energy electrons by fatty acid oxidation, not to mention providing fuel for other tissues.

34. The first oxidation removes two tritium atoms. The hydration adds nonradioactive H and OH. The second oxidation removes another tritium atom from the β-carbon atom.

   Thiolysis removes an acetyl-CoA with only one tritium atom; so the tritium-to-carbon ratio is ½. This ratio will be the same for two of the acetates. The last one, however, does not undergo oxidation, and so all tritium remains. The ratio for this acetate is 3⁄2. The average ratio for all of the acetates is then $(½ + ½ + 3⁄2)/3 = 5⁄6$.

CHAPTER 28

1. 8 acetyl CoA + 7 ATP + 14 NADPH →

   pamitate + 14 $NADP^+$ + 8 CoA + 6 H_2O + 7 ADP + 7 P_i

2. The first reaction is catalyzed by cytoplasmic malate dehydrogenase:

   Oxaloacetate + NADH + H^+ ⇌ malate + NAD^+

   The next reaction is catalyzed by malic enzyme:

   Malate + $NADP^+$ → pyruvate + CO_2 + NADPH

   Finally, oxaloacetate is regenerated from pyruvate by pyruvate carboxylase:

   Pyruvate + CO_2 + ATP + 6 H_2O → oxaloacetate + ADP + 7 P_i + $2H^+$

   The sum of the reactions to generate NADPH from NADH is:

   $NADPH^+$ + NADH + ADP + H_2O → NADPH + $NADH^+$ + ADP + P_i + H^+

3. The committed step in fatty acid biosynthesis is the formation of malonyl-CoA from acetyl-CoA, catalyzed by acetyl-CoA carboxylase.

4. a. 10; b. 1; c. 5; d. 8; e. 3; f. 9; g. 6; h. 7; i. 4; j. 2.

5. By analogy with the balanced equation for synthesis of the 16-carbon palmitate (see text), the balanced equation for synthesis of the shorter 14-carbon myristate is:

$$7 \text{ acetyl CoA} + 6 \text{ ATP} + 12 \text{ NADPH} + 5 \text{ H}^+ \longrightarrow$$
$$CH_3(CH_2)_{12}COOH + 7 \text{ CoA} + 6 \text{ ADP} + 6 \text{ P}_i + 12 \text{ NADP}^+ + 5 \text{ H}_2O.$$

6. By analogy with the synthesis of palmitate and myristate (see problem 5), a balanced equation for synthesis of the still shorter 12-carbon laurate is:

$$6 \text{ acetyl CoA} + 5 \text{ ATP} + 10 \text{ NADPH} + 4 \text{ H}^+ \longrightarrow$$
$$CH_3(CH_2)_{10}COOH + 6 \text{ CoA} + 5 \text{ ADP} + 5 \text{ P}_i + 10 \text{ NADP}^+ + 4 \text{ H}_2O.$$

Therefore, five molecules of ATP and 10 molecules of NADPH are required to synthesize lauric acid (or sodium laurate).

7. The order of steps for synthesis of a fatty acid is:
   (e) formation of malonyl ACP
   (b) condensation
   (d) reduction of a carbonyl group
   (a) dehydration
   (c) release of a complete fatty acid

8. The mutation would inhibit fatty acid synthesis because of a shortage of acetyl-CoA. The enzyme cleaves cytoplasmic citrate to yield acetyl-CoA for fatty acid synthesis.

9. (a) False. Biotin is required for acetyl-CoA carboxylase activity.
   (b) True.
   (c) False. ATP is required to synthesize malonyl-CoA for fatty acid synthesis.
   (d) True. (Palmitate is one of the end-products.)
   (e) True.
   (f) False. Fatty acid synthase is a dimer.
   (g) True.
   (h) False. Acetyl-CoA carboxylase is stimulated by citrate, which also is cleaved to yield the substrate acetyl-CoA.

10. Fatty acids with odd numbers of carbon atoms are synthesized starting with propionyl ACP (instead of acetyl ACP). By starting with a 3-carbon precursor, and then adding 2-carbon units, a product with an odd number of carbons can be achieved. The propionyl ACP is formed from propionyl-CoA by acetyl transacetylase.

11. The avidin in the raw eggs will inhibit fatty acid synthesis by reducing the amount of free biotin that is available as a required cofactor for the acetyl-CoA carboxylase. Cooking the eggs will denature the avidin protein so that it will no longer bind biotin.

12. During the last step of the synthesis, the only acetyl-CoA to be used directly, not in the form of malonyl-CoA, provides the final two carbon atoms at the end of the fatty acid chain. Because palmitic acid is a C16 fatty acid, acetyl-CoA will have provided carbons 15 and 16.

13. The involvement of HCO_3^- is temporary. HCO_3^- is attached to acetyl-CoA to form Malonyl-CoA. Subsequently, when malonyl-CoA condenses with growing acyl-CoA chain to form the keto acyl-CoA that is two carbons longer, the HCO_3^- from malonyl-CoA is lost as CO_2.

14. During fatty acid biosynthesis, the carbon chain grows two carbons at a time by the condensation of an acyl-ACP with malonyl-ACP, with the malonyl-ACP becoming, in every case, the carboxyl end of the new acyl-ACP. Thus, the chain grows from methyl to carboxyl. Since 14C-labeled malonyl-CoA was added a short time before synthesis was stopped, the fatty acids whose synthesis was completed during this short period will be heavily labeled toward the carboxyl end (the last portion synthesized) and less heavily labeled, if at all, on the methyl end.

15. Decarboxylation drives the condensation of malonyl-ACP and acetyl-ACP. In contrast, the condensation of two molecules of acetyl-ACP is energetically unfavorable. In gluconeogenesis, decarboxylation drives the formation of phosphoenolpyruvate from oxaloacetate.

16. The mutant enzyme would be persistently active because it could not be inhibited by phosphorylation. Fatty acid synthesis would be abnormally active. Such a mutation might lead to obesity.

17. The probability of synthesizing an error-free polypeptide chain decreases as the length of the chain increases. A single mistake can make the entire polypeptide ineffective. In contrast, a defective subunit can be spurned in forming a noncovalent multienzyme complex; the good subunits are not wasted.

18. Once glycogen stores are filled, the excess carbohydrates are metabolized to acetyl-CoA, which is then converted to fats. Humans cannot convert fats into carbohydrates, but certainly can convert carbohydrates into fats.

19. Cytoplasmic palmitoyl-CoA provides a signal that fatty acid synthesis is no longer needed. The mechanism of the signaling involves inhibition of the translocase that shuttles citrate from the mitochondria to the cytoplasm. When the citrate shuttle is inhibited, fatty acid synthesis is prevented. Another instance of traffic control is that malonyl-CoA inhibits carnitine acyltransferase I, thereby preventing entry of fatty acids into the mitochondria and inhibiting fatty degradation in times of plenty.

20. Phosphofructokinase is a key regulatory enzyme that controls the flux through the glycolytic pathway. The purpose of glycolysis is to generate ATP and/or building blocks for biosynthesis, depending on the particular tissue. The presence of citrate in the cytoplasm indicates that those needs are met, and there is no need to metabolize additional glucose.

21. (a) Fatty acid oxidation takes place in mitochondria, synthesis in the cytoplasm.
    (b) Coenzyme A is the chain carrier for fatty acid oxidation, acyl carrier protein for fatty acid synthesis.
    (c) FAD and NAD+ are used for fatty acid oxidation, NADPH for synthesis.
    (d) The L isomer of 3-hydroxyacyl-CoA is an intermediate in fatty acid oxidation, the D isomer in synthesis.
    (e) The direction of degradation is from carboxyl to methyl in oxidation of fatty acids. The direction of synthesis is from methyl to carboxyl.
    (f) The enzymes of fatty acid synthesis, but not those of oxidation, are organized in a multienzyme complex.

22. The pyruvate carboxylase reaction (see problem 2, above) is also important in gluconeogenesis. To continue gluconeogenesis, the oxaloacetate produced by pyruvate carboxylase is converted into phosphoenolpyruvate by PEP carboxykinase at the expense of a GTP.

23. The product of the reaction catalyzed by acetyl-CoA carboxylase, malonyl-CoA, inhibits the import of fatty acids into the mitochondria by inhibiting carnitine acyltransferase I.

24. Citrate is an allosteric activator of acetyl-CoA carboxylase. Citrate acts by causing the enzyme to form active filaments (see Figure 28.8). Palmitoyl-CoA causes the filaments to disassemble, thereby inhibiting the enzyme.

25. All of the labeled carbon atoms will be retained. Because we need eight acetyl-CoA molecules and only one carbon atom is labeled in the acetyl group, we will have eight labeled carbon atoms in the 16-carbon palmitic acid.

 One molecule of acetyl-CoA will be used directly and will retain all three tritium atoms. The other seven acetyl-CoA molecules will be used to make malonyl-CoA; each of these will lose one tritium atom on addition of CO_2 and another tritium atom at the dehydration step. Each of the seven malonyl-CoA molecules therefore will retain one tritium atom. Thus, the total number of retained tritium will be (3 + 7) = 10 atoms. The ratio of tritium to carbon is (10/8) = 1.25.

26. The depletion of NAD^+ will inhibit glycolysis. The high concentration of NADH will inhibit gluconeogenesis by preventing the oxidation of lactate to pyruvate while causing the reverse reaction to predominate, leading to lactic acidosis and hypoglycemia. The excess of NADH also inhibits fatty acid oxidation and the citric acid cycle, since the needs for NADH are met by ethanol metabolism. The excess NADH signals that conditions are right for fatty acid synthesis, which leads to the development of "fatty liver."

CHAPTER 29

1. Glycerol + 4 ATP + 3 fatty acids + 4 H_2O → triacylglycerol + ADP + 3 AMP + 7 P_i + 4 H^+

 One ATP is used in the formation of glycerol 3-phosphate and three ATPs are used to convert three fatty acids to acyl-CoAs. The three PP_i formed during fatty acid activation are converted to P_i, hence the total of seven P_i in the equation above.

2. Glycerol + 3 ATP + 2 fatty acids + 2 H_2O + CTP + serine → phosphatidyl serine + CMP + ADP + 2 AMP + 6 P_i + 3 H

3. Glycerol 3-phosphate is formed primarily by the reduction of dihydroxyacetone phosphate, an intermediate in the glycolytic and gluconeogenic pathways, and to a lesser extent by the phosphorylation of glycerol.

4. Three. One molecule of ATP is needed to form phosphorylethanolamine, and two molecules of ATP are used to regenerate CTP from CMP.

5. Each of the three molecules is synthesized from ceramide, and in each case, the terminal hydroxyl group of ceramide becomes modified. In sphingomyelin, the modification involves attachment of phosphorylcholine. In a cerebroside, a glucose or galactose becomes attached to the hydroxyl group. In a ganglioside, oligosaccharide chains are attached to the hydroxyl group.

6. a. 8; b. 4; c. 1; d. 9; e. 3; f. 10; g. 5; h. 2; i. 6; j. 7.

7. (a) A high proportion of fatty acids in the blood are bound to albumin. Cerebrospinal fluid has a low content of fatty acids because it has little albumin.

(b) Glucose is highly hydrophilic and soluble in aqueous media, in contrast to fatty acids, which must be carried by transport proteins such as albumin. Micelles of fatty acids would disrupt membrane structure.

(c) Fatty acids, not glucose, are the major fuel of resting muscle.

8. Either (i) activate the diacylglycerol as CDP-diacylglycerol, or (ii) activate the alcohol to make the CDP-alcohol.

9. Phosphatidic acid phosphatase is the key regulatory enzyme, controlling the extent to which triacylglycerols are synthesized relative to phospholipids, and furthermore regulating the types of phospholipid that are synthesized.

10. Normally, diacylglycerol is acylated to form triacylglycerols. With deficient phosphatidic acid phosphatase activity, there would be a shortage of diacylglycerols that would lead to a severe shortage of triacylglycerols. The amount of adipose tissue would decrease dramatically.

11. Excess activity of phosphatidic acid phosphatase (PAP) would increase the amount of diacylglycerol that is synthesized. Once the phospholipid needs requiring diacylglycerol as a precursor had been met, the excess diacylglycerol would be converted into triacylglycerols. Obesity would result.

12. The three stages of cholesterol synthesis involve: (i) synthesis of activated isoprene (isopentyl pyrophosphate) units, (ii) condensation of six of the activated isoprene units to form the 30-carbon squalene molecule, and (iii) the cyclization of squalene to form cholesterol.

13. (a) None, because the label is lost as CO_2.

(b) None, because the label is lost as CO_2.

14. The hallmark of this devastating genetic disease is elevated cholesterol levels in the blood of even young children. The excess cholesterol is taken up by marcrophages, which eventually leads to the formation of plaques and heart disease. There are many mutations that can cause the disease, all of which result in malfunctioning of the low-density lipoprotein (LDL) receptor.

15. HMG-CoA reductase catalyzes the commited irreversible step in the biosynthesis of cholesterol. Therefore, cholesterol biosynthesis is regulated by the availability and activity the HMG-CoA reductase enzyme. The regulation is implemented at several levels. Transcriptional control is mediated by the sterol regulatory element (SRE) binding protein, a transcription factor. Translation of the reductase mRNA also is controlled. Once formed, the mature reductase may undergo regulated proteolytic degradation. Finally, the activity of the reductase is inhibited by phosphorylation, catalyzed by AMP kinase when ATP levels are low.

16. Statins are competitive inhibitors of HMG-CoA reductase. They are used as drugs to inhibit cholesterol synthesis in patients with high levels of cholesterol.

17. No. Cholesterol is essential for membrane function and as a precursor for bile salts and steroid hormones. The complete lack of cholesterol would be lethal.

18. Five major classes of steroid hormones include the progestagens, glucocorticoids, mineralocorticoids, androgens, and estrogens.

19. Propecia effectively lowers the plasma level of dihydrotestosterone, but dihydrotestosterone is an important embryonic androgen that instigates the development and differeniation of the male phenotype. Pregnant women who had contact with Propecia therefore would risk developmental abnormalities for their unborn male children.

20. A reasonable answer is: "Although it is true that cholesterol is essential and is a precursor to steroid hormones, other aspects of the statement are oversimplified.

    Cholesterol is a component of lipid membranes. While membranes isolate and protect cell components and define cell boundaries, and cells make up tissues, it is nevertheless wrong to say that cholesterol 'makes' cells."

21. The core structure of a steroid is composed of four fused rings, consisting of three cyclohexane rings and one cyclopentane ring. In vitamin D, the second cyclohexane ring (B) is split by ultraviolet light.

22. The apolipoprotein B-100 component of LDL binds to an LDL receptor, an integral membrane protein. The distribution of LDL receptors within the cell membrane is not random, but rather the receptors cluster into regions of the cell surface known as coated pits. On binding, the LDL/receptor complex is internalized by first folding in and then pinching off a small portion of the cell membrane around the coated pit but in a process known as endocytosis, thereby forming an internal vesicle that contains the LDL-bound cholesteryl esters. The vesicle is separated into two components. One component, with the receptor, is transported back to the cell surface where it fuses with the cell membrane, allowing continued use ("recycling") of the receptor.

    The other vesicle component fuses with a lysosome inside the cell. Within the lysozome, the cholesteryl esters are hydrolyzed, and free cholesterol is made available for cellular use. The LDL protein itself is not recycled but rather is hydrolyzed to produce free amino acids.

23. Individual polymorphisms in some of the P450 isozyme genes likely would alter the rates of metabolic degradation (or conversely activation) of particular clinical drugs. Knowledge of the individual differences therefore would help in prescribing appropriately different clinical doses of particular medicines for different individual patients.

24. The small number of cytochrome P450 genes provides an important clue. Indeed, the honey bees may be especially sensitive to environmental toxins, including pesticides.

    With the minimal P450 system, the honey bees may be less able to detoxify such molecules and could therefore be more susceptible to poisoning.

25. Cytidine nucleotides play the same role in phosphoglyceride synthesis as a uridine nucleotide plays in the formation of glycogen. In each case, an activated intermediate (UDP-glucose, or CDP-diacylglycerol, or CDP-alcohol) is formed by reaction of a phosphorylated substrate (glucose 1-phosphate, or phosphatidate, or a phosphorylalcohol) with a nucleoside triphosphate (UTP or CTP). The activated intermediate diphosphate then reacts with a hydroxyl group (the terminus of glycogen; a small alcohol such as, for example, inositol or the side chain of serine; or a diacylglycerol).

    The parallel chemistry involving UTP or CTP is evident at each step.

26. Proteins having such modifications are targeted to membranes. The isoprenoid side chains confer hydrophobic character and insert into lipid bilayer membranes, where they serve to "anchor" a protein to the membrane.

27. When citrate is plentiful in the mitochondria, citrate is transported out of the mitochondria. ATP-citrate lyase breaks the citrate into acetyl-CoA and oxaloacetate. The acetyl-CoA can then be used to synthesize cholesterol.

28. 3-Hydroxy-3-methylglutaryl-CoA is also a precursor for synthesis of ketone bodies. If fuel is needed elsewhere in the body, as might be the case during a fast, 3-hydroxy-3-methylglutaryl-CoA will be converted into acetoacetate, a ketone. If energy needs are met, the liver will synthesize cholesterol.

29. (a) Cholesterol feeding has no effect on the amount of mRNA for HMG-CoA reductase.

   (b) The actin mRNA is a positive control to (1) verify that RNA can be effectively recovered from all samples, and (2) allow normalization of the results, if necessary, to correct for variations in the extent of overall RNA recovery from sample to sample.

   (c) The amount of HMG-CoA reductase protein is greatly reduced when the animals are fed a cholesterol diet.

   (d) Although the amount of specific HMG-CoA reductase mRNA is not affected by cholesterol, the level of HMG-CoA reductase protein decreases to near zero for the cholesterol-fed mice.

   (e) Several mechanisms could explain the presence of the specific mRNA and yet the absence of the specific protein that the mRNA encodes: 1. HMG-CoA reductase could be subject to translational control, so that translation of the message and synthesis of HMG-CoA reductase by ribosomes are inhibited by cholesterol. 2. Alternatively, the protein could be synthesized but then rapidly degraded in the cholesterol-fed mice.

30. The categories of possible mutations in cells from different patients exhibiting familial hypercholesterolemia are:

   (1) no receptor is synthesized. In this case no binding of receptor-specific antibodies would be observed.

   (2) receptors are synthesized but do not reach the plasma membrane because they lack the signals for intracellular transport or do not fold properly. In this case, no binding of antibodies to cell membranes would be observed, but some binding inside the cell might be observed.

   (3) receptors reach the cell surface, but they fail to bind LDL normally because of a defect in the LDL-binding domain. Antibody binding might be observed on membranes if the antibody does not target the LDL recognition domain.

   (4) receptors reach the cell surface and bind LDL, but they fail to cluster in coated pits because of a defect in their carboxyl-terminal regions. Antibody binding will be observed at dispersed sites on cell membranes but not in clustered sites.

31. Benign prostatic hypertrophy can be treated by inhibiting the 5 α-reductase. *Finasteride*, the 4-aza steroid analog of dihydrotestosterone, competitively inhibits the reductase but does not act on androgen receptors. Patients taking finasteride have a markedly lower plasma level of dihydrotestosterone and a nearly normal level of testosterone. The prostate becomes smaller, whereas testosterone-dependent processes such as fertility, libido, and muscle strength appear to be unaffected (see E. Stoner, *Steroid Biochem. Molec. Biol.* 37(1990):375–378). Genetic deficiencies of 5α-reductase are discussed by J. E. Griffin and J. D. Wilson in C. R. Scriver, A. L. Beaudet, W. S. Sly, and D. Valle (eds.), *The Metabolic Basis of Inherited Disease*, 6th ed. (McGraw-Hill, 1989), pp. 1919–1944.

Finasteride

32. As a means of self-defense, it behooves plants to produce a wide array of toxin molecules so as to ward off those who might eat them. Because the plants cannot run from their predators, they employ some extra molecular defense mechanisms.

33. Many hydrophobic odorants are deactivated by hydroxylation. O_2 is activated by a cytochrome P450 monooxygenase. NADPH serves as the reductant. One oxygen atom of O_2 goes into the odorant substrate, whereas the other is reduced to water.

CHAPTER 30

1. (a) pyruvate, (b) oxaloacetate, (c) α-ketoglutarate, (d) α-ketoisocaproate, (e) phenylpyruvate, and (f) hydroxyphenylpyruvate

2. (a) Aspartate + α-ketoglutarate + GTP + ATP + 2 H_2O + NADH + H^+ →
   ½ glucose + glutamate + CO_2 + ADP + GDP + NAD^+ + $2P_i$

    The glucogenic route for aspartate involves transamination to oxaloacetate, conversion of the latter to phosphoenolpyruvate, which is then converted to glucose (see Chapter 17 of the text). PLP and NADH participate as coenzymes in the conversion of aspartate to glucose.

   (b) Aspartate + CO_2 + NH_4^+ + 3 ATP + NAD^+ + 4 H_2O →
   oxaloacetate + urea + 2 ADP + 4 P_i + AMP + NADH + H^+

    This equation represents the summation of the stoichiometry of urea synthesis, the hydrolysis of PP_i, and the conversion of fumarate to oxaloacetate in the citric acid cycle.

3. Most enzymes are specific for either NADH or NADPH (rather than using both of them). Enzymes in catabolic pathways generally use NADH/NAD^+, whereas enzymes in anabolic pathways generally use only NADPH/$NADP^+$. This fundamental distinction in biochemistry enables the catabolic pathways and anabolic pathways to be separately and independently regulated.

4. Aminotransferases transfer the α-amino group of a given amino acid to α-ketoglutarate to form glutamate. The glutamate is then oxidatively deaminated to again form α-ketoglutarate, with release of an ammonium ion.

5. Aspartate is deaminated to form oxaloacetate.

   Glutamate is deaminated to form α-ketoglutarate.

   Alanine is deaminated to form pyruvate.

6. Only serine and threonine can be deaminated directly.

7. Carbamoyl phosphate and aspartate are the sources for the two nitrogen atoms in urea.

8. The statements refer to nitrogen metabolism:

   1. Aspartate provides a second source of nitrogen (c) when arginosuccinate is formed.
   2. Urea is a final product (g).
   3. Ornithine accepts the first nitrogen, which is included within a carbamoyl group from carbamoyl phosphate (f).
   4. Carbamoyl phosphate is formed from NH_4 + (a), together with bicarbonate and phosphate.
   5. Arginine is hydrolyzed to yield urea (b) [and ornithine].
   6. Citrulline reacts with aspartate (d) [to form arginosuccinate].
   7. Cleavage of arginosuccinate yields fumarate (e) [and arginine].

9. $CO_2 + NH_4^+ + 3 ATP + NAD^+ + 3H_2O + $ glutamate $\rightarrow$
    urea $+ 2 ADP + 2 P_i + AMP + PP_i + NADH + H^+ + $ α-ketoglutarate

    The answer in the text is for the conversion of fumarate to oxaloacetate rather than to aspartate. The equation above gives the correct stoichiometry for the synthesis of urea from NH_4^+ and glutamate. It includes a non-energy-requiring transamination reaction. Hence, the number of ~P spent remains at four. Note that aspartate does not appear in this equation, since it is resynthesized. Thus aspartate can be considered a nitrogen-carrying cofactor in the synthesis of urea.

10. The synthesis of fumarate by the urea cycle is important because it links the urea cycle to the citric acid cycle. Fumarate is hydrated to malate, which, in turn, is oxidized to oxaloacetate. Oxaloacetate has several possible fates: (1) transamination to aspartate, (2) conversion into glucose by the gluconeogenic pathway, (3) condensation with acetyl-CoA to form citrate, or (4) conversion into pyruvate. You can collect!

11. The mass spectrometric analysis strongly suggests that three enzymes—pyruvate dehydrogenase, α-ketoglutarate dehydrogenase, and the branched-chain α-keto dehydrogenase—are deficient. Most likely, the common E3 component of these enzymes is missing or defective. This proposal could be tested by purifying these three enzymes and assaying their capacity to catalyze the regeneration of lipoamide.

12. The identities and order of appearance in the urea cycle are:
    (c) ornithine
    (b) citrulline
    (d) arginosuccinate
    (a) arginine

13. Aspartame, a dipeptide ester (aspartylphenylalanine methyl ester), is hydrolyzed to L-aspartate and L-phenylalanine. High levels of phenylalanine are harmful in phenylketonurics.

14. N-acetylglutamate is synthesized from acetyl-CoA and glutamate. Once again, acetyl CoA serves as an activated acetyl donor. This reaction is catalyzed by N-acetylglutamate synthase.

15. The carbon skeletons of ketogenic amino acids can be converted into ketone bodies or fatty acids. Only leucine and lysine are purely ketogenic. Glucogenic amino acids are those whose carbon skeletons can be converted into glucose. Four of the amino acids contain both ketogenic and glucogenic carbon atoms. Fourteen amino acids are purely glucogenic.

16. The end-products of amino acid degradation are:
    * pyruvate (used for glycolysis and gluconeogenesis)
    * acetyl-CoA (used in the citric acid cycle and fatty acid synthesis)
    * acetoacetyl-CoA (used for ketone-body formation)
    * α-ketoglutarate (used in the citric acid cycle)
    * succinyl-CoA (used in the citric acid cycle)
    * fumarate (used in the citric acid cycle)
    * oxaloacetate (used in the citric acid cycle and gluconeogenesis)

17. When one amino acid is missing for protein synthesis, the only source of the essential amino acid will be other proteins. Some proteins therefore would need to be degraded in order to provide the missing amino acid. The nitrogen from the other amino acids in the proteins undergoing degradation would be excreted as urea. Consequently, more nitrogen would be excreted than ingested. Negative nitrogen balance is the result.

18. An appropriate strategy is to bypass fumarate in the urea cycle while still achieving excretion of nitrogen. The defect thereby can be partly bypassed by providing a surplus of arginine in the diet while restricting the total protein intake. In the liver, arginine is split into urea and ornithine, which then will react with carbamoyl phosphate to form citrulline. This urea-cycle intermediate condenses with aspartate to yield argininosuccinate, which is then excreted (because of the enzyme deficiency). As a result, two nitrogen atoms—one from carbamoyl phosphate and the other from aspartate—will be eliminated from the body per molecule of arginine provided in the diet. In essence, the argininosuccinate substitutes for urea in carrying nitrogen out of the body. The formation of argininosuccinate removes the nitrogen. The dietary arginine is needed in order to form the argininosuccinate for the purpose of removing the nitrogen. The restriction on protein intake serves to relieve the aciduria.

19. The enzyme is the "branched-chain α-ketoacid dehydrogenase complex." The complex is required for synthesis of the branched-chain amino acids leucine, isoleucine, and valine.

20. High concentrations of ammonia could increase the ratio of glutamate/α-ketoglutarate (glutamate dehydrogenase reaction) and *increase* the level of glutamate in the brain. Ammonia also could increase the ratio of asparatate/oxaloacetate; the resulting lower level of oxaloacetate would decrease the availability of all citric acid cycle intermediates.

21. The liver is the primary tissue for capturing nitrogen as urea. If the liver is damaged (for instance, by hepatitis or the excessive consumption of alcohol), free ammonia will be released into the bloodstream.

22. The compound should inhibit ornithine transcarbamoylase because it appears to be a nonhydrolyzable analogue of an intermediate that should be formed between ornithine and carbamoyl phosphate. (The CH_2 group in compound A will prevent the release of the phosphate.)

23. (a) The initial surge originates from a need to supply glucose to the brain. When carbohydrates are depleted, mammals cannot resupply glucose from fatty acids. Glycerol provides a small source of carbohydrate, but mammals also must break down amino acids to meet the short-term demands of the brain for glucose. The ammonia byproduct from amino acid degradation accounts for the initial surge of nitrogen excretion.

    (b) Over time, the liver begins to metabolize acetyl-CoA (from fats) to ketone bodies, and the brain adapts to using ketone bodies. During this period, fats can provide many of the energy needs of the brain, and little nitrogen is excreted.

    (c) When lipid stores have been depleted, the organism once again must metabolize amino acids to provide glucose for the brain, and nitrogen excretion again increases.

24. Isoleucine can give its amino group to α-ketoglutarate in a transamination reaction and then be oxidatively decarboxylated and dehydrogenated to form the corresponding (α,β)-unsaturated acyl-CoA derivative. Further reactions (see the figure below) then are identical to fatty acid oxidation until the carbon skeleton is split into acetyl-S-CoA and propionyl-S-CoA. The three subsequent steps for the conversion of the (odd-chain) propionyl-S-CoA to succinyl-S-CoA have been discussed for the oxidation of odd-chain fatty acids (see Chapter 27).

25. In the Cori cycle, the carbon atoms are transferred from muscle to liver as lactate. For lactate to be of any use, it must first be reduced to pyruvate. This reduction requires high-energy electrons from NADH. When the carbon atoms are transferred as alanine, the transamination yields pyruvate directly without a need for high-energy electrons.

CHAPTER 31

1. Nitrogen fixation is the conversion of atmospheric N_2 into ammonium ion, NH_4^+. Only microorganisms possessing the diazotrophic (nitrogen-fixing) capability are able to fix nitrogen.

2. $N_2 + 8e^- + 8 H^+ + 16 ATP + 16 H_2O \rightleftharpoons 2 NH_3 + H_2 + 16 ADP + 16 P_i$

   The fixation of nitrogen is an exergonic reaction. The role of ATP is to reduce the activation energy. When the energy barriers in the reaction pathway are lowered through the coupled hydrolysis of ATP, the reaction becomes kinetically feasible.

3. a. 4; b. 8; c. 10; d. 6; e. 7; f. 9; g. 3; h. 5; i. 2; j. 1.

4. Two main components required for nitrogen fixation are the reductase, which provides electrons with high reducing power, and the nitrogenase, which requires ATP hydrolysis while it uses the electrons to reduce N_2 to NH_3.

5. The statement is false. Nitrogen fixation is thermodynamically favorable. Nitrogenase is required because there is a high activation barrier that renders the process kinetically disfavored.

6. The bacteria provide the plant with a source of vitally necessary reduced nitrogen in the form of ammonia by reducing the atmospheric nitrogen gas (N_2). This reduction is energetically very expensive, and the bacteria use ATP from the plant to accomplish the task.

7. Human beings can synthesize some of the amino acids, but not others. We do not have particular biochemical pathways to synthesize certain amino acids from simpler precursors. Consequently, these amino acids that humans cannot synthesize are "essential" and must be obtained from the diet.

8. The carbon precursors of the 20 amino acids are the keto acids pyruvate, oxaloacetate, and α-ketoglutarate, along with 3-phosphoglycerate, phosphoenolpyruvate, ribose-5-phosphate, and erythrose-4-phosphate.

9. Pyridoxal phosphate is required by all transaminases.

10. Transamination is the main reaction involved here. A reversible transamination reaction will transfer the labeled amino group from aspartate to α-ketoglutarate to form glutamate, with oxaloacetate as the side-product α-keto acid derived from the aspartate. Glutamate then is the principal amino group donor for the synthesis of many other amino acids by means of transamination reactions involving their corresponding α-keto acids.

11. Tetrahydrofolate is a carrier of a variety of one-carbon units.

12. Both of these coenzymes carry one-carbon units. S-Adenosylmethionine has a greater transfer potential for methyl groups. Tetrahydrofolate can transfer carbon atoms in many different oxidation states.

13. The ^{18}O labeling pattern suggests that γ-glutamyl phosphate is a likely reaction intermediate in the synthesis of glutamine.

14. Alanine and aspartate can be synthesized directly from glutamate by transamination of pyruvate and oxaloacetate, respectively. Glutamate is the common intermediate that serves as the amino group donor in these reactions. (α-Ketoglutarate, the side-product, can condense with another molecule of ammonia to regenerate the glutamate for further transamination reactions.)

15. Each final product should inhibit the first *unique* step toward its synthesis, that is, the first step following the branch point of the pathway. Thus, Y should inhibit the conversion of C to D, and Z should inhibit the conversion of C to F. (To avoid wasteful accumulation of C or B if neither Y nor Z is needed, high levels of C should also inhibit the conversion of A to B at the beginning of the pathway.)

16. The effects would multiply so that the net rate would equal ($100 \times 0.6 \times 0.4$ s^{-1}), or 24 s^{-1}.

17. Tetrahydrofolate, S-adenosylmethionine, and biotin are coenzymes that carry activated one-carbon units. Biotin carries CO_2, S-adenosylmethionine carries methyl groups, and tetrahydrofolate can carry single carbon atoms in a variety of different oxidation states. Additionally, vitamin B_{12} is required for some one-carbon transfer reactions (see question 18).

18. In addition to methionine synthase, we have encountered methylmalonyl CoA mutase, an enzyme required for the degradation of odd-chain fatty acids. Indeed, these are the only two mammalian enzymes that require vitamin B_{12}.

19. Lipid biosynthesis also would be affected. Methionine is a component of S-adenosylmethionine, which is the methyl donor for the synthesis of phosphatidylcholine from phosphatidylethanolamine.

20. (a) Asn, Gln, and Gly are affected. Asn is much more concentrated in dark-adapted plants, whereas Gln and Gly are present in somewhat elevated levels in light-adapted plants.

    (b) The transcription of specific mRNA, translation or enzymatic activity of several enzymes, particularly nitrogen-utilizing enzymes such as asparagine synthetase and glutamine synthetase, could be regulated by light.

    (c) From the graph, asparagine would appear to be a likely candidate. (The name of the plant would also suit this interpretation!)

21. Glucose + 2 ADP + 2 P_i + 2 NAD^+ + 2 glutamate → 2 alanine + 2 α-ketoglutarate + 2 ATP + 2 NADH + H^+

    Glucose is converted to pyruvate via glycolysis, and pyruvate is converted to alanine by transamination.

22. Aspartate and glutamate would be synthesized from the citric acid cycle intermediates oxaloacetate and α-ketoglutarate. Increased synthesis of aspartate and glutamate therefore could begin to deplete citric acid cycle intermediates. The cell would need to respond by breaking down carbohydrates to replenish the supply by net synthesis of new cycle intermediates.

23. The strategy is to use the energy from ATP hydrolysis to capture ammonia when it is scarce. Because the value of K_M of glutamate dehydrogenase for NH_4^+ is very high (>> 1 mM), this enzyme is not saturated and is not working effectively when NH_4^+ is limiting. In contrast, glutamine synthase has very high affinity for NH_4^+ and therefore will work when the concentration of NH_4^+ is low. Thus when ammonia is scarce, the combined reactions of glutamine synthase and glutamate synthase are effective.

CHAPTER 32

1. In de novo synthesis, the nucleotides are synthesized from simpler precursor compounds, in essence from scratch. In salvage pathways, preformed bases are recovered and attached to riboses.

2. Glucose + 2 ATP + 2 $NADP^+$ + H_2O → PRPP + CO_2 + ADP + AMP + 2 NADPH + H^+.

    This equation is the summation of the following conversions: glucose → glucose 6-phosphate → ribose 5-phosphate → PRPP.

3. Glutamine + aspartate + CO_2 + 2 ATP + NAD^+ → orotate + 2 ADP + 2 P_i + glutamate + NADH + H^+

4. (a, c) PRPP, (b) carbamoyl phosphate

5. A nucleoside is a base attached to ribose. A nucleotide is a phosphorylated nucleoside in which the ribose ring bears one or more phosphates.

6. (a) Excessive urate can cause gout (9).

    (b) Lack of adenosine deaminase will lead to immunodeficiency (7).

    (c) Lack of GPRT causes Lesch-Nyhan disease (6).

    (d) Carbamoyl phosphate is coupled during the first step in pyrimidine synthesis (10).

    (e) Inosinate is a precursor to both ATP and GTP (2).

    (f) Ribonucleotide reductase is required for deoxynucleotide synthesis (4).

    (g) Lack of folic acid can cause spina bifida (1).

(h) Glutamine phosphoribosyl transferase catalyzes the committed step in purine synthesis (11).

(i) A pyrimidine (8) contains a single aromatic ring.

(j) A purine (3) contains a bicyclic aromatic ring.

(k) UTP (5) is a precursor to CTP.

7. The serine side chain is reduced from CH_2OH to $CH_2/(CH_3)$ as the carbon is transferred first to N^5, N^{10}-methylene-tetrahydrofolate, and then to carbon 5 of the uracil ring in dUMP to form dTMP in the overall net reaction: dUMP + serine + NADPH + $H^+ \rightarrow$ dTMP + glycine + NADP$^+$.

8. There is a deficiency of N^{10}-formyltetrahydrofolate. Sulfanilamide inhibits the synthesis of folate by acting as an analog of p-aminobenzoate, one of the precursors of folate.

9. PRPP is the activated intermediate in the synthesis of (a) phosphoribosylamine in the de novo pathway of purine formation, (b) purine nucleotides from free bases by the salvage pathway, (c) orotidylate in the formation of pyrimidines, (d) nicotinate ribonucleotide, (e) phosphoribosyl-ATP in the pathway leading to histidine, and (f) phosphoribosylanthranilate in the pathway leading to tryptophan.

10. The reciprocal substrate relation refers to the fact that AMP synthesis requires GTP, whereas GMP synthesis requires ATP. These requirements tend to balance the synthesis of ATP and GTP.

11. Seven high-energy phosphate bonds are hydrolyzed during synthesis of CTP:

The synthesis of carbamoyl phosphate requires 2 ATP.

The formation of PRPP from ribose 5-phosphate yields an AMP (equivalent to 2 ATP)*.

The conversion of UMP to UTP requires 2 ATP.

The conversion of UTP to CTP requires 1 ATP.

Total 7 ATP.

* Remember that two high-energy phosphate bonds are expended when AMP is produced because the AMP must be converted first to ADP and then to ATP during the resynthesis.

12. As shown below for cytidylate, ring carbons 4, 5, and 6 in cytosine originate from Asp. C6 from the α-carbon will be labeled with ^{13}C. (Carbon 2 comes from carbamoyl phosphate.)

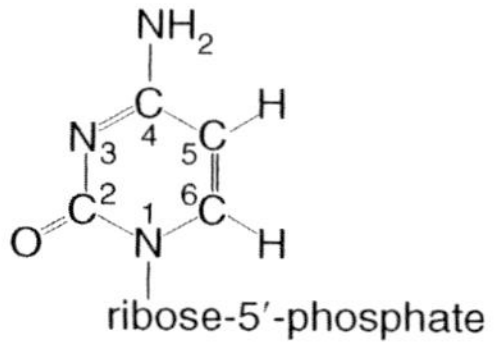

ribose-5'-phosphate

In guanylate (shown below), the bridge carbons #4 and #5 and N7 originate from glycine. C5 from the α-carbon of Gly will be labeled with ^{13}C. These bridge carbons and N^7 originate from glycine. (Carbons 2 and 8 come from formyl-tetrahydrofolate, while carbon 6 comes from bicarbonate.)

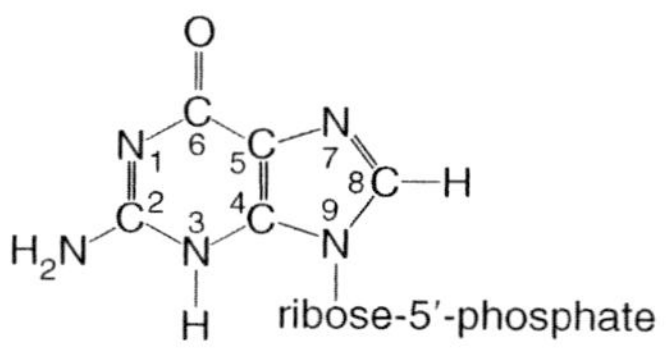

ribose-5'-phosphate

13. Glutamine supplies the nitrogen (via ammonia) for 5-phosphoribosyl-1-amine; this nitrogen becomes atom 9 in the final purine ring (see standard numbering in Figure 32.4). Glutamine also supplies the incoming (third) nitrogen for formation of formyl-glycineamidine ribonucleotide (step 3 in Figure 32.5); this nitrogen becomes atom 3 in the final purine ring. Therefore nitrogen atoms 3 and 9 in the purine ring become labeled.

14. (a) Lack of aspartate will cause carboxyaminoimidazole ribonucleotide to accumulate (blocking step 6 in Figure 32.5).

   (b) Lack of tetrahydrofolate will cause glycinamide ribonucleotide to accumulate (blocking step 2 in Figure 32.5).

   (c) Lack of glycine will cause phosphoribosyl amine to accumulate (blocking step 1 in Figure 32.5).

   (d) Lack of glutamine will inhibit the initial committed step in purine biosynthesis, formation of 5-phosphoribosyl-1-amine, and also will cause formylglycinamide ribonucleotide to accumulate (blocking step 3 in Figure 32.5).

15. Allopurinol, an analog of hypoxanthine, is a suicide inhibitor of xanthine oxidase. Inhibiting this enzyme would help to reduce the oversupply of purine nucleotides.

16. These patients have a high level of urate because of the breakdown of nucleic acids. Allopurinol prevents the formation of kidney stones and blocks other deleterious consequences of hyperuricemia by inhibiting the formation of urate.

17. Because folate is required for nucleotide synthesis, cells that are dividing rapidly would be most readily affected. They would include cells of the intestine, which are constantly replaced, and precursors to blood cells. A lack of intestinal cells and blood cells would account for the symptoms often observed.

18. IMP is the product of the pathway for de novo purine biosynthesis and the precursor of AMP and GMP. With the de novo pathway for purines not working effectively, it would be helpful to stimulate the salvage pathway, perhaps with a diet that is rich in nucleotides that would then be a source of the preformed purine bases hypoxanthine, adenine, and guanine.

19. N^1 in the purine ring of IMP, AMP, ATP, GMP, and GTP will be labeled, following the scheme below:

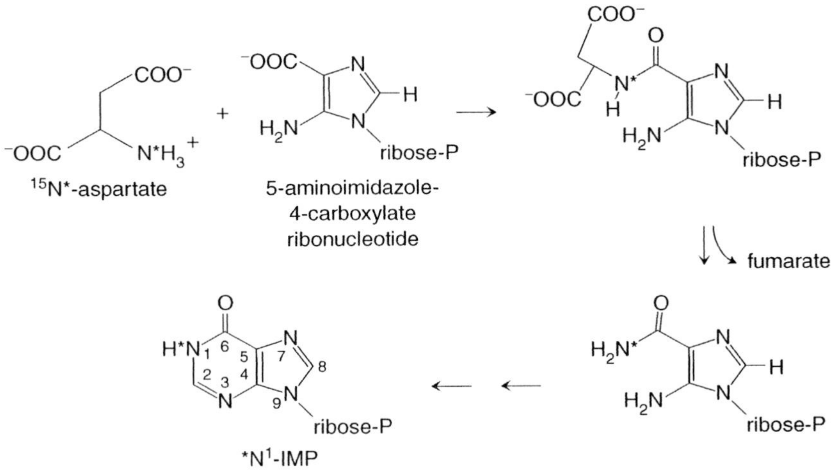

20. By their nature, cancer cells divide rapidly and thus require more frequent DNA synthesis than normal or resting cells that divide infrequently. Inhibitors of TMP synthesis will impair DNA synthesis and therefore will be more toxic to cancer cells than to normal cells. This principle of inhibiting DNA synthesis with minimal impact on cells that are not dividing is one of the strategies for inhibiting cancer growth.

21. (a) Cyclic-(5'-3')-AMP and cyclic GMP influence many intracellular processes.

    (b) ATP is the prototype energy-storage molecule with a high phosphoryl-group transfer potential.

    (c) ATP is a phosphate donor for generating glucose-6-phosphate and fructose-1,6-bisphosphate.

    (d) Flavin adenine dinucleotide (FAD) and nicotinamide adenine dinucleotide (NAD$^+$) participate in the production of acetyl-CoA ("active acetate") from pyruvate by the pyruvate dehydrogenase complex.

    (e) NADH and FADH2 are reduced molecules that have a high electron-transfer potential.

    (f) Synthetic (2',3')-dideoxynucleoside triphosphates serve as chain terminators for DNA sequencing. (The four natural deoxynucleoside triphosphates—dGTP, dCTP, dATP, and dTTP—are the monomers that are precursors for chain elongation.)

    (g) The thymine analogue 5-fluorouracil (converted to 5-fluorodeoxyuridylate in vivo) is a potent anticancer drug.

    (h) ATP and CTP reciprocally regulate the activity of aspartate transcarbamoylase.

22. (i) The formation of 5-aminoimidazole-4-carboxamide ribonucleotide from 5-aminoimidazole-4-(N-succinylcarboxamide) ribonucleotide in the synthesis of IMP (see step 7 in Figure 32.5).

    (ii) The formation of AMP from adenylosuccinate (see Figure 32.6).

    (iii) The formation of arginine from argininosuccinate in the urea cycle (see Figure 30.2 in Chapter 30).

23. The two synthases for carbamoyl phosphate use different sources of nitrogen and fulfill different roles in metabolism. The enzyme that uses ammonia synthesizes carbamoyl phosphate for a reaction with ornithine, the first step of the urea cycle. The enzyme that uses glutamine synthesizes carbamoyl phosphate for use in the first step of pyrimidine biosynthesis.

24. (a) The ADP from muscle contraction is a ready source of additional ATP for additional contraction. Half of the ADP can be converted immediately to ATP at the expense of the other half (being converted to AMP).

    (b) The reactants and products have the same number of high-energy phosphate bonds. The interconversion of (2 ADP) with (ATP + AMP) therefore is essentially isoenergetic.

    (c) In the reaction 2 ADP → ATP + AMP, the removal of one of the products (AMP) will shift the equilibrium to the right and favor the production of additional ATP.

    (d) By first removing and then replacing AMP, the cycle buys time (at the expense of GTP) until aerobic metabolism can "catch up" and reconvert available AMP as well as ADP back into ATP.

25. PRPP and formylglycinamide ribonucleotide accumulate because they are reactions 1 and 2 in the first stage of purine biosynthesis (Figure 32.5 in the text). If these glutamine requiring amidotransferase reactions are inhibited, the precursor molecules will

accumulate. However, since the synthesis of formylglycinamide requires that PRPP be converted to phosphoribosylamine, probably only PRPP will accumulate significantly.

26. (a) Cell A cannot grow in a HAT medium because it cannot synthesize dTMP either from thymidine or from dUMP. Cell B cannot grow in this medium because it cannot synthesize purines by either the de novo pathway or the salvage pathway.

    Cell C can grow in a HAT medium because it contains active thymidine kinase from cell B (enabling it to phosphorylate thymidine to dTMP) and hypoxanthineguanine phosphoribosyl transferase from cell A (enabling it to synthesize purines from hypoxanthine by the salvage pathway).

   (b) Transform cell A with a plasmid containing foreign genes of interest and a functional thymidine kinase gene. The only cells that will grow in a *HAT* medium are those that have acquired a thymidylate kinase gene; nearly all these transformed cells will also contain the other genes on the plasmid.

27. The cytosolic level of ATP in liver falls and that of AMP rises above normal in all three conditions. The excess AMP is degraded to urate. See C. R. Scriver, A. L. Beaudet, W. S. Sly, and D. Vale (eds.), *The Metabolic Basis of Inherited Disease*, 6th ed. (McGraw-Hill, 1989), pp. 984–988, for an illuminating discussion.

28. Succinate can be converted to oxaloacetate by the citric acid cycle. The oxaloacetate can then be transaminated to yield asparate, a key precursor of pyrimidines. The carbons of aspartate then will label positions 4, 5, and 6 in the pyrimidine rings:

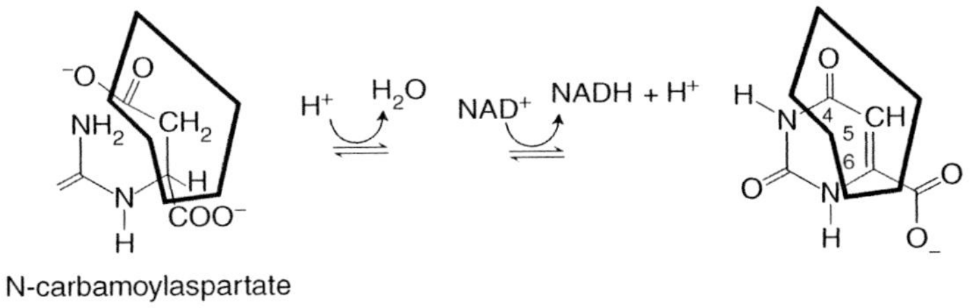

N-carbamoylaspartate

29. Glucose will most likely be converted into two molecules of pyruvate, one of which will be labeled in the 2 position:

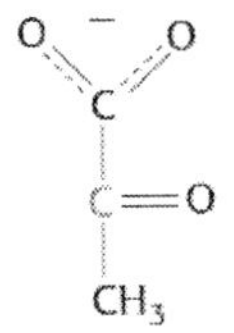

Now consider two common fates of pyruvate—conversion into acetyl CoA and subsequent processing by the citric acid cycle or carboxylation by pyruvate carboxylase to form oxaloacetate. Formation of citrate by condensing the labeled pyruvate with oxaloacetate will yield labeled citrate:

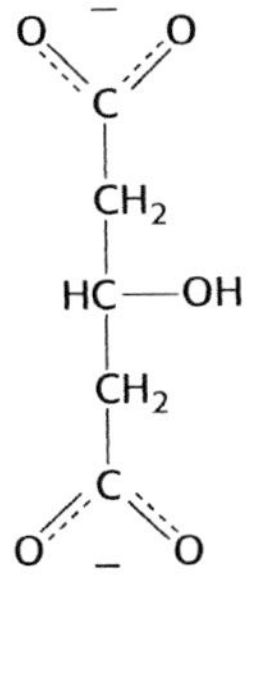

The labeled carbon will be retained through one round of the citric acid cycle but, on the formation of the symmetric succinate, the label will appear in two different positions. Thus, when succinate is metabolized to oxaloacetate, which may be aminated to form aspartate, two carbons will be labeled:

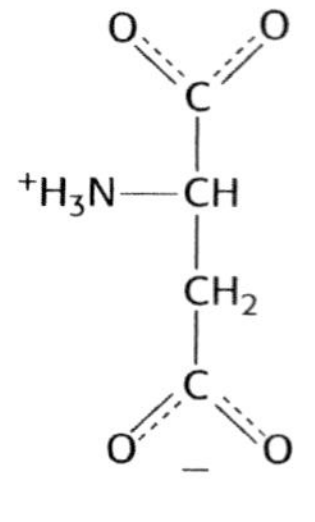

When this aspartate is used to form uracil, the labeled COO$^-$ attached to the α-carbon is lost and the other COO$^-$ becomes incorporated into uracil as carbon 4.

Suppose, instead, that labeled 2-[^{14}C]pyruvate is carboxylated to form oxaloacetate and processed to form aspartate. In this case, the α-carbon of aspartate bears the label.

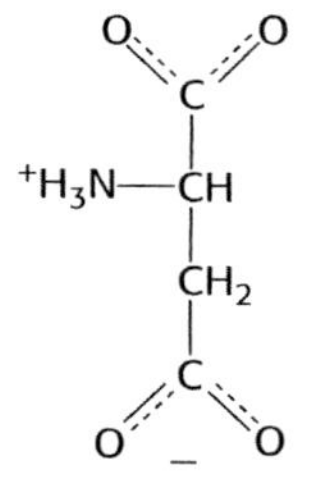

When this aspartate is used to synthesize uracil, carbon 6 bears the label.

CHAPTER 33

1. A nucleoside is a base attached to a ribose sugar. A nucleotide is a nucleoside with one or more phosphoryl groups attached to the ribose.

2. Hydrogen-bond pairing between the base A and the base T as well as hydrogen-bond pairing between the base G and the base C in DNA.

3. (a) 6; (b) 8; (c) 10; (d) 2; (e) 1; (f) 3; (g) 4; (h) 9; (i) 5; (j) 7.

4. The [A] and the [T] are equal. Since the DNA is 20% T, it is also 20% A. The remaining 60% of bases then are divided equally between G and C. Therefore the DNA is 30% G and 30% C.

5. Nothing, because the base-pair rules do not apply to single-stranded nucleic acids.

6. Two purines are too large to fit inside the double helix, and two pyrimidines are too small to form base pairs with each other.

7. By convention, when polynucleotide sequences are written, left to right means 5' → 3'.
   Since complementary strands are antiparallel, if one wishes to write the complementary sequence without specifically labeling the ends, the order of the bases must be reversed.

    (a) TTGATC

    (b) GTTCGA

    (c) ACGCGT

    (d) ATGGTA

8. (a) Since [A] + [G] account for 0.54 mole-fraction units, [T] + [C] must account for the remaining 0.46 (1 − 0.54). However, the individual mole fraction of [C] or [T] cannot be predicted.

    (b) Due to base pairing (A:T, G:C) in the complementary strand, [T] = 0.30, [C] = 0.24, and [A] + [G] = 0.46.

9. The diameter of DNA is 20 Å and 1 Å = 0.1 nm, so the diameter is 2 nm. Because 1 μm = 1000 nm, the length is 20,000 nm. Thus, the axial ratio is (20,000/2) = 10,000.

10. The thermal energy causes the chains to wiggle about, which disrupts the hydrogen bonds between base pairs and the stacking forces between bases and thereby causes the strands to separate.

11. One end of a nucleic acid polymer ends with a free 5′-hydroxyl group (or a phosphoryl group esterified to the hydroxyl group), and the other end has a free 3′-hydroxyl group. Thus, the ends are different. Two chains of DNA can form a double helix only if the chains are running in different directions—that is, have opposite polarity.

12. To answer this question one must know that $2\ \mu m = 2 \times 10^{-6}$ m, that one $Å = 10^{-10}$ m, and that the distance between the base pairs is 3.4 Å. The length of a DNA segment (in this case 2×10^{-6} m) divided by the distance between the base pairs (3.4×10^{-10} m) gives the answer, 5.88×10^{3} base pairs.

13. After 1.0 generation, one-half of the molecules would be ^{15}N-^{15}N, the other half ^{14}N-^{14}N. After 2.0 generations, one-quarter of the molecules would be ^{15}N-^{15}N, the other three-quarters ^{14}N-^{14}N. Hybrid ^{14}N-^{15}N molecules would not be observed.

14. There would be too much charge repulsion from the negative charges on the phosphoryl groups. These charges must be countered by the addition of cations.

15. The nucleosome structure results in a packaging ratio of only seven, which is much less than the compaction ratio of 104 found in metaphase chromosomes. Other structures—such as the chromatin fiber—must form to attain the observed packaging of DNA.

16. The 200-bp segments of DNA are bound to the histones. Consequently, these segments are not readily accessible to DNase. However, when the reaction time is extended or more enzyme is employed, additional DNA from the ends of the 200-bp fragments becomes available for digestion.

17. If one ignores the histidine residues, one counts negative charges for each aspartic and glutamic acid (D and E in the sequences) and positive charges for each lysine and arginine (K and R in the sequences).

    H2A contributes +13 for K, +13 for R, −2 for D, and −7 for E, for a net charge of +17.

    H2B contributes +20 for K, +8 for R, −3 for D, and −7 for E, for a net charge of +18.

    H3 contributes +13 for K, +18 for R, −4 for D, and −7 for E, for a net charge of +20.

    H4 contributes +11 for K, +14 for R, −3 for D, and −4 for E, for a net charge of +18.

    The histone octamer contains two each of H2A, H2B, H3, and H4. The total charge on the histone octamer is therefore estimated to be 2 × (17 + 18 + 20 + 18) = +146. The total charge on 150 base pairs of DNA is −300. Therefore, the histone octamer neutralizes approximately one-half of the charge on the DNA.

18. The faster rate is due to one-dimensional diffusion instead of three-dimensional diffusion. The RNA polymerase holoenzyme will bind initially with low affinity to any random site on the duplex DNA. The polymerase then reaches a promoter site rapidly by sliding along the DNA, rather than needing to diffuse through three-dimensional space.

19. GC base pairs are stabilized by three hydrogen bonds, whereas AT base pairs have only two hydrogen bonds. The graph indicates that DNA with 100% AT base pairs has T_m of approximately 70 °C, DNA with 100% GC base pairs has T_m of approximately 110 °C, and furthermore that there is a linear relationship between the GC content and the T_m of DNA between about 70 °C and 110 °C. The higher content of GC base pairs in DNA leads to more hydrogen bonds and greater helix stability.

20. The C_0t value—representing initial concentration multiplied by time—corresponds to the complexity of the DNA sequence and therefore also to the information content of the DNA sequence. The sample of (poly U)/(poly A) contains a simple sequence with low information content, such that the complementary strands will renature rapidly to form the double helix. The more complex sequences require increasingly longer times (or higher concentrations, hence the "C_0t" parameter) to find their complementary strands and form the double helices.

21. Increasing amounts of salt increase the melting temperature. Because the DNA backbone is negatively charged, there is a tendency for charge repulsion to destabilize the double helix and cause the strands to separate. The addition of salt neutralizes the charge repulsion from the negative phosphate groups, thereby stabilizing the double helix. The results show that, within the parameters of the experiment, more salt results in more stabilization, which gives the DNA a higher melting temperature.

22. The probability that any sequence will appear is 4^n, where 4 is the number of nucleotides and n is the length of the sequence. Using the equation:

$4^n = 3.0 * 10^9$, and solving for n yields:

$n(\log_{10}4) = \log_{10}(3.0 * 10^9)$, or $0.60 n = 9.48$.

$n = (9.48/0.60) = 15.74$, so on average, any particular DNA sequence of length between 15 and 16 bases is likely to appear only once in the human genome. (Many random 15-base sequences will appear slightly more than once (on average), while a random 16-base sequence is likely to appear either once or not at all.)

(Note: For the ratio of logarithms, either the $\log_{10}$ terms or natural logrithms can be used, such that, equivalently: $n = (\ln(3.0 * 10^9))/(\ln 4) = (21.82/1.39) = 15.74$.)

23. (a) From the 4 mononucleotides one can formulate 16 different dinucleotides. If you don't believe it, try it! From these dinucleotides you can make 64 different trinucleotides. Note that 64 is 4^3. There will be 4^4 (256) tetranucleotides. Proceeding in this manner we get to 4^8 (65,536) different octonucleotides (8-mers).

(b) A bit specifies two bases (say A and C), and a second bit specifies the other two (G and T). Hence, two bits are needed to specify a single nucleotide (or base pair) in DNA. An 8-mer stores 16 bits ($2^{16} = 65,535$), the *E. coli* genome (4×10^6 bp) stores 8×10^6 bits, and the human genome (2.9×10^9 bases) stores 5.8×10^9 bits of genetic information.

(c) A high-density diskette stores about 1.5 megabytes, which is equal to 1.2×10^7 bits. A large number of 8-mer sequences could be stored on such a diskette. The DNA sequence of *E. coli*, once known, could be written on a single diskette. Nearly 500 diskettes would be needed to record the human DNA sequence.

24. The instability of RNA in alkali is due to its 2'-OH group. In the presence of OH⁻ the 2'-OH group of RNA is converted to an alkoxide ion (RO⁻) by removal of a proton. Intramolecular attack by the 2'-alkoxide on the phosphodiester in RNA gives a 2',3'-cyclic nucleotide, cleaving the phosphodiester bond in the process. Further attack by OH⁻ on the 2',3'-cyclic nucleotide produces a mixture of 2' and 3'-nucleotides. Since DNA lacks a 2'-OH group, it is quite stable in alkali.

25.

CHAPTER 34

1. A template is the sequence of DNA or RNA that directs the synthesis of a complementary nucleic acid sequence. A primer (usually RNA) is an initial segment of a nucleic acid polymer that is to be extended into a longer DNA or RNA chain and on which elongation depends.

2. DNA polymerase cannot initiate synthesis of a new strand without a pre-existing primer. Consequently, an RNA polymerase, called a primase, synthesizes a short sequence of RNA that then is used as a primer by the DNA polymerase for synthesis of the strand that is complementary to the template.

3. Okazaki fragments are short segments of DNA that are synthesized on the lagging strand during replication of DNA. These fragments subsequently are joined by DNA ligase to form a continuous complementary strand of DNA.

4. When DNA is being synthesized at the replication fork, one strand (the leading strand) is synthesized continuously in the 5'-to-3' direction as the template is read in the 3'-to-5' direction. The other strand (the lagging strand) also is synthesized in the 5'-to-3' direction and therefore must be synthesized as short Okazaki fragments.

5. (a) 5; (b) 4; (c) 8; (d) 1; (e) 10; (f) 2; (g) 6; (h) 7; (i) 3; (j) 9.

6. The nucleotides used for DNA synthesis have the triphosphate attached to the 5'-hydroxyl group with free 3'-hydroxyl groups. Such nucleotides can be utilized only for 5'-to-3' DNA synthesis.

7. The rate of strand separation is because the helix is stabilized by large numbers of hydrogen bonds and stacking forces between bases. Although individually weak, the thousands or millions of such interactions hold the helix together and make spontaneous separation of the strands unlikely.

8. Replication in only one direction from only one fork would take twice as long as bidirectional replication.

9. The unwinding of DNA to expose single-stranded regions at the replication fork causes overwinding (positive supercoils) ahead of the fork. The action of topoisomerase II overcomes this effect by introducing negative supercoils to compensate. Without topoisomerase II, the DNA would become too tightly wound ahead of the fork.

10. Telomerase is required to synthesize the ends of new linear chromosomes during cell division. Because cancer cells are dividing rapidly, it is likely that the telomerase gene must be activated for a cell to become cancerous.

11. The free energy of ATP hydrolysis under standard conditions is -30.5 kJ mol^{-1} (-7.3 kcal mol^{-1}). At 10 kJ mol^{-1} (base pair)$^{-1}$, in principle, the energy of ATP hydrolysis could be used to break a maximum of three base pairs.

12. (a) The nucleotide ddATP is virtually identical in structure with dATP except that it lacks a 3'-OH group. Thus, it will be incorporated into a newly synthesized DNA strand by DNA polymerase when the polymerase first encounters a T residue in the template strand. However, because the incorporated ddAMP has no 3'-OH group, no further nucleotide can be added and synthesis will stop with ddAMP opposite the first T in the template strand.

    (b) Because the ddATP is only 10% of the concentration of dATP, there is a 10% chance that it will be incorporated into the newly synthesized DNA each time that a T is encountered in the template strand. Consequently, a population of fragments of DNA segments of different lengths will be synthesized, in which all of them end in ddAMP. The families of fragments generated in this way by the inability to extend a dideoxy nucleotide forms the basis of the dideoxy chain-termination method of DNA sequencing (Chapter 41).

13. Positive supercoiling resists the unwinding of DNA. The melting temperature of DNA increases in going from negatively supercoiled to relaxed to positively supercoiled DNA. Positive supercoiling is probably an adaptation to high temperature, where the unwinding (melting, denaturing) of DNA is markedly increased.

14. (a) Different supercoiled forms (topological isomers) migrate through the gel at different rates. The highly supercoiled DNA has a compact shape and migrates rapidly. Relaxed DNA has a more extended shape (a larger radius of gyration) and moves more slowly through the gel matrix.

    (b) The bands in lane B represent different supercoiled isomers of DNA. Neighboring bands differ from each other by ±1 superhelical turn.

    (c) With longer exposure to topoisomerase 1 (a "relaxing" enzyme), the population of DNA molecules shifts toward a distribution that is near thermal equilibrium.

15. The high concentration of a particular nucleotide will have the effect of speeding up the polymerization reaction. Consequently, a misformed product (from the previous step) may exit the polymerase active site before it has time to wander into the exonuclease activity site for proofreading. The reverse is true if the next nucleotide is

scarce. The polymerase pauses for a longer time, increasing the likelihood that a mis-formed product will be able to visit the exonuclease site.

16. (a) 1000 nucleotides/s divided by 10.4 nucleotides/turn for B-DNA gives 96.2 revolutions per second.

    (b) 0.34 μm/s. (1000 nucleotides/s corresponds to 3400 Å/s because the axial distance between nucleotides in B-DNA is 3.4 Å.)

17. The activity will be similar to the replacement of an RNA primer with DNA by DNA polymerase I. One makes use of the combined $5' \rightarrow 3'$ exonuclease and $5' \rightarrow 3'$ polymerase activities of DNA polymerase I. From the point of the internal nick (of only one strand) by the endonuclease, polymerase I will extend the free 3'-OH using radioactive dNTPs while at the same time digesting from the internal 5'-phosphate to make room for the newly synthesized DNA. The result is a "nick translation" event in which an unlabeled portion of one DNA strand is replaced with a radioactive stretch of DNA. (Over the section of new synthesis, only one strand becomes labeled. The strand used as the "template" remains unlabeled.)

CHAPTER 35

1. Mutations can be introduced by means of mismatches, insertions, deletions, or breaks in DNA.

2. DNA damage can be caused by oxidizing agents such as reactive oxygen species, and by deamination, alkylation, ultraviolet light or ionizing radiation.

3. First, recognize the damaged base or bases. Second, remove the damaged base(s). Third, repair the gap with DNA polymerase I, and seal the gap using DNA ligase.

4. DNA repair systems include the proofreading ability of DNA polymerase and, additionally, mismatch-repair systems, direct repair, base-excision repair, nucleotide-excision repair, and DNA recombination.

5. The ultraviolet radiation of sunlight causes, in addition to tan lines, thymine dimers in DNA. These thymine dimers, if not repaired, will block replication and gene expression, possibly leading to mutations.

6. Base-excision repair begins with the repair enzyme AlkA in E. coli, which binds to the modified DNA and flips the particular base out of the helix. The enzyme then cleaves the glycosidic bond to release the damaged base. Then AP endouclease nicks the backbone, and another enzyme removes the deoxyribose phosphate unit. DNA polymerase I fills in the gap, and DNA ligase seals the strand.

7. Cytosine in DNA, which pairs with guanine, sometimes undergoes deamination to form uracil, which pairs with adenine. The result would be a mutation (a U–A base pair for a C–G base pair). By using thymine instead of uracil, the repair machinery can immediately recognize the uracil in DNA as a mistake and replace it with cytosine.

8. A T–G base pair is always recognized as a mistaken C–G base pair because 5-methyl-cytosine spontaneously deaminates to form thymine. This results in a T–G base pair. Because the $C \rightarrow T$ mutation is so common, the T (and not the G) in the T–G pair is always treated as the incorrect base and is removed by the base-excision-repair proteins. This repair system allows the methylation of C to serve a role in transcription regulation without resulting in frequent mutations in the DNA.

9. Many misincorporated nucleotides can be corrected. Mistakes in DNA synthesis often are corrected by a subunit of DNA polymerase III, acting as an exonuclease, which removes the offending base. The polymerase activity then makes the correction, and DNA ligase seals the backbone.

10. Each base pair has one purine, which can undergo spontaneous depurination at the rate 3×10^9 depurinations per purine per minute. The human genome contains 6×10^9 base pairs, and so there are $(3 \times 6) = 18$ depurinations per minute. Multiplying 18 by 60 minutes in an hour and by 24 hours in a day reveals that about 26,000 repair events are required per day per cell.

11. Potentially deleterious side reactions are avoided. The enzyme itself might be damaged by light if it could be activated by light in the absence of bound DNA harboring a pyrimidine dimer. The DNA-induced absorption band is reminiscent of the glucose-induced activation of the phosphotransferase activity of hexokinase.

12. (a) 9; (b) 5; (c) 10; (d) 1; (e) 6; (f) 7; (g) 2; (h) 3; (i) 8; (j) 4.

13. (a) The control plate indicates the extent of spontaneous reversion in the absence of an external mutagen.

    (b) The known mutagen is a positive control to show that the procedures are correctly implemented and the test is working.

    (c) The experimental compound by itself (plate C) gives results that are only marginally above background (plate A). The experimental compound itself therefore should be classified as either non-mutagenic or only very slightly mutagenic. However, a metabolic product derived from the experimental compound is mutagenic (plate D).

    (d) One or more enzymes from the liver probably are responsible for the metabolic conversion of the experimental compound into a mutagenic compound.

14. (a) From the graph, the XP group is more susceptible. People with xeroderma pigmentosum develop skin cancer at a much earlier age than do people without it.

    (b) A likely explanation is that people with xeroderma pigmentosum lack a component of the human nucleotide-excision-repair pathway. This pathway is especially important in the repair of ultraviolet-radiation-induced DNA lesions, such as thymidine dimers. Thus, skin cancer readily develops. The actual results are illustrated in the graph.

    (c) The late appearance of skin cancer in normal people suggests that multiple mutations in the DNA must occur and must escape the repair pathways before skin cancer can develop.

CHAPTER 36

1. Transcription is DNA-directed RNA synthesis by RNA polymerase.

2. The template strand is the DNA strand that has a sequence complementary to that of the RNA transcript. The DNA coding strand has the same sequence as that of the RNA transcript except that thymine (T) in the DNA is replaced by uracil (U) in the RNA.

3. Beginning, middle, and end, although strictly true, are not sufficiently precise to describe the stages of transcription. The three stages of RNA synthesis are initiation, elongation, and termination of transcription.

4. RNA polymerase requires a DNA template along with the four nucleotide monomers: ATP, GTP, UTP and CTP; and either Mg^{2+} or Mn^{2+}.

5. The sigma subunit helps the RNA polymerase to locate the promoter sites on the DNA template. After a promoter is located, the sigma subunit leaves the enzyme and assists another molecule of RNA polymerase in finding another promoter.

6. (a) 4; (b) 10; (c) 1; (d) 5; (e) 2; (f) 9; (g) 6; (h) 3; (i) 8; (j) 7.

7. Transcription and replication can be compared and contrasted in several ways:
   - Both processes use a DNA template.
   - Replication copies both strands, whereas transcription copies only one strand.
   - RNA polymerase is the enzyme for transcription, whereas DNA polymerase is the enzyme for replication.
   - The substrates for transcription are ribonucleotides, whereas the substrates for replication are deoxyribonucleotides.
   - Replication requires a primer, but transcription does not.

8. A promoter is a sequence in DNA that directs RNA polymerase to the proper initiation site for transcription.

9. In the closed promoter complex, the DNA is double helical and transcription is not possible. In the open promoter complex, the DNA is unwound and transcription can proceed.

10. The sequence of the coding (+, sense) strand is:

    5′-ATGGGGAACAG CAAGAGTGGGGCCCTGTCCAAGGAG-3′

    and the sequence of the template (−, antisense) strand is:

    3′-TACCCCTTGTCGTTCTCACCCCGGGAC AGGTTCCTC-5′

    Note that the *coding* strand has the same sequence as mRNA (except U → T), whereas the *template* strand is complementary to the coding strand.

11. RNA turns over in the cell, whereas DNA is the "nearly" permanent record of inherited information. The consequences of most errors in RNA synthesis will be short-lived, perhaps a protein synthesized with a mistake in its sequence for a short time during the life of the cell, but then the RNA in question may be degraded and the error will disappear. By contrast, an uncorrected error in DNA replication will be passed to the next generation.

12. RNA synthesis involves copying only short segments of chromosomes, whereas DNA replication must involve copying entire chromosomes at the time of cell division. The length of consecutive nucleotide sequence that must be copied is many times greater for DNA replication than for RNA transcription.

13. This mutant sigma would competitively inhibit the binding of holoenzyme and prevent the specific initiation of RNA chains at promoter sites.

14. The core enzyme without sigma binds more tightly to the DNA template than does the holoenzyme. The retention of sigma after chain initiation would make the mutant RNA polymerase less processive. Hence, RNA synthesis would be much slower than normal.

15. A 100-kd protein contains about 910 residues, which are encoded by 2730 nucleotides. At a maximal transcription rate of 50 nucleotides per second, the protein would be synthesized in 54.6 seconds.

16. Initiation at strong promoters occurs every two seconds. In this interval, 100 nucleotides are transcribed. Hence, centers of transcription bubbles are 34 nm (340 Å) apart (100 × 3.4 Å = 340 Å).

17. A riboswitch is a special secondary structure formed by some mRNA molecules, capable of directly binding small molecules, which determines whether transcription will continue or cease. For instance, a riboswitch controls the synthesis of an mRNA encoding a protein required for FMN synthesis. If FMN is already present, the riboswitch will bind the FMN and trap the RNA transcript in a conformation that favors the termination of RNA synthesis, thereby preventing the production of the full-length, functional mRNA. However, if FMN is absent, an alternative conformation of the riboswitch will allow the production of the full-length mRNA.

18. (a) Without the *lac* repressor gene, the repressor protein will not be produced. Without a repressor, the *lac z, y,* and *a* proteins will be produced constitutively (independently of the presence or absence of lactose, albeit at low levels when glucose is present, due to catabolite repression).

    (b) Provided that the *lac* promoter remains intact, the effect would be the same as in (a): no repression, and constitutive production of the *lac z, y,* and *a* proteins.

    (c) Without CAP to stimulate transcription, the levels of the *lac z, y,* and *a* proteins that are produced will remain low, even in the presence of lactose.

19. With the permease missing, lactose cannot get into the cell and cannot bind to the *lac* repressor. Therefore, the repressor will remain bound to the operator, and the gene for β-galactosidase will not be induced.

20. Because of the σ factor, RNA polymerase binds to DNA at a random location and then slides along the DNA double helix in a one-dimensional search for the promoter. Diffusion in one dimension is much faster than diffusion in three dimensions. The encounter of the two small molecules is governed by diffusion in three dimensions and is therefore a slower process.

21. The three types of post-transcriptional modifications of tRNA are: cleavage of a precursor, addition of CCA to the 3'-end of tRNA, and modifications of bases.

22. The long strand that goes entirely across the picture from left to right is the DNA. The strands of increasing length are molecules of mRNA that are beginning to be transcribed. Transcription begins just ahead of the site on the DNA where the shortest strands of mRNA are seen. Transcription ends just after the site on the DNA where the longest strands of mRNA are attached. (As RNA polymerase passes this site, the primary transcript mRNA is released.) On the page, the direction of RNA synthesis is from left to right. Many different enzymes are simultaneously making many different RNA molecules on a single gene.

23. Heparin, a glycosaminoglycan, is highly anionic. Its negative charges, like the phosphodiester bridges of DNA templates, bind to lysine and arginine residues of β'.

24. A liter contains 1000 cm^3, so a cell volume of about 10^{-12} cm^3 is 10^{-15} liter. One molecule divided by Avogadro's number in 10^{-15} liter corresponds to a concentration of about $1.7 * 10^{-9}$ M.

$$\frac{(1 \text{ molecule})}{(6.02 * 10^{23} \text{ molecules mol}^{-1})(10^{-15} \text{ liter})} = 1.7 * 10^{-9} \underline{M}$$

Since the repressor concentration is much higher than the dissociation constant for the repressor/operator complex (10^{-13} M), the single molecule will be bound to (operator) DNA.

25. The anti-inducer could be a competitive inhibitor of the inducer. As such, the anti-inducer would bind to the repressor at a similar or overlapping site to that of the inducer, but would not cause the conformational change necessary to release the repressor from the operator DNA. Higher concentrations of inducer would then be needed to displace the competitively bound anti-inducer from its site on the repressor.

26. Segments of double helix that are shorter than tetranucleotides (having fewer than about 4 base pairs) are unstable at physiological temperatures due to their small extent of base stacking and small number of inter-strand hydrogen bonds. Until the critical length of RNA is synthesized for a stable RNA/DNA double helix, the short initial di- and trinucleotides are susceptible to release.

27. RNA molecules of different sizes were obtained, designated 10S, 13S, and 17S, when boat was added at initiation, a few seconds after initiation, or 2 minutes after initiation, respectively. If no boat was added, transcription yielded a 23S RNA product. Boat, like ρ, is evidently a termination factor. The template that was used for RNA synthesis contained at least three termination sites that respond to boat (yielding the 10S, 13S, and 17S RNA molecules) and one termination site (yielding 23S RNA) that does not respond to boat. Thus, specific termination at a site producing 23S RNA can take place in the absence of boat. However, boat detects additional termination signals that are not recognized by RNA polymerase alone. Sadly, your search of the literature reveals that someone has already characterized the factor that you named boat—the termination factor ρ.

CHAPTER 37

1. (1) Eukaryotes have more complex transcriptional regulation than that of bacteria.

    (2) RNA, especially mRNA, is more highly processed in eukaryotes than in bacteria.

    (3) Unlike bacteria, RNA synthesis in eukaryotes is localized to a particular organelle—the nucleus. As a result, transcription and translation take place in different cellular compartments in eukaryotes.

2. Eukaryotic RNA polymerase I catalyzes the synthesis of all ribosomal RNA except 5S RNA and is located in the nucleolus. RNA polymerase I is insensitive to α-amanitin inhibition. RNA polymerase II makes mRNA, is located in the nucleoplasm, and is very sensitive to α-amanitin inhibition. RNA polymerase III, also located in the nucleoplasm, synthesizes tRNA and 5S RNA, and can be inhibited by high concentrations of α-amanitin.

3. Three common elements are found in a promoter for RNA polymerase II: (1) the TATA box, (2) the initiator element (Inr), and (3) a downstream promoter element (DPE). Additional elements, such as the CAAT box may be present.

4. The distinguishing feature of RNA polymerase II is a carboxyl-terminal domain that plays a key role in the regulation of RNA polymerase II activity.

5. Cis-acting elements are DNA sequences that regulate the expression of a gene located on the same molecule of DNA. Trans-acting elements, also called transcription factors, may act on different molecules of DNA. The transcription factors are proteins that bind to cis-acting elements and regulate RNA synthesis.

6. Enhancers are DNA sequences that have no promoter activity of their own, yet they can stimulate promoters that are located several thousand base pairs away. An enhancer

can be upstream, downstream, or even in the midst of a transcribed gene and can be effective when present on either strand of DNA. Enhancers are bound by proteins that participate in the regulation of transcription.

7. RNA polymerases I and III produce the same products in all cells. RNA polymerase II, however, produces a wide variety of cell-specific mRNA molecules and furthermore must respond to changes in environmental conditions. Thus, the promoters for the (protein-encoded) genes transcribed by RNA polymerase II must be complex enough to respond to a variety of signals.

8. (a) 2, 6, 9; (b) 1, 4, 5, 7, 8; (c) 3, 4, 10.

9. Cordycepin (3'-deoxyadenosine) is an adenosine analog and, when phosphorylated, is an adenylate nucleotide analog. The absence of a 3'-hydroxyl group means that it cannot form a phosphodiester linkage with another nucleotide. If cordycepin is incorporated into RNA, further elongation of the RNA chain will cease.

10. Phosphorylation of the carboxyl-terminal domain of RNA polymerase II establishes the transition from initiation to elongation. The phosphorylated C-terminal domain facilitates elongation by RNA polymerase II and serves as a binding site for RNA-processing enzymes that act during the course of elongation.

11. The finding of rather constant bubble sizes indicates that DNA is rewound at about the same rate at the rear of RNA polymerase as it is unwound at the front of the enzyme. In essence, the bubble translocates along the DNA strand in a wave-like fashion.

12. (a) 5; (b) 10; (c) 2; (d) 3; (e) 9; (f) 4; (g) 8; (h) 1; (i) 6; (j) 7.

13. Nuclear hormone receptors bind to appropriate response elements in the DNA and then are assisted by coactivators. When a hormone binds to a nuclear hormone receptor, the receptor's structure changes so that the receptor can bind a coactivator (or corepressor), which in turn activates (or inhibits) RNA polymerase.

14. A given regulatory protein may have different effects, depending on the other regulatory proteins that are present at a given time in the particular environment. Therefore, complex regulatory patterns leading to differentiation and development can be obtained with smaller numbers of regulatory proteins.

15. The acetylation of lysine residues on a histone decreases the number of positive charges on the protein and thus reduces the histone's affinity for the negatively charged DNA.

16. Although RNA polymerase II might be rapidly inhibited, there are still many functional mRNAs and proteins in the liver. However, as these proteins and mRNA molecules are damaged, the necessary replacements cannot be provided, so eventually the liver will fail and death will result.

17. An activated amino acid is one that is covalently coupled to its appropriate tRNA molecule.

18. Estradiol, because of its hydrophobic nature, can diffuse across the cell membrane and nuclear membrane, into the nucleus, where it can bind to its receptor. The estradiol-receptor complex can bind directly to DNA. By contrast, the ligands for G-protein-coupled receptors do not enter the cell. Moreover, the G-protein-coupled receptors themselves are confined to the cell membrane, such that any effects on gene regulation must be mediated by additional components of a signal-transduction pathway.

19. The receptor for estradiol is not present in all cells. Because estradiol exerts its effect only in the presence of the estradiol receptor, only tissues having the receptor will recognize the presence of estradiol.

20. One crucial use for zinc is to build zinc finger domains of key proteins. Zinc is a component of zinc fingers, which are the DNA-binding motifs of nuclear hormone receptors.

21. These results suggest that chromatin structure varies locally, depending on the transcription status of each particular gene. If a gene is being transcribed, the chromatin packing is loosened to allow access of proteins such as transcription factors and RNA polymerase to the DNA. In this loosened state, these regions become susceptible to digestion by DNase.

22. (a) The different genes are expressed to differing extents. Only those genes for which mRNA is actively being transcribed will give positive hybridization signals.

    (b) Gene expression patterns differ in the different tissues. Some of the mRNAs are transcribed in some tissues but not others.

    (c) The genes that are expressed in all three tissues could be essential for fundamental metabolic processes that are common to most if not all cells.

    (d) Including the initiation inhibitor allows counting and comparison of the number of ongoing mRNA chains being synthesized among the different gene types and from tissue to tissue at the given moment in time when the cells are broken.
    (Without such an inhibitor, the results could be skewed by differing initiation rates from gene to gene, or by the possibility of some artificial initiation events that could be induced when the cells are broken to isolate the nuclei.)

CHAPTER 38

1. (a) 9; (b) 1; (c) 7; (d) 2; (e) 8; (f) 5; (g) 3; (h) 10; (i) 6; (j) 4.

2. The 5′ cap is a GTP-linked addition to the 5′ end of eukaryotic mRNA that is coupled by means of an unusual 5′-5′ linkage. The basic cap can be further elaborated in some cases.

3. To prepare for the formation of a poly(A) tail, a specific endonuclease recognizes an AAUAAA target sequence and cleaves the precursor RNA. Poly(A) polymerase then adds a string of adenylate residues to the 3′ end of the transcript.

4. The three most common modifications of eukaryotic pre-mRNA primary transcripts are addition of the 5′ cap, addition of the poly(A) tail, and removal of the introns by splicing.

5. The carboxyl-terminal domain of RNA polymerase II allows modification of the newly synthesized RNA.

6. (a) The lack of a 3′-OH group will cause cordycepin to be a chain terminator for RNA synthesis. Cordycepin will be incorporated at the 3′-end of a chain, and further elongation will be blocked.

    (b) The substrate specificity of poly(A) polymerase is higher than that of RNA polymerase because the RNA polymerase uses four nucleotides (ATP, UTP, GTP, CTP), whereas poly(A) polymerase uses only ATP. The result suggests that poly(A) polymerase has a higher apparent affinity for 3′-deoxy-ATP than does RNA polymerase.

    (c) Yes. It must receive a 5′-triphosphate in order to be a substrate for poly(A) polymerase or RNA polymerase.

7. A spliceosome is the splicing machinery in the nucleus. It is composed of snRNPs (U1, U2, U4, U5, and U6) and various protein splicing factors.

8. The carboxyl-terminal domain of RNA polymerase II recruits proteins required for cap formation, splicing, and polyadenylation.

9. Alternative splicing can effectively enlarge the size of the genome because one gene with several introns can be spliced to yield several different mRNAs. These mRNAs will produce different proteins. In essence, one gene can encode more than one protein.

10. Two alternative outcomes exist at each of eight sites. Therefore, a choice between two possible outcomes must be made eight times. The result is $2^8 = 256$ different possible products.

11. The Beadle/Tatum hypothesis, while still generally correct, now needs modification because alternative splicing sometimes allows the formation of more than one protein from one gene.

12. The mechanisms of self-splicing and spliceosome-catalyzed splicing are similar in two respects. First, in the initial step, a ribose hydroxyl group attacks the 5′ splice site. Then the newly formed 3′-OH terminus of the upstream exon attacks the 3′ splice site to form a phosphodiester linkage with the downstream exon. Second, both reactions are transesterifications in which the phosphate moieties at each splice site are retained in the final products. Therefore, the number of phosphodiester linkages remains constant.

13. The possibilities of alternative splicing and of RNA editing allow the final protein products to be more complex and more highly varied than the genes that encode them. Additionally, posttranslational modification of proteins (e.g., glycosylation, phosphorylation) will further enhance the complexity.

14. One could make use of the A–T base pairing potential of the poly-A sequence that is characteristic of eukaryotic mRNAs. One would construct an affinity chromatography column in which an oligo-dT nucleotide is covalently linked to a resin. Eukaroytic mRNAs would bind to this column, whereas other RNAs would not. After washing the other RNAs away from the column, one would elute the eukaryotic mRNAs by weakening the A–T hydrogen bonds, for example, by changing the temperature or by washing the column with a solution containing an excess of soluble oligo-dA (to displace the mRNA).

15. Histones are required in large amounts and in equal quantities only when DNA is being synthesized. The multiple arrays with an equal number of histone types per array will facilitate rapid production of a large number of histones in equal proportions. The lack of posttranscriptional processing may furthermore speed up the synthesis of the histones themselves. The lack of a poly(A) tail may facilitate the degradation of the histone mRNA, which is needed only when DNA synthesis is taking place.

16. If every T is changed to U, the polarity and base sequence of the DNA strands shown are identical with the mRNA synthesized from the complementary strand. Thus, TCTATTTTCCACCCTTAG becomes UCU̲AUUUUC̲CAC̲CCUUAG and encodes Ser-Ile̲-Phe-His̲-Pro-stop̲.

17. A mutation that disrupted the normal AAUAA recognition sequence for the endonuclease could account for this finding. In fact, a change from U to C in this sequence caused this defect in a thalassemic patient. Cleavage occurred at the AAUAAA 900 nucleotides downstream from this mutant AACAAA site. See S. H. Orkin, T.-C. Cheng, S. E. Antonarakis, and H. H. Kazazian, Jr. *EMBO J.* 4(1985):453.

CHAPTER 39

1. Three contiguous bases. Because there are four different bases, a code based on a two-base codon could encode only $4^2 = 16$ amino acids. A three-base codon allows $4^3 = 64$ different combinations, more than enough to account for the 20 amino acids.

2. A mutation that altered the code for the reading of mRNA would change the amino acid sequence of most, if not all, proteins synthesized by that particular organism. Many of these changes would undoubtedly be deleterious. The organism would not survive, and so there would be strong selection against a mutation with such pervasive consequences.

3. (a) 3; (b) 10; (c) 4; (d) 7; (e) 6; (f) 2; (g) 1; (h) 9; (i) 8; (j) 5.

4. A key characteristic of the genetic code is that three consecutive nucleotides encode an amino acid. The code is furthermore nonoverlapping, has no punctuation, and is degenerate.

5. Degeneracy of the code means that, for many of the amino acids, there is more than one codon. This property is valuable because, if the code were not degenerate, only 20 codons would encode amino acids and the rest of the codons could lead to chain termination. Many, and perhaps the majority of, mutations would then likely lead to inactive proteins.

6. The probability is calculated with the equation $p = (1 - \varepsilon)^n$, where p is the probability of synthesizing the error-free protein, ε is the error rate, and n is the number of amino acid residues in the protein.

	Probability of synthesizing an error-free protein	
	Number of amino acid residues	
Frequency of inserting an incorrect amino acid	50	500
10^{-2}	0.605	0.0066
10^{-4}	0.995	0.951
10^{-6}	0.999	0.999

7. An error frequency of one incorrect amino acid every 10^4 incorporations allows for the rapid and accurate synthesis of proteins as large as 1000 amino acids. Higher error rates would result in too many defective proteins. Lower error rates would likely slow the rate of protein synthesis without a significant gain in accuracy.

8. The first two bases in a codon form Watson–Crick base pairs that are checked for fidelity by bases of the 16S rRNA. The third base is not inspected for accuracy, and so some variation is tolerated. Non-canonical base pairs are sometimes permitted in the third position.

9. (a) Because mRNA is synthesized antiparallel to the DNA template and A pairs with U and T pairs with A, the correct sequence is 5′-UAACGGUACGAU-3′.

   (b) Since the 5′ end of an mRNA molecule codes for the amino terminus, appropriate use of the genetic code (see Table 39.1) leads to Leu-Pro-Ser-Asp-Trp-Met.

   (c) Since one has a repeating tetramer (UUAC) and a 3-base code, repetition will be observed at a 12-base interval (3 × UUAC). Comparison of this 12-base sequence with the genetic code leads to the conclusion that a polymer with a repeating tetrapeptide (Leu-Leu-Thr-Tyr) unit will be formed.

10. Note that each complementary strand is missing one of the four bases; d(TAC) lacks G and d(GTA) lacks C. Thus, incubation with RNA polymerase and only UTP, ATP, and CTP led to the synthesis of only poly(UAC), the RNA complement of d(GTA). When GTP was used in place of CTP, the complement of d(TAC), poly(GUA), was formed.

11. Only single-stranded mRNAs can serve as templates for protein synthesis. Since poly(G) forms a triple-stranded helix, it cannot serve as a template for protein synthesis.

12. These alternatives can be distinguished based on the results of studies of the sequences of amino acids in mutants. Suppose that the base C in the given sequence is mutated to C′. In a nonoverlapping code, only amino acid 1 will be changed. In a completely overlapping code, amino acids 1, 2, and 3 will all be altered by a mutation of C to C′. The results of amino acid sequence studies of tobacco mosaic virus mutants and abnormal hemoglobins showed that alterations usually affected only a single amino acid. Hence, the genetic code was concluded to be nonoverlapping.

13. Since three different polypeptides are synthesized, the synthesis must start from three different reading frames. One of these will be in phase with the AAA in the sequence shown in the problem and will therefore have a terminal lysine, since UGA is a stop signal. The reading frame in phase with AAU will result in a polypeptide having an Asn-Glu sequence in it, and the reading frame in phase with AUG will have a Met-Arg sequence in it.

14. Highly abundant amino acid residues have the most codons (e.g., Leu and Ser each have six), whereas the least-abundant amino acids have the fewest (Met and Trp each have only one). Degeneracy (a) allows variation in base composition and (b) decreases the likelihood that a substitution for a base will change the encoded amino acid. If the degeneracy were equally distributed, each of the 20 amino acids would have three codons. Both benefits (a and b) are maximized by the assignment of more codons to prevalent amino acids than to less frequently used ones.

15. The triplets codons 5′-UUU-UGC-CAU-GUU-UGU-GCU-3′ would be translated in sequence as: Phe-Ala-His-Val-Ala-Ala. The codons UGC and UGU encode cysteine but, because the cysteine has been modified to alanine on the aminoacyl-tRNA, alanine is incorporated in place of cysteine at the underlined positions in the sequence.

16. All transfer RNA molecules have these features:
    (i) Each is a single chain of RNA.
    (ii) They contain unusual bases.
    (iii) Approximately half of the bases are base-paired to form double helices. The strands that comprise the double-helical segments are antiparallel to each other.
    (iv) The 5′ end of the tRNA is phosphorylated and is usually pG.
    (v) The 3′ end of the tRNA terminates with the sequence CCA, and the hydroxyl group of the A residue is the acceptor site for attachment of the incoming cognate amino acid.
    (vi) The anticodon is located in a loop near the center of the tRNA sequence.

17. The first step involves the formation of an aminoacyl adenylate, an intermediate that is formed by reaction between an amino acid and ATP, with release of pyrophosphate. The aminoacyl adenylate then reacts with tRNA to form the aminoacyl-tRNA. Both steps are catalyzed by an aminoacyl-tRNA synthetase that is specific for a particular amino acid and its cognate tRNA molecules.

18. Unique features are required so that the aminoacyl-tRNA synthetases can distinguish among the different tRNA molecules and attach the correct amino acid to the proper tRNA. Common features are required because all of the aminoacyl-tRNAs then must interact with the same protein-synthesizing machinery in the ribosomes.

19. An activated amino acid is one that is covalently coupled to its appropriate tRNA molecule.

20. When the single ATP molecule is cleaved to AMP and pyrophosphate, the pyrophosphate is subsequently hydrolyzed to give two molecules of orthophosphate. The effective cost is two high-energy phosphate bonds. A second ATP molecule is then required to convert the AMP into ADP, the substrate for oxidative phosphorylation.

21. Amino acids larger than the correct amino acid cannot fit into the active site of the tRNA. Smaller but incorrect amino acids that may become attached to the tRNA fit into the editing site and are cleaved from the tRNA. For example, serine may become attached to threonyl-tRNA, but the serine will fit into the editing site and be cleaved from the threonyl-tRNA. When the correct threonine is attached, it will not fit the editing site and will not be cleaved.

22. Aminoacyl-tRNA synthetases are the only components that actually match a nucleotide sequence (the three-base RNA anticodon) with a particular amino acid to define the genetic code. All the other interactions of genetic code components involve simply "Watson-Crick" pairing between complementary bases.

23. The instability of RNA in alkali is due to its 2′-OH group. In the presence of OH^- the 2′-OH group of RNA is converted to an alkoxide ion (RO^-) by removal of a proton. Intramolecular attack by the 2′-alkoxide on the phosphodiester in RNA gives a 2′,3′-cyclic nucleotide, cleaving the phosphodiester bond in the process. Further attack by OH^- on the 2′,3′-cyclic nucleotide produces a mixture of 2′ and 3′-nucleotides. Since DNA lacks a 2′-OH group, it is quite stable in alkali.

24. The enzyme-bound Ile-AMP intermediate is necessary for the $^{32}PP_i$ exchange into ATP. Since isoleucine is a requirement, labeled ATP will be formed only in (c).

25. Since there was not enough time to synthesize complete chains after the radioactive leucine was added, the full-length α and β chains that were isolated would need to contain unlabeled leucines in the initial sequences that were started before the radioactivity was added. The observed distribution therefore is the one to be expected if the amino-terminal regions of chains had already been partly synthesized to varying extents before the addition of the radioactive leucine. The existing chains are then extended to their full lengths in the presence of the radioactive leucine, which will be incorporated late in the synthesis of each chain. Thus, protein synthesis begins at the amino terminus and extends toward the carboxyl terminus.

26. AAA encodes lysine, whereas AAC encodes asparagine. Asparagine was the carboxyl-terminal residue and, based on the experiment in problem 25, we know that the carboxyl-terminal sequence was the last to be synthesized. We therefore can conclude that the codon AAC was the last to be read. The mRNA therefore is read in the 5′ to 3′ direction.

CHAPTER 40

1. The *Oxford English Dictionary* defines translation as the action or process of turning one language into another. Protein synthesis converts nucleic acid sequence information into amino acid sequence information.

2. The reading frame for the genetic code involves a set of contiguous, nonoverlapping three-nucleotide codons that begins with a "start" codon and ends with a "stop" codon. The "start" codon establishes the pattern as to which groups of three nucleotides are translated into the respective amino acids in the final protein sequence.

(Insertion or deletion of a single nucleotide within the polynucleotide sequence would confer a "frame shift," as it would interrupt and change the reading frame.)

3. (a) 1, 2, 3, 5, 6, 10; (b) 1, 2, 7, 8; (c) 1, 4, 8, 9.

4. Transfer RNAs need to be rather large to enable specific recognition by particular protein partners. The set of different tRNAs must be specifically recognized by their appropriate cognate aminoacyl-tRNA synthetases. Each tRNA also must interact with the ribosome and, in particular, with the peptidyl transferase.

5. Four bands: light, heavy, a hybrid of light 30S and heavy 50S, and a hybrid of heavy 30S and light 50S. Recall that "ribosomes dissociate into 30S and 50S subunits after the polypeptide product is released." As protein synthesis continues, 70S ribosomes are re-formed from the various heavy and light subunits.

6. About 799 high-energy phosphate bonds are consumed—400 to activate the 200 amino acids, 1 for initiation, and 398 to form 199 pepitide bonds.

7. The sequence GAGGU is complementary to a sequence of five bases at the 3′ end of 16S rRNA and is located several bases on the 5′ side of an AUG codon. Hence this region is a start signal for protein synthesis. The replacement of G by A would be expected to weaken the interaction of this mRNA with the 16S rRNA and thereby diminish its effectiveness as an initiation signal. In fact, this mutation results in a tenfold decrease in the rate of synthesis of the protein specified by this mRNA. For a discussion of this informative mutant, see J. J. Dunn, E. Buzash-Pollert, and F. W. Studier. *Proc. Nat. Acad. Sci.* 75(1978):2741.

8. The error rates of DNA, RNA, and protein synthesis are of the order of 10^{-10}, 10^{-5}, and 10^{-4} per nucleotide (or amino acid) incorporated. The fidelity of all three processes depends on the precision of base-pairing to the DNA or mRNA template. No error correction occurs in RNA synthesis. In contrast, the fidelity of DNA synthesis is markedly increased by the 3′ $\longrightarrow$ 5′ proofreading nuclease activity and by postreplicative repair. In protein synthesis, the mischarging of some tRNAs is corrected by the hydrolytic action of the aminoacyl-tRNA synthetase. Proofreading also takes place when aminoacyl-tRNA occupies the A site on the ribosome; the GTPase activity of EF-Tu sets the pace of this final stage of editing.

9. The Shine–Dalgarno sequence of the mRNA base-pairs with a part of the 16S rRNA of the 30S subunit. This base pairing positions the 30S ribosomal subunit so that the initiator AUG in the mRNA is recognized as distinct from other AUG codons in the sequence.

10. GTP is not hydrolyzed until aminoacyl-tRNA is delivered to the A site of the ribosome. An earlier hydrolysis of GTP would be wasteful because EF-Tu–GDP has little affinity for aminoacyl-tRNA.

11. The translation of an mRNA molecule can be blocked by antisense RNA, an RNA molecule with the complementary sequence. The antisense–sense RNA duplex is degraded by nucleases. Antisense RNA added to the external medium is spontaneously taken up by many cells. A precise quantity can be delivered by microinjection.

    Alternatively, a plasmid encoding the antisense RNA can be introduced into target cells. For an interesting discussion of antisense RNA and DNA as research tools and drug candidates, see H. M. Weintraub. *Sci. Amer.* 262(January 1990):40.

12. (a) Intact protein isolated after only one minute will have been started with unlabeled amino acids. (Only during the last minute of synthesis will label have been

incorporated into the protein.) Therefore, the carboxyl-terminal peptide A_5, the last segment to be synthesized, will be most heavily labeled.

(b) Due to the continuation of previously initiated chains, the order, from most labeled to least, will reflect the reverse order of synthesis:

$$A_5 > A_4 > A_3 > A_2 > A_1$$

(c) Synthesis begins at the amino terminal and proceeds to the carboxyl terminal.

13. The rate of protein synthesis would be slower because the cycling of EF-Tu between its GTP-bound and GDP-bound forms would be slowed.

14.

	Prokaryote	Eukaryote
Ribosome size	60S	80S
mRNA	polycistronic	Not polycistronic
Initiation	Shine–Dalgarno is required	First AUG is used
Protein factors	Required	Many more required
Relation to transcription	Translation can start before transcription is completed	Transcription and translation are spatially separated
First amino acid	fMet	Met

15. Protein translocation across the endoplasmic reticulum membrane usually requires a signal sequence, signal-recognition particle (SRP), SRP receptor, and the translocon.

16. The signal-recognition particle (SRP) binds to the signal sequence and inhibits further translation. The SRP then ushers the arrested ribosome to the endoplasmic reticulum (ER) membrane, where it interacts with the SRP receptor (SR). The SRP–SR complex then binds the translocon and simultaneously hydrolyzes GTP. On hydrolysis of GTP, the SRP and SR dissociate from each other and from the ribosome. Protein synthesis resumes and the nascent protein is channeled through the translocon.

17. The formation of peptide bonds, which in turn is powered by the hydrolysis of the aminoacyl-tRNAs, also drives the co-translational movement of an emerging protein across the endoplasmic reticulum.

18. Without polysomes, the alternative would be to have a single ribosome translating a single mRNA molecule. The use of polysomes is more efficient because polysomes enable more protein synthesis per mRNA molecule in a given period of time. Protein production is thereby enhanced.

19. The addition of an IRE to the 5′ end of the mRNA would be expected to make the translation sensitive to iron, such that translation would be blocked in the absence of iron. The addition of an IRE to the 3′ end of the mRNA would not be expected to block translation, but it could affect mRNA stability.

20. The sequences of all of human mRNAs could be searched to identify those sequences that are fully or nearly complementary to the sequence of the miRNA. Those mRNAs that harbor the (nearly) complementary sequence would be candidates for regulation by the particular miRNA.

21. EF-Ts catalyzes the exchange of GTP for GDP bound to EF-Tu. In G protein cascades, an activated seven-helix receptor catalyzes GTP–GDP exchange in a G protein. For example, photoexcited rhodopsin triggers GTP–GDP exchange in transducin.

22. Many G proteins are sensitive to ADP ribosylation by cholera toxin or pertussis toxin (see Chapter 13). In each case, an ADP-ribose unit is transferred from NAD+, but the acceptor residue varies. For the modification of EF2 by diphtheria toxin, the acceptor is diphthamide (a derivative of histidine; see Figure 40.15 in the text), whereas the acceptors for the cholera toxin or pertussis toxin modifications of G proteins are arginine or cysteine.

23. Type I: b, c, and f; type 2: a, d, and e.

24. The folded protein structure determines its function. The primary structure determines the three-dimensional structure of the protein. Thus, the final phase of information transfer from DNA to RNA to protein synthesis involves the folding of the protein into its functional state.

25. (a) In Graph A, eIF4H exhibits two effects: (1) The higher slope observed at early reaction times shows that the rate of helix unwinding increases. (2) The extent of helix unwinding in the plateau region at late reaction times also increases.

    (b) To establish that eIF4H by itself does not have inherent helicase activity.

    (c) Half-maximal activity was achieved with about 0.11 μM eIF4H, that is, about half of the concentration of eIF4. Depending on the relative kinetics of association and dissociation, this result may suggest a stoichiometric 1:1 binding of the helper to the initiation factor.

    (d) The upward displacement of the straight line indicates that eIF4H enhances the rate of unwinding of all helices. The smaller slope when eIF4H is present indicates that the helper effect is greater for the more stable helices.

    (e) Several answers are possible. Graph A shows that the helper enhances both the rate and extent of helix unwinding. Both of these effects would result if the helper would slow the dissociation of eIF4 from the RNA helix. Such a mechanism would increase the processivity and also would be consistent with the energetics shown in Graph C.

26. (a) The three peaks represent, from left to right, the 40S ribosomal subunit, the 60S ribosomal subunit, and the intact 80S ribosome.

    (b) Not only are ribosomal subunits and the 80S ribosome present, but polysomes of various lengths also are apparent. The individual peaks in the polysome region near the bottom of the tube represent polysomes of discrete lengths. Under the influence of RNase, the polysomes are digested into monosomes (part A).

    (c) Hypoxic conditions significantly inhibited the number of polysomes while increasing the number of free ribosomal subunits. This outcome could be due to lack of mRNA caused by an inhibition of transcription, or to inhibition of the initiation of protein synthesis on mRNA.

27. A frameshift mutation caused by the insertion of an extra base in a protein-coding gene might be suppressed by a mutation that inserts a fourth base into the anticodon of a tRNA gene. For example, UUUC rather than UUU could be read as the codon for phenylalanine by a tRNA that contains 3'-AAAG-5' as its anticodon. In such a case, the longer anticodon could effectively restore the original reading frame for the translation of the rest of the mRNA following the insertion.

28. The nitrogen atom of the deprotonated α-amino group of aminoacyl-tRNA makes a nucleophilic attack on the ester bond of peptidyl-tRNA to form the new peptide bond. As a result, the growing peptide chain is transferred to the tRNA that bears the new amino acid. The tRNA that formerly held the peptide is released:

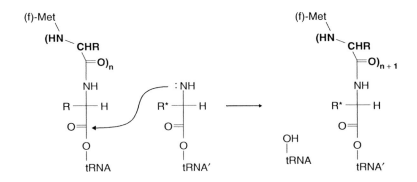

29. Initially Glu-tRNA^{Gln} is formed by misacylation. Then the activated glutamate is subsequently amidated to form Gln-tRNA^{Gln}. In regard to *H. pylori*, a specific enzyme, Glu-tRNA^{Gln} amidotransferase, catalyzes the reaction:

Gln + Glu-tRNA^{Gln} + ATP $\rightarrow$ Gln-tRNA^{Gln} + Glu + ADP + P$_i$

Glu-tRNA^{Glu} is not a substrate for the enzyme; so the transferase must also recognize aspects of the structure of tRNA^{Gln}.

CHAPTER 41

1. A cDNA library is a set of DNA segments that are complementary to mRNA sequences from a given cell type. The total mRNA population from cultured cell is isolated and converted into double-stranded DNA with the use of first reverse transcriptase and then DNA polymerase. The double-stranded DNA molecules are ligated to linker oligonucleotides and then are inserted into some sort of vector. The DNA library can be amplified and propagated in a suitable host organism.

2. A cDNA library is a DNA representation of the set of mRNA molecules expressed in a particular tissue under a specific set of physiological conditions. cDNA libraries vary from cell type to cell type from the same organism. A genomic library is a collection of DNA fragments, inserted into vector molecules, that represents the entire genome of a particular organism. Genomic libraries prepared from any diploid tissue in an organism are therefore identical.

3. Taq polymerase is thermo-stable because it is the DNA polymerase from a thermophilic bacterium that lives in hot springs. Consequently, the enzyme can withstand the cycles of temperature changes, and especially the high temperatures, that are required for PCR without denaturing.

4. (a) 4; (b) 8; (c) 1; (d) 5; (e) 10; (f) 7; (g) 6; (h) 3; (i) 9; (j) 2.

5. The codon(s) for each amino acid can be used to determine the number of possible nucleotide sequences that encode each peptide sequence (see Table 39.1):

Ala—Met—Ser—Leu—Pro—Trp:
$4 * 1 * 6 * 6 * 4 * 1 = 576$ total sequences
Gly—Trp—Asp—Met—His—Lys:
$4 * 1 * 2 * 1 * 2 * 2 = 32$ total sequences
Cys—Val—Trp—Asn—Lys—Ile:
$2 * 4 * 1 * 2 * 2 * 3 = 96$ total sequences
Arg—Ser—Met—Leu—Gln—Asn:
$6 * 6 * 1 * 6 * 2 * 2 = 864$ total sequences

The set of DNA sequences encoding the peptide Gly-Trp-Asp-Met-His-Lys would be most ideal for the probe.

6. Since *E. coli* lack the machinery to excise introns and splice exons, they would make a meaningless mRNA if presented with ovalbumin genomic DNA. Therefore, if you wish to express the ovalbumin gene in *E. coli*, you must use its cDNA, which contains the information in the eight exons, but no introns.

7. The probability of finding a given specific DNA sequence is $\frac{1}{4}^{n}$, where **n** is the number of nucleotides in one strand of the sequence that will be recognized by the restriction enzyme (because any of four nucleotides can be present at any given position in a random sequence). The average distance between cleavage sites in double-stranded DNA therefore is 4^{n} nucleotides along one strand. For *Alu*I, $4^{4} = 256$. For *Not*I, $4^{8} = 65,536$. (The sequence of the second strand of DNA is completely defined by complementary base pairing to the first strand; therefore we need only consider the probability of finding the correct recognition sequence on one strand.)

8. (a) No, because most human genes are much longer than 4 kb. One would obtain fragments containing only a small part of a complete gene.

   (b) No, chromosome walking depends on having *overlapping* fragments. Exhaustive digestion with a restriction enzyme produces nonoverlapping, short fragments.

9. (a) The direction of movement on the gel is from top to bottom, with the smallest fragment, in this case G, moving most rapidly. Since the 5′ end carries the ^{32}P label, the 5′ $\rightarrow$ 3′ sequence is read from bottom to top, opposite the direction of movement. The sequence is 5′-GGCATAC-3′. It should be noted that the fastest-moving spot in the autoradiogram is the radioactive inorganic phosphate resulting from the destruction of the guanine at the 5′ terminus.

   (b) Note that in the Sanger dideoxy method (see Figure 41.11), the new DNA strands that are subjected to electrophoresis are elongated 5′ $\rightarrow$ 3′. Since the larger molecules move more slowly, the results shown below are obtained. The DNA strand serving as template in the Sanger method is the complement of the strand shown here in the figure.

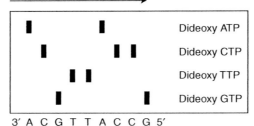

Direction of electrophoresis

Dideoxy ATP
Dideoxy CTP
Dideoxy TTP
Dideoxy GTP

3′ A C G T T A C C G 5′

10. Southern blotting of an *Mst*II digest would distinguish between the normal and mutant genes. The loss of a restriction site would lead to the replacement of two fragments on the Southern blot by a single longer fragment. Such a finding would not prove that GTG replaced GAG; other sequence changes at the restriction site could yield the same result.

11. A number of questions could be asked about the nature of the original sample and the possibility of contamination before DNA amplification by PCR. Even if no contaminants were introduced during the handling of the sample, it is possible that the fossil might have contained remains from microorganisms or other species mixed with

the dinosaur materials. Analysis of the DNA sequence and sequence complexity could be revealing, however, especially in relation to DNA sequences from modern reptiles and other known organisms. If sufficient length and number of DNA sequences would be available from several PCR experiments on the same (fossil) sample, then one would be able to narrow the phylogenetic classification of the type of organism from which the DNA originated with some confidence.

12. Higher hybridization temperatures require greater numbers of complementary base pairs between the primer and target DNAs. Conversely, lower hybridization temperatures are more permissive of sequence mismatch between the primer and the target. Let us suppose that particular yeast gene A indeed has a moderately diverged counterpart (with a moderately different sequence) in humans. If so, no PCR amplification will be observed when the hybridization temperature is too high, but a lower hybridization temperature would allow the target human DNA to be amplified in a PCR experiment that uses the yeast primer. (If the hybridization temperature [stringency] is too low, however, then spurious unrelated artifacts could also be amplified.)

13. These results suggest that the DNA is composed of four repeating units. If these were transcribed into mRNA and the latter translated into protein, one would expect a protein molecule whose linear sequence was composed of four repeating peptides.

14. Within a single species, individual dogs show enormous variation in body size and substantial diversity in other physical characteristics. Therefore, genomic analysis of individual dogs would provide valuable clues concerning the genes responsible for the diversity within the species.

15. On the basis of the comparative genome map shown in Figure 41.13, the region of greatest overlap with human chromosome 20 can be found on mouse chromosome 2.

16. In each PCR cycle, each new DNA strand is synthesized from a complementary strand that was made in the previous cycle. If the synthesis of one strand is inefficient, then the entire process will be inefficient, regardless of the rate of synthesis of the other strand. Because the experiment is performed in a single tube, the same hybridization temperature must be used for the priming of both strands. If the two primers would have very different values of T_M, then one strand could amplify much more readily than the other, and the efficient doubling of DNA at each cycle might not occur.

17. The gels should be read from the bottom to the top. The data indicate the sequence of the coding strand of the DNA. The normal sequence of codons from the first gel is GTG CTG TCT CCT GCC GAC AAG, which encodes Val-Leu-Ser-Pro-Ala-Asp-Lys.

    Hemoglobin Chongqing differs in having CGG instead of CTG as the second codon. The corresponding amino changes from leucine to arginine.

    Hemoglobin Karachi differs in having CCC instead of GCC as the fifth codon. The corresponding amino changes from alanine to proline.

    Hemoglobin Swan River differs in having GGC instead of GAC as the sixth codon. The corresponding amino changes from aspartic acid to glycine.

18. This particular person is heterozygous for this particular mutation: one allele is wild type, whereas the other carries a point mutation at this position. Both alleles are PCR amplified in this experiment, yielding the "dual peak" appearance on the sequencing chromatogram.

19. Individual B is without symptoms because he has one gene that functions normally, even though his X mRNA is smaller than normal. Individual B appears to be heterozygous in the *Hind*III restriction experiment, perhaps having one functional and one nonfunctional gene X. Although B's mRNA for X is shorter than normal, his

Y protein that is produced from this mRNA is of the normal size and apparently is functional because he has no symptoms.

Individuals C and D fail to express mRNA from gene X. Without the mRNA, they cannot make protein Y.

Individual E does express X mRNA but is unable to synthesize protein Y encoded by this mRNA (perhaps a regulatory mutation). (Alternatively, E could possibly make a defective protein Y that does not fold properly or is degraded rapidly and is not recognized by the antibody in the Western blot.)

Individual F makes X mRNA and Y protein of the proper size. Yet the Y protein apparently fails to function properly. This could be due to a point mutation that makes a single change in the amino acid sequence of Y at a location that is critical for function.

20. A few years ago this would have been very difficult, if not impossible. However, the availability of automated solid-phase chemical methods for synthesizing DNA has made the impossible fairly easy. A simple strategy for generating many mutants is to synthesize a group of oligonucleotides that differ only in the sequence of bases in one triplet, or codon. For example, with the 30-mer described in this question, if a mixture of all four nucleotides is used in the *first and second rounds* of synthesis, the resulting oligonucleotides will begin with the sequence XYT (where X and Y denote A, C, G, or T). This will provide 16 different versions of the first triplet (codon) of the 30-mer, which will encode proteins containing either Phe, Leu, Ile, Val, Ser, Pro, Thr, Ala, Tyr, His, Asn, Asp, Cys, Arg, Ser, or Gly at the first position (see Table 39.1 in the text). In similar fashion, one can synthesize oligonucleotides in which two or more codons are simultaneously varied.

21. For PCR to amplify a DNA duplex, the polymerase must be active (primed) in both directions if each strand is to be replicated. If the DNA is linear, known sequences are needed on both sides of the portion to be amplified. To explore DNA on both sides of a single known sequence, one can digest genomic DNA with a restriction enzyme and circularize the fragments. Then, by using a pair of primers that hybridize specifically with portions of the known sequence, one can use PCR to amplify only the fragments containing the known sequence. Note that in a circular DNA a single known sequence can be used to prime polymerase action in *both directions* away from the known sequence, resulting in complete replication of the duplex.

22. Use chemical synthesis or the polymerase chain reaction to prepare hybridization probes that are complementary to both ends of the known (previously isolated) DNA fragment. Challenge clones representing the library of DNA fragments with both of the hybridization probes. Select clones that hybridize to one of the probes but not to the other; such clones are likely to represent DNA fragments that contain only one end of the known fragment, along with the adjacent region of the particular chromosome.